Basic Life Su[...]

D — **Dangers?**

R — **Responsive?**

S — **Send** for help

A — Open **Airway**

B — Normal **Breathing?**

C — Start **CPR**
30 compressions : 2 breaths

D — Attach **Defibrillator (AED)**
as soon as available, follow prompts

Continue CPR until responsiveness or normal breathing return

January 2016

AUSTRALIAN
RESUSCITATION
COUNCIL

NEW ZEALAND
Resuscitation Council
WHAKAHAUORA AOTEAROA

Quick reference

Compiled by Fiona Chow

1 Cardiorespiratory arrest algorithms

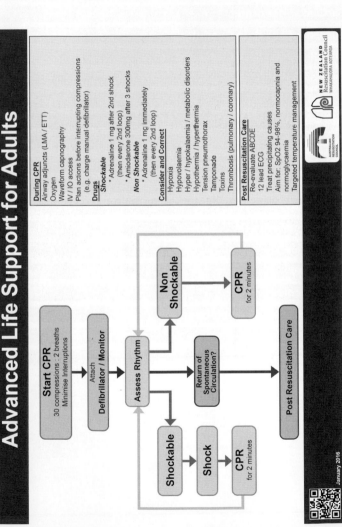

Advanced Life Support for Adults

During CPR
Airway adjuncts (LMA / ETT)
Oxygen
Waveform capnography
IV / IO access
Plan actions before interrupting compressions
(e.g. charge manual defibrillator)

Drugs
Shockable
  * Adrenaline 1 mg after 2nd shock
    (then every 2nd loop)
  * Amiodarone 300mg after 3 shocks
Non Shockable
  * Adrenaline 1 mg immediately
    (then every 2nd loop)

Consider and Correct
Hypoxia
Hypovolaemia
Hyper / hypokalaemia / metabolic disorders
Hypothermia / hyperthermia
Tension pneumothorax
Tamponade
Toxins
Thrombosis (pulmonary / coronary)

Post Resuscitation Care
Re-evaluate ABCDE
12 lead ECG
Treat precipitating causes
Aim for: SpO2 94-98%, normocapnia and
normoglycaemia
Targeted temperature management

Start CPR
30 compressions : 2 breaths
Minimise interruptions

Attach
Defibrillator / Monitor

Assess Rhythm

Non Shockable → CPR for 2 minutes

Shockable → Shock → CPR for 2 minutes

Return of Spontaneous Circulation?

Post Resuscitation Care

January 2016

Figure 1.1 Adult cardiorespiratory arrest algorithm

Reproduced with permission from the Australian Resuscitation Guidelines. Online. Download from: anzcor-adult-cardiorespiratory-arrest-flowchart-jan-2016.pdf (accessed 21 January 2020)

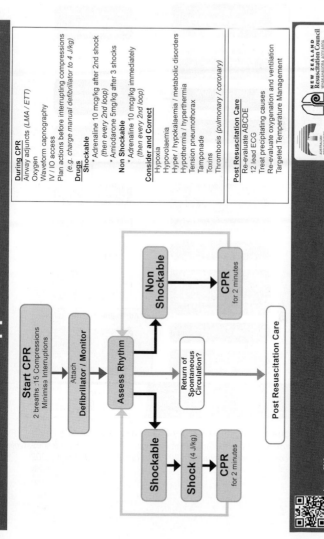

Advanced Life Support for Infants and Children

Start CPR
2 breaths : 15 Compressions
Minimise Interruptions

Attach
Defibrillator / Monitor

Assess Rhythm

Shockable

Shock (4 J/kg)

CPR for 2 minutes

Non Shockable

CPR for 2 minutes

Return of Spontaneous Circulation?

Post Resuscitation Care

During CPR
Airway adjuncts (*LMA / ETT*)
Oxygen
Waveform capnography
I.V / IO access
Plan actions before interrupting compressions
(*e.g. charge manual defibrillator to 4 J/kg*)

Drugs
Shockable
  * Adrenaline 10 mcg/kg after 2nd shock
     (*then every 2nd loop*)
  * Amiodarone 5mg/kg after 3 shocks
Non Shockable
  * Adrenaline 10 mcg/kg immediately
     (*then every 2nd loop*)

Consider and Correct
Hypoxia
Hypovolaemia
Hyper / hypokalaemia / metabolic disorders
Hypothermia / hyperthermia
Tension pneumothorax
Tamponade
Toxins
Thrombosis (*pulmonary / coronary*)

Post Resuscitation Care
Re-evaluate ABCDE
12 lead ECG
Treat precipitating causes
Re-evaluate oxygenation and ventilation
Targeted Temperature Management

NEW ZEALAND
Resuscitation Council
WHAKAHAURA AOTEAROA

AUSTRALIAN
RESUSCITATION
COUNCIL

January 2016

Figure 1.2 Paediatric cardiorespiratory arrest algorithm
Reproduced with permission from the Australian Resuscitation Council Guidelines. Online. Download from: anzcor-paediatric-cardiorespiratory-arrest-flowchart-jan-2016.pdf (accessed 21 January 2020)

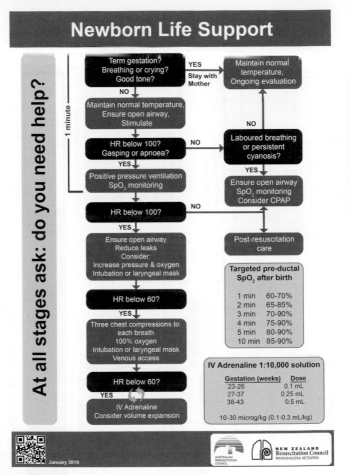

Figure 1.3 Neonatal cardiorespiratory arrest algorithm
Reproduced with permission from the Australian Resuscitation Council Guidelines. Online. Download from: anzcor-neonatal-flowchart-jan-2016.pdf (accessed 21 January 2020)

2 Cardiac arrest drugs

The following tables have been adapted from the Australian Resuscitation Council Guidelines.

Drugs routinely used in ADULT cardiac arrest

Drug	Dose	Indications
Adrenaline	1 mg IV repeat every 2nd loop during CPR	VF/VT Asystole/PEA
Amiodarone	300 mg IV Additional dose of 150 mg IV can be considered that may then be followed by infusion of 15 mg/kg over 24 h	VF/VT

Other drugs to consider in ADULT cardiac arrest

Drug	Dose	Indications
Calcium	5–10 mL IV of 10% calcium chloride	Hyperkalaemia Hypercalcaemia OD of calcium channel blockers
Magnesium	5 mmol IV can be repeated once, then followed with infusion (20 mmol over 4 h)	Torsades de pointes Cardiac arrest associated with digoxin toxicity VF/VT refractory to defibrillation and adrenaline Hypokalaemia Hypomagnesaemia
Potassium	5 mmol IV	Persistent VF due to hypokalaemia
Lignocaine	1 mg/kg IV	VF/VT where amiodarone cannot be used
Sodium bicarbonate	1 mmol/kg	Hyperkalaemia Treatment of documented metabolic acidosis Tricyclic antidepressant OD Prolonged arrest (> 15 min)

Drugs able to be given via endotracheal tube (ETT)
— Lignocaine
— Adrenaline
— Atropine
— Naloxone
Dilution with 0.9% may give better absorption.
If unable to gain intravenous access, consider intraosseous (IO) access.

2

Drugs routinely used in PAEDIATRIC cardiac arrest

Drug	Dose and route of administration
Adrenaline	10 microg/kg IV/IO = 0.1 mL/kg of 1:10 000 (max single dose − 1 mg) 100 microg/kg via ETT
Amiodarone	5 mg/kg IV/IO over 3–5 min
Defibrillation	4 joules/kg

Other drugs to consider in PAEDIATRIC cardiac arrest

Drug	Dose and route of administration
Atropine	20 microg/kg IV/IO (max 600 microg) 30 microg/kg via ETT
Calcium chloride 10% Calcium gluconate 10%	0.2 mL/kg IV/IO 0.7 mL/kg IV/IO
Glucose (dextrose)	0.25 g/kg IV/IO = 0.5 mL/kg of 50% dextrose (via CVC only) = 2.5 mL/kg of 10% dextrose IV/IO
Lignocaine (only if amiodarone is unavailable)	1 mg/kg IV
Magnesium sulfate 50% (= 2 mmol/L)	0.1–0.2 mmol/kg IV/IO bolus 0.3 mmol/kg infusion over 4 h
Potassium	0.03–0.07 mmol/kg IV/IO slow injection
Sodium bicarbonate (8.4%)	0.5–1 mmol/kg IV/IO

3 Miscellaneous drugs—adults

Miscellaneous drugs used in ADULTS

Drug	Dose and route of administration
Acetylcysteine	Initially 150 mg/kg IV 1 h; then 50 mg/kg IV over 4 h; then 100 mg/kg IV over 16 h
Adenosine	Initially 6 mg IV (rapid bolus); if still unsuccessful within 1–2 min give 12 mg IV (rapid bolus) (follow with a rapid saline flush)
Adrenaline For cardiac arrest For anaphylaxis For airway obstruction	 1 mg IV 0.3–0.5 mg of 1:10 000 IV 0.3–0.5 mg of 1:1000 IM 0.5 mL/kg of 1:1000 (max 5 mL) nebulised
Amiodarone (loading dose)	5 mg/kg IV over 1 h
Atropine	0.5 mg IV (max total dose 3 mg)
Benztropine	2 mg IV/IM/PO
Bupivacaine +/− adrenaline For local anaesthesia	Maximum single dose 2 mg/kg SC Do not repeat at intervals less than 4 h Usual dose is 12.5–150 mg (= 5–60 mL of 0.25% = 2.5–30 mL of 0.5%)
Calcium	5–10 mL of 10% calcium chloride IV 10 mL of 10% calcium gluconate IV
Charcoal	50 g PO
Clonazepam	0.5–1 mg IV
Dexamethasone	4–8 mg IV/IM
Dextrose	25–50 mL (12.5–25 g) of 50% slow push
Diazepam	2.5–5 mg IV
Digoxin (loading dose)	Adults: 250–500 microg PO/IV q4–6h to a max of 1500 microg PO or 1000 microg IV Elderly: 250–500 microg PO/IV q4–6h to a max of 500 microg
Digoxin (maintenance dose)	Adults: 125–250 microg PO Elderly: 62.5–125 microg PO
Fentanyl For analgesia/sedation	25–50 microg IV or 50–100 microg SC/IM
Flumazenil	0.2–0.5 mg IV (max total dose 2 mg)
Glucagon	1 mg IV/IM

Continued

3

Miscellaneous drugs used in ADULTS (cont.)

Drug	Dose and route of administration	
Haloperidol	2.5–5 mg IV or IM	
Hydrocortisone	100–200 mg IV	
Hyoscine butylbromide	10–20 mg PO qid 20–40 mg IV/IM up to 100 mg/d	
Ibuprofen	200–400 mg PO tds	
Ketamine For analgesia For anaesthesia	0.3–1 mg/kg IV given slowly over 2 min or 3–4 mg/kg IM 1–2 mg/kg IV or 10 mg/kg IM	
Lignocaine For local anaesthesia	Max single dose 3–4 mg/kg SC (up to 200 mg) Do not repeat max dose at intervals < 1.5 h	
Lignocaine + adrenaline For local anaesthesia	Maximum single dose 7 mg/kg SC (up to 500 mg)	
Loratadine	10 mg PO daily	
Magnesium	2 g IV over 5–15 min depending on clinical setting Eclampsia up to 4 g IV	
Mannitol	1 g/kg IV (= 5 mL/kg of 20% mannitol), max 50 g per dose	
Metoclopramide	10 mg PO/IV/IM q6h	
Midazolam	1–2.5 mg IV 0.07–0.1 mg/kg IM	
Morphine	2.5–5 mg IV 5–10 mg IM/SC	
Naloxone	200–400 microg IV/IM/SC; repeat every 2–3 min to a max 10 mg	
Olanzapine	5–10 mg PO/IM	
Ondansetron	4–8 mg PO/IV	
Oxycodone	2.5–5 mg PO qid	
Pamidronate For hypercalcaemia— dose depends on calcium level (mmol/L)	**Calcium level** < 3.0 3.0–3.5 3.5–4.0 > 4.0	**Dose** 30 mg 30–60 mg 60–90 mg 90 mg

Miscellaneous drugs used in ADULTS (cont.)

Drug	Dose and route of administration
Phenytoin (loading dose)	15–20 mg/kg IV infused at a rate < 50 mg/min
Promethazine For allergy	10–25 mg PO tds 25 mg IM as a single dose
For nausea, vomiting	25 mg PO or 12.5–25 mg IM q6h
Propofol For induction of anaesthesia	1–2 mg/kg IV
For maintenance of sedation during ventilation	1–3 mg/kg/h IV
For conscious sedation	0.5–1 mg/kg IV
Rocuronium For induction	0.6–1 mg/kg IV
For maintenance of paralysis	0.15 mg/kg IV (0.075 mg/kg IV in elderly)
Sugammadex For **immediate** reversal	16 mg/kg IV
For **routine** reversal	2–4 mg/kg IV
Suxamethonium For induction of general anaesthesia	0.5–1.2 mg/kg IV
Thiopentone For induction of general anaesthesia	3–5 mg/kg IV

Commonly used antibiotics in ADULTS

Antibiotic	Dose and route of administration
Amoxycillin	500 mg PO q8h
Amoxycillin/clavulanic acid	500/125 mg PO q8h (Augmentin Duo) 875/125 mg PO q12h (Augmentin Duo Forte)
Ampicillin	1 g IV q6h
Azithromycin	500 mg–1 g PO daily 500 mg IV daily
Ceftriaxone	1–2 g IV daily
Cefepime	1–2 g IV q12h

Continued

Commonly used antibiotics in ADULTS (cont.)

Antibiotic	Dose and route of administration
Cefotaxime	1 g IV q8h 2 g IV q8h (severe infections) up to 6 g/d
Ceftazidime	1–2 g IV q8–12h
Cephalexin	500 mg PO q6h
Cephazolin	1–2 g IV q8h
Ciprofloxacin	250–500 mg PO q12h 400 mg IV q12h
Clarithromycin	500 mg PO q12h
Clindamycin	150–450 mg PO q8h 450–900 mg IV q8h
Dicloxacillin	500 mg PO q6h
Doxycycline	100 mg PO daily
Erythromycin	250 mg PO q6h
Flucloxacillin	500 mg PO q6h 1 g IV q6h
Gentamicin	3–7 mg/kg daily (dosing frequency depends on creatinine clearance and drug monitoring)
Imipenem	1 g IV q6h
Lincomycin	600 mg IV q8h
Meropenem	1 g IV q8h
Metronidazole	400 mg PO tds 500 mg IV bd
Moxifloxacin	400 mg PO/IV daily
Penicillin V (phenoxymethylpenicillin)	500 mg PO q6h
Penicillin G (benzylpenicillin)	1.2–2.4 g IV q6h
Piperacillin + tazobactam	4 + 0.5 g IV q8h
Roxithromycin	300 mg PO daily
Vancomycin	1–1.5 g IV as a stat dose 250 mg PO q6h (dosing frequency depends on creatinine clearance and drug monitoring)

4 Miscellaneous drugs—paediatrics

The following tables have been adapted from the *Australian Medicines Handbook*.

Miscellaneous drugs used in PAEDIATRIC patients

Drug	Dose and route of administration
Adenosine For arrhythmia	< 1 month: initially 0.15 mg/kg IV rapid bolus; increase by 0.05–0.1 mg/kg every 1–2 mins to a max of 0.3 mg/kg 1 month to 1 year: initially 0.15 mg/kg IV rapid bolus; increase by 0.05–0.1 mg/kg every 1–2 mins to a max of 0.5 mg/kg 1–2 years: initially 0.1 mg/kg IV push; increase by 0.05–0.1 mg/kg every 1–2 mins to a max of 0.5 mg/kg (max 12 mg)
Adrenaline For anaphylaxis	0.05–0.1 mL/kg of 1:10 000 IV *or* 0.01 mL/kg (= 0.01 mg/kg) of 1:1000 IM (up to max 0.3 mg)
For croup	0.5 mL/kg of 1:1000 nebulised diluted to 6 mL (max 6 mL)
Calcium chloride 10%	0.2 mL/kg IV (max 10 mL)
Calcium gluconate 10%	0.25–0.5 mL/kg IV (max 20 mL)
Charcoal	1 g/kg PO/NG
Dexamethasone For severe croup	0.15–0.3 mg/kg PO/IM/IV as a single dose 0.6 mg/kg IV/IM (max 20 mg)
Diazepam	0.2–0.3 mg/kg IV (max 10 mg) 0.3–0.5 mg/kg PR (max 10 mg)
Fentanyl	1.5 microg/kg intranasal initially (max 75 microg); subsequent dosing 0.5–1.5 microg/kg at 10-minute intervals (max 75 microg); maximum acute dosing of 3 microg/kg
Glucagon **(1 mg = 1 unit)**	20–30 microg/kg IV (max 1 mg)
Glucose For hypoglycaemia	2 mL/kg IV of 10% dextrose

Continued

4

Miscellaneous drugs used in PAEDIATRIC patients (cont.)

Drug	Dose and route of administration
Hydrocortisone	2–4 mg/kg/dose IV/IM q6h
Ketamine For anaesthesia For analgesia/ sedation	1–2 mg/kg IV or 5–10 mg/kg IM 1–1.5 mg/kg IV or 2–4 mg/kg IM
Loratadine	> 30 kg: 10 mg PO 2–12 y < 30 kg: 5 mg PO 1–2 y: 2.5 mg PO
Midazolam	0.15 mg/kg IV/IM (up to 0.5 mg/kg) 0.2–0.5 mg/kg intranasally
Morphine	0.1–0.2 mg/kg IV
Naloxone	0.01 mg/kg IV/IM (max 0.4 mg) can be repeated every 2 min as necessary
Ondansetron	0.1–0.2 mg/kg PO (usual max 8 mg) 0.1 mg/kg IV over 5 min (max 8 mg)
Phenobarbitone (loading dose)	20 mg/kg IV/IO over 30 min
Phenytoin (loading dose)	20 mg/kg IV (max 1.5 g) over 30 mins
Prednisolone (initial dose)	1 mg/kg PO stat
Propofol	1 month to 8 years: 1–2.5 mg/kg IV
Rocuronium	0.6–1 mg/kg IV for rapid-sequence induction, then 0.15 mg/kg IV boluses for maintenance
Salbutamol—acute asthma attack	< 6 y: 4–6 puffs via spacer > 6 y: 8–12 puffs via spacer < 6 y: 2.5 mg nebulised > 6 y: 5 mg nebulised IV infusion: — initially 5 microg/kg/min for 1 h; — then 1–2 microg/kg/min
Suxamethonium	2 mg/kg IV (neonate/infant) 1 mg/kg IV (child) *Note*: double IV dose for IM
Thiopentone	For neonates: 2–3 mg/kg IV For children: 5–6 mg/kg IV

Commonly used antibiotics in PAEDIATRIC patients

Antibiotic	Dose and route of administration
Amoxycillin	15–25 mg/kg/dose PO q8h
Amoxycillin + **clavulanic acid**	Dose as for amoxycillin
Ampicillin	25–50 mg/kg/dose IV q6h
Cefaclor	10–15 mg/kg/dose PO q8h
Cefotaxime	25–50 mg/kg IV q8h
Ceftazidime	25–50 mg/kg/dose IV q8h
Ceftriaxone For severe infections For epiglottitis	25 mg/kg/dose IV/IM q12–24h 50 mg/kg/dose IV (max 2 g) q12–24h 100 mg/kg (max 2 g) IV (once only)
Cephalexin	6.25–12.5 mg/kg/dose PO q6h
Cephazolin	10–15 mg/kg/dose IV q8h
Dicloxacillin	15–25 mg/kg/dose PO q6h
Flucloxacillin For severe infections	12.5–25 mg/kg/dose PO q6h 25 mg/kg/dose IV q6h > 4-week-old: 50 mg/kg/dose IV q6h
Gentamicin (initial **dose only)**	1 month–10 y: 7.5 mg/kg IV/IM stat (max 320 mg) > 10 y: 6–7 mg/kg IV/IM stat (max 560 mg) *Dose ↓ after initial stat injection*
Penicillin G **(benzylpenicillin)** For serious infections	30 mg/kg/dose q6h IV (max 1.2 g)
Penicillin V **(phenoxy-** **methylpenicillin)**	10–15 mg/kg/dose PO q6h
Roxithromycin	2.5–4 mg/kg PO q12h

5 Cardiology

Reversible causes of cardiac arrest ('4Hs and 4Ts')	
Hypoxia **H**ypovolaemia **H**ypo/**h**yperkalaemia and metabolic disturbances **H**ypo/**h**yperthermia	**T**ension pneumothorax **T**amponade (cardiac) **T**oxins **T**hromboembolism (pulmonary/cardiac)

Post-resuscitation care

Aims:
1. Maximise neurological outcome.
2. Look for and treat the cause of the cardiac arrest.
3. Treat complications (arrhythmias).

Re-evaluate A, B, C, D, E.
Perform ECG and CXR.
4. Look for STE or new LBBB post arrest.
5. Look for trauma related to CPR (e.g. rib fracture).
6. Check placement of tubes (ETT, NGT, OGT)/lines.
Check adequacy of perfusion, oxygenation and ventilation (may require advanced airway if not already placed).
7. Aim for systolic BP $\geq$ 100 mmHg.
8. Aim for O_2 sats 94–98%

Induce hypothermia (32–34°C) for patients who are unresponsive to verbal command (continue for 12–24 h post arrest).
9. Ice packs to neck, axillae, groin.
10. Infuse cold fluids (30 mL/kg 0.9% saline).
11. Cooling mattress.

Monitor BSLs
12. Treat hyperglycaemia (> 10 mmol/L) with insulin but *avoid hypoglycaemia*.

Identify and treat underlying cause of cardiac arrest.
13. See table above (4Hs and 4Ts)
14. PCI may be indicated even in the absence of STE or new LBBB post arrest.

Adapted from Guideline 11.7, Post-resuscitation therapy in adult advanced life support, 2010, Australian Resuscitation Council. www.resus.org.au.

CARDIAC MARKERS

Cardiac markers—approximate time sequence from onset of symptoms

Cardiac marker	Earliest rise (h)	Peak rise (h)	Normalise (d)
CK-MB	4–6	24	2–3
Troponin I	4–6	12	3–10
Troponin T (includes high sensitivity test)	3–12	12	7–10

5

Causes of elevated troponins other than ACS

Cardiovascular	Arrhythmias HOCM Coronary vasospasm CCF Aortic valve disease Aortic dissection LVH
Respiratory	PE Severe pulmonary hypertension
CNS	Acute neurological disease Stroke SAH
Drug toxicity or toxins	Adriamycin Fluorouracil Snake venom
Infiltrative diseases	Amyloidosis Haemochromatosis Sarcoidosis Scleroderma
Inflammatory diseases	Myocarditis Kawasaki disease
Trauma	Cardiac contusion or other trauma/surgery Cardiac surgery Cardiac interventions Pacing Cardioversion Burns, especially if > 25% of BSA
Miscellaneous	Renal failure Critically ill patients Strenuous exercise Rhabdomyolysis with cardiac injury

MANAGEMENT OF STEMI

Thrombolysis/fibrinolysis versus percutaneous coronary intervention (PCI)

- Always consider PCI as the preferred primary reperfusion therapy.
- Primary PCI is superior to thrombolysis **IF** it occurs:
  within 1 hour if the onset of chest pain < 1 hour
  or
  within 90 minutes if a patient presents later.
- PCI or CAGS = preferred treatment options for cardiogenic shock secondary to STEMI.

Contraindications for thrombolysis for AMI
Absolute contraindications
• Any prior ICH
• CVA in the preceding 6 months
• Intracranial neoplasms or cerebral structural vascular lesions (e.g. AVM)
• Recent major trauma/surgery or head injury within the previous 3 weeks
• Active bleeding or known bleeding disorder (excluding menses)
• Gastrointestinal bleeding within the previous month
• Suspected aortic dissection
Relative contraindications
• TIA in the preceding 6 months
• Dementia
• Current anticoagulant therapy
• Pregnancy including 1 week post-partum
• Non-compressible vascular punctures
• Traumatic resuscitation
• Refractory hypertension (SBP > 180 mmHg or DBP > 110 mmHg)
• Advanced liver disease
• Infective endocarditis
• Active peptic ulcer

STEMI high-risk features
• Advanced age
• Hypotension
• Tachycardia
• Heart failure
• Anterior MI

ACUTE CORONARY SYNDROME—
RISK STRATIFICATION
(Adapted from the Australian Resuscitation Council and ANZCOR Guidelines)

High-risk features

Presentation with clinical features consistent with ACS and any of:

History	Signs	Investigations
• Repetitive/prolonged (> 10 min) chest pain • Syncope • LVEF < 40% • Prior PCI within 6 months • Prior CAGS • Diabetes or chronic kidney disease (EGFR < 60 mL/min) with classic chest pain	• Haemodynamic compromise • Sustained VT	• Elevated cardiac marker • Persistent or dynamic ECG changes of ST depression ≥ 0.5 mm or new T wave inversion ≥ 2 mm • Transient ST elevation (≥ 0.5 mm) in more than two contiguous leads

Intermediate-risk features

Presentation with clinical features consistent with ACS and any of the following AND NOT meeting any criteria for high-risk NSTEACS:

History	Investigations

• Chest pain within past 48 h
  — at rest or
  — repetitive or
  — prolonged
• Age > 65 y
• Known IHD
• ≥ 2 of the following risk factors:
  — hypertension
  — family history
  — smoking
  — hyperlipidaemia
• Diabetes or chronic kidney disease with non-classical chest pain
• Prior aspirin use
	• No high-risk ECG changes (see above)

Management of ACS patients

High risk	Intermediate risk
• Aggressive medical therapy — aspirin 300 mg — ticagrelor 180 mg loading dose — heparin/enoxaparin — beta-blocker • Coronary angiography	• Require further investigation to reclassify as high or low risk • Options include: — exercise stress test — sestamibi — CT coronary angiogram

$CHADS_2$ SCORE FOR AF

$CHADS_2$ score: a clinical prediction rule to determine the risk of stroke in a patient with non-rheumatic atrial fibrillation

	Condition	Points
C	Congestive cardiac failure	1
H	Hypertension	1
A	Age $\geq$ 75 y	2
D	Diabetes	1
S_2	Prior stroke/TIA	2

$CHADS_2$ score	Stroke risk %	95% CI
0	1.9	1.2–3.0
1	2.8	2.0–3.8
2	4.0	3.1–5.1
3	5.9	4.6–7.3
4	8.5	6.3–11.1
5	12.5	8.2–17.5
6	18.2	10.5–27.4

Score	Risk	Anticoagulation therapy	Considerations
0	Low	None or aspirin	Aspirin daily
1	Moderate	Aspirin or warfarin	Aspirin daily or raise INR to 2–3
$\geq$ 2	Moderate/high	Warfarin	Raise INR to 2–3, unless contraindicated

6 ECGs
ECG FEATURES

Speed and calibration of the ECG

	Measurement	Duration
Horizontally (width/duration)		
Speed	25 mm/sec	
1 small box	1 mm^2	0.04 s = 40 ms
1 large box	5 mm^2	0.2 s = 200 ms
5 large boxes	25 mm^2	1 s
300 large boxes		1 min
Vertically (amplitude/voltage)		
1 small box	1 mm	0.1 mV
2 large boxes	10 mm	1 mV

6

ECG TERMINOLOGY

Concordance: same polarity—i.e. deflections are occurring in the same direction.

Disconcordance: deflections are occurring in opposite directions.

R wave progression: normally see a relative increase in R wave size and decrease in S wave size when moving from V_1 to V_6.

Transition zone: the chest lead where the R wave approximately equals the S wave—usually V_3/V_4.

Time to onset of intrinsicoid deflection: the time from the beginning of QRS to the peak of the R wave.

Axis:

* Is the average direction of the spread of depolarisation through the ventricles when looking at the front of the patient.
* Leads aVR and II look at the heart from opposite directions.
* Looking at the front of a patient, depolarisation spreads from approx. 11 o'clock to 5 o'clock (i.e. deflections are mainly negative in aVR and positive in II).
* Normal axis is a positive deflection in I, II, III as the depolarising wave is spreading towards these leads.

Normal waves, intervals and complexes in the ECG

	Represents	Duration Width	Duration Amplitude	Features	Special cases/ abnormalities
P wave	Atrial depolarisation	< 120 ms	< 1 mm	Positive in II, negative in aVR, biphasic in V$_1$	Bifid P waves > 120 ms = P mitrale (left atrial enlargement) Peaked P wave amplitude > 2.5 mm = P pulmonale (right atrial enlargement)
PR interval	Time taken for conduction from atria to ventricles	120–200 ms (3–5 small squares)	N/A		PR > 200 ms = 1st degree heart block
QRS complex	Ventricular depolarisation	< 120 ms (< 3 small squares)			
ST segment	Beginning of ventricular repolarisation	N/A	N/A	J point = beginning of the ST segment (i.e. junction of the QRS complex and ST segment)	
T wave	Ventricular repolarisation			Normally is asymmetrical in shape and concordant with QRS	Peaked and symmetrical = hyperacute AMI or hyperkalaemia
QT interval		Average QTc ≤ 440 ms		Bazett's formula QTc = QT (in ms) ÷ √RR —QTc = QT interval corrected for HR —RR = 60/HR	'Abnormal' QTc values > 450 ms (males) > 470 ms (females) Prolongation = increased risk of developing ventricular arrhythmias
U wave	Last phase of ventricular repolarisation		≤ 1 mm or < 25% the amplitude of T wave Looks bigger as the HR ↓	Small rounded deflection following T wave (usually of same polarity as T wave)	↑ amplitude = hypokalaemia, drugs (amiodarone, sotalol, quinidine, procainamice)

ECG AXIS

ECG axis features

Axis		ECG features
Normal	−30° to +90°	Positive in leads I, II and III
Left-axis deviation	< −30°	Positive in lead I, negative in II, III
Right-axis deviation	> +100°	Negative in lead I, positive in II, III
Extreme axis deviation	−100° to +180°	Negative in I and aVF

6

Causes of axis deviation

Deviation	Causes
Right axis	Right ventricular hypertrophy
	MI of lateral wall of LV
	Left posterior fascicular block
	Chronic lung disease
	Acute massive pulmonary embolism
Left axis	Left ventricular hypertrophy
	Left anterior fascicular block
	Inferior MI

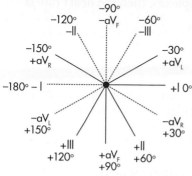

Figure 6.1 Hexaxial lead diagram

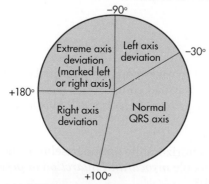

Figure 6.2 Normal QRS axis and axis deviation
Most ECGs show either a normal axis or a left or right-axis deviation. Occasionally, the QRS axis is between −90° and 180°. Such an extreme shift may be caused by marked left or right-axis deviation.

Figures 6.1 and 6.2 adapted from Goldberger AL, Clinical electrocardiography: a simplified approach, 7th edn, Philadelphia: Mosby, 2006: Figs 5-2 and 5-13. Available: www.mdconsult.com/books/bbmapAsset?appID=MDC&isbn=0-323-04038-1&eid=4-u1.0-B0-323-04038-1..50006-8..gr13&assetType=full.

ECG INTERPRETATION
ECG parameters to check

Standardisation.
- Check the paper speed (25 mm/s) and voltage (1 mV = 10 mm).

Rate:
- Count the number of large boxes between successive QRS complexes (use the R–R interval).
- Divide 300 by the above number (e.g. if there are 5 large boxes between successive QRS complexes, then the heart rate is $300 \div 5 = 60$/min).
- < 60/min = bradycardia.
- > 100/min = tachycardia.

Rhythm:
- Regular versus irregular.
- If irregular, is it regularly irregular (*2nd degree heart block, trigeminy*) or irregularly irregular (*atrial fibrillation*)?

P waves:
- Relationship of P waves to QRS complex: is each P wave followed by a QRS complex?
- Is the PR interval the same duration for all complexes?
- If all P waves and QRS complexes are completely unrelated = *AV dissociation*.

QRS complex:
Look at the:
- axis
- amplitude
- duration—short (narrow complex), normal or widened (broad complex)? Broad complexes = *possible bundle branch block (BBB), drug toxicity, electrolyte abnormalities.*

ST segment:
Is the ST segment:
- isoelectric (lies horizontally on the baseline)—*normal*?
- elevated = possible *myocardial infarction or pericarditis* (if widespread)?
- depressed = possible *ischaemia*, drug effect (*digoxin gives 'reverse tick' pattern*)?

T wave:

Look at polarity, *height* and shape:

- Inverted in aVR, upright in I, II
- May be normally inverted in III, V_1
- Inversion in V_1–V_2 'persistent juvenile pattern'
- Examples of patterns:
  - Peaked = hyperkalaemia or hyperacute in early AMI
  - Flattened or inverted = ischaemia
  - Wellen's syndrome = symmetrical deep T wave inversion (usually > 2 mm) in praecordial leads; indicative of critical proximal LAD stenosis

6

Conduction abnormalities

Type	Pattern	Causes
LBBB 'WILLIAM'	QRS > 120 ms Broad, monophasic R waves in I, V_5, V_6 (usually notched/slurred) > 40 ms to peak of R wave in V_5, V_6 (delayed intrinsicoid deflection)	AMI Degenerative Cardiomyopathies Brugada syndrome
RBBB 'MARROW'	QRS > 120 ms rSR' ('M' shape) in V_1 or V_2 Late intrinsicoid deflection in V_1 S wave > 40 ms (or at least longer than R wave duration) in I and V_6 2nd R' is greater in amplitude than 1st r deflection May be associated T wave inversion	Can be normal PE Cor pulmonale Brugada syndrome AMI Myocarditis
Brugada syndrome	RBBB (may be incomplete) with ST ↑ in V_1–V_3 Abnormalities may be transient Normal QT	Channelopathy (Na)—mutation of the *SCN5A* gene in 10–30%
WPW syndrome	Normal P wave axis and morphology PR < 120 ms Delta wave (initial slurring of the QRS)	Alternative conduction pathway

Myocardial infarction localisation

Myocardial infarction	Leads involved
Inferior	II, III, aVF Reciprocal changes in aVL
Anterior	V_1-V_4 Reciprocal changes in III, aVF
Septal	V_1-V_2
Lateral	V_5-V_6, I, aVL
Posterior	ST depression, large R wave in V_1-V_3 ST elevation in posterior leads (V_7-V_9)
Right ventricular	ST elevation > 1 mm in V_4R Associated with 40% of inferior MI

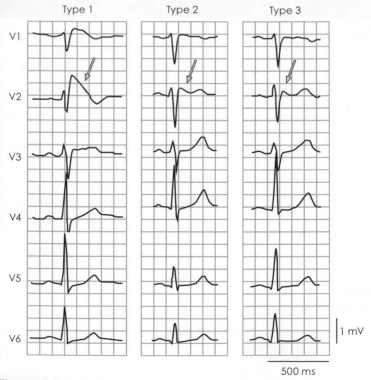

Figure 6.3 Brugada syndrome
(From Wilde AA, Strickberger SA et al: J Am Coll Cardio 47:473–484, 2006, Fig. 3.) In Ferri's Clinical Advisor 2013, 1st ed. Copyright © 2012 Mosby

BBB and AMI

Sgarbossa criteria

ECG criteria that increase specificity of AMI in patients that present with chest pain and new/old LBBB:

- A score ≥ 2 is $> 85\%$ specific for AMI.
- Remember, new LBBB or LBBB with a concordant segment $\rightarrow$ reperfusion recommended.

ECG changes	Points
Concordant ST elevation ≥ 1 mm in one lead	5
Concordant ST depression ≥ 1 mm in one of leads $V_1–V_3$	3
Disconcordant ST elevation ≥ 5 mm	2

6

RBBB

- Any ST elevation, even if disconcordant, is abnormal.
- In $V_1–V_3$, there is often up to 1 mm ST depression, so minimal ST elevation may be seen in an anterior AMI.

Differentiating VT versus SVT with aberrancy

Features making VT more likely	
Clinical features	**ECG features**
• Age > 35 y • IHD • CCF • History of AMI • Positive family history	• AV dissociation • Fusion beats • Capture beats • Extreme 'NW axis' • Concordance of QRS complexes in limb leads (all negative or all positive) • Brugada's sign – > 100 ms from onset of QRS to nadir of S wave • Absence of LBBB or RBBB morphology

7   Respiratory
OXYGEN SATURATION/INSPIRED OXYGEN

Oxygen dissociation curve (approximations)

% Oxygen saturation	Approximate pO_2 (mmHg)
60	30
70	40
80	50
90	60

Correlation between FiO_2 and expected pO_2: 'factor of 5' rule

Examples:
21% FiO_2 = pO_2 ~ 100 mmHg
90% FiO_2 = pO_2 ~ 450 mmHg
100% FiO_2 = pO_2 ~ 500 mmHg

Approximate FiO_2 related to flow rates of semi-rigid masks (i.e. Hudson, non-rebreathing masks)

O_2 flow rate (L/min)	Approximate FiO_2
4	0.35
6	0.50
8	0.55
10	0.60
12	0.65
15	0.70

ALVEOLAR OXYGEN AND A–a GRADIENT
Alveolar gas equation

$$P_AO_2 = PiO_2 - (P_ACO_2 \times 1.25)$$

where:
- P_AO_2 is the alveolar pO_2
- PiO_2 is the inspired pO_2 = $713 \times FiO_2$
- P_ACO_2 is the alveolar pCO_2 (assumed to be equal to the measured arterial blood gas estimation of CO_2)

Example:
If at room air (21% FiO_2) P_ACO_2 = 40 mmHg, then
$$P_AO_2 = (713 \times 0.21) - (40 \times 1.25) \text{ mmHg}$$
$$= 150 - 50 \text{ mmHg}$$
$$= 100 \text{ mmHg}$$

A–a gradient

$$\text{A–a gradient} = P_AO_2 - P_aO_2$$

where:
- P_AO_2 is the alveolar pO_2
- P_aO_2 is the arterial blood gas estimation of O_2

Normal value of A–a gradient:

$$\text{Calculating normal A–a gradient} = (\text{age} \div 4) + 4$$

Note: P_aO_2 decreases with age. As an approximate guide,

$$P_aO_2 \text{ at room air} = [100 - (\text{age} \div 3)] \text{ mmHg}.$$

7

CURB-65 SCORE

A severity scoring system for community-acquired pneumonia.

	Criterion	Score
C	Confusion	1
U	Urea > 7 mmol/L	1
R	Respiratory rate $\geq$ 30/min	1
B	BP (SBP $\leq$ 90 mmHg or DBP $\leq$ 60 mmHg)	1
65	$\geq$ 65 years	1

Score	% 30-day mortality	Treatment considerations
1	2.7 (low risk)	Outpatient
2	6.8 (moderate risk)	Inpatient or close outpatient follow-up
3	14 (severe risk)	Inpatient $\pm$ intensive care admission
4 or 5	27.8 (highest risk)	Inpatient $\pm$ intensive care admission

Risk of death at 30 days increases with increasing score.

SPIROMETRY PATTERNS OF OBSTRUCTIVE AND RESTRICTIVE RESPIRATORY DISEASES

Spirometric values

Definitions	
FVC	Forced vital capacity; the total volume of air that can be exhaled during a maximal forced expiration effort
FEV_1	Forced expiratory volume in one second; the volume of air exhaled in the first second under force after a maximal inhalation
FEV_1/FVC ratio	The percentage of the FVC expired in 1 second

Patterns		
	Obstructive	**Restrictive**
FEV_1	↓	↓ or normal
FVC	Normal or ↓ if very severe	↓
FEV_1/FVC	< 0.70	> 0.70

CLASSIFICATION OF SEVERITY OF COPD

Stage	FEV_1 / FVC*	FEV_1	Clinical features
I (mild)	< 0.70	≥ 80% predicted	Chronic cough, sputum production
II (moderate)	< 0.70	50% ≤ FEV_1 < 80% predicted	Cough, sputum production, SOB
III (severe)	< 0.70	30% ≤ FEV_1 < 50% predicted	↑SOB, ↓exercise tolerance, fatigue, ↑frequency of exacerbations
IV (very severe)	< 0.70	FEV_1 < 30% or < 50% predicted plus chronic respiratory failure	Cor pulmonale, hypoxia, impaired quality of life, life-threatening exacerbations

* Post-bronchodilator measurements are recommended.
Adapted from the Global Initiative on Chronic Obstructive Lung Disease, Table 2.
At-a-glance Outpatient Management Reference for Chronic Obstructive Pulmonary Disease (COPD).

NORMAL VALUES OF PEAK EXPIRATORY FLOW

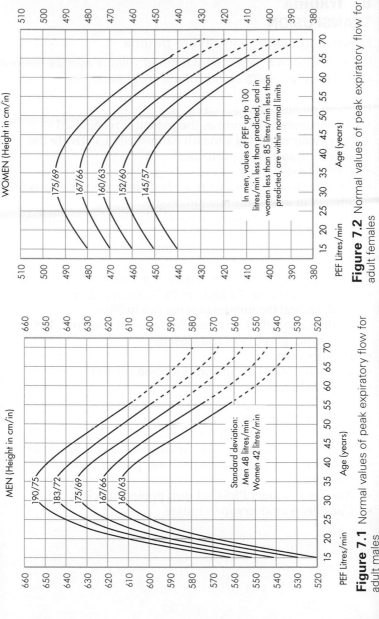

Figure 7.1 Normal values of peak expiratory flow for adult males

Figure 7.2 Normal values of peak expiratory flow for adult females

MEN (Height in cm/in)

190/75
183/72
175/69
167/66
160/63

Standard deviation:
Men 48 litres/min
Women 42 litres/min

WOMEN (Height in cm/in)

175/69
167/66
160/63
152/60
145/57

In men, values of PEF up to 100 litres/min less than predicted, and in women less than 85 litres/min less than predicted, are within normal limits

7

8 Trauma

TRANSFUSION

Massive transfusion in severe trauma

(Replacement of a patient's total blood volume over 24 hours or replacement of > 50% blood volume in 4 hours)

Practical points:
- After 6 units or as soon as the patient is recognised as potentially requiring a massive transfusion, **activate** the massive transfusion protocol.
- Use a blood warmer.
- Priority should be placed in early definitive haemostasis (e.g. surgery or interventional radiology).
- Identify patients who are on anticoagulants or antiplatelet therapy.
- Acidosis and hypothermia can impair coagulation.

Possible complications of massive transfusion:
- Transfusion of 10–12 units of PRBCs can cause:
  — dilutional thrombocytopenia (up to 50%)
  — dilutional effect on coagulation factors (approx. 10% per 500 mL of red cells transfused).
- Hypothermia
- Hypocalcaemia (citrate binds ionised calcium)
- Hyperkalaemia

Other products to use:
- Aim for a ratio of 1 PRBCs:1 FFP.
- Be guided by bleeding visually stopped, haemodynamics.
- Role of factors and plasma probably greater than role of platelets.
- Aim for 4–6 units PRBCs:1 unit pooled platelets.
- Consider 6 units cryoprecipitate.

Monitoring
- Suggest frequently:
  — temperature
  — acid/base sampling
  — FBC, UEC, ionised calcium, coagulation studies, fibrinogen every 3 h.
- Aim for:
  — temperature > 35°C
  — pH > 7.2, lactate < 4 mmol/L, base excess < –6
  — ionised calcium > 1.1 mmol/L
  — platelets > 50 × 10⁹/L
  — fibrinogen > 1 g/L
  — PT, APTT < 1.5 × normal, INR < 1.5
  — Hb > 80 g/L

8

Adjunctive agents to **consider**:
- Tranexamic acid 1 g IV loading dose followed by 1 g infused over 10 mins over 8 h (trauma patients)
- Recombinant factor VIIa
  — Controversial
  — Uncontrolled haemorrhage in a salvageable patient and failed surgical or radiological measures to control bleeding and adequate blood component replacement and pH > 7.2 and temperature > 34°C
- Prothrombinex
- Vitamin K

CANADIAN CT HEAD RULE
Role: to assist in determining who may need CT imaging to determine the presence of intracranial injury.

This rule **only applies** to those with GCS 13–15, witnessed LOC, amnesia to the head injury event or confusion.

GCS < 15 at 2 h after injury	Yes	High risk*
Suspected open or depressed skull fracture	Yes	High risk*
Any sign of base of skull fracture: — Haemotympanum — 'Racoon eyes' — CSF otorrhoea/rhinorrhoea — Battle's sign	Yes	High risk*
Vomiting ≥ 2 episodes	Yes	High risk*
Age ≥ 65 years	Yes	High risk*
Amnesia before impact ≥ 30 min	Yes	Medium risk**
Dangerous mechanism: — Fall from height > 1 m (3 ft) or 5 stairs — Pedestrian struck by motor vehicle — Occupant ejected from motor vehicle	Yes	Medium risk**

* High risk of injury requiring neurosurgical intervention.
** Medium risk of brain injury on CT.

CANADIAN C-SPINE RULE

Canadian C-spine criteria (see Figure 8.1 [below] also):

1 Perform imaging on the patient who has any of the following **high-risk criteria:**
   — Age ≥ 65 years
   — Dangerous mechanism of injury:
     • Fall from 1 m (3 ft) or 5 stairs
     • Axial load to the head, such as diving accident
     • MVA at high speed (> 100 km/h)
     • Motorised recreational vehicle accident
     • Ejection from a vehicle
     • Bicycle collision with an immovable object, such as a tree or parked car
   — Paraesthesiae in the extremities
2 If none of the above, assess for any **low-risk factor** that allows assessment of ROM of the neck:
   — Simple rear end MVC. This excludes:
     • Pushed into oncoming traffic
     • Hit by bus or large truck
     • Rollover
     • Hit by high speed (> 100 km/h) vehicle

— Sitting position in the ED
— Ambulatory at any time
— Delayed onset of neck pain
— Absence of midline cervical spine tenderness

If the patient has none of the low-risk criteria, imaging must be done.

If the patient has any of the low-risk criteria, assess ROM of the neck.

3 Test active ROM of the neck:
— Can the patient rotate their neck actively 45° both left and right?
  • If YES → no imaging is required.
  • If NO → imaging is recommended.

NEXUS CRITERIA FOR C-SPINE IMAGING

C-spine imaging is indicated for all trauma patients UNLESS they have ALL the following criteria:
1 No posterior midline cervical tenderness
2 No evidence of intoxication
3 A normal level of alertness
4 No focal neurological deficit
5 No distracting painful injuries

Based on Hoffman JR et al, Selective cervical spine radiography in blunt trauma: methodology of the National Emergency X-Radiography Utilization Study NEXUS). Ann Emerg Med 1998;32(4):461–9.

8

THE CANADIAN C-SPINE RULE

For alert (GCS = 15) and stable trauma patients where cervical spine injury is a concern

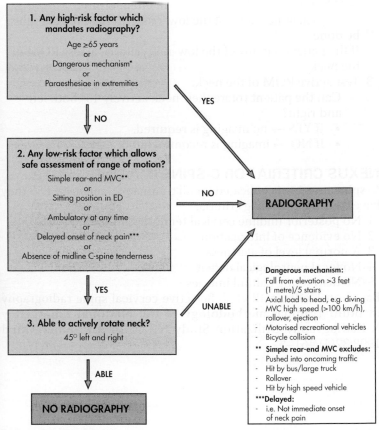

Figure 8.1 Canadian C-spine rule
Adapted from Stiell IG et al. The Canadian CT head rule for patients with minor head injury. Lancet 2001;357:1391–6.

BURNS

Classification of burns

Depth	Structures involved	Clinical features	Healing
Superficial	Epidermis only	Red, painful, dry, blanch with pressure No blisters	Epidermis peels off Heals within 1 week No scarring
Partial thickness—superficial	Epidermis and superficial dermis	Blisters Painful, red, weeping Blanch with pressure	Skin can regenerate Heal by 1–3 weeks Scarring is unusual Pigment changes can occur
Partial thickness—deep (can be difficult to differentiate from full thickness)	As above plus damage to hair follicles/ glandular tissue	Blisters Wet/waxy dry Dark red or yellow-white patches Painful to pressure only Do not blanch	Heal in 3–8 weeks Heal by scarring
Full thickness	All layers of dermis plus often subcutaneous tissue	Charred or leathery grey or waxy white Insensate	Heal by wound contracture and edge epithelialisation Skin cannot regenerate

Eschar

- Dead and denatured dermis
- Can compromise viability of limb/torso if circumferential

Burn treatment tips

- Remove from source of burning
- Remove burnt clothing
- A, B, C assessment
- O_2 (ideally humidified)

Rule of Nines
Ignore simple erythema

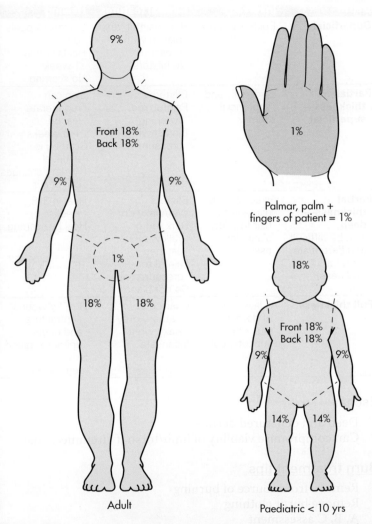

Palmar, palm +
fingers of patient = 1%

Adult

Paediatric < 10 yrs

Figure 8.2 Rule of Nines: determining the percentage total body surface area (TBSA) involved; ignore simple erythema

- Water to cool the burn (only useful in 1st 3 h post injury)
- Cover burn
- Watch for hypothermia and no ice
- Assess % total body surface area (TBSA) affected
- For burns > 15% TBSA:
  — IV access and begin fluid resuscitation
  — IV morphine
  — NBM
  — +/− IDC
- Analgesia
- Check tetanus immunisation status

Parkland formula for fluid requirement

$$4 \text{ mL} \times \text{bodyweight (kg)} \times \% \text{ TBSA burned (adults)}$$

Important points:
- Excludes superficial burns.
- The calculated volume above is to be given over 24 h from the *time of injury*, not the time of presentation.
- Give *half* the total fluid requirements *over the first 8 h from the time of injury*, the rest over 16 h.
- Need to *add maintenance fluid requirements and other losses* (e.g. traumatic blood loss) to the above-calculated volume.
- Fluid resuscitation formulas are *guides only* and the patient's *haemodynamic status must be monitored* continuously (HR, BP, urine output) with fluid management adjusted accordingly.
- Aim for urine output of > 0.5 mL/kg/h (adult) and ≥ 1 mL/kg/h (child).

Consultation/referral criteria to a specialist burns unit

- Partial-thickness burns in adults > 0% TBSA
- Full-thickness burns in adults > 5% TBSA
- Partial/full-thickness burns in children > 5% TBSA
- Burns involving:
  — Face
  — Eyes
  — Ears
  — Hands

8

- — Feet
- — Genitalia
- — Perineum
- — Major joints
- Chemical burns
- Electrical/lightning burns
- Burns associated with inhalational injury
- Circumferential burns to the limbs or chest
- Burns associated with other traumatic injuries
- Burns associated with comorbidities that could affect management and outcome
- Suspected child abuse

8 LOCAL ANAESTHETICS
Types of local anaesthetics

(*Note:* allergies = more common with esters than amides.)

Amides	Bupivacaine
	Levobupivacaine
	Lignocaine
	Prilocaine
	Ropivacaine
Esters	Amethocaine
	Cocaine

Local anaesthesia—buffering

When infiltrating lignocaine subcutaneously for local anaesthesia, buffering with sodium bicarbonate benefits in several ways:
- It reduces the pain of the injection.
- It decreases the time to onset of action.
- It maintains efficacy and duration of the local anaesthetic effect.

To buffer the lignocaine, use 1 part of sodium bicarbonate 8.4% injection (containing bicarbonate 1 mmol/mL) to 9 parts of lignocaine 1%.

Local anaesthetic concentration

Concentrations of local anaesthetics are expressed as a % or in mg/mL.

Multiply by 10 to convert from percentage to mg/mL (e.g. 0.5% = 5 mg/mL).

% Concentration	Concentration in g/100 mL	Dose per mL
0.25%	0.25 g/100 mL	2.5 mg/mL
0.5%	0.5 g/100 mL	5 mg/mL
1%	1 g/100 mL	10 mg/mL
2%	2 g/100 mL	20 mg/mL

8

Local anaesthetics combined with adrenaline

Do not use in:
- nose
- digits
- ears
- genitals.

9 Metabolic equations and electrolytes

ANION GAP (AG)

AG acidosis

$$AG = (Na^+) - (HCO_3^- + Cl^-)$$
$$Normal\ AG = 3\text{--}12$$

Causes of ↑ AG acidosis (mnemonic—'CATMUDPILES'):

C Cyanide
A Alcoholic ketoacidosis
T Toluene
M Methanol, Metformin
U Uraemia
D Diabetic ketoacidosis
P Paraldehyde, Propylene glycol
I Iron, Isoniazid
L Lactic acidosis
E Ethylene glycol
S Starvation ketoacidosis, Salicylates

Causes of normal AG acidosis (mnemonic—'USED CARP'):

U Ureteroenterostomy
S Small bowel fistula
E Extra chloride (hyperchloraemic acidosis)
D Diarrhoea, resolving DKA, Drugs (acetazolamide, cholestyramine)
C Carbonic anhydrase deficiency
A Adrenal insufficiency
R Renal tubular acidosis (type 1, 2, 4)
P Pancreatic fistula

ACID–BASE DISORDERS FORMULAS: COMPENSATORY MECHANISMS

These formulas are used to assess the appropriateness of the compensatory response. Deviations from these values indicate mixed metabolic/respiratory disorders.

Metabolic acidosis (Winter's formula)

$$\text{Expected } PCO_2 = (1.5 \times HCO_3^-) + 8 \text{ mmHg } (+/- 2)$$

If the actual PCO_2 > expected PCO_2, there is a concomitant respiratory acidosis.

Metabolic alkalosis

$$\text{Expected } PCO_2 = (0.7 \times HCO_3^-) + 20 \text{ mmHg } (+/- 5)$$

If the actual PCO_2 < expected PCO_2, there is a concomitant respiratory alkalosis.

Respiratory acidosis

Acute: ↑ 1 mmol HCO_3^- per 10 mmHg ↑ PCO_2 above 40 mmHg

$$\text{Expected } HCO_3^- = 24 + [(\text{actual } PCO_2 - 40) \div 10] \text{ mmol/L}$$

Chronic: ↑ 4 mmol HCO_3^- per 10 mmHg ↑ PCO_2 above 40 mmHg

$$\text{Expected } HCO_3^- = 24 + 4 [(\text{actual } PCO_2 - 40) \div 10] \text{ mmol/L}$$

9

Respiratory alkalosis

Acute: ↓ 2 mmol HCO_3^- per 10 mmHg ↓ PCO_2 below 40 mmHg

$$\text{Expected } HCO_3^- = 24 - 2 [(40 - \text{actual } PCO_2) \div 10] \text{ mmol/L}$$

Note: This rarely leads to a HCO_3^- < 8 mmol/L. If HCO_3^- < 18 mmol/L, a metabolic acidosis co-exists.

Chronic: ↓ 5 mmol HCO_3^- per 10 mmHg ↓ PCO_2 below 40 mmHg

$$\text{Expected } HCO_3^- = 24 - 5 [(40 - \text{actual } PCO_2) \div 10] \text{ mmol/L } (+/- 2)$$

Note: Compensation is limited to HCO_3^- of about 12–15 mmol/L.

OSMOLAR GAP
Calculating the osmolar gap

$$\text{Osmolar gap} = \text{Measured osmolarity} - \text{Calculated osmolarity}$$
$$(\text{Normal osmolar gap} \le 10 \text{ mOsm/L.})$$

$$\text{Calculated osmolarity} = (2 \times Na^+) + \text{Glucose} + \text{Urea}$$
$$(\text{where all parameters are in mmol/L}).$$

Exogenous agents causing ↑ osmolar gap

- Ethanol
- Methanol
- Ethylene glycol
- Isopropyl alcohol
- Propylene glycol
- Mannitol
- Sorbitol
- Glycine
- Glycerol

Non-toxicological conditions associated with ↑ osmolar gap

- DKA
- Alcoholic ketoacidosis
- Severe lactic acidosis
- Chronic renal failure
- Trauma and burns
- Hyperlipidaemia
- Hyperproteinaemia
- Massive hypermagnesaemia

HYPERKALAEMIA

- Severe > 7 mmol/L
- Signs and symptoms:
  — Often asymptomatic
  — Neuromuscular (weakness → paralysis)
  — Arrhythmias (including palpitations, syncope, chest pain)

9

Causes of true hyperkalaemia

↑ cellular release of K⁺	Massive blood transfusion Massive haemolysis Rhabdomyolysis Burns Trauma Tumour lysis syndrome
Shift of K⁺ out of cells	Metabolic acidosis Insulin deficiency Beta blockers Digoxin overdose Suxamethonium
↓ renal excretion of K⁺	Renal failure Mineralocorticoid deficiency: — Hypoaldosteronism — Addison's disease Medications: — ACEIs — Angiotensin receptor blockers — Cyclosporin — Tacrolimus — Spironolactone (K⁺ sparing)

9

ECG changes of hyperkalaemia
• Tall peaked T waves (> 5 mm) • PR prolongation • Small amplitude P waves/loss of P wave • ↑ QRS width • Intraventricular blocks, BBB • Fusion of QRS complex with T wave (→ sine wave) • Bradycardias, AV dissociation, VT, VF, PEA

Treatment options for true hyperkalaemia

Note: Patients with hyperkalaemia and normal ECGs can suddenly go into cardiac arrest. The ECG is not an indicator of how serious the hyperkalaemia is in that particular patient.

Treatment	Dose	Time to onset of effect	Duration of effect
Temporary			
Calcium gluconate 10% (if patient awake)	10 mL IV; can be repeated at 10-min intervals	Should improve ECG within 3 min	30 min
Calcium chloride 10% (if patient in cardiac arrest)	10 mL IV		
Glucose and short-acting insulin (Actrapid)	50 mL 50% dextrose IV, 10 U of Actrapid IV (if BSL > 15 mmol/L dextrose is not required)	Within 15 min (K ↓ by 0.5–1 mmol/L)	4–6 h
Salbutamol	10–20 mg nebulised	Within 30 min (K ↓ by 0.5–1 mmol/L)	2 h
Sodium bicarbonate 8.4% (IF patient is acidotic)	50–100 mmol IV	Within 30 min	2 h
Permanent (removes potassium)			
Resonium	30–60 g PO/PR	Within 1 h (K ↓ by 0.5–1 mmol/L)	6 h
Dialysis		Immediate	3 h

Note: Avoid calcium in hyperkalaemia caused by digoxin toxicity.

HYPOKALAEMIA

* Severe < 2.5 mmol/L
* Signs and symptoms of hypokalaemia
  — Weakness (begins in lower extremities, moves cephalad)
  — Muscle cramps and tenderness
  — Flaccid paralysis
  — Hyporeflexia
  — Ischaemic rhabdomyolysis
  — Paraesthesiae
  — Constipation, ileus
  — Ventricular/atrial ectopic beats
  — Arrhythmias

Causes of hypokalaemia

↑ gastrointestinal loss	Diarrhoea (including laxative abuse) Vomiting Intestinal/pancreatic fistulae Ileostomy
Shift of K^+ into cells	During treatment of DKA Alkalosis Treatment of asthma (frequent beta-agonists)
↑ renal loss	Diuretics (loop, thiazides, carbonic anhydrase inhibitors) Hypomagnesaemia Hyperaldosteronism: • 1° (adrenal hyperplasia, adenoma, cancer) • 2° (renal artery stenosis, CCF, liver cirrhosis) Alkalosis Congenital syndromes (Bartter and Gitelman) Renal tubular damage: • RTA type I, II • Interstitial nephritis • Analgesic nephropathy • Drug toxicity (amphotericin, gentamicin, toluene)

9

ECG changes of hypokalaemia

- Low amplitude, flattened or inverted T waves
- U waves
- ST depression
- Wide PR interval
- Illusion of prolonged QT (T wave disappears, U wave = prominent)
- Ectopic beats and arrhythmias

Useful lab investigations in hypokalaemia

Test	Result	Possible underlying cause
HCO$_3^-$	High	Vomiting Diuretic abuse Mineralocorticoid excess Bartter, Gitelman
	Low	Renal tubular disease Diarrhoea
Na$^+$	High	1° hyperaldosteronism
	Low	Diuretic use Hypovolaemia (GI loss)
Urine K$^+$	< 20 mmol/L	GI loss Intracellular shift of K$^+$ Poor oral intake
	> 40 mmol/L	Renal loss
Urine Na$^+$	< 20 mmol/L (with ↑ urine K$^+$)	2° hyperaldosteronism

Treatment of hypokalaemia

- Replace with IV/PO potassium chloride depending on symptoms, severity and cause of hypokalaemia.
- PO is the safer route.
- IV if:
  — neuromuscular dysfunction
  — arrhythmias
  — ongoing GI losses
  — severe.
- KCl IV at 10 mmol/h is the safest rate. (Higher rates → pain, phlebitis, ventricular arrhythmias)

HYPERNATRAEMIA

- Severe > 155 mmol/L
- High mortality rate (~50%)

Causes of hypernatraemia

Hypovolaemic (most common)	Loss/deficiency of water or Loss of Na+ and water with Na+ losses > water losses	Inability to drink/obtain water Impaired thirst mechanism Osmotic diuresis: — Glycosuria — Mannitol Extreme sweating Severe watery diarrhoea Vomiting Burns
Euvolaemic	Water loss without Na+ loss	Diabetes insipidus: — Hypothalamic — Nephrogenic
Hypervolaemic	Gain of Na+ and water with Na+ gain > water gain	Iatrogenic (NaCl tablets, hypertonic saline, administration of $NaHCO_3$, hypertonic dialysis) Hypertonic medicines (ticarcillin) Cushing disease Adrenal hyperplasia Primary aldosteronism Sea water drownings

Treatment of hypernatraemia

Volume resuscitation if hypovolaemic	0.9% NS IV bolus
Calculate water deficit	Free water deficit (in L) = bodyweight (kg) × %TBW* × (actual Na+ ÷ desired Na+] – 1)
Correct slowly (rapid correction precipitates seizures)	↓ by < 1 mmol/L/h

*%TBW = percentage total body water

%TBW	Population group
0.6	Young men
0.5	Young women Elderly men
0.4	Elderly women

9

HYPONATRAEMIA
- Concerning level: < 130 mmol/L
- Symptoms occur when the fall in sodium occurs rapidly or when adaptive responses fail to develop.

Useful investigations
- Serum
  — Osmolality
  — Uric acid
  — TSH, cortisol
- Urinalysis
  — Electrolytes
  — Uric acid
  — Urea
  — Creatinine
  — Osmolality

Treatment of hyponatraemia
- **Hypertonic saline** (3%) IV for CNS dysfunction (altered mental state, coma, seizures):
  — 100 mL IV (can go through peripheral IV access) over 10–20 min (for seizure)
  — Can repeat once (10 min between doses)
  — Send repeat Na^+
  — Each bolus will raise Na^+ 2 mmol
- *Note:* Risk of osmotic demyelination with treatment.
- **Fluid restrict** unless hypotensive
- **Monitor urine output**
- **'Rule of 6s':**
  — For those with CNS dysfunction, no more than 6 mmol correction in 6 h
  — Then no more than 6 mmol correction over 24 h

HYPERCALCAEMIA
Serum calcium:
- 45% ionised = physiologically active form of Ca^{2+}
- 40% bound to albumin
- 15% bound to other ions (citrate, phosphate, carbonate)

Causes of hypercalcaemia

- Primary hyperparathyroidism
- Malignancy
- Vitamin D excess
- Granulomatous disease (sarcoidosis)
- Renal failure
- Milk–alkali syndrome
- High bone turnover rates
  — Paget's
  — Prolonged immobilisation
  — Multiple myeloma

Symptoms of hypercalcaemia

Stones	Renal Biliary
Bones	Bone pain
Abdominal groans	Abdominal pain Nausea Vomiting Anorexia Pancreatitis
Psychiatric overtones	Confusion Depression Anxiety Coma

9

Useful lab investigations

- UEC
- Ionised calcium, phosphate
- BSL
- LFTs (albumin)
- PTH level

ECG changes of hypercalcaemia

- Prolongation of PR interval
- Shortening of QT interval
- QRS widening
- Sinus bradycardia
- BBB, AV block
- Cardiac arrest

Treatment of hypercalcaemia

Treatment option	Dose
Hydration (0.9% saline)	Titrate
Diuretics—e.g. frusemide	10–40 mg IV
Bisphosphonates—e.g. pamidronate	60–90 mg IV
Calcitonin	4 U/kg IM/SC q12h

HYPOCALCAEMIA

- Severe: total $Ca^{2+} < 2.175$ mmol/L (8.7 mg/dL)
- If ionised Ca^{2+} normal, then asymptomatic
- Symptoms when ionised $Ca^{2+} < 0.8$ mmol/L
- $\uparrow$ 0.1 unit of pH $\rightarrow$ $\downarrow$ ionised Ca^{2+} by 3–8%

Causes of hypocalcaemia

Factitious	Hypoalbuminaemia
$\downarrow$ PTH	Hypoparathyroidism Pseudohypoparathyroidism Parathyroid/thyroid surgery Radical neck dissection Radiation therapy for head/neck cancer
$\downarrow$ Vitamin D	Nutritional malabsorption $\downarrow$ Intake Renal disease Pronounced hypophosphataemia
$\uparrow$ Calcitonin	Medullary thyroid ca
$\uparrow$ Phosphate	Tumour lysis syndrome Rhabdomyolysis CRF
$\uparrow$ Citrate in serum	Massive blood transfusion Plasmapheresis
$\uparrow$ Bone formation/turnover	Malignancy (prostate, breast, lung, chondrosarcoma) Osteomalacia
Medications	Phenytoin Phenobarbitone Colchicine Cisplatin
Others	Sepsis Severe burns Pancreatitis (calcium complex formation)

Symptoms and signs of hypocalcaemia

Symptoms dependent on the absolute value and rate of fall in Ca^{2+}.

Neuromuscular	Paraesthesiae Hyperreflexia Muscle spasm Tetany Chvostek's sign (facial N tap) Trousseau sign (BP cuff pumped up) Laryngeal stridor Seizures Choreoathetosis
Cardiovascular	Arrhythmias Hypotension Impaired contractility (heart failure)
Psychiatric	Anxiety, irritability Psychosis Depression Confusion Delusions

Chvostek's sign:
- Tap 0.5–1 cm below zygomatic process, 2 cm anterior to ear lobe.
- Positive if see twitching of circumoral Ms and orbicularis oculi.

Trousseau's sign:
- Inflate BP cuff to above systolic BP for several minutes.
- Positive if see carpopedal spasm.

ECG changes of hypocalcaemia
• Bradycardia • Prolongation of QT interval • Heart block • T wave inversion • Torsades de pointes

9

DIFFERENCES BETWEEN CA CHLORIDE AND CA GLUCONATE

Ca chloride	Ca gluconate
3 times more potent	⅓ potency of Ca chloride
Ca^{2+} ions immediately available post injection	Requires liver to metabolise gluconate component and release Ca
Can be given as a slow push	Given over 10 min due to sugar load (gluconate) which can cause hypotension
Highly irritant to veins	Less irritant
10% solution → 0.70 mmol/mL	10% solution → 0.22 mmol/mL

ION CORRECTION FORMULAS

Sodium corrected for hyperglycaemia

corrected Na^+ = measured Na^+ + [glucose (mmol/L) ÷ 4]

Calcium corrected for hypoalbuminaemia

corrected Ca^{2+} (mmol/L) = measured Ca^{2+} (mmol/L)
+ [40 − measured albumin (g/L)] × 0.02

9

10 Thromboembolism and coagulopathy

Pulmonary embolism rule-out criteria (PERC)

- Age < 50 years
- HR < 100/min
- O_2 sats on room air $\geq 95\%$
- No prior history of DVT/PE
- No trauma or surgery requiring hospitalisation within 4 weeks
- No haemoptysis
- No exogenous oestrogen
- No unilateral leg swelling

Note: Low clinical suspicion for PE + ALL the above criteria = < 2% probability of PE and no further work-up is required.

WELLS' CRITERIA FOR PE

Determines the pre-test probability of PE. This can then be used in conjunction with a D-dimer assay to determine the need for imaging.

Clinical feature	Points
Clinical symptoms of DVT	3
Other diagnosis less likely than PE	3
Heart rate > 100/min	1.5
Immobilisation or surgery in past 4 weeks	1.5
Previous DVT/PE	1.5
Haemoptysis	1
Malignancy	1

Risk score (probability of PE)	
Points	**Risk of PE at 3 months**
> 6	High (40.6% chance of PE in the ED population)
2–6	Moderate (16.2% chance of PE in the ED population)
< 2	Low (1.3% chance of PE in the ED population)

Based on Wells PS et al. Excluding pulmonary embolism at the bedside without diagnostic imaging: management of patients with suspected pulmonary embolism presenting to the emergency department by using a simple clinical model and D-dimer. Ann Intern Med 2001;135(2):98–107.

10

WELLS' CRITERIA FOR DVT

Clinical feature	Points
Active cancer (treatment within past 6 months, palliation)	1
Paralysis, paresis or immobilisation of lower extremity	1
Bedridden for more than 3 days and/or surgery within 4 weeks	1
Localised tenderness along distribution of deep veins	1
Entire leg swollen	1
Unilateral calf swelling > 3 cm (measured below tibial tuberosity)	1
Unilateral pitting oedema	1
Collateral superficial veins	1
Alternative diagnosis as likely or more likely than DVT	−2

Risk score (probability of DVT)	
Points	**Risk of DVT**
≥ 3	High
1–2	Moderate
< 1	Low

10

MANAGEMENT OF THROMBOLYTIC-INDUCED MAJOR BLEEDING

1 Ensure large bore IV access.
2 Draw bloods for FBC, platelet count, PT/INR, APTT, G&H.
3 Volume resuscitation—including packed RBCs.
4 Stop heparin/LMWH: consider protamine.
5 6–12 U cryoprecipitate.
6 Stop antiplatelet therapy.
7 If the patient is still bleeding, check fibrinogen level:
    — if fibrinogen > 1 g/L → FFP 2 U
    — if fibrinogen < 1 g/L → cryoprecipitate 8–12 U.
8 If patient is still bleeding, consider tranexamic acid 1 g IV, reverse antiplatelet effect.
9 Reverse antiplatelet effects—platelets, DDAVP 0.3 microg/kg.
10 Recheck PT/INR, APTT, fibrinogen, bleeding time.
11 Haematology consult.

St Vincent's Hospital
GUIDELINES FOR THE MANAGEMENT OF AN ELEVATED INTERNATIONAL NORMALISED RATIO (INR) IN ADULT PATIENTS WITH OR WITHOUT BLEEDING

Note:
- *Prothrombinex-HT* can only be prescribed after consultation with a haematologist.
- The anticoagulant effect of warfarin may be difficult to re-establish for some time after vitamin K is used. Use the lowest dose possible and, if possible, consult the treating specialist prior to using vitamin K.
- Small oral doses of vitamin K are obtained by measuring the dose from the injectable formulation and administering orally. Vitamin K effect on INR can be expected within 6–12 hours; however, the full effect of vitamin K in reducing the INR can take up to 24 hours.

Table 1 Guidelines for the management of an elevated international normalised ratio (INR) in adult patients with or without bleeding

Clinical setting	Action
INR higher than the therapeutic range but < 5; bleeding absent	Lower the dose or omit the next dose of warfarin. Resume therapy at a lower dose when the INR approaches therapeutic range. If the INR is only minimally above therapeutic range (up to 10%), dose reduction may not be necessary.
INR 5–9; bleeding absent	Cease warfarin therapy; consider reasons for elevated INR and patient-specific factors. Bleeding risk increases exponentially from INR 5 to 9; INR ≥ 6 should be monitored closely. If bleeding risk is high (see Table 2), give vitamin K (1–2 mg orally or 0.5–1 mg intravenously). See the notes above for further information about vitamin K. Measure INR within 24 hours and resume warfarin at a reduced dose once INR is in therapeutic range.
INR > 9; bleeding absent	Where there is a low risk of bleeding, cease warfarin therapy, give 2.5–5 mg vitamin K orally or 1 mg intravenously. Measure INR in 6–12 hours, resume warfarin therapy at a reduced dose once INR < 5.0. Where there is high risk of bleeding (see Table 2), cease warfarin therapy, give 1 mg vitamin K intravenously. Consider Prothrombinex-HT (25–50 IU/kg) and fresh frozen plasma (150–300 mL), measure INR in 6–12 hours, resume warfarin therapy at a reduced dose once INR < 5. *Prothrombinex-HT can only be prescribed after consultation with a haematologist.* See the notes above for further information about vitamin K.

10

Figure 10.1 St Vincent's Hospital guidelines for the management of an elevated INR in adult patients with or without bleeding (continues)
FFP, fresh frozen plasma; INR, international normalised ratio; PTX, Prothrombinex
Based on Tran HA, Chunilal SD, Harper PL et al, on behalf of the Australasian Society of Thrombosis and Haemostasis. An update of consensus guidelines for warfarin reversal. Med J Aust 2013;198(4):198–9

Continued

Clinical setting	Action
Any clinically significant bleeding where warfarin-induced coagulopathy is considered a contributing factor	Cease warfarin therapy, give 5–10 mg vitamin K intravenously, as well as Prothrombinex-HT (25–50 IU/kg) and fresh frozen plasma (150–300 mL), assess patient continuously until INR < 5, and bleeding stops. OR If fresh frozen plasma is unavailable, cease warfarin therapy, give 5–10 mg vitamin K intravenously, and Prothrombinex-HT (25–50 IU/kg), assess patient continuously until INR < 5, and bleeding stops. OR If Prothrombinex-HT is unavailable, cease warfarin therapy, give 5–10 mg vitamin K intravenously, and 10–15 mL/kg of fresh frozen plasma, assess patient continuously until INR < 5, and bleeding stops. ***Prothrombinex-HT can only be prescribed after consultation with a haematologist.*** In all situations carefully reassess the need for ongoing warfarin therapy.

10

Table 2 Risk factors for bleeding complications of anticoagulation therapy

Risk factor category	Specific risk factors
Age	> 65 years
Cardiac	Uncontrolled hypertension
Gastrointestinal	History of gastrointestinal haemorrhage, active peptic ulcer, hepatic insufficiency
Haematological/oncological	Thrombocytopenia (platelet count < 50 × 10^9/L), platelet dysfunction, coagulation defect, underlying malignancy
Neurological	History of stroke, cognitive or psychological impairment
Renal	Renal insufficiency
Trauma	Recent trauma, history of falls (> 3 within previous treatment year, or recurrent, injurious falls)
Alcohol	Excessive alcohol intake
Medications	Aspirin, non-specific non-steroidal anti-inflammatory drugs (COX-2 inhibitors do not impair platelet function, but can influence warfarin effect), 'natural remedies' that interfere with haemostasis. Careful monitoring of warfarin effect is critical to minimise risk in patients taking multiple medications.

Figure 10.1, cont'd

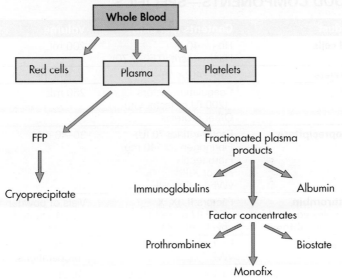

Figure 10.2 Blood components flow chart

REVERSING ANTICOAGULATION: PROTAMINE
- SLOW IV infusion (if rapid → hypotension, anaphylactoid reaction)

Protamine vs enoxaparin:
- 1 mg protamine will approximately neutralise 1 mg enoxaparin.
- Time since last dose of LMWH also determines protamine dose.

Time elapsed since last enoxaparin dose	Dose
< 8 h	1 mg protamine per 1 mg enoxaparin
> 8 h	0.5 mg protamine per 1 mg enoxaparin
> 12 h	Protamine may not be required

Protamine vs heparin:
- 10 mg protamine over 10 min followed by 10–20 mg protamine over 10–20 min.
- This will neutralise 2000–3000 U of heparin (approximately 1 mg protamine for every 100 U of heparin).

BLOOD COMPONENTS—SPECIFICS

Product	Contents (per unit)	Volume
Red cells	Hb (> 40 g) Haematocrit (0.50–0.70)	200 mL
Platelets	200–240 × 10^9	> 160 mL
FFP	Coagulation factors (200 IU of factor VIII) Other proteins	250 mL
Cryoprecipitate	Factor VIII (≥ 70 IU) Fibrinogen (≥ 140 mg) Fibronectin Factor XIII vWF (≥ 100 IU)	30–40 mL
Prothrombin complex concentrate (Prothrombinex)	Factors II, IX, X (500 IU of each) Low levels of VII	Vials of powder reconstituted to 20 mL
Biostate	Factor VIII vWF	Variety of preparations
MonoFIX	Factor IX concentrate	Variety of preparations

Adapted from the Australian Red Cross.

BLEEDING DISORDERS

Disorder	Defect	Treatment options
Haemophilia A *Mild* *Moderate* *Severe*	Absence/low factor VIII *6–25% factor VIII* *1–5%* *< 1%*	Desmopressin for mild (> 15%) Recombinant factor VIII Biostate
Haemophilia B	Absence/low factor IX	Recombinant factor IX MonoFIX
Von Willebrand	Quantitative +/− qualitative defect in vWF	Desmopressin Biostate
Coagulopathy 2° liver disease		Vit K FFP Platelets Cryoprecipitate
Thrombolytic drugs	Systemic fibrinolysis	Cryoprecipitate FFP

Note: Treatment should be guided by a specialist haematologist.

11   Neurology
ADULT CEREBROSPINAL FLUID (CSF) STUDIES

CSF studies in adults in normal and infected fluid

CSF studies	Normal	Bacterial	Viral	TB/fungi
Pressure (cmH$_2$O)	7–25	↑↑↑	Normal / ↑	Variable
WCC (per mm^3)	< 5	> 200–20 000	< 100	< 1000 ?variable
Predominant cell type	Lymphocytes, no polymorphs	Polymorphs (10% lymphocytes)	Lymphocytes	Lymphocytes
Glucose	≥ 0.6 × serum	↓ / normal	↑ / normal	↑ / normal
Protein (mg/L)	< 400 mg/L	↑ / normal	↑ / normal	↑
Organisms	0	+ve Gram stain in 80%		+ve India ink stain with cryptococcal

Causes of increased protein in CSF
• Inflammation
• Tumour
• Demyelinating disorders
• Subarachnoid haemorrhage
• Traumatic TAP

TRAUMATIC LUMBAR PUNCTURE (TAP)

Differences between traumatic lumbar puncture (TAP) and pathological bleeding

Traumatic TAP	Pathological bleeding
Decreasing blood in subsequent tubes	Same amount of blood in all tubes
Clear supernatant	Xanthochromia
Clots	No clots

Calculation to correct for falsely elevated WBC count due to a traumatic TAP

WBC artificially introduced =
WBC in blood × [RBC in CSF ÷ RBC in blood]

11

Therefore:

$$\text{WBC in CSF (predicted)} = \text{WBC in CSF (measured)} - \text{WBC artificially introduced}$$

COMMON UPPER LIMB NERVE PALSIES

Inspection and signs

Nerve	Inspection	Motor signs	Sensory signs	Pearls
Median	Thenar atrophy	Weak pronation of forearm	Numbness of radial 3½ digits and corresponding portions of the palm	Superficial branch of median supplies thenar eminence—distinguishes low from high lesion
	'Ape-hand' deformity (thumb lies in the same plane as the palm)	Weak flexion of wrist and fingers (especially index and middle) Unable to make a fist or close hand around a bottle Unable to flex or oppose thumb		
Ulnar	'Claw-hand' deformity (ring and little fingers curl up)	Froment's sign—testing thumb adduction causes thumb to flex instead of remaining straight	Numbness of entire little finger and ulnar half of ring finger	Less clawing in a high lesion Low lesion at level of wrist will have normal sensation Check intrinsic function by crossing middle finger over index finger
Radial	Wrist drop	Weak elbow extension Weak extension at wrist/digits Weak forearm supination	Dorsum of the hand	If weak elbow extension present then high lesion

Autogenous zones for median, ulnar and radial nerves

Nerve	Zone
Median	Volar aspect of the index finger
Ulnar	Volar aspect of the little finger
Radial	Dorsal aspect of 1st web space

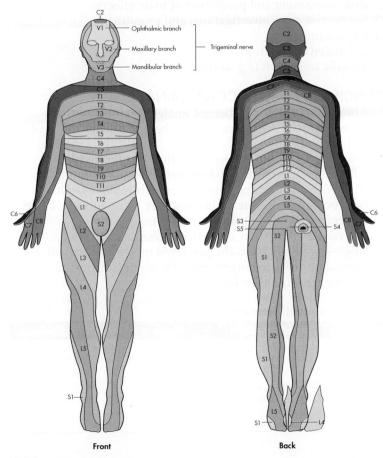

Figure 11.1 Dermatome maps

Reproduced with permission from Standring S, Gray's anatomy, 40th edn. Philadelphia: Churchill Livingstone, 2008: Fig 15.2A.

13 Toxicology
POISONS INFORMATION
Call 131126 (nationwide in Australia).

PRINCIPLES OF MANAGEMENT OF POISONINGS
1 Resuscitation
2 Risk assessment and prediction of toxic effects
3 Supportive care, investigations and monitoring
4 Decontamination
5 Enhanced elimination
6 Specific treatment (e.g. antidotes)

PRINCIPLES OF GI DECONTAMINATION
- Always perform a risk–benefit analysis—risks from the decontamination process vs likely benefit for that particular toxicity and patient.
- Not routinely used—depends on time of presentation following ingestion and risk of toxicity.
- Not recommended for non-toxic or sub-toxic ingestions.
- Not recommended for toxins that may → seizures or ↓ LOC.
- Not recommended for hydrocarbon ingestions.
- Not recommended for corrosive ingestions.
- Single-dose charcoal is the preferred modality. Use will depend on risk assessment and safe administration as opposed to strict time limits.

Decontamination methods

Modality	Agent/method	Dose	Contraindications
Activated charcoal (AC)	Place in cup Mix with ice cream for children Can give via OGT/ NGT once tube placement confirmed	1 g/kg (children) 50 g (adults)	As text above plus: — ↓ LOC — Toxin does not bind to AC*

Decontamination methods (cont.)

Modality	Agent/method	Dose	Contraindications
Gastric lavage	Patient position left lateral, head down 36–40 G lavage tube inserted into oesophagus Aspirate gastric contents Instil 200 mL warm water into stomach Drain fluid into dependent bucket Continue instilling/draining until effluent is clear Finish with administering AC		As text above plus: — Unprotected airway — Small children
Whole-bowel irrigation**	Polyethylene glycol electrolyte solution (PEG) Place NGT and administer PEG at rate of 2 L/h (adults) or 25 mL/kg/h (children) Give metoclopramide (minimise vomiting and ↑ gastric emptying) Easy access to toilet/commode Continue until effluent is clear or packages/drug preparations apparent Monitor for abdominal distension or ↓ bowel sounds		

* See table below: Drugs not well adsorbed by activated charcoal
** See box below: Poisonings where whole-bowel irrigation MAY be useful

13

Drugs not well adsorbed by activated charcoal

Drug group	Examples
Alcohols	Ethanol, methanol, isopropyl alcohol, ethylene glycol
Metals	Lithium, iron, mercury, potassium, lead, arsenic
Acids and alkalis	
Hydrocarbons	Turpentine, kerosene, eucalyptus oil, benzene

Poisonings where whole-bowel irrigation MAY be useful

- Life-threatening ingestions of sustained-release preparations (e.g. verapamil, diltiazem, potassium)
- Life-threatening ingestions of enteric-coated preparations
- Agents that do not bind to charcoal (e.g. lead, arsenic)
- 'Body packers/stuffers' (illicit drug 'mules')
- Iron overdose

Complications associated with GI decontamination

- GI trauma or perforation
- Bowel obstruction
- Nausea, vomiting
- Aspiration pneumonitis
- Laryngospasm
- Hypoxia

Measurable (serum) toxin levels useful in assessing toxicity

- Alcohol
- Carbamazepine
- Carboxyhaemoglobin
- Digoxin

- Iron
- Lithium
- Methaemoglobin
- Paracetamol

- Phenytoin
- Salicylate
- Sodium valproate
- Theophylline

Enhanced elimination techniques

	Multiple-dose activated charcoal	Urinary alkalinisation	Haemodialysis
Toxins technique may be used in	Carbamazepine Dapsone Phenobarbitone Quinine Theophylline	Phenobarbitone Salicylates	Alcohols Lithium Metformin Potassium Salicylate Theophylline Valproate

13

RISK-ASSESSMENT CHART FOR COMMON OVERDOSES

This table highlights *approximate* doses associated with significant toxicity requiring observation, treatment and discussion with a toxicologist or Poisons Centre.

Drug	Adult	Children
Aspirin	150 mg/kg $>$ 300 mg/kg = severe intoxication	
Carbamazepine	20–50 mg/kg	
Carbon monoxide	$>$ 10%	
Chlorpromazine	$>$ 5 g	1 tablet

Drug	Adult	Children
Cocaine	> 1 g = potentially lethal	
Colchicine	> 0.2 mg/kg Any intentional OD = potentially lethal	
Digoxin—acute ingestion	> 10 mg = potentially lethal	> 75 microg/kg > 4 mg = potentially lethal
Ibuprofen	> 100 mg/kg	> 300 mg/kg
Iron	20–60 mg/kg	> 60 mg/kg
Lithium—acute ingestion	> 25 g	
Metformin	> 10 g	> 1700 mg
Olanzapine	40–100 mg	> 0.5 mg/kg
Opioids		> 2 mg/kg codeine PO
Paracetamol—acute single ingestion	> 150 mg/kg *or* > 10 g	> 200 mg/kg
Phenelzine	> 2 mg/kg 4–6 mg/kg potentially lethal	1–2 tablets
Phenytoin	> 20 mg/kg	> 200 mg
Quetiapine	> 3 g	> 100 mg
Quinine	> 1 g	600 mg = potentially lethal
Risperidone		> 1 mg
Salicylates	150–300 mg/kg	> 5 mL of methyl salicylate (oil of wintergreen)
Sulfonylureas	1 tablet (especially if non-diabetic)	1 tablet
Tramadol	> 1.5 g	> 10 mg/kg
Tricyclic antidepressants (TCAs)	> 10 mg/kg	> 5 mg/kg
Valproate	> 400 mg/kg	> 200 mg/kg

13

RATIO OF ACUTE EQUIPOTENCY OF OPIOID ANALGESICS

When changing opioid start at 50%, the equipotent dose, then titrate according to response.

Drug	Oral dose	Parenteral dose	Approximate duration of action
Buprenorphine	0.8 mg sublingual	0.4 mg IM	6–8 h
Codeine	200 mg	120–130 mg IM/SC	3–4 h
Fentanyl	–	100–150 microg IV/SC	0.5–1 h
Methadone	Complex	–	8–24 h
Morphine	30 mg	10 mg IM/SC	2–3 h 12–24 h (controlled release)
Oxycodone	15–20 mg	–	3–4 h 12–24 h (controlled release)
Pethidine	–	75–100 mg IM	2–3 h
Tramadol	150 mg	100–120 mg IM/IV	

Based on the *Australian Medicines Handbook*, 2011. Online. Available: www.amh.hcn.com.au

ANTIDOTES

Drug	'Antidote'
Benzodiazepines	Flumazenil
Beta blockers	High-dose insulin therapy
Calcium channel blockers	Calcium chloride Calcium gluconate High-dose insulin therapy
Carbon monoxide	Oxygen (enhances elimination)
Cyanide	Hydroxocobalamin (Cyanokit) = 1st line Sodium thiosulfate = 2nd line
Digoxin	Digoxin immune Fab (antibody fragments)

Drug	'Antidote'
Heparin	Protamine
Hydrofluoric acid (skin exposure)	Calcium gel 2.5% Calcium gluconate 1 g/10 mL DO NOT USE CALCIUM CHLORIDE (it causes tissue damage)
Insulin	Glucose
Iron	Desferrioxamine
Isoniazid	Pyridoxine
Lead	Dimercaptosuccinic acid (DMSA) Sodium calcium edetate (for lead encephalopathy/severe poisoning)
Lignocaine	Intralipid 20%
Methanol, ethylene glycol	Ethanol
Methaemoglobinaemia	Methylene Blue
Opiates	Naloxone
Organophosphates	Atropine Pralidoxime
Paracetamol	N-acetylcysteine
Sulfonylureas	Octreotide + glucose
Tricyclic antidepressants	Bicarbonate
Warfarin	Vitamin K Prothrombin complex concentrates (e.g. Prothrombinex, FFP)

13

15 Paediatrics
PAEDIATRIC FORMULAS

Formulas for approximate weight (kg) based on age

Age	Approximate calculated weight
< 12 months	(age in months ÷ 2) + 4
1–5 years	(2 × age in years) + 8
6–12 years	(3 × age in years) + 7

BP

Approximate systolic BP (mmHg) = 80 + (age in years × 2)

Formulas for ETT size

Age > 1 year	
ETT size (mm)	(age ÷ 4) + 4 (uncuffed)
	(age ÷ 4) + 3 (cuffed)
ETT length (cm) at lips	(age ÷ 2) + 12
ETT length (cm) at nose	(age ÷ 2) + 15

For the newborn	
Weight	ETT size (mm)
< 1 kg	2.5
1–3.5 kg	3.0
> 3.5 kg	3.5

PAEDIATRIC VITAL SIGNS: NORMAL RANGES

Age (years)	Heart rate (beats/min)	Systolic BP (mmHg)	Respiratory rate (breaths/min)
< 1	110–160	70–90	30–40
1–2	100–150	80–95	25–35
2–5	95–140	80–100	25–30
5–12	80–120	90–110	20–25
> 12	60–100	100–120	15–20

PAEDIATRIC MODIFIED GLASGOW COMA SCALE

Eyes open			
Any age			**Score**
Spontaneously			4
To speech			3
To pain			2
No response			1

Best verbal response			
> 5 y	**2–5 y**	**0–23 mths**	**Score**
Orientated and converses	Appropriate words and phrases	Smiles, coos, cries appropriately	5
Confused	Inappropriate words	Cries but consolable	4
Inappropriate words	Cries and/or screams	Persistent cries and/or screams	3
Incomprehensible sounds	Grunts	Grunts	2
No response	No response	No response	1

Best motor response		
> 1 y	**< 1 y**	**Score**
Obeys command	Spontaneously moves	6
Localises pain	Localises pain	5
Flexion–withdrawal	Flexion–withdrawal	4
Flexion–abnormal (decorticate rigidity)	Flexion–abnormal (decorticate rigidity)	3
Extension (decerebrate)	Extension (decerebrate)	2
No response	No response	1

15

PAEDIATRIC PEAK EXPIRATORY FLOW

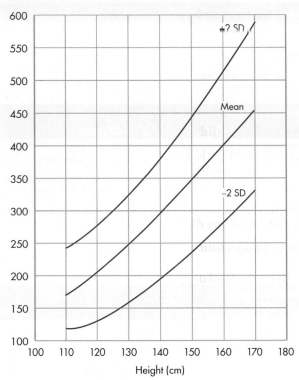

Figure 15.1
Peak expiratory flow chart for children 5–18 y (male and female)

PAEDIATRIC FLUID THERAPY

Bolus for resuscitation: 20 mL/kg IV with usually 0.9% saline
Maintenance fluids:
— 10% dextrose +/− 0.18% saline in neonates
— plasmalyte or 0.9% saline with 5% glucose for children

Weight in kg	mL/kg/day	mL/kg/h
0–10	100	4
11–20	50	2
> 20	20	1

Example 1: 3-kg child

$$\text{Maintenance fluids} = (3 \times 100) \text{ mL/day}$$
$$= 300 \text{ mL/day}$$

Example 2: 13-kg child

$$\text{Maintenance fluids} = (10 \times 100) + (3 \times 50) \text{ mL/day}$$
$$= 1000 + 150 \text{ mL/day}$$
$$= 1150 \text{ mL/day}$$

Example 3: 25-kg child

$$\text{Maintenance fluids} = (10 \times 100) + (10 \times 50) + (5 \times 20) \text{ mL/day}$$
$$= 1000 + 500 + 100 \text{ mL/day}$$
$$= 1600 \text{ mL/day}$$

Note: This formula does not include any losses or additional fluid requirements. Add any deficits and ongoing losses to the above.

Example 4: 11-kg child with 5% dehydration

$$\text{Maintenance fluids} = (10 \times 100) + (1 \times 50) \text{ mL/day}$$
$$= 1000 + 50 \text{ mL/day}$$
$$= 1050 \text{ mL/day}$$

$$\text{Deficit} = 5\% \times 11 \text{ kg}$$
$$= 0.05 \times 11\,000 \text{ mL}$$
$$= 550 \text{ mL}$$

$$\text{Total fluids required} = 1050 + 550 \text{ mL/day}$$
$$= 1600 \text{ mL/day}$$

15

16 Pathology

Haematology

Anaemia type	Laboratory findings	More common causes
Iron deficiency	Hb = N/ ↓ MCV = N/ ↓ (microcytic) MCH = N/ ↓ (hypochromic) Fe ↓ ferritin ↓ TIBC ↑ Transferrin ↑	Blood loss, diet low in iron, poor absorption of iron
Pernicious and vitamin B deficiency	Hb ↓ MCV ↑ (macrocytic) Reticulocyte count ↓ B₁₂ or folate level ↓ if deficient	Intrinsic factor antibodies Diet low in vitamin B₁₂, folate
Haemolytic	Hb ↓ MCH ↑ Reticulocyte count ↑ Abnormal forms of RBC in peripheral smear (spherocytes, elliptocytes, spur cells, tear drops, inclusions) Unconjugated (indirect) bilirubin ↑ LDH ↑ Haptoglobin ↓	Sickle-cell anaemia, thalassaemia, autoimmune diseases, transfusion reaction, drugs
Aplastic	Hb ↓ RBC and WBC counts ↓ Platelet count ↓ MCV, MCH usually N WBC differential usually shows ↓ all white cell types except lymphocytes Reticulocyte count ↓	Cancer therapy, toxins, autoimmune, viral infections

Fe = iron; Hb = haemoglobin; LDH = lactate dehydrogenase; MCH = mean corpuscular haemoglobin (average amount of Hb in RBCs); MCV = mean corpuscular volume (average size of RBCs); N = normal; RBC = red blood cell; TIBC = total iron-binding capacity; WBC = white blood cell.

PLEURAL FLUID
What tests to order:

- Differential cell count
- Protein
- LDH

- Glucose
- Culture (also put fluid into blood culture bottles—this improves yield of anaerobic organisms)
- Cytology

Note: There must be simultaneous measurement of the equivalent serum values of protein, LDH and glucose in order to do the calculations below.

Normal pleural fluid

Colour	Clear
pH	7.60–7.64
Protein content	< 2% (1–2 g/dL)
Cell count	< 1000 WBC per mm^3
Glucose	Similar to that of plasma
LDH	< 50% that of plasma

Exudate if:

Pleural fluid protein:serum protein > 0.5	Light's criteria
Pleural fluid LDH:serum LDH > 0.6	
Pleural LDH > ⅔ the upper limit of the normal serum value	
Pleural fluid LDH > 0.45 the upper limit of the normal serum value	Additional criteria
Pleural fluid cholesterol level > 45 mg/dL	
Pleural fluid protein level > 2.9 g/dL	

Transudates Low protein and LDH	Exudates Relatively high protein or LDH, pH < 7.2
• CCF • Cirrhosis, ascites • Hypoalbuminaemia • Nephrotic syndrome • Peritoneal dialysis • Myxoedema • Constrictive pericarditis	• Parapneumonic causes • Malignancy • PE • Infection • Pancreatitis • Sarcoidosis • Autoimmune (RA, SLE) • Chylothorax • Haemothorax • Intra-abdominal abscess

16

Laboratory result on pleural fluid	Possible cause
LDH > 1000 IU/L	Empyema Malignancy RA
Low glucose (1.7–2.8 mmol/L)	Malignancy TB Oesophageal rupture SLE
Very low glucose (< 1.7 mmol/L)	RA Empyema
pH < 7.30 with a normal serum pH	Malignancy TB Oesophageal rupture SLE
> 85% lymphocytes	Lymphoma TB Sarcoidosis Chronic rheumatoid pleurisy Yellow nail syndrome Chylothorax
50–70% lymphocytes	Malignancy
Eosinophilia (> 10%)	Air/blood in pleural space PE/pulmonary infarction Benign asbestos disease Parasitic disease Fungal infection Drugs

SYNOVIAL FLUID ANALYSIS

16

	Appearance	WBCs/mm³	PMN%	Crystals
Normal	Clear	< 200	< 25%	None
Non-inflammatory	Clear	< 400	< 25%	None
Acute gout	Cloudy	2000–5000	> 75%	Negative birefringence
Pseudogout	Cloudy	5000–50 000	> 75%	Positive birefringence
Septic arthritis	Purulent	15 000–> 50 000	> 75% (> 90% = very suggestive)	None
Inflammatory (e.g. RA)	Cloudy	5000–50 000	50–75%	None

17   Orthopaedics
SYSTEMATIC APPROACH TO DESCRIBING A FRACTURE

1 **Age** and **sex** and **occupation** of patient $+/-$ hand dominance if upper limb
2 Name the **bone(s) involved**
3 **Open versus closed** injury—if open, describe the wound (e.g. abrasion, full-thickness laceration) and its relationship to the fracture site
4 **Location** of the fracture
   a   Is it in the proximal, middle or distal part of the bone?
   b   Is it at a junction?
      Examples:
      • Junction of the proximal ⅔ and distal ⅓
      • Junction of the proximal ¼ and distal ¾
      • Junction of the lateral ⅓ and medial ⅔
   c   Is it involving the head, neck, shaft or base of the bone?
      Examples:
      • Head of the 5th metacarpal
      • Middle part of the shaft of the humerus
   d   Is it involving an anatomical part of the bone?
      Examples:
      • Greater trochanter of the femur
      • Greater tuberosity of the head of the humerus
5 **Pattern/direction** of the fracture (horizontal, spiral, oblique, comminuted [more than 2 pieces], segmental [several large fragments in one bone], T-shaped, Y-shaped etc)
6 **Alignment**
   a   Is it displaced or undisplaced?
   b   Is it straight or angulated (estimate degree of and anatomical direction)?
7 **Special features**
   a   Number of malleoli in ankle (unimalleolar/bimalleolar/trimalleolar)
   b   Medial and lateral plateau of tibia
   c   Named fracture patterns (e.g. Colles' [distal radius]; Weber A, B, C [lateral malleolus])
   d   Neck of femur—subcapital, transcervical, pertrochanteric, intertrochanteric

17

Common fracture patterns

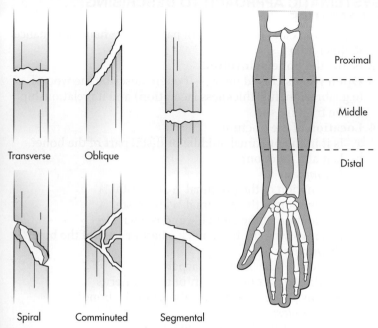

Transverse Oblique

Proximal

Middle

Distal

Spiral Comminuted Segmental

Figure 17.1 Common types of fractures

OTTAWA ANKLE RULES
An ankle X-ray is required if:

17

There is any pain in the malleolar region and one of the following:
- bone tenderness at the posterior edge of the distal 6 cm of the fibula or the tip of the lateral malleolus *or*
- bone tenderness at the posterior edge of the distal 6 cm of the tibia or the tip of the medial malleolus *or*
- inability to weight bear both immediately and in emergency department.

A foot X-ray is required if:

There is any pain in the midfoot region and one of the following:
- bone tenderness over the base of the 5th metatarsal *or*
- bone tenderness over the navicular *or*
- inability to weight bear both immediately and in emergency department (not applicable to < 18 y).

Clinical judgement is required for those intoxicated, uncooperative, ↓ sensation in leg or with distracting injuries.

Classification	Location of fracture line	Integrity of syndesmosis	Stability
A	Below the level of the ankle joint	Intact	Usually stable; occasionally needs ORIF
B	At the level of the ankle joint	Disruption in 50%	Variable
C	Above the level of the ankle joint	Always disrupted	Unstable ORIF

Syndesmosis is made up of anterior–inferior tibiofibular ligament, interosseous ligament and posterior–inferior fibular ligaments, inferior transverse tibiofibular ligament and interosseous ligament.
ORIF = open reduction internal fixation.

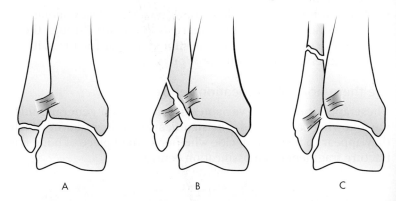

Figure 17.2 Weber classification of ankle (fibular) fractures

17

OTTAWA KNEE RULES
A knee X-ray is required if:

- Age > 55 y
- Unable to transfer weight for 4 steps both immediately after injury and in emergency department
- Unable to flex to 90°
- Tenderness over fibular head
- Isolated tenderness of patella

INTERPRETATION OF ELBOW FRACTURES IN CHILDREN
Is there a joint effusion?

- Fat pad sign—present with effusion
- Look for upward displacement of anterior fat pad
  or
- a visible posterior fat pad (almost always abnormal).

Is there normal alignment of the bones?

- Radiocapitellar line—line drawn through the centre of the proximal radius should pass through the centre of the capitellum on all views. If not, the radial head is subluxed or dislocated.
- Anterior humeral line—line drawn on a lateral view along the anterior border of the humerus should pass through the middle ⅓ of the capitellum—in supracondylar fractures, it often intersects with anterior ⅓ or beyond.

Are there normal ossification centres?

These appear at highly variable times but, as a general guide, the following can be used. The significance is the order in which they appear to help you decide whether a small piece of bone is a fracture fragment or an ossification centre.

17

Elbow ossification order—CRITOE

	Ossification centre	Age of appearance
C	Capitellum	1 y
R	Radial head	3 y
I	Internal (medial) epicondyle	5 y
T	Trochlea	7 y
O	Olecranon	9 y
E	External (lateral) epicondyle	11 y

X-ray changes to look for

Features to look for	What it means	Likely cause
Elevation of anterior fat pad	Joint effusion	Fracture or dislocation of radial head in elbow joint
Presence of a posterior fat pad (not normally visible at all)	Joint effusion	Fracture or dislocation of radial head in elbow joint
Radiocapitellar line (evident on all views)	Displacement of radial head	Subluxation or dislocation of the radial head
Anterior humeral line (use a TRUE lateral view)	Displacement of the distal part of the humerus	Supracondylar fracture

Supracondylar fractures

- Represent 60% of paediatric elbow fractures
- Commonly distal fragment angulates and displaces posteriorly
- Pay close attention to neurovascular status of the limb—10% incidence of nerve injury—radial most commonly then median and finally ulnar

17

SALTER-HARRIS CLASSIFICATION OF PHYSEAL (GROWTH PLATE) FRACTURES IN CHILDREN

- Grades I–V (see also Figure 17.3)
- Significance: higher grades have greater risk of growth abnormalities

Grade	Description	Pearls and pitfalls
I	Fracture within the growth plate	May not be visible on X-ray or may see widening or displacement of the growth plate on X-ray
II	Involves metaphysis and growth plate	Most common Rarely cause future functional limitations
III	Involves epiphysis and growth plate	Intra-articular therefore can cause chronic disability but rarely significant deformity
IV	Intra-articular fracture which involves the metaphysis, growth plate and epiphysis	Can cause deformity due to premature fusion of bones
V	Compression injury	Difficult to see on X-ray Cause functional limitations due to growth disturbance History of axial load injury might be only clue to diagnosis

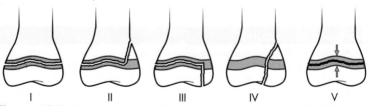

I II III IV V

17 **Figure 17.3** Salter-Harris classification of physeal (growth plate) fractures in children

18   Obstetrics and gynaecology
BETA-HUMAN CHORIONIC GONADOTROPHIN (beta-hCG)

- In normal pregnancy, levels double every 2 days.
- Transvaginal ultrasound (TVUS) will detect:
  — gestational sac at ~4.5–5 weeks gestation
  — yolk sac at 5–6 weeks (until 10 weeks)
  — fetal pole with cardiac activity (5.5–6 weeks).
- Discriminatory zone:
  — This is the serum beta-hCG level at which a gestational sac should be visualised by ultrasound if the pregnancy is intrauterine.
  — For TVUS, this is 1500–2000 IU/L.
  — For transabdominal ultrasound (TAUS), this is 6500 IU/L.
  — These may vary according to individuals/multiple gestation.

Rh D IMMUNOGLOBULIN (ANTI-D) ADMINISTRATION
Dose:

- If < 12 weeks gestation → 250 IU IM
- If > 12 weeks gestation → 625 IU IM

Indications:

- Possible fetomaternal haemorrhage (see box below)

Indications for Anti-D administration

- Antenatal haemorrhage
- Induced abortion
- Miscarriage
- Ectopic pregnancy
- Maternal abdominal trauma
- Delivery
- Partial molar pregnancy
- Chorionic villus sampling, amniocentesis
- Cordocentesis
- Percutaneous fetal procedures (e.g. fetoscopy)
- External cephalic version
- Abruptio placenta
- Manual removal of the placenta

18

PRETERM LABOUR SUPPRESSION

- Between 24 and 34 weeks.
- Accounts for only 10% of births but is associated with 75% of neonatal morbidity and mortality.
- To prevent respiratory distress syndrome, administer betamethasone 11.4 mg IM. Repeat the dose 24 h later, unless delivery has occurred.
- Tocolytic agent (see table) = *nifedipine is preferred; salbutamol may also be used*

Tocolytic agent	Nifedipine	Salbutamol infusion
Initial dose	20 mg PO (onset of tocolysis = 30–60 mins)	6 mL/h of 10 mg in 100 mL 0.9% saline*
Subsequent dosing	20 mg PO at 30-minute intervals for 2 more doses (if required)	↑ rate by 3 mL/h every 10 min until response (maximum dose 30 mL/h)
Maintenance dose	20–40 mg PO q6h depending on uterine activity and side effects (max 160 mg/24 h)	If contractions cease, maintain infusion rate for 6 h and then ↓ by 3 mL/h each hour until maintenance level reached
Side effects	Hypotension Tachycardia Palpitations Flushing Headache Nausea	Tremor Anxiety Nausea Palpitations
Tips	Do not use if hypotensive, established cardiac disease BP reduction may be potentiated by other antihypertensives Caution using magnesium concurrently	Cease if maternal chest pain, SOB, vomiting Slow rate if maternal HR > 140/min or FHR > 180/min

* To make up infusion, withdraw 10 mL from a 100-mL bag of 0.9% saline and replace with 10 mL (10 mg) of obstetric salbutamol. This results in 100 microg/mL. FHR = fetal heart rate

18

19 Dental

Dental trauma

Trauma	Definition	Treatment
Concussion	Tooth is immobile and undisplaced, normal X-ray; sensitive to percussion	Rest (no biting)
Subluxation	Loosening of tooth but no displacement; sensitive to percussion	Use local anaesthetic Return tooth to correct anatomical position without further damage to tissues and bone and secure to adjacent teeth with a periodontal splint Analgesia Antibiotic cover Early dental follow-up
Avulsion	Complete extraction of tooth	
Intrusive luxation	Forcing of tooth into its socket (in apical direction)	
Extrusive luxation	Tooth forced in axial direction out of socket	
Lateral luxation	Tooth is forced into a sideways direction	
Dental fracture	Ellis class I: enamel only; non-tender, no colour change, rough edges	File rough edges if necessary
	Ellis class II: enamel and dentin involved; tender to touch and air exposure; may see yellow layer of dentin	Cover exposed site with calcium hydroxide composition Analgesia Antibiotic cover
	Ellis class III: pulp involved; tender as with class II and pink/red or blood seen in centre of tooth	Cover exposed site with calcium hydroxide composition Analgesia Antibiotic cover

19

Figure 19.1 Ellis fracture classification

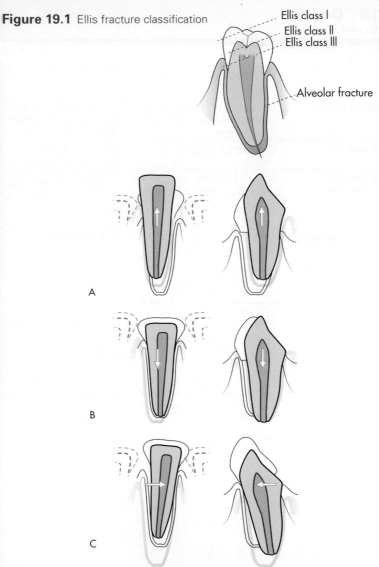

Ellis class I
Ellis class II
Ellis class III

Alveolar fracture

A

B

C

Figure 19.2 Patterns of luxation **A,** Extrusive luxation. **B,** Intrusive luxation. **C,** Lateral luxation.

19

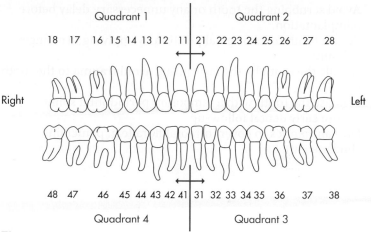

Figure 19.3 Dental chart—nomenclature and universal numbering system for permanent (adult) dentition

LOCAL ANAESTHESIA—SUPRAPERIOSTEAL INFILTRATION

This technique is useful for a single tooth or closely clustered group of teeth.

- Place the needle in the mucobuccal fold with the bevel facing the bone.
- Direct the needle tip towards the apex of the desired tooth (usually several millimetres deep).
- If bone is contacted, withdraw slightly to avoid periosteal infiltration.
- Inject anaesthetic once satisfied the needle is in the correct place (i.e. not intravascular).
- Generally 1–2 mL of local anaesthetic is sufficient.
- It may take up to 10 min to achieve complete anaesthesia.

REIMPLANTATION OF AVULSED TOOTH

- Gently clean tooth in either normal saline or sterile auxiliary solution (e.g. Hank's balanced salt solution).

19

- Avoid scrubbing the tooth or any unnecessary delay before reimplantation.
- Return tooth to its original position by applying firm finger pressure.
- Handle the tooth by the crown, and avoid trauma to the tooth root.
- Stabilise the tooth with a temporary periodontal splint.
- Ensure early dental follow-up.
- Give antibiotics to cover intraoral flora (e.g. penicillin, clindamycin).

22 Normal values
(Approximate reference ranges)

Blood chemistry

Sodium	137–146 mmol/L
Potassium	3.5–5.0 mmol/L
Chloride	95–110 mmol/L
Bicarbonate	24–31 mmol/L
Urea	3.0–8.5 mmol/L
Creatinine	Male: 60–120 micromol/L Female: 40–90 micromol/L
Glucose	3.0–7.8 mmol/L
Phosphate	0.70–1.40 mmol/L
Magnesium	0.70–1.05 mmol/L
Calcium	2.10–2.60 mmol/L
Albumin	36–52 g/L
Total protein	66–82 g/L
Total bilirubin	0–18 micromol/L
ALT	0–30 U/L
AST	0–30 U/L
ALP	30–100 U/L
GGT	0–35 U/L
Lipase	< 60 U/L
Troponin T (hs)	0–14 ng/L

Full blood count

Haemoglobin	130–180 g/L (men) 115–165 g/L (women)
MCV	76–96 fL
Platelets	$150–400 \times 10^9$/L
WCC	$4.0–11.0 \times 10^9$/L
APTT	25–35 s
PT	11–15 s

22

Abbreviations

1°, 2° primary, secondary
3D three-dimensional
AAA abdominal aortic aneurysm
AAI acute arterial insufficiency
ABC or ABCs airway, breathing, circulation (the ABCs of resuscitation)
ABCDE (in medical retrieval) airway, breathing, circulation, disability, exposure/expectations
ABG arterial blood gas
AC acromioclavicular; alternating current
ACE angiotensin-converting enzyme
ACEM Australasian College for Emergency Medicine
ACI acute cardiac ischaemia
ACL anterior cruciate ligament
ACLS advanced cardiac life support
ACS acute coronary syndrome
ACTH adrenocorticotrophic hormone
AD Addison's disease, atopic dermatitis
ADC AIDS dementia complex
ADH antidiuretic hormone
ADHF acute decompensated (chronic) heart failure
ADL or ADLs activities of daily living
ADT adult diphtheria tetanus
AED automatic external defibrillator
AF atrial fibrillation
AG anion gap
AGE arterial gas embolism
AGEP acute generalised exanthematic pustulosis
AGVHD acute graft-versus-host disease
AHF acute heart failure
AIDS acquired immune deficiency syndrome
AIR assessment, intervention, reassessment
ALS (adult) advanced life support

ALT alanine aminotransferase
AMC area medical coordinator
AMI acute myocardial infarction
AML acute myelocytic leukaemia
AMTS Abbreviated Mental Test Score
ANUG acute necrotising ulcerative gingivitis
AP anteroposterior
APLS advanced paediatric life support
APO acute pulmonary oedema
APTT activated partial thromboplastin time
ARDS acute respiratory distress syndrome
ARF acute renal failure
ARS adjective rating scale (for pain)
ART antiretroviral therapy
ASCOT a severity characterisation of trauma
ASD atrial septal defect
ASET aged service emergency team
AST aspartate aminotransferase
ATLS advanced trauma life support
ATN acute tubular necrosis
ATP adenosine triphosphate
ATS Australasian Triage Scale
AV arteriovenous; atrioventricular
AVM arteriovenous malformation
AVN avascular necrosis
AVNRT AV nodal re-entry tachycardia
AVRT AV re-entry tachycardia
AWS alcohol withdrawal scale
AXIS electrical pathway mapping
BAC blood alcohol concentration
BD, bd, bid twice daily
BBB bundle branch block
beta-hCG beta-human chorionic gonadotrophin
BiPAP bi-level positive airway pressure
BLS basic life support
BNP B-type natriuretic protein

BP blood pressure
bpm beats per minute
BPV benign positional vertigo
BPPV benign paroxysmal positional vertigo
BSA body surface area
BSL blood sugar level
BURP backward, upward, rightward pressure
BVM bag–valve–mask
Ca calcium
CABG coronary artery bypass graft
CAL (acute-on)-chronic airflow limitation, chronic airway limitation
CA-MRSA community-acquired methicillin-resistant *Staphylococcus aureus*
CAM Confusion Assessment Method
CAPD continuous ambulatory peritoneal dialysis
CAS coloured analogue scale (for pain)
CBR chemical, biological, radiological
CCF congestive cardiac failure; chronic cardiac failure
CCO casualty clearing officer
CCR5 chemokine (C–C motif) receptor 5 (blockers)
CCU coronary care unit
CHB complete heart block
CIN clinical initiatives nurse
COPD chronic obstructive pulmonary disease
CHB complete heart block
CIAP Clinical Information Access Program
CIN clinical initiatives nurse
CJD Creutzfeldt–Jakob disease
CK creatine kinase
CLL chronic lymphocytic leukaemia
CMC central medical coordinator
CML chromic myeloid leukaemia
CMO career medical officer
CMV cytomegalovirus
CNS central nervous system

CO carbon monoxide; cardiac output
CO₂ carbon dioxide
COAD chronic obstructive airways disease
COLD chronic obstructive lung disease
COPD chronic obstructive pulmonary disease
CPAP continuous positive airway pressure
CPK creatine phosphokinase
CPP cerebral perfusion pressure
CPR cardiopulmonary resuscitation
CRAG cryptococcal antigen
CRF chronic renal failure
CRP C-reactive protein
CSF cerebrospinal fluid
C-spine cervical spine
CSL Commonwealth Serum Laboratories
CT computed tomography
CTA computed tomography angiography
CTCA CT coronary angiography
CTG cardiotocography
CTPA computed tomography pulmonary angiogram
CTR cardiothoracic ratio
CVA cerebrovascular accident
CVC central venous catheter
CVP central venous pressure
CVS cardiovascular system
CXR chest X-ray
D&C dilation and curettage
DBP diastolic blood pressure
DC direct current
DD differential diagnosis/diagnoses
DFA direct fluorescent antibody
DI diabetes insipidus
DIC disseminated intravascular coagulation
DIP distal interphalangeal
DISPLAN medical response plan
DKA diabetic ketoacidosis
DM diabetes mellitus
DNA deoxyribonucleic acid

DPL diagnostic peritoneal lavage

DRESS drug reaction/rash with eosinophilia and systemic symptoms

DRS disability rating scale

DSA digital subtraction angiography

DTP diphtheria, tetanus, pertussis (vaccine)

DTaP, DTPa diphtheria, tetanus, acellular pertussis (vaccine)

DTs delirium tremens

DUB dysfunctional uterine bleeding

DVT deep vein thrombosis, deep venous thrombosis

EB epidermolysis bullosa

EBV Epstein–Barr virus

ECC emergency control centre

ECF extracellular fluid

ECG electrocardiogram, electrocardiography

ECMO extracorporeal membrane oxygenation

ED emergency department

EDH extradural haematoma

EDIS Emergency Department Information System

EER external emergency response

EEG electroencephalogram, electroencephalography

EF ejection fraction

eFAST extended FAST (focused assessment with sonography in trauma)

eGFR estimated glomerular filtration rate

EGFRI epidermal growth factor receptor inhibitor

EIA enzyme immunoassay

ELISA enzyme-linked immunosorbent assay

ELS emergency life support

EM erythema multiforme

EMA Emergency Management Australia

EMD electromechanical dissociation

EMR electronic medical record

EMLA trade name for topical anaesthetic

EMST early management of severe trauma (guidelines)

EOC emergency operation centre

ENT ear, nose, throat

EOC emergency operation centre

EPAP expiratory positive airway pressure

EPS electrophysiological study

ERCP endoscopic retrograde cholangiopancreatography

ESR erythrocyte sedimentation rate

ESWL extracorporeal shock-wave lithotripsy

EtCO$_2$ end-tidal carbon dioxide

ETT endotracheal tube

EUC electrolytes, urea and creatinine (also UEC)

EVD external ventricular drain

FAS facial affective scale (for pain)

FAST focused assessment with sonography in trauma

FBC full blood count

FBE full blood examination

FDP fibrin degradation products; flexor digitorum profundus (deep digital flexor)

FDS flexor digitorum superficialis (superficial digital flexor)

FEV$_1$ forced expiratory volume in the 1st second

FFP fresh frozen plasma

FIM functional independence measure

FiO$_2$ fraction of inspired oxygen

Fr French gauge

FRC functional residual capacity

FSH follicle-stimulating hormone

FVC forced vital capacity

G&H group and hold (blood)

GABA gamma-aminobutyric acid

GBHS group B beta-haemolytic *Streptococcus*

GCS Glasgow Coma Scale
GDR Geriatric Depression Scale
GFR glomerular filtration rate
GHB gamma-hydroxybyturate
GI gastrointestinal
GIT gastrointestinal tract
GM-CSF granulocyte–macrophage colony-stimulating factor
GNR Gram-negative rods
GORD gastro-oesophageal reflux disease
GP general practitioner
GTN glyceryl trinitrate
GVHD graft-versus-host disease
HAART highly active antiretroviral treatment
HADS Hospital Anxiety and Depression Scale
HAPE high-altitude pulmonary (o)edema
HAV hepatitis A virus
HA-MRSA hospital-acquired methicillin-resistant *Staphylococcus aureus*
Hb haemoglobin
HBC hepatitis B core antibody
HBO hyperbaric oxygen therapy
HBS hepatitis B surface antibody
HBV hepatitis B virus
hCG human chorionic gonadotrophin
HCM hypertrophic cardiomyopathy
Hct haematocrit
HCV hepatitis C virus
HDL high-density lipoprotein
HDV hepatitis delta agent
HEV hepatitis E virus
HF hydrofluoric acid
HFMD hand, foot and mouth disease
HGV hepatitis G virus
HHNS hyperosmolar hyperglycaemic non-ketotic state
HHS hyper-osmolar hyperglycaemic syndrome
HIDA hepatobiliary iminodiacetic acid (scan)

Hib *Haemophilus influenzae* type b
HIDA hepatobiliary iminodiacetic acid scan
HITH hospital in the home
HITTS heparin-induced thrombotic thrombocytopenia syndrome
HIV human immunodeficiency syndrome
HLA human leucocyte antigen
HOCM hypertrophic cardiomyopathy
HONK hyperosmolar non-ketosis
HPI history of present illness
HPV human papillomavirus
HR heart rate
HRT hormone replacement therapy
HSV herpes simplex virus
HTLV-1 human T-lymphotropic virus type 1
HZ herpes zoster
IABC intra-aortic balloon counterpulsation
IBS irritable bowel syndrome
ICC intercostal catheter
ICD implantable cardiac defibrillator
ICF intracellular fluid
ICH intracerebral haemorrhage
ICP intracranial pressure
ICRP International Commission on Radiological Protection
ICS intercellular space
ICU intensive care unit
IDC indwelling (urinary) catheter
IDU injecting drug user
IIOC immediate initiation of care
Ig immunoglobulin
IHD ischaemic heart disease
ILCOR International Liaison Committee on Resuscitation
IM intramuscular(ly)
IMI intramuscular injection
IMV intermittent mandatory ventilation
IN intranasal, nasally
INH isoniazid
INR international normalised ratio (for prothrombin time)

Abbreviations

IO intraosseous(ly)
IOP intraocular pressure
IP intraperitoneal
IPAP inspiratory positive airway pressure
iPEEP intrinsic PEEP (positive end-expiratory pressure)
IPPV intermittent positive-pressure ventilation
IRIS immune reconstitution inflammatory syndrome
IRT incident response team
ISS Injury Severity Score
IT information technology
ITN ischaemic tissue necrosis
ITP idiopathic thrombocytopenia, idiopathic thrombocytopenic purpura
IUD, IUCD intrauterine (contraceptive) device
IV intravenous(ly)
IVC inferior vena cava
IVDU intravenous drug use/user
IVI intravenous injection
IVP intravenous pyelogram
IVS intravascular space
IVT intravenous therapy
JRA juvenile rheumatoid arthritis
JVP jugular venous pressure
JVT jugular venous distension
K potassium
KPI key performance indicator
KS Kaposi's sarcoma
KUB kidneys–ureters–bladder (X-ray or CT)
L litre, left
LAD left-axis deviation (in ECG); left anterior descending
LAFB left anterior fascicular block (anterior hemiblock)
LAP left atrial pressure
LBBB left bundle branch block
LBFB left posterior fascicular block (posterior hemiblock)
LCA left coronary artery
LCL lateral collateral ligament; lateral cruciate ligament

LDH lactate dehydrogenase
LDL low-density lipoprotein
LFT liver function test
LH luteinising hormone
LIF left iliac fossa
LMA laryngeal mask airway
LMO local medical officer
LMP last (normal) menstrual period
LMWH low-molecular-weight heparin
LOC level of consciousness; loss of consciousness
LP lumbar puncture
LPFB left posterior fascicular block
LR likelihood ratio
LSD lysergic acid diethylamide
LTBI latent tuberculosis infection
LV left ventricular
LVEF left ventricular ejection fraction
LVF left ventricular failure
LVH left ventricular hypertrophy
m, mo, mths months
M/C/S or M&S microculture and sensitivity (both used)
MAC *Mycobacterium avium–intracellulare* complex
MAOI monoamine oxidase inhibitor
MAP mean arterial (blood) pressure
MAST military antishock trousers
MCH mean corpuscular haemoglobin
MCI mass-casualty incident
MCL medial collateral ligament
MCP metacarpophalangeal
MCU micturating cystourethrogram
MCV mean corpuscular volume
MDI metered-dose inhaler
MDMA 3,4-methylene dioxymethylamphetamine (ecstasy)
MET mobile emergency team
Mg magnesium
MILS manual in-line stabilisation/immobilisation
MIMMS major incident medical management support
MMR measles, mumps, rubella
MMSE Mini Mental State Examination

MODS multi-organ dysfunction syndrome
MR magnetic resonance
MRA magnetic resonance angiography
MRI magnetic resonance imaging
MRSA multi-resistant *Staphylococcus aureus*; methicillin-resistant *Staphylococcus aureus*
MS mitral stenosis
MSM men who have sex with men
MSU midstream urine
MVP mitral valve prolapse
N/2 half normal
N/4 quarter normal
N₂O nitrous oxide
Na sodium
NAAT nucleic acid amplification testing
NAC *N*-acetylcysteine
NAD nothing abnormal detected
NAPA *N*-acetylprocainamide
NAPQI *N*-acetyl-*p*-quinone imine
NAT nucleic acid testing
NBM nil by mouth
NFR not for resuscitation
NG nasogastric
NGO non-government organisation
NGT nasogastric tube
NHL non-Hodgkin's lymphoma
NIBP non-invasive blood pressure (monitoring)
NIPPV non-invasive positive-pressure ventilation
NIV non-invasive ventilation
NMDA *N*-methyl-D-aspartate
NMR nuclear magnetic resonance
NMS neuroleptic malignant syndrome
NNRTI non-nucleoside reverse transcriptase inhibitor
NO nitric oxide
NOACN non-vitamin K antagonist oral anticoagulant
NOF neck of femur
NORSA non-multiresistant oxacillin-resistant *Staphylococcus aureus*

NP nurse practitioner
NRS numeric rating scale (for pain)
NRTI nucleoside reversion transcriptase inhibitor
NSA normal serum albumin
NSAID non steroidal anti-inflammatory drug
NSTEACS non-ST-segment elevation acute coronary syndrome
NSTEMI non-ST-elevation myocardial infarction
NT *N*-terminal
NTT nasotracheal tube
O&G obstetrics and gynaecology
O₂ oxygen
OCP oral contraceptive pill
od once daily
OI opportunistic infection
OM occipitomental
OPG orthopantomogram
ORIF open reduction internal fixation
OT occupational therapy; operating theatre
PA posteroanterior
PACO₂ partial pressure (tension) of alveolar carbon dioxide
PaCO₂ partial pressure of arterial carbon dioxide
PACS Patient Archiving and Communication System
PAN polyarteritis nodosa
PAWP pulmonary artery wedge pressure
PBL problem-based learning
PC platelet count
PCA patient-controlled analgesia; percutaneous coronary angioplasty
PCI percutaneous coronary intervention
PCL posterior cruciate ligament
PCO₂ partial pressure of carbon dioxide (may be arterial or venous)
PCP *Pneumocystis jiroveci (carinii)* pneumonia
PCR polymerase chain reaction

PCV packed cell volume

PDN paroxysmal nocturnal dyspnoea

PE pulmonary embolism

PEA pulseless electrical activity

PEEP positive end-expiratory pressure

PEFR peak expiratory flow rate

PEP post-exposure prophylaxis

PERC PE Rule-out Criteria

PET positron emission tomography

PG prostaglandin

PGL persistent generalised lymphadenopathy

PI product information (drugs); protease inhibitor

PID pelvic inflammatory disease

PiO₂ partial pressure of inspired oxygen

PIOPED prospective investigation of pulmonary embolism diagnosis

PIP peak inspiratory pressure; proximal interphalangeal

PML progressive multifocal leucoencephalopathy

PND paroxysmal nocturnal dypnoea

PNS peripheral nervous system

PO per orem, by mouth

POP plaster of Paris

POSI position of safe immobilisation

Posm plasma osmolarity

PPE personal protective equipment

PPI proton-pump inhibitor

PPNG penicillinase-producing *Neisseria gonorrhoeae*

PPV patency, protection, ventilation

PR per rectum, rectally

PrEP pre-exposure prophylaxis

PRVC pressure-regulated volume control

PSA prostate-specific antigen

PSI Pneumonia Severity Index

PSVT paroxysmal supraventricular tachycardia

PT prothrombin time

PTCA percutaneous transluminal coronary angioplasty

PTH parathyroid hormone

PTHrp parathyroid hormone related protein

PTSD post-traumatic stress disorder

PTT partial thromboplastin time

PUD peptic ulcer disease

PUO pyrexia of unknown origin

PUVA psoralen ultraviolet A (therapy)

PV per vaginam, vaginally

q4h every 4 hours (etc)

QID, qid 4 times daily

R respiratory quotient; right

RA radiofrequency ablation; rheumatoid arthritis

RAA renin–angiotensin–aldosterone (system)

RAD right-axis deviation (in ECG)

RAP right atrial pressure

RAT rapid assessment team

RBBB right bundle branch block

RBC red blood cell

RCA right coronary artery

RF radiofrequency

RLQ right lower quadrant

RICE rest, ice, compression and elevation

RMO resident medical officer

RNA ribonucleic acid

ROM range of movement

ROSC return of spontaneous circulation

RPFB right posterior fascicular block

RPR rapid plasma reagin (test)

RR relative risk

RSI rapid-sequence induction, rapid-sequence intubation

RSV respiratory syncytial virus

RTA road traffic accident

rTPA tissue plasminogen activator

RTS Revised Trauma Score

RUQ right upper quadrant

RV right ventricle

RVH right ventricular hypertrophy

SA sinoatrial

SAED semi-automated external defibrillator

SAH subarachnoid haemorrhage

SaO₂ peripheral oxygen saturation

SARS severe acute respiratory syndrome

SBP systolic blood pressure

SBT skin bleeding time

SC subcutaneous(ly)

SCA sickle-cell anaemia

SCAR serous cutaneous adverse reaction

SCD sickle-cell disease

SCID severe combined immune deficiency

SCIWORA spinal cord injury without radiological abnormality

SDH subdural haematoma/haemorrhage

SF-36 a 36-item health survey (Medical Outcomes Study)

SFFS sitting fetal feet supported

SGOT serum glutamic oxaloacetic transaminase

SIADH syndrome of inappropriate antidiuretic hormone

SIDS sudden infant death syndrome

SIMV synchronised intermittent mandatory ventilation

SIRS systemic inflammatory response syndrome

SJS Stevens–Johnson syndrome

SK streptokinase

SLE systemic lupus erythematosus

SLS sodium lauryl sulfate

SMA superior mesanteric artery

SNRI serotonin and noradrenaline reuptake inhibitor

SOB shortness of breath

SOL space-occupying lesion

SPC suprapubic catheter

SpO₂ peripheral oxygen saturation

SR sinus rhythm

SSD silver sulfadiazine

SSLR serum-sickness-like reaction

SSRI selective serotonin reuptake inhibitor

SSSS staphylococcal scalded skin syndrome

stat at once

STI sexually transmitted infection

STEMI ST-elevation myocardial infarction

SV stroke volume

SVC superior vena cava

SvO₂ central venous oxygen saturation

SVT supraventricular tachycardia

TAC tetracaine, adrenaline and cocaine in a gel preparation

TASER Thomas A Swift Electric Rifle

TB tuberculosis

TBI traumatic brain injury

TBSA total body surface area

TED thromboembolism

TCA tricyclic antidepressant

TDS, tds 3 times daily

TEN toxic epidermal necrolysis

TENS transcutaneous electrical nerve stimulation

TFT thyroid function test

TGA Therapeutic Goods Administration

THC tetrahydrocannabinol

TIA transient ischaemic attack

TIG tetanus immunoglobulin

TIMI thrombolysis in myocardial infarction (score)

TIPS transjugular intrahepatic portosystemic shunt

TLS tumour lysis syndrome

TMJ temporomandibular joint

TNF tumour necrosis factor

TPHA *Treponema pallidum* haemagglutination assay

TOE transoesophageal echocardiogram/echocardiography

TORCH toxoplasmosis, rubella, cytomegalovirus, herpes simplex and HIV

TOV trial of void

TPA tissue plasminogen activator

TPHA Treponema pallidum haemagglutination assay (syphilis test)

TPN total parenteral nutrition

TPR total peripheral resistance

TRALI transfusion-related acute lung injury

TRISS Revised Trauma Score and Injury Severity Score combined

TRTS Triage Revised Trauma Score

TSH thyroid-stimulating hormone

TSST toxic shock syndrome toxin

TT thrombin time

U/A urinalysis

UA urinalysis; unstable angina

U&E urea and electrolytes

UEC urea, electrolytes and creatinine (also EUC)

UNH unfractionated heparin

URTI upper respiratory tract infection

US ultrasound

UTI urinary tract infection

VAS Visual Analogue Scale (for pain)

VBG venous blood gas

vCJD variant Creutzfeldt–Jakob disease

VDK venom detection kit

VDRL venereal disease reference laboratory (test)

VEB ventricular ectopic beat

VF ventricular fibrillation

VP ventriculoperitoneal

V/Q ventilation–perfusion

VSD ventricular septal defect

VT ventricular tachycardia

VTE venous thromboembolism

vWF von Willebrand's factor

VZIG varicella zoster immune globulin

VZV varicella zoster virus

WBC white blood cell

WCC white (blood) cell count

WHO World Health Organization

WPW Wolff-Parkinson-White (syndrome)

y, yrs years

emergency medicine
the principles of practice

emergency
medicine
the principles of practice

SEVENTH EDITION

Edited by
Sascha Fulde

MBBS, BSc (Med), FACEM
Emergency Specialist, St Vincent's Hospital,
Sutherland Hospital, Sydney, NSW
Royal North Shore Hospital, St Leonards, NSW
Senior Lecturer, University of New South Wales

Gordian Fulde

AO, MBBS, FRACS, FRCS (Edin),
FRCS/RCP (A&E) (Edin), FACEM
Director of Emergency The Sydney Hospital, Sydney, NSW
Stream Director, Critical Care, South Eastern Sydney Local
Health Care District
Professor, Emergency Medicine, Notre Dame and
New South Wales Universities
Former Director, Emergency, St. Vincent's Hospital,
Sydney, NSW

ELSEVIER

ELSEVIER

Elsevier Australia. ACN 001 002 357
(a division of Reed International Books Australia Pty Ltd)
Tower 1, 475 Victoria Avenue, Chatswood, NSW 2067

ISBN: 978-0-7295-4301-9

National Library of Australia Cataloguing-in-Publication Data

A catalogue record for this
book is available from the
National Library of Australia

NATIONAL
LIBRARY
OF AUSTRALIA

Senior Content Strategist: Larissa Norrie
Content Project Manager: Kritika Kaushik
Edited by Leanne Peters, Letterati Publishing Services
Proofread by Tim Learner
Cover and Internal design by Georgette Hall
Index by SPi Global
Typeset by GW Tech
Printed in Singapore by Markono Print Media Pte Ltd

Last digit is the print number: 9   8   7   6   5   4   3   2   1

Preface

Since the first edition of this book in 1988 and following editions in 1992, 1998, 2004, 2009 and 2014, emergency medicine has—fortunately—continued to advance. In this edition much new information, many new approaches and extensive refinements of existing clinical management have been incorporated. Again, current and respected practising clinicians have been chosen as authors for their clinical expertise and experience, so that they can compact their knowledge into the pocket-sized format. As healthcare resources continue to be stretched, the first hours of a patient's illness or initial contact with healthcare providers, outside and inside a hospital, are even more critical to the outcome. It is also very pertinent given the challenge of re-engineering patient flow (e.g. COVID-19, the '4-hour rule'), the many key performance indicators (KPIs) and expeditious competent care which can be coupled to funding. This book aims to help with this initial contact. Any suggestions for improving this will be much appreciated.

Acknowledgments

Once again I am very grateful to the busy clinician authors for their excellent contributions. Also, the support and stimulation from many doctors, nurses, students and other professionals who use this book and have helped with ideas are greatly appreciated.

How do I adequately thank my wife, Lesley, for her unfailing encouragement and support?

Sophia Espinosa, with the help of her daughter Sierra and son Emilio, typed, collated, chased up details and much more; I most sincerely thank her.

Also to all the fabulous staff of the emergency departments and back up who are so great to work with—not only are the patients lucky to have such people care for them, but also the way they support and care for each other is wonderful.

Disclaimer:

Every effort has been made to ensure that all the information contained in this book is correct and accurate. However, the publisher, editor and authors accept no responsibility for the clinical decisions, management or dosages given. The final responsibility rests with the treating doctor.

Gordian and Sascha Fulde

Contents

Contents

Contents

Contents

Contents

Contents

Contents

Contents

Editors note on COVID-19

Dear fellow healthcare workers,

First and foremost, THANK YOU to you and your family, loved ones and friends who support you.

This is not an update on COVID-19, nor is it an excuse for the delay of this 7th edition appearing.

The world is being devastated by the pandemic; it is global war. We still know very little about the virus. For example: What medications will be effective? When will a vaccine bring up the 'herd immunity' across the world?

Much more is unknown. We are responding, adapting and changing, and making difficult decisions on the spot while facing shortages to keep healthcare staff and the population protected.

Among the main enemy is anxiety and fear of death or loss, which is very much exacerbated by all the unknown.

Emergency medicine workers, responders and all those caring for others are in the frontline and you are amazing to be putting yourselves first while at definite risk to yourselves and those around you. This is especially amazing with the risk that in the line of duty you face the possibility of exposure to infected COVID-19 people who may be, although asymptomatic, infectious for days. Let alone caring for the full spectrum of sick patients up to full resuscitation, with the high risk of aerosol-generating procedures such as intubation.

Sadly, besides so many really good deeds and behaviours, this crisis also brings out the worst in some.

COVID-19 will pass with unimaginable consequences at so many levels. Healthcare workers will be among the unfathomable statistics. We all know the true toll will be incalculable. It is definitely not just dollars and deaths, but also the stress and scars to the mind, body and soul over generations.

Please keep well, safe and sane because what you do really matters and makes such a difference. We all owe you and need you! Thank you again.

Sincerest best wishes,
Gordian and Sascha Fulde
Sydney, April 2020

Contributors

Gonzalo Aguirrebarrena, MB, BS, FACEM
Staff Specialist, Emergency Medicine
St Vincent's Hospital, Sydney, NSW

Judy Alford, MBBS, FACEM, Grad Cert Clinical Teaching
Senior Staff Specialist, Emergency Medicine, St Vincent's Hospital,
  Sydney, NSW

Glenn Arendts, MBBS, MMed, PhD, FACEM
Emergency Medicine Physician, Fiona Stanley Hospital, Murdoch,
  Western Australia; Associate Professor, University of Western
  Australia

Shalini Arunanthy, MBBS, FACEM
Senior Staff Specialist, Emergency Department, Westmead Hospital,
  Westmead, NSW

Neil Ballard, MBBS, FACEM
Senior Staff Specialist, Aeromedical Operations, NSW Ambulance;
  Senior Staff Specialist, Paediatric Emergency Medicine, Sydney
  Children's Hospital, Randwick, NSW; Visiting Medical Officer,
  Emergency Medicine, Royal Prince Alfred Hospital, Randwick,
  NSW

Melinda Berry, MBBS, FACEM, CCPU
Senior Staff Specialist Emergency Physician, St Vincent's Hospital,
  Sydney, NSW and Sydney Children's Hospital, Randwick, NSW;
  Conjoint Senior Lecturer University of New South Wales and The
  University of Notre Dame

Sophie Blake, BSW
Social Worker, Violence Abuse and Neglect Service, Northern NSW
  Local Health District, Lismore, NSW

Professor Anthony FT Brown, AM, FRCP, FRCSEd, FRCEM, FACEM
Professor, Consultant Emergency Medicine Physician, Affiliation
    Emergency and Trauma Centre, Royal Brisbane and Women's
    Hospital, Brisbane, Qld

Bonita Byrne, BEd, MEd
Aboriginal Liaison Officer, Aboriginal Elder Wiradjuri People of NSW

Mark Byrne, BMed, FACRRM
Remote Medicine Specialist, Indigenous Doctor of the Wiradjuri
    People of NSW

Bill Croker, MBBS, BMedSci, MMedEd, FACEM, MMedEd
Senior Staff Specialist, The Sanitarium Hospital, Wahroonga, NSW;
    Emergency Department, Nepean Hospital, Penrith, NSW

Michael R Delaney, MBBS, FRACO, FRACS
Visiting Ophthalmic Surgeon, St Vincent's Hospital, Sydney, NSW;
    Clinical Lecturer in Ophthalmology, University of New South Wales

Pauline Deweerd
Director, Aboriginal Health, St Vincent's Hospital, Sydney, NSW

Stephen Dunjey, MB, BS, FACEM, DDU
Staff Specialist, Emergency Medicine, Royal Perth Hospital, St John of
    God Midland, WA; Professor, Emergency Medicine, St John of God
    Murdoch Hospital, Perth, WA

Rob Edwards, MBBS, FACEM
Senior Staff Specialist in Emergency Medicine, Westmead Hospital,
    Westmead, NSW

Peter Foltyn, BDS
Consultant Dentist, Dental Department, St Vincent's Hospital, Sydney,
    NSW

Lesley Foster, AM, MBBS, MHP, FRACMA, Dip Ind Rel and Lab Law, FAFPHM
Professor and Dean of Medicine, Charles Sturt University

Gordian W O Fulde, AO, MBBS, FRACS, FRCS (Ed), FRACS/RCP (A&E) Ed, FACEM
Director of Emergency The Sydney Hospital, Sydney, NSW; Stream Director, Critical Care, South Eastern Sydney Local Health Care District; Professor, Emergency Medicine, Notre Dame and New South Wales Universities; Former Director, Emergency, St. Vincent's Hospital, Sydney, NSW

Sascha Fulde, MBBS, BSc (Med), FACEM
Emergency Specialist, St Vincent's Hospital, Sutherland Hospital, Royal North Shore Hospital, St Leonards, NSW; Senior Lecturer, University of New South Wales

Tiffany Fulde, MBBS (Hons), FRANZCA
Anaesthetic Fellow, Royal Prince Alfred Hospital, Randwick, NSW

Daniel Gaetani, FACEM, MBBS, BSc (Pharm)
Co-DEMT and Staff Specialist in Emergency Medicine, Campbelltown Hospital, Camden Hospital, Sydney, NSW

Julie Gawthorne, BNurs, MNur (Critical Care)
Clinical Nurse Consultant, Emergency Department, St Vincent's Hospital, Sydney, NSW; Clinical Fellow, Nursing and Midwifery, Australian Catholic University

Mark Gillett, MBBS, DipRACOG, FRACGP, FACEM, MClinEd, GradCertSono
Senior Staff Specialist and Director Emergency Research, Emergency Department, Royal North Shore Hospital, St Leonards, NSW

Jessica Green, MB, ChB, FACEM, FRCEM, Grad Cert Clinical ED
Emergency Physician and Director of Prevocational Education and Training, St Vincent's Hospital, Sydney, NSW

Tim Green, MBBS, FACEM
Senior Staff Specialist, Former Director, Emergency Department, Royal
Prince Alfred Hospital, St Leonards, NSW

Shahrzad Jahromi, MBBS, FRACP
Senior Staff Specialist, Geriatric Medicine, St Vincent's Hospital,
Sydney, NSW

Jackie Huber, MBBS (Hons), BSc (Hons 1), MPsychMed,
FRANZCP
Staff Specialist Psychiatrist, Psychiatry, St Vincent's Hospital, Sydney,
NSW

Nadine Huddle, BPharm (Hons), BMBS, FACEM
Emergency Physician, WA Country Health Service and St John of God
Hospital Midland, Western Australia

Farzad Jazayeri, FACEM, CCPU
Staff Specialist, Emergency Medicine, St Vincent's Hospital, Sydney,
NSW; Conjoint Lecturer, Clinical School of Medicine, University of
New South Wales

Anthony D Kelleher, PhD, MBBS, FRACP, FRCPA
Director and Professor of Medicine, Kirby Institute, University of New
South Wales; Senior Staff Specialist, HIV and Immunology Unit, St
Vincent's Hospital, Sydney, NSW

Marian Lee, MBBS, DCH, FACEM, MHA, Cert Clin Teach
Emergency Physician, Senior Staff Specialist, Prince of Wales Hospital,
Randwick, NSW

Julie Leung, MBBS, FACEM, DDU
Emergency Physician, Emergency, St Vincent's Hospital, Sydney, NSW;
Conjoint Lecturer, University of New South Wales

Derek Louey, MBBS, FACEM
Emergency Physician, Emergency Department, Flinders Medical
Centre, Bedford Park, SA

Kevin Maruno, MBBS, FACEM, BMedSc (Hons)
Staff Specialist, Emergency Medicine, St Vincent's Hospital, Sydney,
NSW; Academic Coordinator, Senior Conjoint Lecturer, The
University of Notre Dame; Conjoint Lecturer, Faculty of Medicine,
University of New South Wales

Greg McDonald, MBBS, FACEM
Director of Emergency Care, Sydney Adventist Hospital, Wahroonga,
NSW

Stephen Macdonald, PhD, BSc (Hons), MB, ChB (Edin), FACEM,
FRCP (MRCGP)
Associate Professor, Consultant Emergency Physician, Royal Perth
Hospital, Perth, WA

Chris Mobbs, MBBS, FACEM
Senior Staff Specialist, University Hospital Geelong, Geelong, Vic.

David Murphy, BSc (Med), MBBS, FACEM
Acting Director of Emergency Medicine, Prince of Wales Hospital,
Randwick, NSW

Alicia O'Connor, MBBS, BAppSc (Phty), MPH, FACD
Department of Dermatology, Liverpool Hospital, Liverpool, NSW;
Conjoint Senior Lecturer, University of New South Wales

Andrew Orr, MBBS, FACEM
Emergency Physician, Emergency Department, Port Macquarie Base
Hospital, Port Macquarie, NSW

Bronwyn Orr, MBBS (Hons), BSci (Hons), FACEM, DCH
Emergency Physician, Emergency Department, Port Macquarie Base
Hospital, Port Macquarie, NSW

Edmond Park, MBBS (BSc), FACEM
Senior Staff Specialist in Emergency Medicine, Liverpool Hospital,
Liverpool, NSW

Kevin Phan, MD
Paediatric Dermatology Fellow, Sydney Children's Hospitals Network,
Randwick and Westmead, NSW; Department of Dermatology,
University of New South Wales, Liverpool Hospital, Liverpool,
NSW

John Raftos, MBBS (Hons), FACEM
Senior Specialist in Emergency Medicine, St Vincent's Hospital, Sydney,
NSW; Conjoint Associate Professor, Faculty of Medicine, University
of New South Wales

Arjun Rao, MBBS, MAppSci, FRACP
Paediatric Emergency Physician, Sydney Children's Hospital, Randwick,
NSW

Drew Richardson, BMedSc, MBBS(Hons), Grad Cert HE, MD,
FACEM
Chair of Road Trauma and Emergency Medicine, Medical School,
Australian National University, Canberra, ACT; Senior Staff
Specialist, Emergency Department, Canberra Hospital and Health
Services, Garran, ACT

John Roberts, MBBS, FACEM
Critical Care Consultant
Conjoint Senior Lecturer, University of New South Wales Rural Clinical
School, Port Macquarie, NSW

Kent Robinson, MBChB, FACEM
Emergency Physician, Associate Professor, Liverpool Hospital,
Liverpool, NSW

Contributors

Patricia Saccasan, MBBS, FACEM
Emergency Physician, Director of Critical Care, Critical Care Unit, Murrumbidgee and Southern NSW Local Health Districts, Goulburn, NSW

Iromi Samarasinghe, MBBS, FACEM
Emergency Physician, Sydney Hospital and St Vincent's Hospital, Sydney, NSW; Conjoint Lecturer, University of New South Wales

Rahul Santram, MBChB, FACEM
Emergency Medicine Staff Specialist, St Vincent's Hospital, Sydney, NSW

Sarah C Sasson, PhD, BA, BSc (Hons), MBBS (Hons), FRACP, FRCPA
The Kirby Institute, University of New South Wales; Westmead Hospital, Westmead, NSW

Deshan Sebaratnam, MBBS (Hons), MMed (Clin Epi), FACD
Staff Specialist, Department of Dermatology, Liverpool Hospital, Liverpool, NSW; Visiting Medical Officer, The Skin Hospital, Westmead, NSW; Senior Lecturer, University of New South Wales

E S Seelan, MBBS, FRANZCR
Managing Radiologist, Healthcare Imaging, Miranda, NSW; Former Director of Radiology, Sutherland Hospital, Caringbah, NSW

Kate Sellors, BMed, Grad Cert Clin Tox, FACEM
Emergency Staff Specialist, Prince of Wales Hospital, Randwick, NSW

Ania Smialkowski, MBBS, BMedSci (Hons)
NSW Plastic and Reconstructive Surgery Trainee, St Vincent's Hospital, Sydney, NSW

Emma Spencer, MBBS, BSc (Med), FRACP, Dip Tropical Health and Hygiene, Cayetano Heredia University, Lima, Peru
Infection Disease Consultant, Royal Darwin Hospital, Darwin, NT

Jennifer Stevens, MBChB, FANZCA, FFPMANZCA
VMO Anaesthesia and Pain Medicine, St Vincent's Hospital, Sydney,
NSW; Conjoint Senior Lecturer, University of New South Wales

Richard Sullivan, MBBS (Hons), FRACP
Staff Specialist Infectious Diseases, Department Infectious Diseases,
Immunology & Sexual Health, St George Hospital, Kogarah, NSW;
Conjoint Lecturer, St George and Sutherland Clinical School,
University of New South Wales

Alan Tankel, BSc, MBChB, FACEM, FRCP
Director, Emergency Medicine, Coffs Harbour Base Hospital, Coffs
Harbour, NSW; Network Director, Emergency Medicine, Coffs
Clinical Network, Coffs Harbour, NSW; Conjoint Senior Lecturer,
University of New South Wales

Tad Tietze, MBBS (Hons), FRANZCP
Senior Staff Specialist Psychiatrist, Psychiatric Emergency Care Centre,
St Vincent's Hospital, Sydney, NSW; Conjoint Lecturer, School
of Psychiatry, University of New South Wales; Adjunct Senior
Lecturer, School of Medicine, The University of Notre Dame

Wayne Varndell, MN, BSc, Grad Dip, PGCE
Clinical Nurse Consultant, Emergency Department, Prince of Wales
Hospital, Randwick NSW

John Vinen, MBBS, FACEM, MHP, FIFEM, FACBS
Emergency Physician and Medicolegal Consultant, Calvary Health
Care, ACT

Rebecca Walsh, BSc, MBBS, FRACP, FRCPA
Genomicist and Staff Specialist Haematologist, Prince of Wales
Hospital, Randwick, NSW

Anthony Whelan, MBBS, FRACP
General and Thoracic Physician, Goulburn Base Hospital, Goulburn,
NSW

Contributors

Luis Winoto, BA, BSc(Med), MBBS, FACEM
Staff Specialist Emergency Physician, Emergency Department,
St Vincent's Hospital, Sydney, NSW

Christopher Wong, MBBS, FRCS, FAMS
Consultant in Emergency Medicine, Woodlands Health Campus,
Singapore

Nikki Woods, MBBS, FACEM
Consultant in Emergency Medicine, Director of Emergency Medicine
Training, St Vincent's Hospital, Sydney, NSW

Chapter 1
Cardiopulmonary resuscitation
Melinda Berry and Gordian WO Fulde

Basic life support

The principles of basic life support (BLS) are the same in children and adults, and the Australian Resuscitation Council recommends the same BLS algorithm (Figure 1.1) for all ages. This allows for ease of learning and retention for lay people in the community (as well as many healthcare workers!).

There are obviously differences in anatomy, physiology and pathology between children and adults, and this is reflected in the recommendations for healthcare workers providing more-advanced life support for these different groups (see following sections).

BLS commences with looking for danger, quickly assessing the response of the patient and calling for help. If there is life-threatening external bleeding, it must be stopped by applying direct pressure and elevating the wound above the level of the heart.

Open the airway with a head tilt, chin lift and/or jaw thrust. Any visible obstructing material can be removed, but a routine finger sweep is not recommended. Look, listen and feel for normal breathing.

Commence chest compressions if the patient is unresponsive and not breathing normally. Healthcare workers may feel for a pulse, but this has been found to be alarmingly unreliable and can cause delays in commencing chest compressions. No more than 10 seconds should be spent feeling for a pulse before moving on to start chest compressions. Chest compressions are commenced prior to delivering ventilations.

Chest compressions are delivered at a rate of 100/min to the lower half of the sternum and to a depth of at least one-third of the depth of the chest. After 30 compressions, pause briefly to deliver 2 ventilations. Early, effective and uninterrupted chest

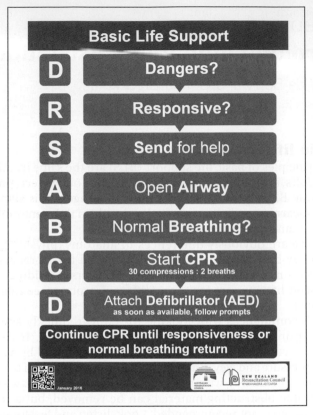

Figure 1.1 Basic life support
AED = automatic external defibrillator; CPR = cardiopulmonary resuscitation
From Australian Resuscitation Council; reproduced with permission.

compressions have been shown to improve survival outcomes from cardiac arrest.

Chest compressions to an adult are delivered with a two-handed technique. For infants and small children, only one hand may be needed; and for babies, two fingers or the thumb/hand encircling technique. In late pregnancy, position the arrested patient supine but with something under the right buttock to provide sideways pelvic tilt to lift the gravid uterus off the inferior vena cava.

Performing chest compressions is tiring, even in a paediatric patient, and effectiveness declines over time with the same compressor. Change compressors every 2 minutes wherever possible, but with minimal interruption to the compressions.

Ventilations can be delivered by mouth-to-mouth expired air (mouth-to-nose in babies and infants), mouth-to-mask or by bag-and-mask. The volume delivered just needs to be enough to see the chest wall rise. Overventilation causes hyperinflation of the chest which impairs venous return to the heart, limiting cardiac output. Overventilation can also cause gastric distension, predisposing to regurgitation of stomach contents and aspiration of this into the lungs.

Early defibrillation improves outcome. Automatic external defibrillators (AEDs) allow early defibrillation in community areas and low-acuity hospital areas where advanced life support is not immediately available. If an AED is available, it should be used as soon as possible.

Editorial Comment

Lack of an airway pre-hospital and in hospital continues to be a main cause of preventable death in an unconscious patient! The lateral position on the ground is very effective, also allowing stomach contents to drain out the mouth—not into the lung.

Cardiac arrest management is a core skill of emergency departments. Nursing and medical staff should all be familiar with the delivery of advanced life support and how to work together as a team.

Defibrillation of a shockable rhythm is the most significant intervention that we can provide to cardiac arrest patients. Early defibrillation makes the biggest impact on patient outcome of any intervention in cardiac arrest.

Strategies in the community attempt to provide early defibrillation. This includes insertion of automatic implantable cardioverter defibrillators (AICDs) in at-risk patients. There are also increasingly more AEDs in the community but despite this, there are still avoidable delays. Reasons for delays in the community include unrecognised cardiac arrest due to agonal breathing, bystanders unwilling or unable to perform basic life support and unwilling or unaware of the use of the AED. Increasing community education programs could reduce these delays further.

Uninterrupted, effective chest compressions have also been shown to improve outcome from cardiac arrest. This is not to delay defibrillation, but to support the circulation while defibrillation or other causes of the arrest are addressed.

Effective chest compressions are provided at a rate of 100–120/ minute on the lower half of the sternum to one-third the depth of the patient's chest. This equates to 5–6 cm in adults. Depth and full recoil are just as important as rate of compressions.

Chest compressions should be commenced immediately in patients who are unresponsive and not breathing normally. The defibrillator and further help are sent for. The airway is opened and cleared. Two breaths are delivered (by mouth-to-mask or bag-to-mask) for every 30 chest compressions. Defibrillation is delivered for patients in a shockable rhythm.

Advanced life support

Advanced life support (ALS; Figure 1.2) aims to get return of spontaneous circulation (ROSC) by working on three interrelated objectives:

- rhythm control
- oxygen delivery to the heart and brain
- reversal of any contributing causes.

RHYTHM CONTROL

Rhythm control is reversion of the patient from ventricular fibrillation (VF) or pulseless ventricular tachycardia (pVT) into a coordinated rhythm. Time to defibrillation is the single most important factor in improving survival from cardiac arrest and the chance of successful defibrillation decreases rapidly with each passing minute.

Defibrillation pads are placed on the patient with the heart sitting in between them as much as possible. In cardiac arrest, the most convenient position is usually right parasternal and left mid axilla.

Chest compressions need to pause briefly for staff to be able to see the rhythm, or the machine to analyse it. If the rhythm is VF or pVT, a shock of maximum joules is delivered. It is recommended that all staff stand away from the patient during shock delivery and any free-flowing oxygen be removed temporarily.

Chest compressions are recommenced after shock delivery regardless of success. The heart is 'stunned' after defibrillation and cardiac output is often initially poor, even if defibrillation has been successful. Unless the patient has obvious signs of a good cardiac output (moving or talking!), chest compressions continue for 2 minutes and then the rhythm is checked again. If it is a co-ordinated rhythm, the patient is examined for a pulse. If a pulse is not detected after 10 seconds, chest compressions are resumed.

Rhythm analysis occurs every 2 minutes and one shock of maximum joules is delivered if VF or pVT are present. The defibrillator can be charged leading up to the 2-minute mark, before chest compressions are paused. Shock can then be delivered immediately following rhythm analysis, in the same pause in compressions. The charge can be dumped if the rhythm is non-shockable (pulseless electrical activity [PEA] or asystole).

If 3 shocks have been delivered and the patient remains in VF or pVT, amiodarone 300 mg intravenous (IV) (5 mg/kg in paediatrics) is administered. A further dose of 150 mg may be considered after the fifth unsuccessful defibrillation attempt.

Editorial Comment

Venous blood gases (VBG) correlation to arterial blood gases:
- VBG PH 0.03–0.05 LOWER
- VBG HCO_3 1.5–2.0 mEq LOWER
- VBG CO_2 6 mmHg HIGHER

OXYGEN DELIVERY TO THE HEART AND BRAIN

Chest compressions are a key factor in maintaining oxygen delivery to the heart and brain. The use of chest compression devices is becoming more common. They allow easy transport and access to the patient, but have not yet proven to be better than manual chest compressions.

Placement of an advanced airway (laryngeal mask airway [LMA] or endotracheal tube [ETT]) means that chest compressions can be continuous at 100–120/min with ventilations delivered at 6–10/min. Overventilation is harmful in cardiac arrest, mainly due to rising intra-thoracic pressure impeding venous return.

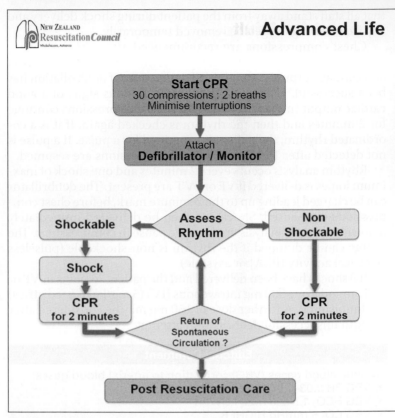

Figure 1.2 Advanced life support for adults
ABCDE = airway, breathing, circulation, disability, exposure algorithm;
CPR = cardiopulmonary resuscitation; ETT =endotracheal tube; IO =
intraosseous; IV = intravenous; LMA = laryngeal mask airway

Editorial Comment

- Minimise interruptions to compression.
- Supraglottic airways may be initially adequate simulation and practice.

Placement of an endotracheal tube allows measurement of end-tidal CO_2. Circulation is required to deliver CO_2 to the airways, so in addition to confirming tracheal placement of the tube,

Support for Adults

AUSTRALIAN
RESUSCITATION
COUNCIL

During CPR
Airway adjuncts (LMA / ETT)
Oxygen
Waveform capnography
IV / IO access
Plan actions before interrupting compressions
(e.g. charge manual defibrillator)
Drugs
Shockable
* Adrenaline 1 mg after 2nd shock
(then every 2nd loop)
* Amiodarone 300 mg after 3rd shock
Non Shockable
* Adrenaline 1 mg immediately
(then every 2nd loop)

Consider and Correct
Hypoxia
Hypovolaemia
Hyper / hypokalaemia / metabolic disorders
Hypothermia / hyperthermia
Tension pneumothorax
Tamponade
Toxins
Thrombosis (pulmonary / coronary)

Post Resuscitation Care
Re-evaluate ABCDE
12 lead ECG
Treat precipitating causes
Re-evaluate oxygenation and ventilation
Temperature control (cool)

From Australian Resuscitation Council; reproduced with permission.

end-tidal CO_2 gives feedback about circulation. The end-tidal CO_2 reading is low in cardiac arrest due to the low output state and it can rise suddenly with ROSC. Likewise, a fall in end-tidal CO_2 can indicate loss of cardiac output. The initial end-tidal CO_2 reading in cardiac arrest may prove to have prognostic value, as it seems that the higher the reading, the more likely is ROSC achieved.

Adrenaline IV 1 mg (10 microg/kg in paediatrics) is administered to direct more blood flow to the heart and brain. If the patient is not in a shockable rhythm, adrenaline is administered immediately. If the rhythm is shockable, adrenaline is administered after the second unsuccessful shock. Adrenaline is then given every second 2-minute cycle.

Where intravenous access is not attainable, the intraosseous route is recommended. Endotracheal administration of medications is no longer recommended. Intraosseous access devices for adults (drills) are becoming more widely available.

REVERSAL OF ANY CONTRIBUTING CAUSES

Working through a checklist of 'reversible causes' is important in every arrest in order that contributing causes are not overlooked. Most people are familiar with the 'four Hs and four Ts' mnemonic:

H Hypoxia—respiratory arrest, airway obstruction
H Hypovolaemia—haemorrhage, sepsis
H Hyper/hypo electrolytes—mainly K, Mg, Ca, glucose
H Hypothermia— temperature below 35°C
T Tension pneumothorax
T Tamponade—post cardiothoracic surgery, trauma
T Toxins—ingestions, envenomations, anaphylaxis
T Thromboembolus—pulmonary embolus, AMI

Bedside ultrasound is being increasingly used in cardiac arrest. It can assist in looking for reversible causes such as cardiac tamponade, volume status, abdominal free fluid and tension pneuomothorax. Ultrasound will also demonstrate whether there is cardiac motion in pulseless electrical activity.

POST-RESUSCITATION CARE

Ongoing cardiac and neurological function can be improved by the quality of post-resuscitation care. It includes airway management, achieving normal oxygen levels while avoiding hyperoxia, maintaining perfusion to the vital organs and a normal blood glucose level. The underlying cause of the arrest needs to be addressed, including considering the need for percutaneous coronary intervention in many adult cases.

It is impossible to predict accurately the degree of neurological recovery during or immediately after cardiac arrest. Relying on the neurological examination during or immediately after cardiac arrest to predict outcome is not recommended and should not be used.

In cases where there is no return of spontaneous circulation, senior medical staff may decide to stop resuscitation efforts and declare the person deceased. This decision is made in the context of the duration and nature of the arrest, the premorbid state of the patient and the likelihood of significant neurological recovery.

In some cases, it may be appropriate to place the patient on venoarterial extracorporeal membrane oxygenation (VA-ECMO) if this is available. Patients are only suitable if there has been minimal cerebral hypoxia as a result of the arrest and the cause for the arrest is reversible.

Paediatric advanced life support

There are only a few but important differences in providing ALS to children. Cardiac arrest in paediatrics is usually secondary to hypoxia or hypovolaemia so these are the issues that need to be addressed. Cardiac rhythm is usually non-shockable pulseless electrical activity or asystole.

In the community, the BLS algorithm is the same for children as it is for adults. In the emergency department (ED), we are able to appreciate the differences for children, and use the paediatric ALS algorithm (Figure 1.3). More emphasis is placed on ventilation—2 breaths are given for every 15 chest compressions.

In infants, the airway is held in a neutral position and ventilation with a bag/mask on 100% oxygen is the priority. A ~500 mL self-inflating bag is an appropriate size for most babies to ~8 years old before moving on to an adult size. An oropharyngeal airway (sized from the middle of the gum/incisors to angle of mandible) can be inserted directly and gently to lift the tongue off the back of the pharynx. If foreign body aspiration is thought to be the cause of the arrest, prompt laryngoscopy might be appropriate.

Chest compressions are the same as adults; that is, 100–120/min to the lower half of the sternum to one-third the depth of the chest. VF and VT can occur in children and so rhythm analysis and defibrillation of shockable rhythms is still done. Defibrillation dose is 4 J/kg for the first and all subsequent shocks.

Adrenaline 10 microg/kg IV (or IO) is administered immediately in cases of asystole or PEA and after the second unsuccessful

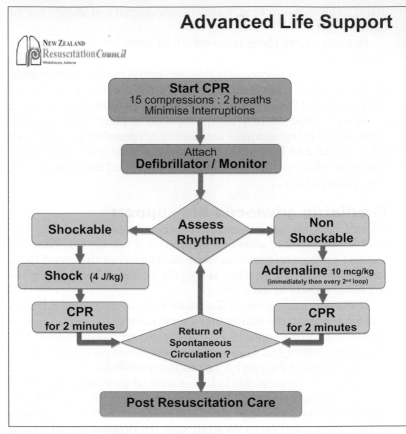

Figure 1.3 Advanced life support in children

defibrillation in VF or pVT with the recommencement of chest compressions. Amiodarone 5 mg/kg is recommended for refractory VF or VT after the third unsuccessful defibrillation attempt.

IV access is the first-line route of drug administration. No more than 90 seconds should be spent attempting IV access before resorting to intraosseous access.

The checklist for reversible causes is the same as for adults, but come causes are more pertinent than others. Hypoxia is addressed

for Infants and Children

AUSTRALIAN
RESUSCITATION
COUNCIL

<u>**During CPR**</u>
Airway adjucts (LMA / ETT)
Oxygen
Waveform capnography
IV / IO access
Plan actions before interrupting compressions
    (e.g. charge manual defibrillator to 4 J/kg)
Drugs
    Shockable
        * Adrenaline 10 mcg/kg after 2nd shock
          (then every 2nd loop)
        * Amiodarone 5mg/kg after 3rd shock
    Non Shockable
        * Adrenaline 10 mcg/kg immediately
          (then every 2nd loop)

<u>**Consider and Correct**</u>
Hypoxia
Hypovolaemia
Hyper / hypokalaemia / metabolic disorders
Hypothermia / hyperthermia
Tension pneumothorax
Tamponade
Toxins
Thrombosis (pulmonary / coronary)

<u>**Post Resuscitation Care**</u>
Re-evaluate ABCDE
12 lead ECG
Treat precipitating causes
Re-evaluate oxygenation and ventilation
Temperature control (cool)

From Australian Resuscitation Council; reproduced with permission.

with the most priority. Sepsis is commonly involved so a fluid bolus of 20 mL/kg (0.9% sodium chloride) is usually administered. Blood sugar level should be tested early on with administration of dextrose 10% 5 mL/kg if hypoglycaemic.

Parents or carers are usually present during the resuscitation. Senior nursing or medical staff member should be allocated solely to provide support and information.

Newborn resuscitation

A small percentage of newborn babies (< 3%) require some resuscitation at birth, usually initial breathing assistance (Figure 1.4). Deliveries in the ED are unexpected or precipitous and so carry

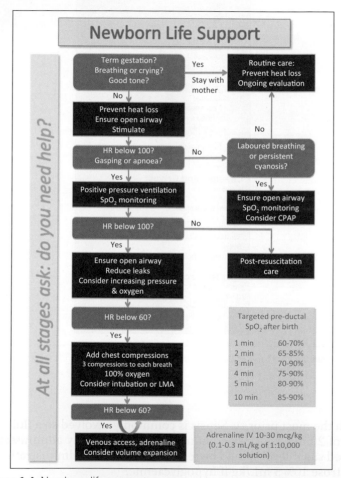

Figure 1.4 Newborn life support
CPAP = continuous positive airway pressure; HR = heart rate; LMA = laryngeal mask airway; SpO₂ = peripheral oxygen saturation
From Australian Resuscitation Council; reproduced with permission.

a higher risk of neonatal complications. All deliveries in the ED warrant preparations for full neonatal resuscitation with a dedicated team that is separate from the team dedicated to assisting the mother.

The healthy term baby can be placed directly on the mother's bare chest or abdomen and a warm blanket placed over them both. Cord clamping can be delayed 1–3 minutes provided this doesn't interfere with any required resuscitation.

Assessment of the newborn begins immediately after birth and involves tone, breathing and heart rate. Good tone means that all the limbs are moving, generally in a flexed posture. Breathing should commence spontaneously within 30–45 seconds and not require chest recession. Heart rate should be 110–160/min and can be assessed by feeling the pulse at the base of the umbilical stump or listening to the heart with a stethoscope. Keep in mind that it can take up to 10 minutes for oxygen saturations to rise above 90% in normal newborns and even brief exposure to excessive oxygenation can be harmful.

If the baby is floppy, not breathing or heart rate is < 100/min, they should be placed on the neonatal resuscitation bed under a radiant heater and provided with stimulation by drying with a soft towel. Ensure the airway is open. Routine suctioning is not recommended, but if there are secretions causing obstruction, these can be very gently and briefly suctioned.

If the baby has not started breathing or the heart rate is < 100/min, provide positive pressure ventilation with air via a self-inflating 240–500 mL paediatric self-inflating bag or T piece using room air. Use a soft-rimmed mask that covers the mouth and nose, but not the eyes. Keep the head in a neutral position as extension or flexion can kink and obstruct the airway.

Deliver breaths at a rate of 40–60/min with just enough volume to see the chest wall rise. The heart rate should rise above 100/min. Persistent bradycardia is usually due to hypoxia and inadequate ventilation. Oxygen can be added if there is no improvement in heart rate.

If the heart rate is < 60/min after adequate assisted ventilation for 30 seconds, commence chest compressions. Use both hands encircling the chest with both thumbs on the lower half of the sternum. Compress the chest to one-third of its depth at a rate of

13

90/min, pausing after 3 compressions to deliver 1 breath. Intubation can be performed if there is an experienced operator available.

Drugs and IV fluids are rarely required. If the heart rate remains below 60/min despite adequate ventilation, oxygenation and chest compressions, adrenaline 10–30 microg/kg IV may be administered but must not detract from the above measures. Intravenous access is usually readily available through the umbilical vein.

Choking

Sudden onset of noisy breathing, stridor and coughing can be signs of partial airway obstruction by a foreign body. The patient's own coughing can be the most effective way of relieving the obstruction, but if coughing is inadequate, call an ambulance or cardiac arrest team and move on to the manoeuvres outlined below and in Figure 1.5.

The conscious patient who is unable to cough and clear her or his own airway needs assistance. Deliver up to 5 back blows with the heel of the hand to the middle of the back between the shoulder blades, checking after each if it has been successful in clearing the airway. If this is unsuccessful, up to 5 chest thrusts can be performed. This is a sharp blow with the heel of the hand delivered to the same area of the chest as chest compressions. Continue 5 back blows and 5 chest thrusts until the obstruction is relieved.

If it is a baby or infant, they can be placed prone and head down across your lap. Firm blows are delivered with the heel of your hand to the baby's back between the shoulder blades. Deliver up to 5 blows, checking in between to see if the airway has been cleared. If not successful, turn the infant over and perform up to 5 chest thrusts. Again, these are sharp blows delivered to the same location as for chest compressions. Continue 5 chest thrusts and 5 back blows until the obstruction is relieved.

If the patient becomes unconscious, commence basic life support while waiting for the ambulance or arrest team to arrive.

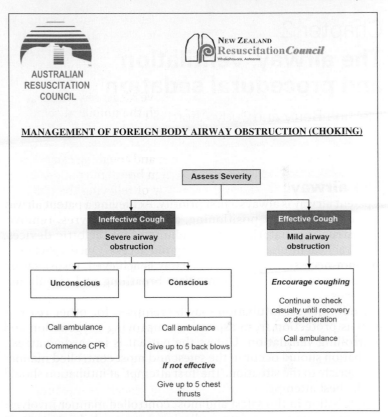

Figure 1.5 Management of foreign body airway obstruction (choking)
From Australian Resuscitation Council; reproduced with permission.

Online resources

International Liaison Committee on Resuscitation (ILCOR)
    www.ilcor.org
Australian Resuscitation Council (ARC)
    www.resus.org.au

Chapter 2
The airway, ventilation and procedural sedation

Melinda Berry and Judy Alford

The airway

A patent airway is always a first priority. Achieving a patent airway may require patient positioning, airway manoeuvres, removal of obstructing material, airway adjuncts, supraglottic devices, endotracheal intubation or cricothyroid access. Once a PATENT (but not necessarily protected) airway is achieved, resuscitation can move to addressing immediate breathing and circulation concerns.

Endotracheal intubation may be required for other reasons such as protection from aspiration, improving oxygenation and controlling ventilation. Unless the patient is in cardiac arrest, intubation should occur in the safest and most controlled manner appropriate to the situation. The 'first attempt' at intubation should be 'the best attempt'.

Intubation in the safest and most controlled manner involves:
1 summoning appropriate medical and nursing help
2 assessing the airway for potential difficulties and preparing to deal with these
3 maximising resuscitation and oxygenation beforehand
4 choosing sedating and paralysing agents and doses appropriate for the patient and condition
5 using some form of checklist to ensure everything is prepared.

Airway management is time critical. There may not be time to make extensive preparations and a difficult airway may be unexpected. The risk to each patient may be minimised by having routine safe practices, using a checklist and rehearsing difficult airway drills.

Airway assessment

Traditional predictors of a difficult airway have not been validated in the ED setting. Although these predictors are still useful, there are many factors unique to the ED situation that renders all airways potentially difficult:

- history taking is often limited
- physical examination is often limited
- pre-oxygenation may be impossible or ineffective
- positioning may be difficult as a result of trauma/restricted neck motion
- airway may be partially obstructed by trauma, blood or vomit
- patient may be uncooperative
- patient may already be hypoxic or haemodynamically compromised
- increased risk of aspiration due to fasting status, pain or opiates.

A difficult airway may or may not be anticipated. Every intubation should involve some degree of 'preparing for the worst'.

- Personnel: utilise the most experienced operators and assistants, or delay until they are available
- Equipment: 'difficult airway' trolley at the bedside with equipment and staff ready to use it
- Communication: articulate the difficult airway plan all the way through to cricothyroidotomy
- Time out: consider the risks versus the benefits of intubation; it may be judged safer to postpone intubation and move the patient to the operating theatre and have the airway managed by our anaesthetic colleagues.

There are three considerations to airway assessment:

1 ability to bag-mask ventilate
2 ability to intubate
3 ability to perform surgical airway.

DIFFICULT BAG-MASK VENTILATION

Six risk factors for difficult mask ventilation have been defined: beard, age > 57 years, snoring, BMI > 26, Mallampati III/IV and limited mandibular protrusion. A commonly used mnemonic for a quick assessment of ventilation difficulty is 'BONES'.

B Beard
O Obesity

N No teeth
E Elderly
S Stiffness

DIFFICULT INTUBATION

The LEMON mnemonic can be used as a reminder.

L Look externally: Gestalt view—trauma, trismus, obesity
E Evaluate 3:3:2 rule (below)
M Mallampati score (below)
O Obstruction
N Neck immobility: cervical collar, rheumatoid arthritis, surgery

DIFFICULT SURGICAL AIRWAY

Look for factors that may obscure surgical landmarks. These can be remembered using the mnemonic SHORT.

S Surgery/Scar
H Haematoma
O Obesity
R Radiation
T Trauma/Tumour

3:3:2 rule

• Interincisor distance = mouth opening > 3 fingers
    — Measure with the mouth fully open and head extended (Figure 2.1)

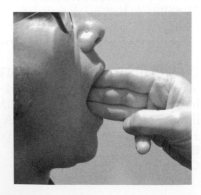

Figure 2.1 Interincisor distance

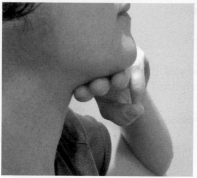

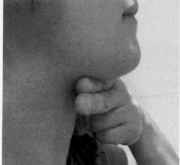

Figure 2.2 Hyo-mental distance   **Figure 2.3** Thyrohyoid distance

* Hyo-mental distance ≥ 3 fingers
  — Measure from mental process to the hyoid (Figure 2.2)
* Thyro-hyoid distance ≥ 2 fingers
  — Measure from the thyroid cartilage to the base of the mouth (Figure 2.3)

Mallampati examination

The patient needs to be sitting upright, head neutral, mouth fully opened, tongue extended and not talking. We can rarely ascertain a true Mallampati score in an ED patient requiring intubation but it should be done prior to procedural sedation (see Figure 2.4).

* Class I: soft palate, fauces, uvula, anterior and posterior pillars
* Class II: soft palate, fauces, uvula

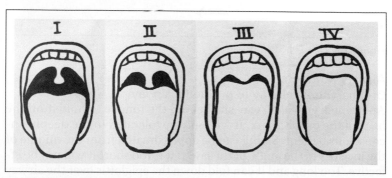

Figure 2.4 Mallampati score

- Class III: soft palate, base of uvula
- Class IV: hard palate

Neck immobility
Short thick necks and conditions of the cervical spine, such as arthritis and previous surgery, can limit neck extension and make laryngoscopy difficult.

Ability to prognath
The patient should be asked to put their lower teeth in front of their upper teeth.

BASIC AIRWAY MANAGEMENT
Airway manoeuvres
Head tilt, chin lift and jaw thrust help to open the airway by pulling the tongue off the back of the oropharynx (Figure 2.5). In patients with suspected cervical spine injury, this is limited to jaw thrust.

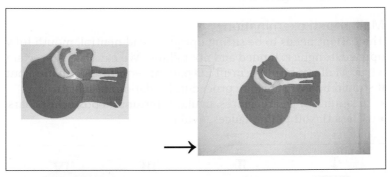

Figure 2.5 Head tilt

Airway adjuncts
Oropharyngeal airway (e.g. Guedel airway)
An oropharyngeal airway sits behind the tongue to hold it off the back of the oropharynx. It will only be tolerated in the deeply unconscious patient. Sizing can be approximated from the middle of the incisors to the angle of the jaw. If it is too short it will not be effective. Too long and it can fold down the epiglottis over the airway

or touch the vocal cords and stimulate laryngospasm. Insertion in adults is by initially curving upwards to get over the tongue, then twisting 180° while advancing. Jaw thrust while simultaneously completing insertion can help ensure the oropharyngeal airway gets behind the tongue. If any resistance is met, or it makes the airway more obstructed, it should be removed.

Nasopharyngeal airway

A nasopharyngeal airway (NPA) is a soft pliable tube, with a slight concave curvature and proximal flange. It is designed to sit with the proximal flange just outside the nostril and the pharyngeal end above the level of the epiglottis, but under the base of the tongue. Patients don't need to be deeply unconscious to tolerate an NPA. Insertion can cause significant bleeding so needs to be done gently with lots of lubricant and avoided in patients with bleeding disorders. A vasoconstrictor spray prior to insertion may minimise bleeding.

NPA insertion in a patient with a base of skull fracture has the potential to pass through the fracture and so this is a relative contraindication.

The correct size is estimated from the nostril to the tragus. It is inserted through the nostril and angled directly posterior, not upwards. The bevelled tip should slide against the nasal septum. If resistance is encountered, a smaller airway or the other nostril may need to be used.

Suction

The Yankauer suction tip is a hard, plastic device used to clear liquid from the oropharynx. It must be passed with care to avoid tissue damage and bleeding. It may cause gagging in conscious patients if inserted too far, and dental damage if patients bite on it. A Y-suction catheter is a soft, pliable tube that can be used for suctioning through an oral or nasopharyngeal airway or, more commonly, down an endotracheal tube. Suction is applied when the side port is occluded.

Face masks

A clear plastic single-use mask is well suited to the ED as vomit or secretions from the patient's mouth can be readily visualised.

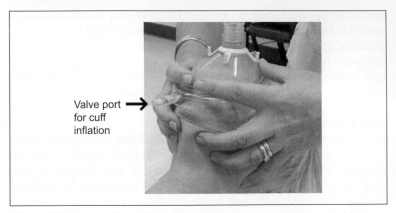

Valve port for cuff inflation →

Figure 2.6 Face mask application

The inflatable cushion seal allows a low-pressure seal to be made with the patient's face. Some face masks will have a hook ring attached at the connector, which may be used for various harnesses (e.g. for non-invasive ventilation). The pointed end of the mask sits across the bridge of the nose and the rounded end comes down to sit between the lower lip and the chin. The thumb and index finger of the non-dominant hand are placed either side of the universal connector. The other three fingers are placed on the mandible and make a seal by pulling the face up to the mask (Figure 2.6). The best seal is achieved when both hands are used to apply the mask, and an assistant squeezes the bag.

Self-inflating bag

With the oxygen tubing connected to oxygen, the reservoir bag will fill with oxygen. After being compressed, the self-inflating bag spontaneously reforms its shape and refills with the 100% oxygen in the reservoir bag. If the reservoir bag is empty, room air is drawn in. When the self-inflating bag is squeezed, gas is forced through the one-way valve to the patient via an applied facemask or airway device. Expired gas flows to the atmosphere via an expiratory valve (Figure 2.7).

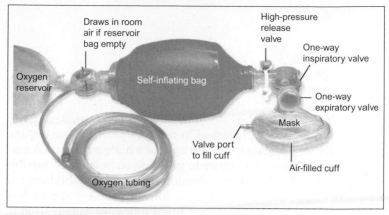

Draws in room air if reservoir bag empty

High-pressure release valve

One-way inspiratory valve

Oxygen reservoir

Self-inflating bag

One-way expiratory valve

Mask

Valve port to fill cuff

Air-filled cuff

Oxygen tubing

Figure 2.7 Self-inflating bag and valve

ENDOTRACHEAL INTUBATION

A simple way to remember indications for intubation and ventilation is ABC.

- **A** Airway
  - — Protection (e.g. reduced level of consciousness)
  - — Patency – airway burns, angio-oedema, airway trauma
- **B** Breathing
  - — Inadequate oxygenation
  - — Inadequate ventilation
  - — Tracheal toilet
- **C** Course of current condition
  - — Expected to deteriorate (lung contusion, multi-trauma, burns etc.)
  - — Haemodynamically unstable
  - — Patient transfer (radiology/other institution etc.)

Equipment preparation

A mnemonic for the equipment required is MALES.

M Mask + bag

Monitoring: oximetry, non-invasive blood pressure (monitoring) (NIBP), ECG, waveform capnography

Medication: induction agent, muscle relaxant, post-intubation drugs

A Airway: oropharyngeal, NPA

L Laryngoscope
E ETT
S Suction
Stylet or bougie
Stethoscope
Securing mechanism (tie or tapes)

The endotracheal tube

The size of the tube is expressed in mm of internal diameter. The average size for a female is 7.5 mm and for a male is 8.5 mm. A narrower tube increases resistance to gas flow, so as large as possible that is suitable for the patient should be selected. In children, the ETT size can be estimated with the formula age/4 + 4 with half sizes above and below available. Cuffed tubes are usually used in children these days, which means a half size smaller than predicted is required.

Cuff inflation post insertion

The cuff should be inflated with the minimal volume that will allow it to seal against the trachea with peak inspiratory pressure. Listening for an audible inspiratory leak assesses this. Inflating the cuff further may lead to tracheal wall pressure and ischaemia. Withdrawing the tube without deflating the cuff can result in herniation of the cuff over the tip of the tube and cause obstruction.

Intubation adjuncts

Stylets are malleable rods used to mould endotracheal tubes into a position and aid control during tube insertion. They are made of aluminium with a plastic cover. The stylet is inserted so that its tip DOES NOT protrude past the end of the tube to avoid trauma from the tip of the stylet. The tube can then be shaped, such as with a bend at the distal end like a hockey stick (Figure 2.8). When the endotracheal tube and stylet are placed through the vocal cords, an assistant holds the stylet in place while the endotracheal tube is advanced further into the trachea. The stylet can then be removed while holding the endotracheal tube in place.

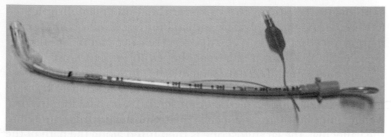

Figure 2.8 Stylet moulded with a bend in the distal end, the 'hockey stick' position

Bougie

The Eschmann tracheal tube introducer (also known as the blue bougie; see Figure 2.9) is not made of gum and is not elastic. The tip can be bent to approximately 35° to facilitate passing around the back of the epiglottis. The tip of the bougie can run along the inside of the trachea, and the bumps of the tracheal rings felt, confirming position. The bougie is inserted into the trachea first and then with the laryngoscope still in position, the ETT can be railroaded over it. The ETT may need to be rotated to facilitate this. Remove the bougie, while holding onto the endotracheal tube, so as to avoid pulling out the endotracheal tube.

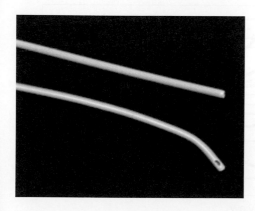

Figure 2.9 Bougie

The laryngoscope

Laryngoscopes have a handle and blade. The handle contains the battery or connection to power source. The blades are usually detachable and come in different shapes and sizes.

The most commonly used shape is the curved Macintosh blade. The Macintosh blade is inserted into the right side of the patient's mouth. A flange on the left side of the blade is used to push the tongue out of the way to the left. The tip of the blade is inserted to the vallecula. The laryngoscope is then lifted along the path of the long axis of the handle (anterior and caudal), indirectly lifting the epiglottis up and exposing the vocal cords.

The straight Miller blade is often used in children. The blade is narrow and so fits into smaller mouths for a given length. The blade is inserted beyond the epiglottis and lifts it up to expose the vocal cords.

Laryngoscopic view

There are four grades of laryngoscopic view (Figure 2.10) as per Cormack and Lehane.

Grade I: entire length of vocal cords are seen

Grade II: only a portion of the vocal cords are seen

   IIa: arytenoids and a portion of the cords

   IIb: arytenoids only

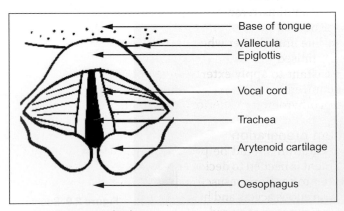

Figure 2.10 Laryngoscopic view

Grade III: epiglottis only
Grade IV: palate and tongue only

Video laryngoscopy
Video laryngoscopy can greatly improve the view of the larynx. Assistants and supervisors can also see what the intubator is seeing, enabling teaching and assistance. A very curved blade on a video laryngoscopy can visualise a very anterior larynx. To then be able to insert the tube around this curve, it usually needs a curved stylet in place.

PREPARATION FOR INTUBATION
A checklist is a useful tool to aid preparation for intubation. Preparation can be divided into five headings.
1 Team assembly
2 Patient preparation
3 Drugs
4 Equipment
5 Difficult airway plan

Team assembly
Ideally the team comprises the following:
- team leader
- intubator
- airway assistant
- drug administrator
- scribe
- in-line immobiliser when cervical motion needs to be minimised
- assistant to apply external laryngeal manipulation if required
- cricothyroidotomy performer if required.

Patient preparation
Resuscitation should be provided prior to intubation. Clinical judgment is needed to decide at what point intubation is necessary in order to continue resuscitation. Ideally, the patient has two sites of intravenous access and has had correction of shock with volume and inotropes as required.

27

Positioning the patient correctly can make tremendous improvement to the laryngoscopic view achieved. The patient should be in the 'sniffing' position, with the neck flexed and the head extended at the atlanto-occipital joint. This position provides the straightest possible line from the mouth to the trachea. This position can usually be achieved in an adult by placing a folded towel behind the head. In an infant, the towel is placed under the shoulders rather than the head to make room for their large occiput. In addition, the reverse Trendelenburg position (slightly head up) is very useful for obese patients.

Monitoring should always be applied including 2-minutely blood pressure readings, pulse oximetry and waveform capnography.

Oxygenation of the patient must be maximised prior to intubation and continued during intubation. This maximises the oxygen reservoir and lengthens the time to desaturation during the induced apnoea. Pre-oxygenation can be achieved with a firmly fitting high-flow oxygen reservoir mask for spontaneously breathing patients. Hypoxic patients may benefit from non-invasive ventilation prior to intubation. Sometimes sedation with a drug like ketamine is needed to facilitate this.

Nasal prongs need to be applied to the patient in this preparation phase. High-flow (> 15 L/minute) oxygen is then delivered via these nasal prongs during intubation to allow continued oxygenation of the apnoeic patient.

Drugs

Intubation drugs are required for all intubations unless the patient is in cardiac arrest (Table 2.1). Even for patients with a GCS 3, sedation and paralysis are required to prevent gagging and to maximise the laryngoscopic view. Medications for post-intubation sedation should be prepared prior to intubation. Other drugs to consider preparing are inotropes or vasopressors. Metaraminol for sedation-induced vaso-relaxation can be very handy.

Equipment

Preparing equipment involves selecting the appropriate endotracheal tube size. Adjuncts should also be selected such as a bougie,

Table 2.1 Drugs in airway management

Drug	Dose	Important effects
Induction agents		
Thiopentone	3–5 mg/kg Less (0.5–1 mg/kg) in elderly or unstable	Hypotension, especially in hypovolaemia Respiratory depression Reduces cerebral metabolism, ICP Increases laryngeal sensitivity
Propofol	1–2.5 mg/kg	Decreases BP, especially in hypovolaemia Respiratory depression Reduces cerebral metabolism
Ketamine	1–2 mg/kg IV 3–5 mg/kg IM	Raises BP Raises HR Airway reflexes maintained Respiration not depressed Bronchodilation Raises ICP and IOP Hallucinations more common in adults
Fentanyl	2–3 microg/kg	Dose-related respiratory depression Analgesia Large doses may cause chest wall rigidity Relative cardiovascular stability
Midazolam	0.1–0.4 mg/kg	Some decrease in BP Respiratory depression
Muscle relaxants		
Suxamethonium	1 mg/kg	Drug of choice for RSI Raises K by 0.5 mEq/L, more in burns (> 48 hours old), paralysis and denervation (> 3 days old), crush injury Raises IOP (avoid in open eye injury) Triggers malignant hyperthermia Prolonged apnoea (rare, inherited)
Rocuronium	1 mg/kg for RSI 0.6 mg/kg for non-RSI 0.15 mg/kg PRN	Use for RSI when suxamethonium contraindicated Use for maintaining paralysis

BP = blood pressure; HR = heart rate; K = potassium; ICP = intracranial pressure; IOP = intraocular pressure; PRN = as needed; RSI = rapid sequence induction oropharyngeal airway, NPA and laryngeal mask airway. Suction needs to be turned on and within easy reach. The assistant will need a syringe for inflating the endotracheal tube cuff. Trachy tape can be passed under the patient's neck ready to tie the tube in place.

Difficult airway plan

The team should clearly and deliberately discuss what actions are to be taken if intubation is not possible and then if oxygenation is not possible. Oxygenation 'rescue' devices, such as a laryngeal mask airway, should be ready. Cricothyroidotomy equipment should be readily available with a doctor able to perform this if needed. Practising 'Can't intubate, Can't oxygenate' drills regularly as a team prepares everyone for this situation. Figure 2.11 is an example of an easy-to-follow algorithm for 'Can't Intubate, Can't Oxygenate' situation.

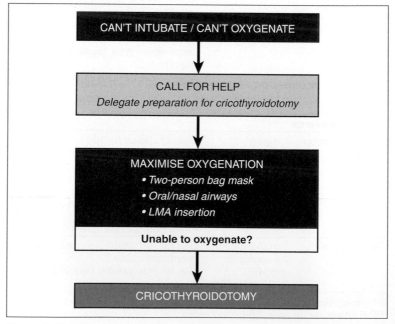

Figure 2.11 Difficult airway plan

Laryngeal mask airway

The laryngeal mask airway (LMA) is an important airway 'rescue' device in the ED. The inflatable mask sits over the glottis and can provide oxygenation that wasn't possible with airway manoeuvres and adjuncts. This may prevent the need for cricothyroidotomy. However, patients that have been difficult to intubate and oxygenate are often also difficult to fit with an LMA.

Cricothyroidotomy

Refer to Chapter 3 Resuscitation Procedures.

Confirmation of endotracheal tube position

Waveform capnography is a reliable and objective marker of tracheal placement of the endotracheal tube and should be used in all patients. It doesn't indicate if the tube has been inserted too far, so listening for air entry on both sides of the chest should still be performed to detect bronchial intubation. Length of insertion of an endotracheal tube is 20–22 cm in females and 22–24 cm in males. In children it can be calculated from $12 + age/2$. On chest X-ray the tip of the endotracheal tube should be above the aortic knuckle, as we know that the aorta passes over the left main bronchus, and hence above the carina.

Securing the endotracheal tube

An ED patient is more likely to have endotracheal tube dislodgement than elsewhere in the hospital for a number of reasons. Trachy tape needs to be tied tightly around the endotracheal tube, not just looped, and this tied firmly around the patient.

Ventilators

Ventilators are used in the ED to assist or control the respiration of patients. Patients needing invasive ventilation need an artificial airway, most commonly an endotracheal tube. The level of ventilatory support needed by a patient varies widely. Some have essentially normal lungs (e.g. sedative overdose), while others have severe respiratory failure.

Indications for ventilation fall into three broad categories.

1 **Respiratory failure**
   — Airway obstruction

- Neuromuscular weakness (spinal cord injury, myasthenia gravis, organophosphate poisoning, exhaustion)
- Chest wall disorders (deformity, flail chest, morbid obesity)
- Pleural disease (massive effusions, pneumothorax or haemothorax)
- Parenchymal lung disease (infection, adult respiratory distress syndrome [ARDS], pulmonary oedema, fibrosis, asthma, chronic airflow limitation [CAL])

2 **Central nervous system (CNS) disease**
- Poisoning
- Trauma
- Cerebrovascular accident (CVA)
- Infections

3 **Circulatory failure**
- Hypovolaemia
- Sepsis
- Cardiogenic shock

The type of ventilator used in the ED is usually small and portable. The range of ventilatory modes available varies, but is usually less than is available on more complex machines in the ICU. Nonetheless most patients can be managed in the short term.

Choosing initial settings for ventilation
Initially, ventilator settings are estimated; adjustments should be made according to the patient's clinical progress and serial blood gas measurements.

Is the patient breathing spontaneously?
Spontaneously breathing patients are ventilated using a mode that assists each inspiratory effort by providing extra pressure or volume. Examples are continuous positive airway pressure (CPAP) and pressure support. Some ventilators and their circuits increase the work of breathing significantly and spontaneous breathing may not be tolerated. In these cases, the patient may need to be sedated and fully ventilated.

The patient who is not breathing adequately needs a mode that does all the work for them. Intermittent positive pressure ventilation (IPPV) or intermittent mandatory ventilation (IMV) provides a breath at a preset rate regardless of the patient's respiratory effort. Some ventilators can deliver a breath synchronised to an inspiratory effort; this is known as synchronised intermittent mandatory ventilation (SIMV).

How much oxygen does the patient need?

In most cases, start ventilation with 100% oxygen and titrate downwards as soon as possible according to the patient's arterial blood gases (ABG) results. Prolonged ventilation with high levels of inspired oxygen may be associated with complications such as absorption atelectasis and oxidative injury.

Some ventilators have limited options in selecting an inspired oxygen level. In patients who are inadequately oxygenated, positive end-expiratory pressure can increase the arterial oxygen tension for a given level of inspired oxygen.

How much gas should the patient receive?

The minute volume is the amount of gas moved every minute:

$$\text{minute volume} = \text{respiratory rate} \times \text{tidal volume}$$

The arterial tension of carbon dioxide is sensitive to changes in minute volume. Increasing the minute volume reduces the partial pressure of CO_2 ($PaCO_2$) and decreasing the minute volume raises $PaCO_2$. In patients with raised intracranial pressure, it may be necessary to deliberately hyperventilate to maintain a modest decrease in $PaCO_2$. In some patients with lung injury, trying to deliver a 'normal' minute volume may pose a risk of barotrauma. In these cases, the $PaCO_2$ may be allowed to rise quite significantly, an approach called permissive hypercapnia.

The ventilators in common use apply positive pressure to the lungs to enable gas movement. The amount of gas moved per breath depends on the ventilator settings and the lung compliance.

Ventilators can be set to deliver a given tidal volume at each breath. This mode is called volume control and is available on even the most basic machines. It may be possible to limit the delivery of the set volume if the airway pressures exceed a limit chosen by the operator (pressure-regulated volume control [PRVC] mode).

Pressure control is a mode commonly used in the ICU but not always available on smaller ventilators. A constant airway pressure is provided during inspiration, with the tidal volume varying. This approach is often used where barotrauma is a concern.

Lung compliance is the change in lung volume for a given change in transpulmonary pressure. Diseased lungs often have abnormal compliance (e.g. in pulmonary oedema the lung is less compliant or 'stiffer'). Trying to deliver a 'normal' tidal volume to a poorly compliant lung can cause high airway pressures, increasing the risk of pneumothorax. Over-distension can worsen lung damage. The approach to ventilating is usually one of providing limited tidal volumes (6–8 mL/kg, sometimes less) with PEEP. This can be done using either volume or pressure control.

The choice of initial tidal volume depends on the clinical situation. In patients with respiratory failure or shock, a volume of 6–8 mL/kg is safest, as this will minimise barotrauma and volutrauma. Inspiratory pressures should not exceed 30 cmH$_2$O.

Positive end-expiratory pressure (PEEP)

PEEP leaves a constant pressure on the lungs at the end of expiration, preventing the collapse of alveoli. Constant opening and closing of alveoli can damage them. Using PEEP may prevent further lung injury as well as maintain functional residual capacity. As noted earlier, PEEP has a positive effect on oxygenation. However, PEEP has a negative effect on cardiac output because high intrathoracic pressures impede venous return. High levels of PEEP may not be tolerated in haemodynamically unstable patients. Another factor to be considered is 'auto-PEEP'. This is the pressure difference between the alveoli and the proximal airway at end-expiration, which can be raised in conditions with air-trapping, such as severe asthma. 'Auto-PEEP' can contribute to haemodynamic instability in some patients. Prolonging expiration may help to reduce air-trapping in affected patients.

Choosing a level of PEEP

PEEP of 5 cmH$_2$O is tolerated by most patients. In patients with severe lung disease, increases in PEEP up to about 12 cmH$_2$O may be needed. PEEP may not be tolerated in patients with haemodynamic instability. Another group of patients who may not tolerate PEEP have raised intracranial pressure. In some cases the reduction in cerebral venous return may be enough to exacerbate the increase in intracranial pressure.

SPECIAL SITUATIONS
Asthma
Use low respiratory rates with a prolonged expiratory phase to limit gas trapping. Auto-PEEP may be significant, so additional PEEP may lead to hypotension. Avoid large tidal volumes. Permissive hypercapnia may be needed.

Raised intracranial pressure
Avoid hypercapnia. Maintain $PaCO_2$ between 30 and 35, using end-tidal monitoring and ABG. High levels of PEEP should be avoided.

Adult respiratory distress syndrome (ARDS)
ARDS is a difficult problem. The ideal ventilatory strategy is controversial. In the ED the key points are: 1. to avoid barotrauma by using small tidal volumes and avoiding high airway pressures; 2. to use PEEP as tolerated and tolerate a high $PaCO_2$. Paralysis may be necessary. Frequent adjustments to tidal volume and respiratory rate may be needed, along with recruitment manoeuvres to reopen collapsed alveoli. Specialised techniques such as prone ventilation and high-frequency oscillatory ventilation may be undertaken in the ICU. In the rapidly deteriorating patient with refractory hypoxaemia, early referral for consideration of extracorporeal membrane oxygenation (ECMO) may be life-saving.

Troubleshooting
+ Ask for advice early.
+ Never assume the monitor is at fault.
+ If there is difficulty ventilating the patient, immediately remove the patient from the circuit and commence bag ventilation with 100% oxygen. Check the endotracheal tube for kinking, displacement (in or out), obstruction and leaking. Examine the patient for equal and adequate breath sounds. Check the trachea is midline. If breath sounds are

diminished, suction for mucous plugs and consider treating for a pneumothorax. Treat bronchospasm or pulmonary oedema if present. Get a chest X-ray. Consider bronchoscopy.
* If all of the above are normal, the problem may be with the machine. The ventilator may have become disconnected (from the circuit, the gas supply or the power supply). There may be leaks in the tubing or valves, or tubing may be obstructed. Consider changing the circuit.

Non-invasive ventilation

Non-invasive ventilation (NIV) is widely used in EDs. It is used to improve both oxygenation and ventilation in patients and can avoid the need for intubation in some patients. It can also be used to improve oxygenation prior to intubation.

There are a number of acronyms involved in NIV that are very simple once explained. NIV can be referred to as non-invasive positive pressure ventilation (NIPPV). All our ventilation is with positive pressure, so it is the same as NIV. CPAP (continuous positive airway pressure) is where the pressure delivered is the same in both inspiration and expiration. If a higher pressure is used during inspiration, it is called BiPAP (bilevel positive airway pressure). BiPAP therefore has both an inspiratory pressure (inspiratory positive airway pressure [IPAP]) and an expiratory pressure (expiratory positive airway pressure [EPAP]). IPAP is always greater than or equal to EPAP. If IPAP and EPAP are equal, it is the same as CPAP.

EFFECTS OF NIV

In CPAP the positive pressure has the effect of holding the alveoli open larger—like a balloon with more air in it is larger in size. This results in a greater surface area for gas exchange, and so improves oxygenation. The increased pressure prevents some alveoli from closing during expiration, so the surface area is available during expiration as well as inspiration and hence better oxygenation, and less work of breathing to open alveoli.

BiPAP has the benefits of CPAP plus inspiratory support. This reduces the work of breathing and gives a bigger inspiratory breath (tidal volume). A bigger tidal volume means an increase in ventilation for the same respiratory rate. An increase in ventilation directly reduces $PaCO_2$.

INDICATIONS FOR NIV

- Acute respiratory failure: chronic obstructive pulmonary disease [COPD], asthma, pulmonary oedema
- Acute on chronic respiratory failure: COPD, neuromuscular disease
- Obstructive sleep apnoea

CONTRAINDICATIONS

- Apnoea or impending cardiorespiratory arrest
- Inability to protect airway (relative contraindication)
- Copious secretions/airway bleeding/vomiting
- Significant hypotension
- Airway obstruction
- Facial fractures
- Untreated tension pneumothorax
- Uncooperative patient, not tolerating the mask

COMPLICATIONS OF NIV

- Hypotension from the increased intrathoracic pressure
- Barotrauma
- Pressure sores
- Conjunctivitis
- Gastric over-distension and gastro-oesophageal reflux
- Aspiration (rare)
- Dry mucous membranes and thick secretions

STARTING NIV

A clear explanation to the patient is the key to compliance. Decide on a communication strategy with the patient as it is difficult to talk while undergoing NIV. The best ventilation is with the patient sitting up. Starting with low pressures can make it easier for the patient to tolerate. The pressure can then be gradually increased as needed. The mask can be held on to the patient's face initially, before applying the straps so that the patient doesn't feel suddenly tied in. FiO_2 can be high initially, but this should be weaned down as soon as possible according to the patient's oxygen saturation levels.

STRATEGIES DURING THERAPY

Patients may develop hypotension due to the increased intrathoracic pressure, particularly if they were hypovolaemic beforehand. Blood pressure needs to be monitored and IV fluid boluses may be needed.

Pressure settings should be titrated to the patient's response. Tidal volumes should be 5–8 mL/kg.

If this is too low, IPAP should be increased relative to EPAP. If tidal volumes are too high, IPAP should be decreased relative to EPAP.

Oxygenation should be improved by increasing CPAP/EPAP in order that FiO_2 can be weaned down quickly.

Patients on NIV need to be reviewed regularly. The pressure settings and oxygen levels should be titrated to their response. Nebulisers can be administered through the circuit as indicated.

Procedural sedation

Procedural sedation (also known as conscious sedation) refers to administration of sedative drugs to facilitate performance of a distressing or painful procedure. The level of sedation required varies with the procedure and the individual patient. The level of sedation falls short of general anaesthesia. The patient should retain the ability to respond to stimulus and airway reflexes should be maintained.

INDICATIONS

Procedures involving significant pain and/or anxiety are tolerated to varying degrees by individual patients. For example, a child may require sedation for wound suturing where an adult may not.

PROCEDURES REQUIRING SEDATION IN NEARLY ALL PATIENTS

- Reduction of dislocations of large joints
- Reduction and splinting of long bone fractures
- Cardioversion

PROCEDURES REQUIRING SEDATION IN SOME PATIENTS

- Lumbar puncture
- Central line insertion

- Wound suturing
- Foreign body removal
- Burn dressing
- Chest drain insertion

REQUIREMENTS

Procedural sedation should be undertaken in an area with working suction and oxygen. Pulse oximetry should be used. Continuous ECG and blood pressure monitoring may be used in selected patients (e.g. older or with cardiac history). Ready access to resuscitation equipment and emergency drugs is essential. At least one person should be present who has skills to manage any complications, including airway obstruction and cardiac arrest. All patients should have details recorded on a standard form (e.g. Figure 2.12). Fasting status does not necessarily preclude the use of sedation, but does influence the depth of sedation induced.

DRUGS

The ideal drug for procedural sedation has rapid onset and offset, has no significant side effects, preserves airway reflexes and is easily titrated. Some commonly used agents are found in Table 2.2.

AFTERCARE

The patient should be monitored until they have emerged from sedation. It is not uncommon for patients to become more deeply sedated once painful stimulus has ceased. Patients should not be discharged from the ED until they have returned to their baseline mental state, are ambulant and have safe transport and supervision. Patients with poor social circumstances may require a longer period of observation.

St Vincent's Hospital
EMERGENCY DEPARTMENT

Anaesthetic/Procedural
Sedation Assessment Form

MRN			SURNAME	
OTHER NAMES				
DOB	SEX	AMO	WARD/CLINIC	

(Please enter information or affix patient information label)

Reason for intubation/procedural sedation:_____

Emergency procedure (unable to complete form)   (tick if applicable)

Reason_____

HISTORY

Allergies:_____

Medications:_____

Past health   Comorbidities (tick if present)   Diabetes   COPD

                                                        Asthma   IHD

Other significant history:_____

_____

Anaesthetic history:_____

Tobacco: _____   Alcohol:_____   Other: _____

Fasting time (in hours):_____

EXAMINATION

BP:_____   PR:_____   SpO$_2$: _____

Mallampati: Class I   Class II   Class III   Class IV

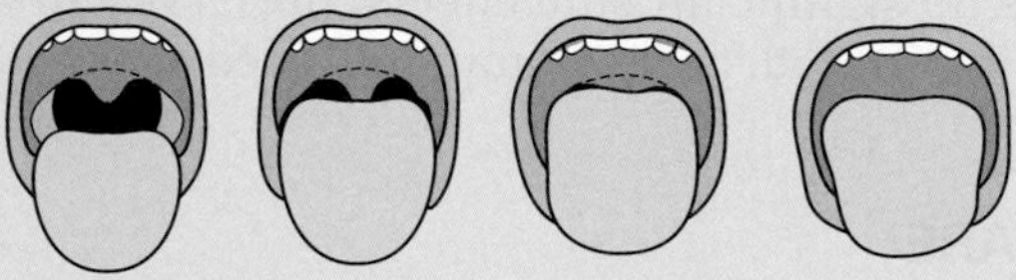

Teeth: _____
Neck mobility:_____
Other relevant physical findings: _____

INVESTIGATIONS

_____
_____

Consent obtained: Yes ☐   No ☐   If no, reason _____

MEDICAL OFFICER

Name: _____   Signature:_____

Designation: _____   Date:_____

Name of supervising medical officer (if applicable): _____

ANAESTHETIC/PROCEDURAL SEDATION ASSESSMENT FORM

Figure 2.12 Anaesthetic procedural sedation assessment

Table 2.2   Drugs used in procedural sedation

Drug	Dose	Duration
Midazolam	0.02–0.1 mg/kg IV 0.05 mg/kg PO (onset about 20 minutes)	30 minutes IV 45–60 minutes PO
Fentanyl	2–3 microg/kg IV	20–30 minutes
Propofol	0.5–1 mg/kg IV	10 minutes
Ketamine	1–2 mg/kg IV 3–5 mg/kg IM	15 minutes IV 30 minutes IM
Nitrous oxide	Given as 30–50% mix in oxygen Causes expansion of gas-filled structures (e.g. pneumothorax)	5 minutes

Chapter 3
Resuscitation procedures

Drew Richardson

Overview
- Intravenous access techniques
- Arterial access techniques
- Chest drainage procedures
- Pericardiocentesis
- Urinary catheterisation
- Suprapubic cystostomy
- Cricothyroidotomy
- Lumbar puncture
- Emergency department thoracotomy

Introduction

This chapter gives a brief overview of major procedures which may be carried out in the emergency department. It is designed to be used as a reminder for a doctor who has already been trained in these techniques, and not as a training manual. The common procedures should be practised under supervision, and the uncommon procedures should be formally taught before they are attempted solo. Some procedures require both training and experience, and some institutions require formal accreditation for operators (e.g. for focused assessment with sonography in trauma or FAST scanning). Many procedures and their integration into complex, team-based resuscitation are best learned in a simulator laboratory rather than in an ED.

For all procedures, the following is essential.

1 Appropriate sterile technique and standard precautions. Minimally invasive procedures such as peripheral intravenous access require only gloves and a clean technique, but more invasive procedures mandate formal sterile technique with a sterile field, appropriate drapes, gown, gloves, mask and eye protection. Lesser technique may

be acceptable only when the procedure is required within seconds (e.g. cricothyroidotomy or ED thoracotomy) and full protection for the staff must still be observed.

2 Obtain the patient's informed consent whenever possible. The level of explanation obviously varies with the invasiveness of the procedure and the urgency of the patient's condition, but all conscious patients must give their consent (even if only implied).

3 Ensure patient comfort and safety of all parties by using appropriate analgesia, and, if necessary, sedation. Do not attempt difficult procedures on patients who are unable or unwilling to lie still.

4 Utilise a 'time out routine': stop and reflect at least for a moment to ensure that the right procedure is being undertaken on the right patient at the right site—look again at any relevant imaging to confirm it is the right way around. In the case of team-based procedures, verbally confirm that all members understand the plan (for endotracheal intubation this commonly involves a checklist).

5 Ensure continuing care and resuscitation of the patient, particularly during long procedures, utilising other staff and patient monitoring throughout.

6 Document the time, operator and result of the procedure appropriately in line with local practice. Even minor procedures such as insertion of an intravenous cannula normally require a standardised form of documentation such as a date written on the dressing.

Editorial Comment

Ask: Can I do this procedure more safely with ultrasound guidance?

Intravenous access techniques

There are four basic intravascular access techniques.

1 Indwelling metal needle, now used only rarely and in peripheral sites (e.g. 'a butterfly').

2 Catheter over needle technique, such as common intravenous cannula.

3 Catheter through needle technique is used infrequently. A large-bore needle is inserted into the relevant vessel, and

a smaller catheter advanced up the needle, usually into a central vein. The metal needle is then withdrawn and rendered safe in a plastic guard. This technique carries the disadvantage of a small-bore catheter and the risks of catheter tip embolisation with poor technique and ongoing ooze due to the diameter difference.

4 Seldinger technique, widely accepted for all large or long intravascular lines. The vessel is punctured with a long needle on a syringe, and a flexible guidewire passed down the needle (sometimes through the syringe). The syringe and needle are removed, the skin incised, and appropriate dilators passed over the wire and then removed. The catheter is passed over the wire into the vessel, and the wire then removed. With this technique it is important to:

a check and understand the equipment before starting (various sets are available)

b have cardiac monitoring in place if the wire is to be near the heart

c secure the catheter properly (usually by stitching)

d above all, never let go of the wire.

Ultrasound guidance

All of the following techniques benefit from appropriate ultrasound guidance. If small veins cannot be seen or palpated, then ultrasound assists in location. Large deep veins are beyond vision, so skin marking using ultrasound before the procedure and/or direct visualisation using ultrasound (with sterile technique) during the procedure increases success and decreases complications. In settings where large, deep vessels are regularly cannulated, availability of ultrasound is now considered 'standard of care'.

Editorial Comment

Ultrasound guidance is increasingly being used for all access and is considered very desirable for any central access procedures.

INTRAVENOUS LINES—PERIPHERAL

Indications

- Administration of fluid—resuscitative and/or maintenance
- Administration of drugs or IV contrast
- Obtaining blood (rare)

Contraindications

- Overlying skin damage (e.g. burns) or infection
- Venous damage proximal to the site insertion
- Arteriovenous fistula in the limb

Technique

1 Apply a venous tourniquet.
2 Identify a suitable vessel, ideally as peripheral as possible. Start looking on the back of the hands. Use cubital fossa veins only when large-volume resuscitation is required or other sites have proven unsuitable.
3 Prepare the area with a disinfectant-soaked swab, swabbing in a distal direction.
4 Stretch the skin slightly over the vein.
5 Insert the needle, bevel upwards, until a flushback is obtained.
6 Advance the catheter over the needle all the way—in most modern cannulas this locks away the 'sharp'.
7 Remove the needle, attach IV line or bung, and secure catheter.
8 Check the position and patency by infusion or injection to clear blood from the catheter.
9 Mark the time and date in accordance with local protocol.

Complications

- Haematoma
- Subcutaneous extravasation of fluid
- Damage to nearby structures
- Inter-arterial cannulation

INTRAVENOUS (IV) LINES—PAEDIATRIC

The selection of a site for IV infusion in the neonate or young child should include consideration of the femoral vein in the groin and the scalp veins.

Of these, the femoral vein is probably the best to use in the critically ill child. Although no tourniquet can be applied, the vein is reliably located medial to the femoral artery pulse just below the inguinal ligament.

The scalp veins can be rendered more visible by use of a rubber band tourniquet around the head and entered in the usual fashion. Always inject saline and check for blanching to exclude arterial puncture. Careful strapping and often use of a protector (e.g. plastic cup) are essential to avoid displacement of the scalp vein catheter.

INTRAOSSEOUS (IO) INFUSION— PAEDIATRIC OR ADULT

This is a rapid technique for reliably obtaining vascular access in sick, small children. It can be used in patients of all ages, but the thicker bones of older children and adults mandate the use of a drill rather than manual insertion. Blood can usefully be drawn for biochemistry (not haematology and check with your laboratory) and large volumes of fluid or drug infused. It is highly recommended this technique be practised on animal bones or simulators before it is attempted on a patient. As always, be familiar with the equipment used in your ED.

Indications
- Critically ill patient (especially small child) in urgent need of drug or fluid administration
- No other vascular access readily available

Editorial Comment

IOs are becoming standard use in some acute resuscitations and problematic access. Practise with a kit available to you on a simulation trainer/bone to get the feel. Also ensure you know laboratory limitations for any blood tests, care of the IO site and safe length of use.

Contraindications
- Infection at puncture site
- Fracture of the bone
- Osteogenesis imperfecta
- Recent nearby intraosseous puncture (relative contraindication that is likely to lead to extravasation)

Technique
1 Identify infusion site: preferably upper medial surface of the tibia, 1–2 cm distal to the tibial tuberosity, but the

lower tibia (at the junction of the medial malleolus and the shaft) may be suitable. The antero-lateral femur just above the femoral condyle can be used and in larger children and adults the humerus (abducted and internally rotated) just above the surgical neck gives the fastest access to the central circulation.

2 Prepare the area with an iodine swab.

3 Use an intraosseous drill with the appropriate needle at 90° to the bone, first penetrating the skin then squeezing the trigger until cortical penetration is felt. If working manually in small children, insert intraosseous needle (16- to 18-gauge special needle with stylet) into the bone at 45° aiming away from the epiphyseal plate (distally in upper tibia) with a rotary 'grinding' motion until a 'crunch' is felt as the cortex is penetrated. Using a drill, progress is faster, but the definite penetration is still felt.

4 Remove stylet and attempt to aspirate marrow contents. Success clearly indicates correct placement, but failure sometimes occurs despite placement.

5 In a conscious large child or adult patient, inject 2 mL of 2% lignocaine for comfort.

6 Begin infusion or injection of fluids and drugs. Flow should be relatively free.

7 Secure and protect the infusion site.

Complications
1 Extravasation of fluid
2 Needle blockage
3 Infection (rare, reduced by good technique and removal as soon as practicable).

INTRAVENOUS LINES—CENTRAL
Indications
- Central venous pressure monitoring
- Infusion of concentrated/irritant solutions (e.g. inotropes, parenteral nutrition)
- Insertion of specialised equipment (e.g. plasma exchange catheter, Swan-Ganz catheter, transvenous pacemaker)
- Emergency venous access when peripheral access impossible

Contraindications
- Distorted local anatomy
- Known or suspected vessel damage (current trauma, previous radiation therapy, previous surgery)
- Coagulopathy or vasculitis
- Inability to provide cardiac monitoring
- Pneumothorax in central venous access on the opposite side (risk of bilateral pneumothoraces)

Technique—general
All of the following techniques carry different risks and benefits. All require ongoing cardiac monitoring but the choice of technique should depend on operator experience and on the technique favoured in the particular hospital. Remember: the ICU may have to care for 'your' catheter for days or weeks so, if a choice is available, use the method preferred by the inpatient team.

1 Use local anaesthesia liberally, following down the intended track.
2 Have cardiac monitoring in place, and always withdraw the catheter/wire slightly when arrhythmias (usually ventricular ectopics) occur.
3 After catheter placement, always aspirate each part then inject adequate saline to clear the line.
4 Secure the catheter by stitching and apply dressing.

Complications
- Arterial puncture: when detected, remove the needle or catheter and apply pressure over the site for a full 10 minutes, followed by arterial observation of the limb.
- Pneumothorax: always obtain chest X-ray (CXR).
- Malposition of catheter tip: always check X-ray.
  — Wrong vein: passing into jugular vein to subclavian vein instead of superior vena cava (SVC). This is difficult to reposition without an image intensifier and may require repuncture.
  — Excessive length: in right atrium or ventricle rather than SVC. The CXR should show that the tip is not below the carina. If it is too low the catheter can be easily withdrawn.

- Damage to mediastinal contents: haemothorax, hydrothorax, arteriovenous fistula and perforation of any structure in the chest may occur (even an endotracheal cuff has been reported).
- Infection
- Embolism: of air, wire or catheter parts
- Knotting/kinking of catheter

SUBCLAVIAN CANNULATION
Infraclavicular technique
1 Position the patient supine in 15° Trendelenburg with the arm adducted.
2 Enter at the junction of the middle and medial thirds of the clavicle.
3 Aim along the inferior surface of the clavicle towards the suprasternal notch, with a needle bevel facing inferomedially.
4 Advance 1–2 mm after the first flush of blood to obtain reliable flow back into the syringe.

Complications
- Pneumothorax
- Arterial puncture
- Others as described above

Supraclavicular technique
1 Position the patient supine in 15° Trendelenburg.
2 Enter the neck just lateral to the lateral border of the clavicular head of sternocleidomastoid and just above the clavicle.
3 Aim approximately at the contralateral nipple with the bevel of the needle towards the patient's toes.
4 Advance 1–2 mm after the first flush of blood to obtain reliable flow back into the syringe.

Complications
Although the full range of complications is as described previously, they occur significantly less frequently with the supraclavicular approach.

INTERNAL JUGULAR CANNULATION
Technique
1 Position the patient's head down 10°, with the head turned slightly away from the side of entry.
2 Enter just above the point of the triangle formed by the two heads of sternocleidomastoid and 1 cm lateral to the internal carotid pulsation.
3 Aim parallel to the carotid artery ('straight down the neck').

Complications
- Arterial puncture
- More easily displaced by movement than subclavian lines
- Others as above (rare)

Arterial access techniques
The same basic types of cannula used for venous access are available for arterial access, often again in specialised kits. Note that arterial puncture is painful, and for a single sample puncture the smallest practical needle should be used: usually 25 gauge (radial) or 23 gauge (femoral). Indications for arterial blood gas measures are few in the emergency setting: the venous pH and PCO_2 are normally close enough to the arterial values for diagnostic purposes, and the peripheral oxygen saturation (SaO_2) is usually a good measure of gas exchange.

INDICATIONS
1 Arterial blood gas measurement (see earlier this chapter)
2 Need for recurrent (e.g. hourly) blood sampling—normally patients going to ICU
3 Ongoing monitoring of arterial blood pressure—also ICU and theatre patients

---
Editorial Comment
Even in the critically ill we should be doing fewer arterial punctures and more VBG; see VBG values.

CONTRAINDICATIONS
- Overlying skin damage (e.g. burns) or infection
- Arteriovenous fistula in the limb
- Clotting diathesis (relative)

RADIAL ARTERY CANNULATION

1 With the wrist in mild extension, palpate the radial arterial pulse over the distal radius.
2 Insert the catheter or needle into the centre of the pulsation parallel to the long axis of the forearm with the bevel forward.
3 Pulsatile flushback into the syringe or cannula indicates successful puncture. If inserting a cannula, proceed another 1–2 mm to ensure the tip of the needle is entirely within the artery.
4 If puncture fails, apply pressure to the site to reduce haematoma formation.

FEMORAL ARTERY CANNULATION

1 Palpate the femoral pulse at the mid-point of the inguinal ligament.
2 Insert the catheter or needle into the centre of the pulsation parallel to the thigh.
3 Pulsatile flushback into the syringe or cannula indicates successful puncture. If inserting a cannula, proceed another 1–2 mm to ensure the tip of the needle is entirely within the artery.
4 If puncture fails, apply pressure to the site to reduce haematoma formation.

Complications
• Haematoma or haemorrhage (apply pressure)
• Venous cannulation (check for pulsation, pressure wave)
• Thrombosis or embolism (rare and usually late)
• Infection

Chest drainage procedures

Any chest drainage procedure for pleural fluid also benefits from ultrasound guidance.

NEEDLE THORACOSTOMY

This is performed either with a soft flexible catheter 'over a needle' such as an IV cannula, or a specialised drainage which may utilise a catheter through needle or Seldinger technique. The location depends on the setting and urgency. For a tension pneumothorax, the procedure is performed rapidly and without anaesthetic over the anterior chest wall. For therapeutic drainage of an effusion, it is performed posteriorly. For aspiration of a simple pneumothorax, laterally or posteriorly. Note that many readily available IV cannulae are too short for emergency drainage in an obese population.

Indications
- Tension pneumothorax: drain direct to air
- Simple pneumothorax (spontaneous) up to 75% collapse
- Pleural effusion: drainage or sampling

Contraindications
- Traumatic pneumothorax (unless tension is present) since tube thoracostomy indicated
- Haemothorax
- Bleeding diathesis (relative)

Technique
1 Check equipment: for drainage of fluid or simple pneumothorax, either a large syringe and three-way tap or an underwater seal drain set in addition to the soft catheter; a syringe is normally attached if an IV cannula is being used.
2 Position the patient:
   a lying flat for anterior puncture of tension pneumothorax—2nd interspace, mid-clavicular line
   b head of bed elevated with shoulder abducted for lateral puncture of simple pneumothorax—4–5th interspace, mid-axillary line
   c leaning forwards over a pillow for posterior puncture of pleural effusion—8–10th interspace, mid-scapular line.
3 Inject local anaesthetic if needed.
4 Insert the needle just over the lower rib of the interspace (in order to avoid the neurovascular bundle that lies beneath the rib above).
5 Aspiration of air/fluid through a cannula or a 'pop' into the pleural space indicates correct placement—advance the catheter and remove the needle or follow the technique appropriate to the individual kit.

6 For a tension pneumothorax leave open and undertake subsequent tube thoracostomy.
7 For other drainage connect a three-way tap and syringe or an underwater seal drain to the catheter.
8 Aspirate air or fluid as needed, emptying the syringe and sealing the catheter by means of the tap.
9 Small catheters are removed after aspiration or when a tube thoracostomy is in place. Larger catheters (e.g. 'pigtail') can be left in situ and managed like a tube thoracostomy.
10 Always obtain repeat chest X-ray.

<u>Complications</u>
- Damage to local structures: neurovascular bundle, internal thoracic artery (anterior approach)
- Inadequate drainage due to small size of catheter, adhesions or blockage
- Underlying lung damage: a pneumothorax will be created if one is not already present
- Infection at the site

FINGER THORACOSTOMY

This is an emergency procedure for drainage of a pneumothorax or suspected pneumothorax in a ventilated patient. It is carried out as for intercostal catheter insertion (next section) but the wound is left open with no catheter, allowing free drainage. By allowing free drainage it avoids the risks of blocked tubes, and so it is often favoured in the pre-hospital environment. In the ED it is only ever used as a temporising measure. Great care should be taken to confirm correct location before converting a preexisting field finger thoracostomy to a tube thoracostomy.

INTERCOSTAL CATHETER—TUBE THORACOSTOMY
<u>Indications</u>
- Tension pneumothorax: only after needle thoracostomy
- Traumatic pneumothorax
- Simple pneumothorax which has not responded to needle drainage or is causing significant respiratory compromise
- Haemothorax
- Haemopneumothorax

- 'Prophylactic' use in the chest trauma patient who is to receive positive pressure ventilation or aeromedical transport; this indication depends on available skills and circumstance

Contraindications (all relative)
- Multiple adhesions
- Need for immediate thoracotomy
- Coagulopathy

Technique
1 Provide appropriate sedation/analgesia—the majority of conscious patients will tolerate narcotics well and should receive them.
2 Position the patient.
    a Elevate head of bed 45° if possible.
    b Raise the arm on the relevant side over the head and place the fingers behind the head.
    c Tilt the patient slightly away.
3 Select and mark the site, the 4th or 5th interspace and the mid-axillary line (i.e. at the level of the nipple just behind the muscle bulk of the anterior chest wall muscles).
4 Select appropriate tube size, in general the largest reasonable tube (32 Fr to 36 Fr) should be used in adults with haemothorax, but much smaller tubes are appropriate if only air is to be drained.
5 Prepare drainage system—normally disposable plastic underwater seal drain sets, but bag drainage with some form of flutter valve is often used in the field.
6 Prepare the area and inject local anaesthetic down to the pleura over the line of the rib below.
7 Incise skin 3–4 cm along the line of the rib below.
8 Bluntly dissect through the subcutaneous tissue and muscle layers to the pleura passing just above the rib to avoid the neuromuscular bundle. A hiss will normally be heard when the pleural space is entered.
9 Enlarge the tract with a finger and insert the finger into the chest cavity to ensure full penetration and check for adhesions.

10 Insert tube without stylet in one of three ways.
   a Hold tube and advance through hole manually.
   b Grasp tip of tube in curved forceps and advance through hole.
   c Use specially designed forceps (Pollard forceps) to open a path through which the tube is passed.
   d Advance the tube to at least 3 cm beyond the last lateral hole.
11 Immediately connect the tube to the drainage system. If there is to be any delay then the tube should be clamped for a spontaneously breathing patient, but must not be clamped for a patient who is ventilated. 'Fogging' of the tube normally confirms its location inside the chest cavity.
12 Check that the underwater seal drain is bubbling or swinging; ask the patient to cough to confirm position. If it is not swinging, rotate the tube or remove and re-insert.
13 Close the skin wound with sutures and stitch the tube in place. Dress the wound and anchor the dressing to the tube.
14 X-ray to check position of tube and re-expansion of pneumothorax or drainage of haemothorax.

Complications

- Blockage or failure to drain due to blood clots, position against chest wall, multiple adhesions or kinks
- Puncture of solid organs—should not occur if stylet is not used and technique is followed, even in the presence of diaphragmatic hernia
- Reverse flow—keep drainage bottle below patient
- Re-expansion pulmonary oedema
- Local injury or infection
- Persistent bubbling or failure of re-expansion due to leakage in circuit, ICC hole outside pleural cavity, or (rare) oesophageal rupture/bronco-pleural fistula

Pericardiocentesis

This is an emergency procedure for the treatment of pericardial tamponade, a diagnosis usually made on ultrasonography (either FAST or formal echocardiography) or sometimes clinically, on the basis of high central venous pressure, hypotension, tachycardia and muffled heart sounds. It is relatively common after penetrating chest trauma, relatively uncommon after blunt chest trauma, and is seen in left ventricular free wall rupture after myocardial infarction. In any setting where pericardiocentesis is expected to occur it should be done with ultrasound guidance, but lack of ultrasound is not a contraindication to a potentially life-saving procedure. Survival is poor unless the patient is reasonably fit and access to cardiothoracic surgery facilities is available.

INDICATIONS

- Diagnostic: if the patient is stable, this is not indicated in the ED
- Pericardial tamponade or suspicion in deteriorating patient
- Electromechanical dissociation in cardiac arrest when other causes excluded; this indication has a low success rate as tamponade is a rare cause of cardiac arrest unless there is a sizeable hole in the ventricular wall

CONTRAINDICATIONS

- Immediate need for thoracotomy, particularly in cases of trauma
- Stable patient: seek echocardiographic evidence before proceeding
- Prolonged cardiac arrest when good outcome is not possible

TECHNIQUE

1 Position patient with head up at 45°.
2 Pass a nasogastric tube if abdominal distension present.
3 Prepare equipment: syringe, three-way tap and large needle. Ideally an insulated 10 cm needle, purpose-designed for such taps, or a pericardial catheter ('catheter over a needle') should be used. However, when the diagnosis is clear or when the patient is in cardiac arrest, then any large needle or large-bore IV catheter may be used. The metal hub of the needle should be attached to the V lead of the ECG monitor, and monitoring must be ongoing through the procedure.
4 Approach. Insert the needle between xiphoid process and left costal margin at 30–45° advancing towards the left shoulder.
5 The pericardium is normally entered 6–8 cm below the skin, and any fluid will be aspirated. If the needle touches the

epicardium, an injury current with high ST segment should be seen on the ECG. In this case, withdraw the needle a few millimetres.

6 Aspirate with a syringe, using the three-way tap to disperse the contents if necessary. If a catheter has been inserted, withdraw the needle and re-connect the catheter to the tap.

7 Withdraw whatever fluid can be obtained, but if blood continues to flow freely, suspect ventricular penetration. Pericardial fluid may have a lower haematocrit than blood and may not clot, but neither of these tests is absolutely reliable nor helpful within the first few minutes of aspiration.

8 If a response is obtained, leave the catheter in place and be prepared to re-aspirate prior to a thoracotomy.

9 Repeat ultrasound for size of effusion and obtain CXR to check for a pneumothorax.

COMPLICATIONS

- Myocardial damage: ventricular puncture or coronary artery laceration
- Arrhythmias: ventricular ectopics, ventricular fibrillation, cardiac arrest
- Pneumothorax or lung laceration
- Air embolism if accidental injection of air occurs
- Local infection

Urinary catheterisation
INDICATIONS

- Urinary retention
- Monitoring of urinary output
- Drainage of neurogenic bladder
- Diagnostic urinary specimen
- Pre-operative procedure for pelvic surgery
- Management of the unconscious patient

Editorial Comment

Hospital-acquired urinary tract infections (e.g. from catheters) now have financial penalties.

CONTRAINDICATIONS

• Clinical suspicion of urethral injury: if there is a perineal haematoma and blood at the meatus, then an ascending urethrogram should be performed to identify urethral damage and/or a suprapubic catheter used as an alternative

• Urinary tract infection (UTI): relative contraindication as introducing a foreign body to an infected area is undesirable

TECHNIQUE—MALES

1 Patient position is supine; stand on the side of the patient corresponding to the operator's dominant hand.
2 Prepare penis using no-touch technique, retracting the foreskin in and swabbing the glans and surrounding areas. Drape with a fenestrated sheet and repeat swab.
3 Instil lignocaine gel into urethral opening while holding the penis in the 'dirty' hand. From this point on, the hand holding the penis should be considered 'dirty' and only the other hand should touch the tray and catheter equipment.
4 After a delay for the gel to take effect, hold the catheter in forceps and insert into the bladder to a distance of 20–25 cm.
5 Inflate the catheter balloon using 5–10 mL of sterile saline.
6 Ensure foreskin is returned.
7 Check for free flow of urine and collect a specimen if necessary.
8 Connect an appropriate drainage bag.

Editorial Comment

Ensure the foreskin is fully replaced after every catherisation.

TECHNIQUE—FEMALES

1 Position patient supine with heels drawn up and thighs abducted.
2 Prepare external genitalia by swabbing and drape with a fenestrated sheet. Separate labia with gauze squares and identify urinary meatus and re-swab.
3 Apply sterile lubricant liberally to the catheter.
4 Insert catheter into bladder using forceps, to a distance of 10–12 cm.

5 If catheter is to be left indwelling, inflate balloon with 5–10 mL sterile saline.

6 Collect any specimens necessary and connect appropriate drainage bag.

COMPLICATIONS—BOTH SEXES

• Failure to catheterise.
  — Inability to identify urethra (females): the urinary orifice is frequently displaced by gynaecological surgery or obscured by oedematous tissue. A more thorough examination, repositioning and better light are appropriate.
  — Strictures of the urethra: excessive force should not be used, but a smaller catheter may be tried.
  — Prostatic obstruction: this is commonly the indication for catheterisation. Once again, a small catheter, and possibly an introducer, should be tried.
• Trauma: creation of false passage, partial or complete urethral tear, long-term risk of stricture.
• Infection: urethritis, epididymitis, pyelonephritis.
• Haemorrhagic cystitis: rare complication of rapid decompression of a chronically distended bladder.
• Paraphimosis in males: always replace a retracted foreskin.

REMOVAL OF TRAPPED URINARY CATHETER

Doctors in the ED may be called upon to remove a urinary catheter which is either blocked and unable to be removed, or simply 'stuck' at a time of routine removal. The usual cause is a 'flap valve' in the balloon tubing which prevents balloon deflation.

Various techniques are described. Cutting the catheter is rarely effective, since the blockage is usually proximal. If the patient's bladder is not excessively distended and the catheter balloon definitely lies within the bladder, then the balloon may be over-inflated with sterile water or saline until it bursts. If there is doubt about the position of the balloon, then ultrasound should be used to identify it, since it must not be over-inflated in the urinary tract. The balloon within the bladder can also be punctured using a suprapubic needle.

Suprapubic cystostomy
INDICATIONS

- As for urinary catheter but catheter cannot be passed due to a suspected or definite urethral trauma
- Failed catheterisation, usually strictures or prosthetic disease
- Other reasons such as blockage of an existing catheter

CONTRAINDICATIONS

- Previous lower abdominal surgery/scarring/radiation
- Inability to palpate the bladder (or visualise on ultrasound)
- Bleeding diathesis
- Urinary tract infection

TECHNIQUE

1 Check equipment: a number of suprapubic catheter sets are available, mostly relying on a variant of the 'catheter over the needle' technique.
2 Position the patient supine.
3 Inject local anaesthetic starting 2–3 cm above the symphysis pubis and heading down the expected track at approximately 20° towards the pelvis. When urine is drawn back into the anaesthetic syringe, the bladder has been reached.
4 Incise the skin with an appropriate scalpel blade.
5 Puncture the bladder down the same track used for the anaesthetic.
6 Follow appropriate technique to secure the catheter in the bladder. This varies between suprapubic catheter sets.
7 Collect any necessary specimens and connect the catheter to an appropriate drainage bag.
8 Apply adhesive and/or sutures as appropriate to maintain the catheter in place.

COMPLICATIONS

- Failure to catheterise the bladder
- Bowel perforation
- Extravasation of urine: intra peritoneal or extra peritoneal
- Local bleeding: intraperitoneal, extraperitoneal or into bladder

- Infection
- Obstruction

Cricothyroidotomy

There are many different kits available for cricothyroidotomy—this is the final common pathway of all 'difficult airway' algorithms and so it is critical that anyone who undertakes endotracheal intubation is familiar with the equipment available in their ED. However, it can be done with any scalpel and hollow tube—lack of equipment is never a reason not to undertake a life-saving procedure.

INDICATIONS

- Supralaryngeal airway obstruction when tracheal intubation not possible (e.g. epiglottitis, burns, facial trauma)
- Ventilatory support required (e.g. apnoea) and tracheal intubation failed ('Cannot intubate, Cannot ventilate')

TECHNIQUE

1. Position the patient supine with the neck extended if possible.
2. Identify the cricothyroid membrane as a horizontal depression in the midline anteriorly between the notch of the thyroid cartilage and the cricoid cartilage. Prepare the area.
3. Make a 1.5 cm incision across the lower half of the cricothyroid membrane, then incise the membrane. This is best done with a guarded scalpel blade, usually supplied in cricothyroidotomy kits. However, it can be accomplished with any scalpel.
4. Open the cricothyroidotomy by dilating with artery forceps or gently twisting the scalpel blade.
5. Insert the tube (either a 6 mm cuffed endotracheal tube for an adult, or a 4.5 mm uncuffed cricothyroidotomy tube) in a downward direction.
6. Remove any trochar, secure the tube and ventilate the patient.
7. Check ventilation in the same way as for endotracheal intubation.

COMPLICATIONS

- Local bleeding: external or into the airway
- Creation of a false passage

- Damage to larynx, trachea, oesophagus
- Local infection

Lumbar puncture
INDICATIONS

- Clinical suspicion of CNS infection, particularly meningitis
- Clinical suspicion of subarachnoid haemorrhage when CT scan unavailable or CT scan negative
- Sample of cerebrospinal fluid (CSF) required for non-emergent evaluation (e.g. Guillain-Barré Syndrome)
- Therapeutic: drainage of CSF or installation of chemotherapy

CONTRAINDICATIONS

- Clinical or CT evidence of raised intracranial pressure or localising signs
- Infected site of puncture
- Coagulopathy

Editorial Comment

Always explain, and obtain consent (preferably written), as complaints frequently follow.

TECHNIQUE

1 Position the patient: if measurement of CSF pressure is indicated, in the lateral recumbent position with knees drawn up; otherwise sitting up leaning forwards with the feet over the side of the bed on a chair ('sitting fetal feet supported'). Mark the L4 spinous process which is palpable in a line connecting the posterior and superior iliac crests.
2 Prepare and drape the area.
3 Infiltrate local anaesthetic in L3/L4 or L4/L5. Gently insert a spinal needle in the midline. A non-cutting needle with side port is preferred, in which case the skin may need to be punctured first with a sheath. If a cutting needle is used, position the bevel horizontal. After penetrating the skin, aim approximately for the patient's umbilicus.

4 Advance, feeling for the loss of resistance as the needle penetrates the ligamentum flavum.
5 Remove the stylet to check for CSF flow. If the subarachnoid space has not been reached, carefully re-insert the stylet and continue.
6 When CSF is obtained, connect a manometer to measure CSF pressure and then collect a sample, normally into three sterile bottles.
7 Remove the needle and dress the site.

COMPLICATIONS
- CSF infection—rare but potentially fatal.
- Spinal cord or corda equina damage—should not occur if performed at the correct level.
- Uncal herniation is described after lumbar puncture in cases with raised intracranial pressure.
- Post lumbar puncture (LP) headache.

Emergency department thoracotomy
ED thoracotomy should only be considered if the operator is experienced, there is some hope of meaningful survival based on the patient's presentation and facilities exist for rapid removal of the patient to a thoracic operating facility.

INDICATIONS
- Penetrating chest trauma with all of the following:
  — signs of life present during pre-hospital phase
  — any pneumothorax drained
  — pericardiocentesis undertaken
  — fluid load given
  — continued poor response: in cardiac arrest or cardiac arrest clinically imminent
- Blunt trauma: only when signs of life have been present in the ED, no other lethal injuries (e.g. severe head injury) present, no response to standard resuscitation and electrical cardiac activity still present
Note: Even in these circumstances, the response rate to ED thoracotomy in blunt trauma is exceedingly low. The aim of ED thoracotomy is to drain pericardial tamponade, repair cardiac

lacerations or cross-clamp the aorta. Internal cardiac massage or internal defibrillation may be performed, but do not constitute indications for thoracotomy alone.

CONTRAINDICATIONS

- Inadequately skilled personnel
- Thoracic operating theatre not available
- 'Medical' cardiac arrest

TECHNIQUE

1 Patient is normally supine, intubated, undergoing CPR.
2 Prepare the left side of the chest.
3 Incise along the top of the left 6th rib (5th intercostal space) down to the chest wall muscles. Begin 2 cm lateral to the sternum and extend beyond the posterior axillary line.
4 Dissect through the intercostal muscles into the pleura with Mayo scissors, stopping ventilation so that the lung collapses momentarily. Divide the intercostal muscles with a sweep of the Mayo scissors along the top of the 6th rib.
5 Insert rib spreaders with a handle and ratchet bar downwards and retract the ribs.
6 If extending to the right ('clamshell thoracotomy') then cut through the sternum with heavy scissors or a saw (this will cut the inferior mammary arteries which will require ligation later) and use the same incision technique on the other side.
7 If pericardiotomy is required (history consistent with pericardial tamponade, pericardium swollen and tense) perform it with scissors starting at the diaphragm and moving upwards, 1 cm anterior to the phrenic nerve. Use fingers to gently sweep clots of blood from the pericardium.
8 If direct cardiac compression is required, use two hands anterior and posterior to the heart to gently compress.
9 If aortic cross-clamping is required, this is difficult to perform with a vascular clamp since the aorta must be separated from the oesophagus. It is easier to apply pressure through the pleura to compress the aorta against the thoracic spine.

10 Repair of lacerations in the myocardium is particularly difficult in the emergency setting but may be attempted if necessary.
11 Proceed immediately to the operating theatre for further definitive treatment.

Editorial Comment

Most problems arise when procedures are ill prepared, ill explained and performed with inadequate analgesia and in haste.

Chapter 4
Trauma
Judy Alford

Acknowledgment

The author wishes to acknowledge the content used from the previous edition of *Emergency Medicine* which was provided by Martin Duffy, Karon McDonnell, Anthony Grabs.

Trauma in Australia and New Zealand is the leading cause of death in the first four decades of life. Fortunately, injury-related deaths have declined over the past 20 years; however, they continue to be a significant burden on health resources. The major causes of death remain brain injury and haemorrhage.

Definition of major injury

Numerous trauma scoring systems are presently used throughout the world in an attempt to define the severely injured patient. Unfortunately, all have their advantages and disadvantages, with one of the key problems being the need to collect data 'after the fact'. Scoring at the time of presentation may underestimate the severity of the injury and lead to under-triage. Major injury has previously been defined as having an Injury Severity Score (ISS) in excess of 15, as it was associated with a chance of dying in excess of 10%. Most trauma centres would now define major injury as one of:

- ISS > 15
- requirement for urgent surgery
- intensive care admission
- inpatient stay longer than 3 days
- head injury requiring assisted ventilation for more than 24 hours
- death.

Patients with major injuries need to be triaged early, with activation of a coordinated trauma response from emergency, anaesthetics, intensive care and surgery.

Pre-hospital triage

Pre-hospital assessment and management by ambulance services now enables the initial triage of patients to regional or major trauma services. The overriding goal is to get the *right patient* to the *right hospital* at the *right time*. Patients meeting the criteria should be considered as having potentially life-threatening injuries requiring the services of an appropriately designated trauma centre and thus allowing a trauma call to be put out pre-arrival after notification by the ambulance. Major trauma centres are able to talk directly via radio or phone with the paramedics.

On arrival at the ED, these features indicate a potentially critically ill trauma patient:

- respiratory distress—rate < 10/min or > 30/min, or cyanosis
- systolic BP < 90 mmHg or no palpable radial pulse in children
- reduced level of consciousness (LOC)
- serious trauma to any region of the body
- burns (partial or full thickness) > 20% in adults or > 10% in children.

The definition of **serious trauma** to any body region includes the following.

- Penetrating injury of:
  — head
  — neck
  — chest
  — abdomen
  — perineum
  — back.
- Head injury with:
  — one or both pupils dilated
  — open head injury
  — severe facial injury.
- Abdominal injury with:
  — distension
  — rigidity.
- Spinal injury with:
  — weakness
  — sensory loss.

- Limb injury with:
  — vascular injury with ischaemia of limb
  — amputation
  — crush injury
  — bilateral femur fractures.

Preparation

Effective communication between the pre-hospital personnel and the receiving hospital is paramount. The history of the injury and pre-hospital management is extremely important and this should be relayed via the IMIST-AMBO system shown in Table 4.1.

Pre-hospital information enables the activation of a team response to a trauma patient with defined roles for nursing and medical staff, along with planning for specific urgent interventions such as intubation and transfusion.

Editorial Comment

If a massive transfusion (i.e. > 1 whole blood volume in 24 hours or > 50% of blood volume loss in 3 hours) is required, the local massive transfusion guideline (see Figure 4.1) should be implemented immediately to avoid morbidity and mortality.

Table 4.1   The IMIST-AMBO system

I	IDENTIFICATION	Patient's name and details
M	MECHANISM	Mechanism of injury
I	INJURIES	ABCDEF
S	SIGNS	Vital signs and GCS
T	TREATMENT/ TRENDS	Interventions Response to treatment
A	ALLERGIES	Does the patient have any allergies?
M	MEDICATIONS	Are the medications with the patient?
B	BACKGROUND	Medical history
O	OTHER ISSUES	Characteristics of the scene Social Advance care order Belongings/valuables

Adapted from the Centre for Health Communication Ambulance/ED Handover Protocol.

St Vincent's Hospital

MASSIVE TRANSFUSION GUIDELINE

Definition	**Massive Transfusion** is when greater than one whole blood volume is given to a patient within 24 hours, or replacement of >50% blood volume loss in 3h.
Notify Blood Bank	**Phone 9148 or 9150** As soon as a patient is recognised as potentially requiring massive transfusion and baseline bloods have been taken, the **blood bank should be notified** of the clinical situation and the anticipated demand, so that they can plan and call for help as required. A **named senior clinician** must take responsibility for communication with the blood bank and completing the tally sheet.
Maintain Homeostasis	Consider early definitive haemostasis eg surgery or interventional radiology. Measures should be taken to prevent and correct hypothermia (with the use of fluid warmers and external warming devices), acidosis and electrolyte abnormalities eg: aim ionised Ca > 1.1.
Pre-Treatment Status	It is important to recognise patients on anti-platelet drugs, warfarin or other anticoagulants or those who have a known coagulopathy, as clotting components and adjuvants may be required immediately. Trauma patients arriving in ED may have already lost a significant blood volume and may also require clotting components as soon as they are available.

Order 4 units of Packed Red Blood Cells (PRBC).

In an **emergency**, if there is **no current group and hold**,
uncrossmatched group 0 blood may be issued

(Rh −ve for **premenopausal females**, otherwise Rh +ve is acceptable).

If bleeding is considered to be severe and ongoing, blood components other than
PRBC should generally be given after 4 units have been transfused.

Order subsequent products as required in groups alternating as follows:

4–6 units PRBC 4 units Fresh Frozen Plasma (FFP) 1 pooled Platelets	4–6 units PRBC 4 units Fresh Frozen Plasma (FFP) 6 units Cryoprecipitate

Mixture of components may vary aiming for:
- Platelet count >50 x 10⁹/L or >100 x 10⁹/L with head injury
- Fibrinogen >1g/L
- PT, APTT <1.5 x mean control
- Hb > 80g/L (may vary depending on scenario)

Monitor:
- Arterial or venous blood gases every 60–90 min during the resuscitation
- Monitor FBC, EUC, Coags and Fibrinogen every 3h
- Samples should be labelled urgent and sent immediately to the lab.

Consider adjunct medications:
- Protamine (Heparin reversal)
- Vit K (Warfarin reversal)
- Prothrombinex (Warfarin reversal)
- Antifibrinolytics
- Desmopressin
- Recombinant Factor VIIa

Consider seeking advice via switch, of the haematologist-on-call at any time.

Figure 4.1 Massive transfusion guideline
Reproduced with permission from St Vincent's Hospital.

The use of ABCDE algorithms as taught in the early management of severe trauma (EMST) or advanced trauma life support (ATLS) courses allows a systematic approach to an unknown patient. Knowledge of the mechanism of injury enables some prediction of possible injury/injuries. It is important to note that management of the airway, breathing and circulatory systems must occur concurrently rather than sequentially, and occasionally control of one system must be gained before safe definitive management of another is possible (e.g. control of exsanguinating bleeding before intubation).

Standard precautions are a must—goggles, mask, impervious gown and gloves. The early donning of lead gowns enables potentially crucial X-rays to be performed in a timely and appropriate fashion without significant interruption to resuscitation efforts once the patient arrives.

Editorial Comment

Code Crimson
A badly injured trauma patient can exsanguinate from major internal bleeding quickly. It has been shown that a direct transfer of the patient to a waiting operating theatre suite, with anaesthetics, ICU, etc. ready to receive the patient and get the patient into theatre for the surgeon to stem the blood loss, saves lives and morbidity (e.g. major vessel, cardiac injury). It also allows prompt, effective resuscitation (e.g. avoids hypovolaemic arrest with its poor results, avoids massive transfusions). It is a criteria-based, practised organisational innovation, at times even avoiding stopping in the ED. It must be called and supervised by senior staff. It works.

Systematic assessment and management

The care of an injured patient by a trauma team is somewhat different to traditional medicine, with diagnosis, investigations and management frequently occurring simultaneously and performed by more than one doctor. A team leader should direct the overall management, including:

1 primary survey
2 resuscitation
3 history

4 secondary survey
5 definitive care.

When caring for the paediatric trauma patient, the priorities are the same as for the adult patient. Allowances must be made for the child's size and physiology, but the approach to assessment and management is otherwise identical. Beware of differences in injury patterns and the child's ability to compensate. Don't forget the parents—modify your approach to include family in the resuscitation room.

Care of the pregnant patient follows a similar line. Again, allowing for differences due to the anatomical and physiological changes of pregnancy, assessment and management are the same as for the non-pregnant patient. Positioning of the mid–late pregnant woman is important, as the gravid uterus may compress the vena cava. To avoid this position, try tilting the pelvis to the left side using a rolled towel underneath, if not contraindicated. Early use of fetal monitoring is important, but good care of the mother equals good care of the fetus, so remain focused on the following priorities as outlined for the adult patient.

Primary survey

During the primary survey you need to simultaneously identify and manage immediately life-threatening injuries. The priorities of the primary survey, in order, are:

1 Airway maintenance with cervical spine protection
2 Breathing and oxygenation
3 Circulation and control of external haemorrhage
4 Disability—brief neurological examination
5 Exposure with environment control.

The primary survey needs to be continually repeated throughout the initial phase of management. The key to good trauma care is directed assessment, followed by appropriate and timely intervention and subsequent directed reassessment—the AIR (assessment, intervention, reassessment) approach.

Six key injuries that need to be excluded during the primary survey can be remembered by the mnemonic **At This Moment Find Ominous Conditions.**

A Airway obstruction
T Tension pneumothorax

M Massive haemothorax
F Flail chest
O Open pneumothorax
C Cardiac tamponade

1 AIRWAY MAINTENANCE WITH CERVICAL SPINE PROTECTION

Patients with a decreased level of consciousness or inadequacy of protective reflexes are prone to airway obstruction and aspiration. All patients should be considered to have a cervical spine injury until proved negative—this has significant implications for airway management. The head and neck should be supported at all times, especially during log-rolling.

The first priority is to establish a patent airway, allowing for oxygenation. This may require:

- the removal of blood, vomitus and foreign bodies by posturing, suction or Magill's forceps
- jaw thrust and chin lift manoeuvres
- the insertion of an oropharyngeal airway
- endotracheal intubation
- supraglottic devices such as a laryngeal mask
- establishment of a surgical airway.

A high concentration of oxygen should be administered to all patients. Patients with a decreased LOC associated with a traumatic brain injury should be considered for early endotracheal intubation. Patients with a relatively high GCS may require intubation for the management of agitation or pain, as may patients with the potential for deterioration in their airway due to swelling or local haemorrhage, as well as progressive respiratory injury or shock.

A surgical airway should be anticipated in cases with adverse anatomical features, facial or neck trauma and burns, with a dedicated member of the resuscitation team tasked to intervene should the patient be unable to be oxygenated by other means.

Drug choice and dose will be influenced by the patient's physiological parameters, baseline level of consciousness and injuries, with care taken to avoid compromise of cerebral perfusion due to iatrogenic hypotension. While a rapid sequence induction technique remains suited to most cases, selected patients benefit from a delayed sequence approach, with sedation to enable pre-oxygenation and optimal positioning before full induction of anaesthesia.

2 BREATHING AND OXYGENATION

Once the airway has been deemed patent and protected, the adequacy of ventilation should be assessed. This is achieved by:

- exposure of the chest
- inspection for cyanosis, tachypnoea, chest movement and chest wall integrity
- palpation of the tracheal position, subcutaneous emphysema and chest wall integrity
- auscultation for the presence and symmetry of air entry
- oxygen saturation $\pm$ end-tidal carbon dioxide measurement
- visualisation of bilateral lung sliding using ultrasound.

The team should identify and provide immediate management for the following life-threatening injuries well before a chest X-ray has been obtained:

- tension pneumothorax
- large haemothorax
- large flail segment
- open pneumothorax.

Use of needle decompression of tension pneumothorax may fail due to a large chest wall, so immediate finger thoracotomy using sterile technique is recommended, with insertion of a chest tube once tension has been relieved.

Early chest X-ray may provide vital warning of a potentially life-threatening chest injury not yet detected by clinical examination.

3 CIRCULATION AND CONTROL OF EXTERNAL HAEMORRHAGE

The maintenance of adequate tissue perfusion, especially of the brain, is the primary objective of the circulation component of the primary survey. Hypotension is almost always due to blood loss in the trauma setting. Tachycardia precedes hypotension in most patients; however, the elderly can be less able to increase their heart rate in response to blood loss.

The common sites for bleeding include the thoracic cavity, the peritoneal cavity, the retroperitoneum or the pelvis. You must **stop the bleeding**. This may simply require the application of pressure to a site of external haemorrhage, or it may necessitate transfer to the operating suite for an immediate laparotomy. Early application of a pelvic binder or limb tourniquet in the appropriate setting may be life-saving.

Severely injured patients may present with established co-agulopathy due to massive tissue trauma, and with the increasing numbers of elderly injured patients, therapeutic anticoagulation adds to the difficulty of haemorrhage control. Early assessment of clotting using thromboelastography (TEG) or rotational throm-boelastometry (ROTEM) may allow targeted management. These are dynamic clot studies to help target therapy.

Examination

Assessment of a patient's circulatory status does not require waiting for the blood pressure reading. Information gained from examination of the patient's pulse, skin and level of consciousness is enough to make immediate resuscitation decisions, and the only equipment required is your eyes and your fingers. Remember to interpret your findings in the context of each individual you are assessing—the young, fit male who can compensate well despite considerable blood loss versus the elderly female with multiple comorbidities on numerous physiology-altering medications are two entirely different scenarios. Beware of pa-tients who are hypotensive in the supine position—they have lost in excess of 30–40% of their blood volume and will require urgent resuscitation (Table 4.2).

- **Pulse.** The pulse rate and character should be determined as an initial assessment of the circulatory status. Tachycardia with a small volume pulse is due to hypovolaemia until proven otherwise. Patients with systolic blood pressure (SBP) less than 80 mmHg frequently have absent peripheral pulses.
- **Skin perfusion.** Pale, cool, clammy skin with a capillary refill time greater than 2 seconds is an early indicator of hypovolaemia.
- **Level of consciousness.** A decreased LOC is an indicator of poor cerebral perfusion and, again, is presumed to be due to hypovolaemia until proven otherwise.

The presence of pre-hospital hypotension is an important predictor of bleeding, and the patient who responds to relatively

Table 4.2 **Estimated fluid and blood losses based on patient's initial presentation (for a 70 kg patient)**

	Class 1	Class 2	Class 3	Class 4
Blood loss (mL)	Up to 750	750–1500	1500–2000	> 2000
Blood loss (% blood volume)	Up to 15%	15–30%	30–40%	> 40%
Pulse rate (bpm)	< 100	> 100	> 120	> 140
Blood pressure	Normal	Normal	Decreased	Decreased
Pulse pressure	Normal or increased	Decreased	Decreased	Decreased
Respiratory rate (breaths/minute)	14–20	20–30	30–40	> 35
Urine output (mL/h)	> 30	20–30	5–15	Negligible
CNS/mental status	Slightly anxious	Mildly anxious	Anxious, confused	Confused, lethargic

small volumes of pre-hospital fluid may harbour significant internal bleeding.

Priorities

1 **Control of external haemorrhage.**

This may require direct digital pressure over a wound, suturing/stapling of briskly bleeding scalp wounds, the reduction of facial fractures and nasopharyngeal packing.

The application of tourniquets to uncontrolled arterial limb haemorrhage may be life-saving; however, their inappropriate use will worsen venous bleeding. The time of application must be clearly documented, as excessive ischaemic time is associated with limb-threatening complications.

2 **Establishment of intravenous access.**

Two large-bore cannulas (14 or 16 gauge) should be inserted, usually into the cubital fossa of each arm. In patients with severe upper limb or chest trauma, one large-bore cannula should be above the diaphragm and one below the diaphragm.

Intraosseous needles can be placed in an uninjured limb, with the proximal humerus being the best choice in torso trauma.

Large-bore cannulas may also be placed in the subclavian or jugular position or into the femoral vein if necessary. The use of ultrasound to find appropriate intravenous access in the difficult patient is becoming more common.

3 **Resuscitation fluids.**

Warmed intravenous fluids should be given at a rate appropriate for the clinical situation at hand. Dilution of clotting factors and red blood cells by the excessive infusion of crystalloid or colloid should be avoided. Minimal volume resuscitation may be appropriate in some circumstances, such as penetrating trauma before surgical control of bleeding has been achieved, where mentation or palpable central pulses may be the goal, rather than normotension.

Anticipate the need for transfusion early, as fully cross-matched blood takes at least 40 minutes to organise. Be prepared to use group-specific or un-cross-matched group O blood in urgent cases.

The use of protocolled massive transfusion packs containing red cells, platelets and fresh frozen plasma in a 1:1:1 ratio avoids the development of coagulopathy associated with the transfusion of red cells alone.

Early use of tranexamic acid in significant haemorrhage has been shown to improve outcomes. In patients with acute coagulopathy of trauma or a hypofibrinolytic state, the early use of cryoprecipitate may be indicated.

Specialist haematology advice should be sought for patients taking anticoagulant therapy.

4 **Stop the bleeding.**

Fluid resuscitation does not replace the need to control ongoing bleeding—get the patient to the operating suite at the **right time**. In selected cases, embolisation in an interventional radiology or hybrid suite may be indicated to control haemorrhage, particularly from the pelvis.

'**Code Crimson**' is a protocol designed to facilitate the rapid transfer to operating theatres (OTs) of massive exsanguinating trauma or vascular emergencies. This involves bypassing resuscitation cubicles, where valuable time may be wasted while carrying out monitoring and radiology. It has been shown that, although each minor task may individually consume barely minutes, together they accumulate some 20 minutes to ready the patient.

Deteriorating haemodynamic status may be due to:

• ongoing blood loss
• tension pneumothorax
• cardiac tamponade.

Immediate directed re-examination for tension pneumothorax and cardiac tamponade should be performed. Frequently neck veins will be collapsed in hypovolaemia; however, if the jugular venous pressure is raised, this suggests increased intrathoracic pressure. Having clinically ruled out these two conditions, you are then faced with the challenge of determining the source of ongoing blood loss.

Major blood loss can occur from the following five sites:

1 external haemorrhage
2 long-bone fracture(s)
3 chest
4 pelvis
5 abdomen/retroperitoneum.

Focus on these sites, particularly when dealing with the trauma patient who remains hypotensive despite intravenous fluid resuscitation and other appropriate measures. It is imperative to remember that, at this stage of the resuscitation, determining the site of blood loss is far more important than trying to determine which specific organ is bleeding.

External haemorrhage can be visualised and then controlled with appropriate pressure. Long-bone fractures can be determined by clinical examination and then splinted to limit further blood loss. Significant blood loss into the chest can be ruled out by clinical examination and with the aid of an early chest X-ray. Likewise, significant blood loss from the pelvis can be ruled out by clinical examination and with the aid of an early pelvic X-ray. The abdomen/retroperitoneum is, by default, the only other site of blood loss left to contend with and, in the context of haemodynamic instability, this usually means an emergency laparotomy is in order.

Always remember, however, that the patient may bleed into multiple sites simultaneously, making such an 'orderly' assessment difficult in practical terms. The role of bedside ultrasonography as an adjunct to the clinical examination in the trauma patient has been developing for many years throughout the world and is routine in Australia. It has the advantage of being rapid, safe, non-invasive and, most importantly, repeatable.

Code Crimson activation can be simplified to four steps:

1 Pre-hospital notification by ambulance service of major trauma ('batphone').
2 Switchboard sends a major trauma page to trauma team.
3 Team leader (most senior emergency doctor) upgrades to Code Crimson on patient arrival, in consultation with surgical registrar.
4 Switchboard sends Code Crimson page to surgical and anaesthetic teams.

The use of **ultrasound** in a directed and limited manner by performing a focused assessment with sonography in trauma (FAST) examination is now commonplace. Its primary role is to look for free fluid in the abdomen by examining the hepatorenal, splenorenal and retrovesical regions. In the appropriate circumstances, examination for fluid in the pericardial sac may also be carried out. It should be performed by an experienced team member and should not distract the trauma team from the other components of the primary survey. Extended FAST examination continues to evolve, detecting thoracic injuries such as pneumothorax/haemothorax with potentially greater accuracy than plain chest radiography, not to mention its role in assessment of a patient's volume status and response to resuscitation. *Remember:* It is a **rule-in** test—if it is negative all bets are off.

4 DISABILITY: BRIEF NEUROLOGICAL EXAMINATION

A decreased level of consciousness is due to hypoxia or hypovolaemia until proven otherwise. Beware of hypoglycaemia. However, once these issues have been addressed, the priority is to determine the presence or absence of an intracranial injury that requires urgent neurosurgical intervention. The pupils should be assessed for size, symmetry and response to light and the patient's level of consciousness should be quickly assessed using the **AVPU** method; that is, is the patient:

A Alert?
V responding to Verbal stimuli only?

P responding to Painful stimuli only?
U Unresponsive?

The **Glasgow Coma Scale (GCS)** may also be used to assess the LOC at this stage, or can be deferred until the secondary survey is performed. In conscious patients, all limbs should be assessed for movement and sensation to detect possible spinal injury.

All patients with a GCS score of less than 12 should have aggressive ABC management, including consideration for early intubation. This will enable controlled ventilation/oxygenation and allow the team to focus on the circulatory status, thus attending to two key factors responsible for adverse outcomes in traumatic brain injury: hypoxaemia and hypotension.

5 EXPOSURE WITH ENVIRONMENT CONTROL

Patients who have sustained a major injury should have all their clothing cut off without delay to allow adequate assessment of the entire body. Remember, however, that hypothermia kills trauma patients. Unless your resuscitation room has dedicated temperature-control capabilities, as soon as your examination and any required procedures have been performed the patient needs to be covered. A warming mattress and a Bair Hugger may also be needed to control the patient's temperature.

Investigations

While placing intravenous lines, **draw blood** for the following investigations. Note that not all will be necessary in every situation.

- Full blood count
- Electrolytes/urea/creatinine
- Glucose
- Liver function tests
- Lipase
- Coagulation studies including fibrinogen
- Group and hold/cross-match
- Blood alcohol level—including an appropriate sample for the police when required
- Beta-human chorionic gonadotrophin (hCG)
- Creatine kinase (CK) in crush injuries

The timing of **radiological studies** will vary depending on the urgency of the situation. In major trauma patients, however, the early performance of a trauma series (chest and pelvis X-rays) is appropriate and usually takes place as the team is performing the primary survey. The most logical order for the films is:

1 chest X-ray—as an adjunct to 'B' and 'C' assessment
2 pelvis—as an adjunct to 'C' assessment.

An E-FAST exam is performed at a similar time if available.

During the resuscitation phase, a **urinary catheter** should be passed to assess urine output. A urinary catheter is contraindicated if there is blood at the external meatus, blood in the scrotum or rectum or the prostate cannot be palpated or is high riding. In general, a urethrogram is indicated in these circumstances and an urgent urological opinion should be sought. A suprapubic bladder catheter is an option in the presence of significant urethral trauma, but should not delay resuscitative procedures.

An **orogastric tube** should be placed in all intubated patients and patients who have sustained significant abdominal trauma. This is to prevent gastric aspiration and the development of acute gastric dilation.

The **relief of discomfort** is an important component of trauma care, and analgesia should be provided in an appropriate form and amount depending on the clinical state of the patient. In most circumstances this will equate to the provision of an intravenous opioid delivered in small aliquots and titrated to effect while monitoring for adverse events. Ketamine and the use of local anaesthetic infiltration may be indicated in some cases.

Consider tetanus immunisation and prophylactic antibiotics as required.

The **ongoing resuscitation status** should be monitored by:

* respiratory rate and effort
* pulse oximetry
* capnography
* peripheral perfusion
* pulse rate/ECG rhythm
* blood pressure—with particular attention to pulse pressure
* GCS score
* blood gases—base deficit and lactate

- urine output
- temperature.

The development of hypothermia, acidosis and coagulopathy is an ominous sign and may herald irreversible shock.

Persistent haemodynamic instability should again raise the possibility of:

- continued blood loss
- tension pneumothorax
- cardiac tamponade
- other conditions (e.g. myocardial injury, spinal cord injury, etc.)
- equipment problems (e.g. blocked or displaced intercostal catheter, dislodged peripheral or central access resulting in extravasation of fluids, malfunction of ventilation equipment, and so on).

At this stage the trauma team leader should decide whether the patient should be transferred immediately to the operating suite for a resuscitative thoracotomy and/or laparotomy.

Management of life-threatening conditions

As previously stated, life-threatening conditions should be suspected and identified during the primary survey. The management of these conditions may be based in the ED or may require immediate transfer to the operating suite.

TENSION PNEUMOTHORAX

The critical initial step is to decompress the pleural space. Classic teaching is to insert a 12- or 14-gauge cannula into the 2nd intercostal space in the mid-clavicular line. Quoted success/failure rates have generated controversy, prompting recommendations to instead perform blunt thoracostomy via a lateral approach. The bottom line—regardless of method used—is to make sure you have *decompressed* the chest! This should be followed by an intercostal catheter in the 4th or 5th intercostal space just anterior to the mid-axillary line.

OPEN PNEUMOTHORAX

A large combine should be placed over the defect and secured in position with a transparent dressing (Opsite). At the same time, a large intercostal catheter needs to be inserted to treat the now 'closed' pneumothorax and to prevent the possible development of a tension pneumothorax.

MASSIVE HAEMOTHORAX

A large intercostal catheter (minimum 28 Fr) should be inserted into the 4th or 5th intercostal space just anterior to the mid-axillary line and directed posteriorly. An initial drainage of greater than 1500 mL should signal the team to consider early thoracotomy, especially in penetrating trauma.

All intercostal catheters should be connected to an underwater sealed drain and have low wall suction applied. A stat dose of prophylactic antibiotics (a first-generation cephalosporin for the non-allergic patient) should reduce the risk of an infective complication.

FLAIL SEGMENT

Flail segments frequently result in inadequate ventilation/oxygenation and are prone to the collection of air or blood in the pleural cavity. Associated pulmonary contusions are the major cause of morbidity and can result in progressive deterioration in respiratory function. Adequate drainage of the pleural cavities should be ensured by a large intercostal catheter; otherwise the management remains largely supportive with adequate analgesia via an appropriate route (including such options as a thoracic epidural) and assisted ventilation/oxygenation (ranging from non-invasive techniques such as bi-level positive airway pressure [BiPAP] to endotracheal intubation).

ONGOING BLOOD LOSS

These patients should be considered for early transfer to the operating suite for a resuscitative thoracotomy and/or laparotomy. If pelvic bleeding is suspected, the immediate application of a pelvic binder for pelvic stabilisation and early angiography should be considered.

CARDIAC TAMPONADE

The diagnosis should be suspected clinically and confirmed with FAST if possible. Management revolves around adequate resuscitation and performing a left anterolateral thoracotomy to release the fluid within the pericardial sac. This should be undertaken by the most experienced trauma team member.

Needle pericardiocentesis should only be considered in smaller hospitals if experienced staff are not available. Needle pericardiocentesis may be life-saving but rarely drains the pericardial sac adequately and is associated with significant complications.

PULSELESS ELECTRICAL ACTIVITY (PEA)

In the context of trauma, PEA is usually caused by exsanguination, tension pneumothorax, massive haemothorax or cardiac tamponade. PEA should be managed by immediate establishment of a patent airway and ventilation, bilateral thoracotomies or chest drains, the administration of at least 3 L of intravenous fluids (ideally blood) and consideration for an open thoracotomy and pericardial release. This is of special importance in penetrating chest injuries. Some centres are using endovascular aortic occlusion (REBOA), which has had both success and significant complications in experienced centres. In patients in advanced pregnancy, resuscitative hysterectomy may be helpful at this point.

Traumatic cardiorespiratory arrest may result from craniocervical trauma. A prompt response to CPR is expected in survivable cases, although respiratory support may need to be prolonged.

Cardiac compressions (external or open) are of limited efficacy in the hypovolaemic patient. Where an acute medical catastrophe is suspected to have led to the traumatic event, standard cardiopulmonary resuscitation should be considered.

History

A nominated member of the trauma team should obtain further information that will allow the acute event to be managed in the context of the patient's pre-morbid state. A simple way to cover most of the important areas is to use the AMPLE approach.

A Allergies

M Medications—particularly anticoagulants!

P Past history—particularly diseases that alter clotting ability; pregnancy

L Last food/fluid; last tetanus injection

E Event details

This history may not be available directly from the patient and other sources may need to be questioned (e.g. pre-hospital personnel, relatives, friends, the local doctor, old medical records). In the unconscious patient always remember to look for a medical alert bracelet or any pertinent information on the person or in a wallet/handbag.

Details of the **mechanism of injury** are vitally important. Conceptually, injury is the result of a transfer of energy to the body's tissues. The severity of injury is dependent on the amount and speed of energy transmission, the surface area over which the energy is applied and the elastic properties of the tissues to which the energy transfer is applied. In the Australian setting, the most common cause is blunt trauma; however, penetrating trauma is on the increase. Common causes of blunt trauma include:

- motor vehicle crashes
- pedestrian–motor vehicle accidents
- falls
- industrial accidents
- assaults.

Specific injuries may be predicted from the mechanism of injury.

INJURIES IN MOTOR VEHICLE CRASHES

- Frontal impact: cervical spine fracture, anterior flail chest, traumatic aortic disruption, pneumothorax, myocardial contusion, ruptured spleen or liver, posterior dislocation/ fracture of hip/knee.
- Lateral impact: cervical spine fracture, lateral flail chest, traumatic aortic disruption, pneumothorax, diaphragmatic injury, ruptured spleen or liver, renal injury, fractured pelvis.
- Rear impact: cervical spine injury.
- Ejection: increased risk for any injury.
- Rollover: increased risk for any injury.

Important information from pre-hospital personnel that provides some idea of the energy transfer involved includes details of the estimated speed, impact, damage to vehicle, entrapment, use of restraint devices, deployment of airbags, and so on. Nowadays, digital photos of the scene are an invaluable source of information.

INJURIES IN PEDESTRIAN–MOTOR VEHICLE ACCIDENTS

Remember the injury triad—impact with the bumper, impact with the bonnet and windscreen, and subsequent impact with the ground.

* Bumper: lower-limb fractures, fractured pelvis, torso injuries in children.
* Bonnet/windscreen: head injury, torso injuries.
* Ground: head injury, spinal injuries.

Again, pre-hospital information that gives some idea of the energy transfer involved is important.

INJURIES IN FALLS

* The predominant underlying mechanism of injury is deceleration.
* Important considerations include the height of the fall, the landing surface and the position of the patient on impact.
* Injuries include head, spine, torso, pelvis and multiple fractures (calcaneus, ankle, tibial plateau, hip and vertebral column).

The elderly and frail may sustain life-threatening trauma from low falls.

INJURIES IN INDUSTRIAL ACCIDENTS

* May be blunt or penetrating.
* Other mechanisms need to be considered: blast, thermal, chemical.
* Injuries will depend on the above mechanisms.

INJURIES IN ASSAULTS

* Unfortunately a common cause.
* May be blunt or penetrating.
* Determine the energy transfer: weapon, fists, stomping.
* Injuries will depend on the above mechanisms.
* Stabbings are low-energy injuries: severity determined by organs injured (e.g. major vascular injury versus muscle).
* Gunshot injuries vary in energy level: increased bullet velocity equals increased injuries secondary to cavitation.

Knowledge of the mechanism of injury provides 'advance warning' regarding possible injuries—it is a useful guide, but remember there are always exceptions.

Secondary survey

The secondary survey is a detailed systematic head-to-toe examination in order to detect all injuries and enable planning of definitive care. This should not commence until the primary assessment and management have stabilised the patient. During the secondary survey all components of the primary survey should be repeated and the team should be responsive to any new findings. Unless the patient has been transferred immediately to the operating suite, the secondary survey should be undertaken in the ED.

- **Head.** Assess the scalp for lacerations, contusions, fractures and burns. Examine the ears for haemotympanum and cerebrospinal fluid (CSF) leakage. Check the eyes for visual acuity, pupil symmetry and response to light, movements, lens injury; always check for the presence of contact lenses and remove them early.
- **Face.** Assess for lacerations, contusions, fractures and burns. Check cranial nerve function. Examine the mouth for bleeding, loose teeth and soft-tissue injuries.
- **Cervical spine and neck.** Assess for tenderness, bruising, swelling, deformity, subcutaneous emphysema and tracheal deviation. Beware of carotid dissection.
- **Chest.** Assess for evidence of rib fracture, subcutaneous emphysema, open wounds, haemothorax and pneumothorax. Check for evidence of myocardial injury, and perform a 12-lead ECG.
- **Abdomen.** Assess for bruising of the anterior abdominal wall, distension, tenderness and guarding, rebound, rectal and vaginal examinations.
- **Back.** All trauma patients need to undergo a log-roll with cervical spine immobilisation to examine the entire length of the spine, looking for tenderness, bruising or deformity. This should be done early so the patient can be removed from the spinal board, improving patient comfort and decreasing the risk of pressure injuries in patients with spinal cord injuries and altered sensation/awareness. A rectal examination should be done at this time.

• **Limbs.** All limbs need to be examined for fractures, lacerations, haematomas, peripheral pulses and neurological deficits. All fractures should be reduced and splinted and consideration given for intravenous antibiotics and tetanus prophylaxis.

Specific injuries
HEAD TRAUMA
(See also Chapter 27 Neurosurgical Emergencies.)

Traumatic brain injury is common. Unfortunately, despite this fact, there is limited good evidence in the literature upon which to base investigation and management decisions, particularly with regard to the patient with mild head injury. The NSW Health Institute of Trauma and Injury Management (ITIM) has published the adult trauma clinical practice guideline *Initial Management of Closed Head Injury in Adults* in an ongoing effort to fill this void and provide clinicians with evidence-based advice.

It is important to determine at an early stage whether your facility can provide the appropriate care necessary for the patient's severity of injury or whether urgent transfer to another hospital will provide the best possible care. There has been the re-release of the ITIM guidelines which advocates the use of the Abbreviated Westmead Post Traumatic Amnesia Screen (A-WPTAS). Recent studies have shown this to be an effective screening tool to identify a brain injury being present.

Classification systems abound and all have their limitations, but the following GCS-based system is a useful guide.

• Mild head injury: GCS 14–15
• Moderate head injury: GCS 9–13
• Severe head injury: GCS 3–8.

Editorial Comment

The management of concussion is complex and still evolving. There is increasing awareness, especially in sports injury and research using amnesia scales. Doctors need to keep up to date on recommendations as to when people can return to sports/contact sports/work after a concussive episode.

Mild head injury

Fortunately the majority of patients you deal with will have only a mild injury, usually characterised by an awake patient who may have a history of a brief loss of consciousness and some degree of amnesia about events surrounding the injury. Often the history of loss of consciousness is unclear and, despite information from bystanders and pre-hospital personnel, it can be difficult to determine the true details of the event.

In general, if there is a history of more than a brief loss of consciousness, persistent posttraumatic amnesia, significant headache or vomiting following the injury, then a CT scan of the head should be performed. If the CT scan is normal, subsequent deterioration is unlikely and the majority of patients can expect an uneventful recovery.

Importantly, all patients with mild head injury should be screened for posttraumatic amnesia with the abbreviated Westmead PTA Scale (see Figure 4.2). Persistent posttraumatic amnesia not only raises the suspicion for significant intracranial injury (prompting CT imaging if not already performed), but may also signal an increased risk for post-concussion symptoms, prompting appropriate referral.

Most patients with mild head injury may be discharged to the care of a responsible adult provided the home circumstances are adequate. Prior to discharge a discussion with the patient and carer regarding important symptoms and signs to look out for should take place—and this information should also be provided in written form by way of a head injury advice card.

Moderate head injury

Patients with this degree of head injury require more-aggressive management and further investigation. Remember to keep in mind the different needs of patients, depending on where they lie on the disease spectrum.

Early endotracheal intubation and controlled ventilation/oxygenation should be considered. Appropriately aggressive fluid resuscitation in the hypovolaemic patient is also vitally important. Having performed a primary and secondary survey and responded appropriately to the findings, the next priority is to determine

St Vincent's Hospital

MRN			SURNAME	
OTHER NAMES				
DOB	SEX	AMO	WARD/CLINIC	

ABBREVIATED WESTMEAD PTA SCALE (A-WPTAS)
GCS & PTA TESTING OF PATIENTS
WITH MTBI FOLLOWING MILD HEAD INJURY

(Please enter information or affix Patient Information Label)

USE OF A-WPTAS AND GCS FOR PATIENTS WITH MTBI
The A-WPTAS combined with a standardised GCS assessment is an objective measure of post traumatic amnesia (PTA). Only for patients with **current GCS of 13–15 (<24 hrs post injury)** with impact to the head resulting in confusion, disorientation, anterograde or retrograde amnesia, or brief LOC. **Administer both tests at hourly intervals** to gauge patient's capacity for full orientation and ability to retain new information. **NB:** *This is a screening device, so exercise clinical judgment. In cases where doubt exists, more thorough assessment may be necessary. If GCS deteriorates by >2 then cease A-WPTAS and commence neurological observations on emergency patient assessment sheet.*

ABBREVIATED WESTMEAD PTA SCALE (A-WPTAS) AND GLASGOW COMA SCALE (GCS)

ADMINISTRATION AND SCORING

1. ORIENTATION QUESTIONS

Question 1: WHAT IS YOUR NAME?

The patient must provide their full name.

Question 2: WHAT IS THE NAME OF THIS PLACE?

The patient has to be able to give the name of the hospital. For example: St Vincent's Hospital. (NB: The patient does not get any points for just saying 'hospital'.) If the patient can not name the hospital, give them a choice of 3 options. To do this, pick 2 other similar sized hospitals in your local area or neighbouring region. The three choices are 'Royal Prince Alfred, Royal North Shore or Prince of Wales'.

Question 3: WHY ARE YOU HERE?

The patient must know why they were brought into hospital, e.g. they were injured in a car accident, fell, assaulted or injured playing sport. If the patient does not know, give them three options, including the correct reason.

Question 4: WHAT MONTH ARE WE IN?

For emphasis the examiner can ask what month are we in now? The patient must name the month. For example, if the patient answers 'the 6th month', the examiner must ask the further question 'What is the 6th month called?'.

Question 5: WHAT YEAR ARE WE IN?

It is considered correct for patients to answer in the short form '08', instead of '2008'. Also, an acceptable alternative prompt (for the rest of the 2000's) is 'The year is 2000 and what?'

2. PICTURE RECOGNITION

Straight after administering the GCS (standardised questions), administer the A-WPTAS by presenting the 3 Westmead PTA cards. Picture Cards the first time—T1: Show patients the target set of picture cards for about 5 seconds and ensure that they can repeat the names of each card. Tell the patient to remember the pictures for the next testing in about one hour. Picture Cards at each subsequent time T2–T5: Ask patient, 'What were the three pictures that I showed you earlier?'.

SCORING

- For patients who free recall all 3 pictures correctly, assign a score of 1 per picture and add up the patient's GCS (out of 15) and A-WPTAS memory component to give the A-WPTAS score (total = 18). Present the 3 target pictures again and re-test in 1 hour.

- For patients who can not free recall, or only partially free recall, the 3 correct pictures, present the 9-object recognition chart. If patient can recognise any correctly, score 1 per correct item and record their GCS and A-WPTAS score (total = 18). Present the target set of pictures again and re-test in 1 hour.

- For patients who neither remember any pictures by free recall nor recognition, show the patient the target set of 3 picture cards again for re-test in 1 hour.

ADMISSION AND DISCHARGE CRITERIA
A patient is considered to be out of PTA when they score 18/18. Both the GCS and A-WPTAS should be used in conjunction with clinical judgment. Patients scoring 18/18 can be considered for discharge. For patients who do not obtain 18/18 re-assess after a further hour. Patients with persistent score <18/18 at 6 hours post time of injury should be considered for admission. If abnormal PTA was present or patient's pain score is greater than 4.5/10 on discharge please refer patient to the Friday mild brain injury rehabilitation clinic. Patients who reside in outer metropolitan or rural areas refer to their GP. Please provide patient with a head injury advice sheet.

Figure 4.2 Westmead Post-Traumatic Amnesia (PTA) Scale
Reproduced with permission from St Vincent's Hospital.

Continued

St Vincent's Hospital

ABBREVIATED WESTMEAD PTA SCALE (A-WPTAS)
GCS & PTA TESTING OF PATIENTS
WITH MTBI FOLLOWING MILD HEAD INJURY

MRN			SURNAME	
OTHER NAMES				
DOB	SEX	AMO	WARD/CLINIC	

(Please enter information or affix Patient Information Label)

Date: Time:		T1	T2	T3	T4	T5	T6	T7	T8	T9	T10	T11	T12
Motor	Obeys commands	6	6	6	6	6	6	6	6	6	6	6	6
	Localises	5	5	5	5	5	5	5	5	5	5	5	5
	Withdraws	4	4	4	4	4	4	4	4	4	4	4	4
	Abnormal flexion	3	3	3	3	3	3	3	3	3	3	3	3
	Extension	2	2	2	2	2	2	2	2	2	2	2	2
	None	1	1	1	1	1	1	1	1	1	1	1	1
Eye Opening	Spontaneously	4	4	4	4	4	4	4	4	4	4	4	4
	To speech	3	3	3	3	3	3	3	3	3	3	3	3
	To pain	2	2	2	2	2	2	2	2	2	2	2	2
	None	1	1	1	1	1	1	1	1	1	1	1	1
Verbal	Oriented ** (tick if correct)	5	5	5	5	5	5	5	5	5	5	5	5
	Name	☐	☐	☐	☐	☐	☐	☐	☐	☐	☐	☐	☐
	Place	☐	☐	☐	☐	☐	☐	☐	☐	☐	☐	☐	☐
	Why are you here	☐	☐	☐	☐	☐	☐	☐	☐	☐	☐	☐	☐
	Month	☐	☐	☐	☐	☐	☐	☐	☐	☐	☐	☐	☐
	Year	☐	☐	☐	☐	☐	☐	☐	☐	☐	☐	☐	☐
	Confused	4	4	4	4	4	4	4	4	4	4	4	4
	Inappropriate words	3	3	3	3	3	3	3	3	3	3	3	3
	Incomprehensible sounds	2	2	2	2	2	2	2	2	2	2	2	2
	None	1	1	1	1	1	1	1	1	1	1	1	1
GCS	Score out of 15	/15	/15	/15	/15	/15	/15	/15	/15	/15	/15	/15	/15
	Picture 1												
	Picture 2												
	Picture 3												
A-WPTAS	Score out of 18	/18	/18	/18	/18	/18	/18	/18	/18	/18	/18	/18	/18

** must have all 5 orientation questions correct to score 5 on verbal score for GCS, otherwise the score is 4 (or less).

Pain Score on Discharge
No pain = 0
Worst Pain Imaginable = 10
Patient Score _____

PUPIL ASSESSMENT	T1		T2		T3		T4		T5		T6		T7		T8		T9		T10		T11		T12	
	R	L	R	L	R	L	R	L	R	L	R	L	R	L	R	L	R	L	R	L	R	L	R	L
Size																								
Reaction																								

+	REACTS BRISKLY
SL	SLUGGISH
C	CLOSED
–	NIL

TARGET SET OF PICTURE CARDS

PUPIL SIZE

Figure 4.2, cont'd

whether a neurosurgically correctable lesion is present by proceeding to urgent CT scanning.

Further management will depend on the findings, with a number of patients requiring urgent transfer to the operating suite for evacuation of a haematoma. The majority of other patients will require admission for ongoing neurological observations.

Severe head injury

Patients with severe head injury are fortunately in the minority. However, when faced with such a patient a coordinated team approach with meticulous attention to the prevention of secondary brain injury is paramount. Early notification of the neurosurgical team is important. The ABCs must be appropriately and aggressively resuscitated. Key points in the management include the following.

1 Endotracheal intubation with controlled ventilation/ oxygenation. Prior to sedating and paralysing the patient, every attempt should be made to perform and document a limited neurological examination—the GCS and pupillary responses. It is important to note these findings in the context of the patient's blood pressure at the time because of its potential influence on cerebral perfusion/function. Also, remember it is the best motor response that is the more accurate predictor of outcome.

2 Mild hyperventilation to a pCO_2 of 30–35 mmHg in the patient showing signs of raised intracranial pressure from an expanding haematoma—as a 'stop gap' to make it to the operating suite. The patient's end-tidal CO_2 should be monitored closely, having confirmed the accuracy of the readings by performing a formal ABG measurement.

3 Fluid resuscitation with normal saline, Hartmann's or blood (no glucose-containing solutions) as required to maintain a mean arterial pressure of greater than 90 mmHg in the patient suspected of raised intracranial pressure.

4 Mannitol 0.5–1 g/kg given as an infusion over approximately 5 minutes in the patient showing signs of raised intracranial pressure from an expanding haematoma—as a 'stop gap' to make it to the operating suite; frusemide 20–40 mg IV may also be used, often in addition to mannitol.

5 Prophylactic anticonvulsants. At the discretion of the treating neurosurgeon—usually phenytoin 15 mg/kg administered intravenously at a rate no faster than 50 mg/min in adult patients.

6 Meticulous nursing care. Positioned head up 30°. Avoidance of constricting endotracheal ties, etc.

The management of the patient with head injury with intercurrent hypotension can be a real challenge. Therefore, it is important to keep a few key principles in mind:

1 head injury + hypotension = worse outcome
2 determine the cause of the hypotension
3 treat the cause of the hypotension

then

4 treat the head injury.

Neck injuries

The accurate assessment and management of neck injuries is important, not only because of the potentially devastating effects of cervical spine/spinal cord injuries, but also because of the life-threatening potential of injuries to other vital structures such as the airway/ larynx and vascular anatomy. A detailed search for swelling, expanding haematoma formation, subcutaneous emphysema, tracheal deviation, hoarseness, stridor and carotid bruits should be performed.

Key points in management include the following.

1 Ensure airway patency. Repeated examinations are essential and early intubation may be life-saving.
2 Blunt injury to vascular structures can be 'occult'. Maintain a high degree of suspicion and proceed to further investigation (e.g. ultrasound, angiography).
3 Beware of penetrating injuries. If the platysma is breached, the right place for the patient to be further examined and treated is in the operating suite with on-table angiography facilities.
4 Clear the cervical spine. Patients suffering blunt trauma who meet the following five criteria can be classified as having a low probability of cervical spine injury and can be cleared on clinical grounds. No radiological imaging is required if the patient has:
— normal alertness
— no intoxication
— no painful, distracting injury

— no midline cervical tenderness
— no focal neurological deficit.

An alternative guideline for clearing the cervical spine is the Canadian C-spine rule; see Figure 4.3.

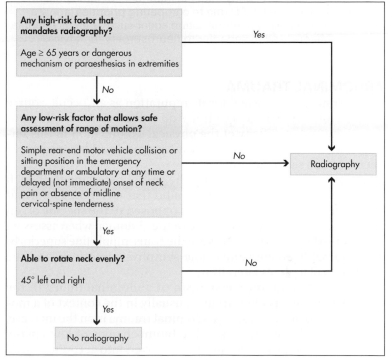

Figure 4.3 The Canadian C-spine rule. For patients with trauma who are alert (as indicated by a score of 15 on the GCS) and in a stable condition and in whom cervical spine injury is a concern, the determination of risk factors guides the use of cervical spine radiography. A dangerous mechanism is considered to be a fall from an elevation of ≥ 3 feet (1 metre) or five stairs; an axial load to the head (e.g. diving); a motor vehicle collision at high speed (> 100 km/h) or with rollover or ejection; a collision involving a motorised recreational vehicle; or a bicycle collision. A simple rear-end motor vehicle collision excludes being pushed into oncoming traffic, being hit by a bus or a large truck, a rollover and being hit by a high-speed vehicle.

Editorial Comment

Foam collars are increasingly used in the initial management of injured adults and children requiring cervical spine immobilisation being transported by ambulance and presenting to health facilities. If cervical bony injury is identified, or if the patient cannot be cleared in ED due to competing priorities, apply a locally agreed cervical immobilisation collar such as a Philadelphia or Miami J collar, and refer to neurosurgery for advice.

ABDOMINAL TRAUMA

The abdomen is renowned for its reputation as an 'occult' source of blood loss in the trauma victim. Add to this reputation the poor sensitivity and specificity of the physical examination in this setting, and it is not hard to see why investigation and management decisions can seem daunting.

As stated previously, during the initial assessment of such patients it is important to keep in mind that it is more important to determine the site of bleeding as opposed to the specific organ injured. Remember the full 'extent' of the abdomen when assessing a patient—the anterior borders are the trans-nipple line superiorly, the inguinal ligaments and pubic symphysis inferiorly and the anterior axillary lines laterally.

The most common mechanism of abdominal injury in the Australian setting is blunt trauma, usually in the context of a motor vehicle crash. Penetrating abdominal trauma is on the increase, though, and the differences in the biomechanics of low-energy versus high-energy injuries need to be taken into account.

However, regardless of the mechanism, the initial assessment and management need to follow the same principles of airway, breathing, cardiovascular, drug therapy (the ABCDs).

Blunt abdominal trauma

Key points in the management include the following.

1 Remember that the physical examination is **unreliable**.

2 By a process of elimination the abdomen/retroperitoneum can be diagnosed as the site of blood loss—if it is not external, long bones, chest or pelvis, the abdomen/retroperitoneum is the only site left.

3 If the patient is haemodynamically stable, a CT scan is an appropriate investigation to confirm your clinical suspicion (Table 4.3).

4 If the patient is haemodynamically unstable do not go to CT—go to the operating suite!

5 For the patient 'in between', a FAST examination or a diagnostic peritoneal lavage may be invaluable (Table 4.3).

6 Remember that a FAST examination can only *rule in* the presence of free fluid. If it is negative, all bets are off.

7 Be appropriately aggressive with resuscitation fluids—the **right amount** for the **right patient** at the **right temperature**.

8 **Stop the bleeding**—for some patients this will mean immediate transfer to the operating suite.

Table 4.3   Imaging in abdominal trauma

	Ultrasound	Diagnostic peritoneal lavage	Computed tomography
Indication	Document free fluid if decreased BP	Document bleeding if decreased BP	Document organ injury if BP normal
Advantages	Early diagnosis; performed at the bedside; non-invasive; repeatable; 86–97% accurate	Early diagnosis; performed at the bedside; 98% accurate	Most specific for injury; 92–98% accurate
Disadvantages	Operator dependent; bowel gas and subcutaneous air distortion; misses diaphragm, bowel and some pancreatic injuries	Invasive; misses injury to diaphragm and retroperitoneum	Cost and time; transfer to medical imaging department; misses diaphragm, bowel tract and some pancreatic injuries

Penetrating abdominal trauma

Advice regarding resuscitation and imaging is as for blunt trauma (see above). Other important points include the following.

- The entry wound can be a misleading predictor of the trajectory of penetration and potential underlying injury/ies—**do not** rely on it.
- Anterior abdominal stab wounds with hypotension, peritonitis or evisceration of omentum or small bowel require no further imaging or investigation—they need to go to the operating suite for a laparotomy.
- Local exploration of stab wounds under sterile conditions and local anaesthesia may be performed by the skilled surgeon in stable patients, searching for a breach in the anterior fascia. If a breach is present the patient is at increased risk of an intraperitoneal injury, and common practice in Australia is to proceed to laparoscopy.
- The value of repeated examinations should not be underestimated.

THORACIC TRAUMA

The majority of chest injuries can be managed in the ED with the use of supplemental oxygen, an appropriately placed intercostal catheter and the judicious use of analgesics via an appropriate route. Hence, it is important that doctors working in such an environment develop the skills to assess and manage these patients correctly.

Often when the patient first arrives, the examination and chest X-ray are performed in the supine position, and allowances must be made for this in terms of exam technique and film interpretation. For example, percussion should be performed in an anterior to posterior direction for detecting the presence of a haemothorax—and the chest X-ray will have a generalised increase in radiodensity on the affected side as compared to the usual meniscus on an erect film. Watch out for the patient with a widened mediastinum on chest X-ray suspicious for a contained rupture of the aorta—if you don't have cardiothoracic facilities, transfer the patient without delay so further investigation and treatment can take place at the right hospital.

Keep in mind the presence of common intercurrent diagnoses that may impact on a patient's ability to cope with their chest injury, such as chronic airflow limitation and asthma, not to mention smoking status.

Given the important structures within the chest, it is not surprising that patients can suffer a large number of possible life-threatening injuries, including those previously discussed under the primary survey, as well as the following.

- **Pulmonary contusion.** Commonly associated with many of the other injuries and is often the main cause of deteriorating lung function. Develops over hours to days. May require increasing supplemental oxygen, non-invasive ventilatory support or subsequent intubation/ventilation.

- **Haemothorax.** Drainage via an appropriately sized and placed intercostal catheter is important, as noted previously. Transfer to the operating theatre needs to be considered in any patient who drains more than 1500 mL immediately or continues to drain more than approximately 200 mL/h for 2–4 hours.

- **Simple pneumothorax.** There is some controversy as to how some of these injuries should be managed depending on such factors as the size of the pneumothorax, associated injuries, need for positive-pressure ventilation, need for transfer to another facility, and co-existent respiratory diseases; most would still advocate drainage via an appropriately sized intercostal catheter.

- **Blunt cardiac injury.** Suspect in the patient who remains haemodynamically unstable. There is no single clear diagnostic test—the ECG, cardiac markers and other imaging modalities such as echocardiography are all adjuncts to the clinical examination.

- **Traumatic aortic disruption.** Most patients die at the scene. If they survive to reach hospital, there is a window of opportunity to investigate and treat them at a facility with cardiothoracic capabilities. Signs to look for on the chest X-ray include a widened mediastinum, obliteration of the aortic knob, deviation of the trachea to the right, obscuration of the aortopulmonary window, depression of the left main stem bronchus, deviation of the oesophagus (nasogastric tube) to the right, widened paratracheal stripe, widened paraspinal interfaces, presence of a pleural or apical cap, left haemothorax or fractures of the first and second ribs or the scapula. Early surgical consultation is important.

- **Tracheobronchial tree disruption.** An unusual injury; patients usually die at the scene. Suspect if a large air leak persists after placement of an intercostal catheter for a pneumothorax. Early surgical consultation is important.
- **Traumatic diaphragmatic injury.** Often missed; interpret X-rays with care. Early surgical consultation is important.
- **Traumatic oesophageal disruption.** Rare; fatal if missed because of subsequent mediastinitis. Suspect if there is a left pneumothorax or haemothorax without a rib fracture, pain or shock out of proportion to the injury (usually a blow to the lower sternum or epigastrium) or if there is particulate matter in the intercostal catheter. Early surgical consultation is important.

However, having noted the above injuries, do not underestimate the significant morbidity and potential mortality associated with the most common of chest injuries—**rib fractures**! Important points in the management of this everyday problem include the following.

1. The ability of X-rays to detect rib fractures is poor—even if the films are read accurately!
2. If the patient has a good history and significant pain, rib fracture is probably the diagnosis.
3. The role of the chest X-ray is to help exclude complications such as a pneumothorax, haemothorax, pulmonary contusion, atelectasis, subsequent pneumonia.
4. It is clear from the above that 'rib views' are not necessary.
5. The presence of intercurrent disease may influence management decisions.
6. Adequate analgesia that allows deep breathing and coughing is paramount to the successful management of patients with the following injuries.
   — Start with simple oral therapy—paracetamol.
   — Add other oral options—NSAIDs/oxycodone, being alert for respiratory depression.
   — Use parenteral therapy—opioids, again being alert for respiratory depression.
   — The use of patient-controlled analgesia may be appropriate in many circumstances.

   — Consultation with the anaesthetic/pain management service with the view to other alternatives—intercostal blocks/epidural anaesthesia.

7 Paramedical services play an important role—physiotherapy.

8 Use non-invasive ventilatory support such as BiPAP early.

9 Closely monitor the patient's progress—respiratory rate and effort, pulse oximetry, ABGs.

10 Be prepared for the patient who, despite the above measures, continues to struggle—intubation with controlled ventilation/oxygenation may be necessary.

11 With few exceptions, elderly patients with fractured ribs require inpatient care.

PELVIC TRAUMA

Pelvic injuries can range in severity from simple pubic rami fractures to unstable injuries with associated life-threatening exsanguination. It is important to appreciate the magnitude of the force required to fracture the pelvis—and hence the high association with other potentially life-threatening injuries.

   Three common mechanisms of injury are:

1 anteroposterior compression (e.g. crushing injury)

2 lateral compression (e.g. motor vehicle crash)

3 vertical shear (e.g. fall from a height).

   Be suspicious of significant pelvic injury with the above mechanisms and perform a careful clinical examination, noting any lower-limb shortening or rotation (in the absence of a lower-limb fracture) and any pain or movement on palpation of the pelvic ring. Compression-distraction of the pelvic ring is controversial and at most should be performed *once* **with compression** *only* as part of this examination because of the risk of exacerbating any bleeding. The early performance of a pelvic X-ray as part of the trauma series will assist decision-making.

   Important points in the management of these injuries include the following.

1 Major pelvic disruption with haemorrhage should be suspected from the mechanism of injury (e.g. motorcycle crash, pedestrian–motor vehicle crash, fall from a height or a direct crushing injury).

2 Significant injuries are usually clinically apparent.

3 Be alert for and understand the potential for major blood loss—from the ends of fractured bones, from injured pelvic muscles and from the pelvic veins/arteries—and fluid-resuscitate the patient appropriately.

4 Simple measures to control bleeding in the ED include:
— bringing the lower limbs back out to length with traction
— internally rotating the lower limbs and strapping them together
— the application of a pelvic binder—this may be as simple as wrapping a sheet around the pelvis.

5 Early consultation with the angiography/orthopaedic teams is paramount.

Always remember the possibility of associated **urological injury**. Suspicious examination findings include blood at the external urethral meatus, scrotal or perineal bruising and an impalpable or high-riding prostate on rectal exam (all contraindications to catheterisation, as previously noted). In the multi-injured patient with a significant pelvic fracture, the bladder and/or urethra may be injured. In this setting the urethra is more commonly injured above the urogenital diaphragm. The patient is often in 'retention'. The usual approach to management includes the following.

1 Assess and treat for other life-threatening conditions.
2 Perform a urethrogram and treat accordingly.
3 Suprapubic catheterisation in selected patients.
4 Urological consultation.

MUSCULOSKELETAL TRAUMA

Musculoskeletal trauma is very common. Fortunately most injuries are neither limb- nor life-threatening, although they can on occasion look very dramatic. It is important not to be distracted by the injury and to manage all these patients in an orderly fashion with meticulous attention to the ABCs first. Some important points in the management of such injuries include the following.

1 Musculoskeletal injuries that are potentially life-threatening need to be recognised early and managed appropriately.
— **Major arterial haemorrhage.** These injuries may be as obvious as an avulsed limb or as subtle as the bleeding associated with a long-bone injury or major joint dislocation. Do not blindly clamp open injuries—use

direct pressure. Limb realignment and splinting are important measures that help reduce blood loss. Carefully assess the limb for the presence of distal pulses—absence equals arterial injury until proven otherwise. It is important to contact the surgical team early with a view to transfer to the operating suite for urgent exploration and/or angiography on the operating table.

— **Crush syndrome.** Be alert for this potential problem in any patient who has had a significant portion of a limb trapped for a period of time. The associated rhabdomyolysis and release of toxic by-products can lead to life-threatening hyperkalaemia, hypovolaemia, metabolic acidosis, hypocalcaemia and disseminated intravascular coagulation (DIC). Resuscitate the patient with large volumes of normal saline, aiming for a urine output of approximately 200 mL/h in an adult. Alkalinisation with sodium bicarbonate and the use of osmotic diuretics have also been advocated, although evidence is limited.

2 Most other injuries can be diagnosed and treated as part of the secondary survey.

3 Carefully examine the limb—skin integrity, colour, bruising, haematoma formation, neurovascular status, bony tenderness, function.

4 Be thorough—it is easy to overlook extremity injuries; therefore repeated examination is important.

5 Only proceed to imaging once the patient is stable and all life/limb threats have been addressed. Image the joints above and below the suspected fracture site.

6 Limb realignment and splinting reduces movement at the injury site, limits further bleeding and reduces pain. Always re-examine the neurovascular status of a limb if you have performed manipulation or applied a splint.

7 Early elevation of the injured limb reduces oedema formation.

8 Provide adequate analgesia, usually in the form of intravenous opioids titrated to effect.

9 Consider tetanus and antibiotic prophylaxis for open injuries.

10 Always be on the alert for complications—any site where muscle is contained within a closed fascial space has the potential to develop compartment syndrome.

Compartment syndrome

- This is a time-critical diagnosis—you have 4–6 hours at most to save the ischaemic contents of the compartment! It is potentially devastating if missed.
- Commonly occurs in the leg, forearm, foot, hand, gluteal region and thigh.
- Suspect the diagnosis in any patient who has pain greater than expected and that typically increases when the involved muscles are passively stretched—most of the other clinical signs are insensitive or develop late in the disease process.
- Warning—the distal pulse is usually present!
- Measure compartment pressures—greater than 35 mmHg in a normotensive patient is abnormal (lower pressures in the hypotensive patient may be significant). The trend in repeated measurements is generally more helpful than a one-off reading.

Treatment
1 Release any constricting bandages, casts, etc.
2 Urgent fasciotomy if no improvement.
3 Treat complications (e.g. rhabdomyolysis).

Definitive care

Definitive care in all trauma patients needs to be directed by the trauma surgeon or the team leader.

Definitive care involves:
1 specific investigations (e.g. CT scan of the head/chest)
2 consultation with specialty teams
3 documentation of all injuries and treatment
4 specific management plans from all appropriate teams
5 definitive placement to appropriate specialty team.

TERTIARY SURVEY

The tertiary survey is a complete review of the patient performed within the first 24 hours of their admission to hospital, aimed at detecting any further injuries or problems that may have been overlooked in the excitement of the initial resuscitation. It includes a further thorough head-to-toe clinical examination as well as a complete review of all investigations and treatments performed thus far.

Trauma service performance improvement

Care of the injured patient requires the services and skills of many different individuals. Trauma service performance improvement refers to the evaluation of the quality of care provided by a trauma service. Hospital-based performance improvement programs generally focus on the following aspects of healthcare.

- Safety: the extent to which risks and inadvertent harm are minimised.
- Effectiveness of care: does the treatment/intervention achieve the desired outcomes?
- Appropriateness: is the selected treatment/intervention likely to produce the desired outcome?
- Consumer participation: engaging consumers in planning and evaluating healthcare services.
- Efficiency: maximal total benefit is derived from the available treatments/resources.
- Access: the extent to which an individual or population can obtain healthcare services.

Performance improvement in trauma relies on the continual efforts of the multidisciplinary trauma team to measure, monitor, assess and improve both processes and outcomes of care. Trauma performance improvement programs are based on the following elements:

- a trauma registry/database to identify problems and the results of corrective actions
- multidisciplinary peer review of care, including morbidity and mortality analysis
- incident monitoring
- use of specific statistical methods for mortality analysis (e.g. Revised Trauma Score and Injury Severity Score [TRISS} and A Severity Characterisation of Trauma [ASCOT])
- classification of deaths and complications as preventable, potentially preventable, non-preventable
- clinical indicators to measure current practice against accepted benchmarks
- use of evidence-based clinical guidelines, protocols and pathways
- evidence of 'loop closure'—that is, evidence that the process/ outcome needing improvement is remeasured following corrective action and that improvement is demonstrated.

CLINICAL PRACTICE GUIDELINES AND PROTOCOLS

Clinical practice guidelines and protocols are outlines of accepted management approaches based on best available evidence and are designed to assist clinical decision-making. Clinical pathways are multidisciplinary plans of best clinical practice for specified groups of patients with a particular diagnosis that aid the coordination and delivery of high-quality care.

CLINICAL INDICATORS

Clinical indicators are measures of the process or outcomes of care. They are not designed to be exact standards, but rather act as 'flags' to alert clinicians to possible problems in the system or opportunities for improvement. For clinical indicators to be effective they must be relevant and clearly defined. Development of a set of clinical indicators is interactive. Indicators are reviewed on an ongoing basis with reference to the usefulness of the data and the resources required to collect it. Trauma service indicators are used to monitor process and outcomes of care from the pre-hospital phase through to rehabilitation and discharge. Close analysis of data is required, as there may be valid reasons why an event occurs differently from an expectation.

Examples of trauma service clinical indicators are:

- proportion of patients with a documented GCS < 9 who do not receive an endotracheal tube (ETT) within 10 minutes of documentation of that score
- proportion of head-injured patients with a documented GCS < 12 who do not have a CT scan of the head within 4 hours of arrival in the ED
- proportion of trauma patients transported to hospital by ambulance (not entrapped at the scene) who have a documented scene time of > 20 minutes.

OUTCOME MEASURES

Historically, trauma services have focused on the issue of preventable deaths as the main outcome measure. Outcome analysis in trauma is slowly expanding. Trauma services are now beginning to analyse other outcomes such as morbidity, functional impairment, quality of life and patient satisfaction. Comparison of outcomes across different sites relies on use of standardised, reliable outcome measures. Similarly, morbidity analysis requires tight definitions of problems, with rate comparisons potentially confounded by demographic differences between hospitals.

A large number of measures exist for outcomes analysis in trauma. These include:

• Glasgow Outcome Scale (GOS) for head-injured patients
• Disability Rating Scale (DRS)
• Short Form (SF)-36 survey
• sickness impact profile
• Hospital Anxiety and Depression Scale (HADS)
• functional independence measure (FIM).

Conclusion

The patient suffering multiple injuries is often a distressing sight and can at times seem like an overwhelming challenge to manage. By approaching care of such patients in a directed manner, prioritising the assessment and management of life-threatening injuries as outlined in this chapter, hopefully both you and your patients can look forward to the best outcomes possible. Appropriate and timely intervention is the key.

Online resources

American Trauma Society
www.amtrauma.org
Australasian Trauma Society
www.traumasociety.com.au
Brain Trauma Foundation
www.braintrauma.org
Eastern Association for the Surgery of Trauma
www.east.org
Liverpool Hospital Trauma Department
www.swslhd.health.nsw.gov.au/liverpool/Trauma/
National Trauma Research Institute
www.ntri.org.au
NSW Institute of Trauma and Injury Management (ITIM)
www.aci.health.nsw.gov.au/get-involved/
institute-of-trauma-and-injury-management
Youth and Road Trauma Forum at Westmead
www.bstreetsmart.org/index.php

Chapter 5
Shock

Stephen Macdonald and Steve Dunjey

Shock is a clinical condition, commonly encountered in practice, with multiple causes which share the final common pathway of inadequate tissue perfusion. The consequence of inadequate perfusion is that insufficient metabolic substrates (primarily oxygen) are provided to sustain cellular homeostasis. The challenge for the clinician is to manage the shock, and to simultaneously seek and treat the cause.

Timely recognition of this state of inadequate perfusion reduces mortality. However, haemodynamic abnormalities, particularly hypotension, are insensitive markers of early shock. Clinical assessment should also include assessment for tachypnoea and for signs of end-organ hypoperfusion such as altered mental status, poor skin perfusion and oliguria.

Causes and effects

Causes of shock are broadly grouped as follows:

- hypovolaemic (inadequate circulating volume; e.g. major haemorrhage)
- cardiogenic (inadequate cardiac output; e.g. myocardial infarction, ruptured papillary muscle)
- distributive (adequate volume, which is maldistributed; e.g. sepsis, anaphylaxis)
- obstructive (adequate volume, with impedance of flow; e.g. massive pulmonary embolus, cardiac tamponade).

A more complete list of causes is given in Table 5.1. A patient in shock will manifest signs of:

- the cause of the shock
- inadequate tissue perfusion, with end-organ dysfunction (e.g. confusion, agitation, acidosis, decreased urine output, reduced capillary return, and so on); see Box 5.1

Table 5.1 Types of shock, causes and signs

Type of shock	Causes	Signs
Hypovolaemic	Haemorrhage Vomiting/diarrhoea Dehydration Addisonian crisis	Obvious external blood loss/ signs of trauma/signs of concealed blood loss Skin turgor Dry mucous membranes ↓ JVP
Cardiogenic	Myocardial infarction (especially anterior, right ventricular) Myocardial contusion Acute valvular lesion Cardiomyopathies Arrhythmias	Extremes of pulse rate ↑ JVP ECG evidence of AMI, arrhythmias New murmurs
Distributive	Neurogenic/spinal cord injury Anaphylaxis Sepsis	Flaccid paralysis, warm peripheries, relative bradycardia, priapism Urticaria, angio-oedema, wheezes Febrile, warm peripheries, evidence of focus
Obstructive	Pulmonary embolism Cardiac tamponade Tension pneumothorax	Evidence of DVT, pulmonary hypertension, ↑ JVP Distant muffled heart sounds, pulsus paradoxus, electrical alternans Subcutaneous emphysema midline shift trachea, ↓ breath sounds

AMI = acute myocardial infarction; DVT = deep vein thrombosis; JVP = jugular venous pressure

- compensation; the sympathetic nervous system predominates, and is marked by tachycardia, peripheral vasoconstriction (sweaty, pale, cold peripheries with decreased capillary return), central vasoconstriction (narrowed pulse pressure) and decreased blood flow through non-vital structures, such as abdominal viscera (manifested by decreased urine output, decreased bowel sounds).

Box 5.1   Adverse effects of shock

- CNS: confusion, restlessness and decreased level of consciousness
- Myocardium: may impair myocardial function in severe shock
- Lung: hypoxia and sustained shock may induce adult respiratory distress syndrome in survivors
- Liver: elevation of hepatic transaminases and bilirubin
- Gastrointestinal tract: ischaemia, ileus, diarrhoea, stress ulceration and bacterial translocation into the systemic circulation
- Kidney: oliguria and renal failure
- Coagulopathy
- Other tissue damage: all tissues are impaired by sustained underperfusion, but the processes involved are difficult to quantify

---

Haemodynamic compensation can be so effective in young patients that the underlying shock state is manifest only by tachycardia, and more fully revealed by measuring postural BP drop (greater than 20 mmHg systolic). Younger patients are able to maintain an increased heart rate and cardiac output, but may suddenly deteriorate when they are unable to compensate further. Elderly patients may be incapable of mounting a tachycardic response to shock because of medications (especially beta-blockers) or underlying heart disease.

Overview of management

Shocked patients should be managed in a fully monitored area. The assessment and treatment of the shocked patient should occur in parallel. Initial treatment focuses on resuscitation, monitoring (to assess response to treatment) and seeking a specific cause (history, examination and investigations). Once the cause of shock has been determined, specific therapy should be considered. What follows is a description of initial management, then a description of specific therapies once the cause is known.

AIRWAY AND BREATHING

1 Ensure adequate airway.
2 Enhance oxygenation. All patients will benefit from supplemental oxygen: initially provide the highest level of inspired O_2 available.
3 Support ventilation if necessary.

CIRCULATION

1 Control accessible haemorrhage.
2 Gain intravenous access with a minimum of two large-bore peripheral IV lines.
3 Begin fluid replacement. The volume of fluid replacement required will depend to a great degree on the type of shock being treated. Hypovolaemic shock commonly requires large volumes of fluid replacement, whereas patients with cardiogenic shock may require very little, if any at all. It is reasonable to begin with 250–500 mL boluses of isotonic crystalloid fluid, and to review the response.
4 If the patient demonstrates ongoing signs of shock despite adequate volume replacement, the use of inotropic/vasopressor support should be considered.

MONITORING

Monitoring should include pulse rate, non-invasive blood pressure, urine output, temperature, pulse oximetry and ECG. If the blood pressure remains low, or the patient is perceived to be unstable, invasive arterial monitoring should be considered. Central venous access may be required for administration of drugs; however, central venous pressure (CVP) monitoring is of limited use for guiding haemodynamic resuscitation.

INVESTIGATIONS

The cause of shock should be sought, and investigations appropriate to make a diagnosis should be performed on the basis of the history and exam findings.

• Initial investigations should include blood tests (full blood count [FBC], electrolytes, group and hold or cross-match if blood loss is the likely cause, coagulation profile), ECG and CXR.
• Lactate testing is available in most EDs. The sources of lactate elevation in shock are complex and it may be produced aerobically due to adrenergic stimulation or by anaerobic metabolism in hypoperfused tissues. A lactate level above 2 mmol/L confers increased mortality risk. The measured level, however, reflects both production and removal from the circulation, so it is important to understand that a normal lactate does not exclude the diagnosis of shock.

- Bedside ultrasound is becoming an essential tool in the assessment of shocked patients in the ED. It is useful both in rapid evaluation of the cause of shock and in ongoing management (e.g. assessment of inferior vena cava [IVC] diameter and right ventricle [RV] filling give some indication of volume status). Bedside echocardiography by a suitably trained practitioner can identify features of tamponade, cardiac wall motion/valvular abnormalities, pulmonary embolism or a hyperdynamic left ventricle in sepsis. It is cheap, non-invasive and easy to repeat, and current literature supports the view that bedside ultrasound plays a crucial role.

Hypovolaemic shock

Hypovolaemic shock involves the loss of intravascular volume. Among the most common causes in patients presenting to the ED are blood loss (external, internal) and dehydration. The aims of management are to limit further fluid loss and replenish circulating intravascular volume.

External haemorrhage is best controlled with direct pressure on the bleeding source. In trauma, early stabilisation of possible major fractures (e.g. pelvic binder, splinting of femoral shaft fractures) limits further blood loss and is an essential component of haemorrhage control, as is application of a tourniquet if the bleeding source is from a limb injury.

Adequacy of fluid resuscitation can be judged by the response of measured cardiovascular parameters (pulse rate, blood pressure, CVP, urine output) and by a reduction in serum lactate, but no single measure provides a comprehensive marker of response. Current evidence supports the use of isotonic crystalloids over synthetic colloids. Balanced crystalloid solutions may be preferable to 0.9% saline for ongoing fluid resuscitation to avoid hyperchloraemic acidosis. Albumin should be avoided in trauma patients with brain injury, while in septic shock, despite a beneficial effect being postulated, it has not been proven to reduce mortality.

MANAGEMENT

1. Assess and treat airway, breathing and circulation (ABCs).
2. The initial fluid of choice is usually an isotonic crystalloid (normal saline/Hartmann's), which is best delivered as

250–500 mL aliquots rapidly infused (or 20 mL/kg aliquots for children).

3 Consider the early use of blood products if blood loss is the primary cause of shock. If necessary (e.g. in established shock, with ongoing loss of blood) transfuse O-negative blood until either group-specific or fully cross-matched blood is available. Excessive use of crystalloids results in haemodilution and worsens coagulopathy. Control of haemorrhage is the priority and resuscitation end points are dictated by the need for and timing of possible surgical interventions. Where ongoing resuscitation is indicated, packed red blood cell (RBC) transfusions should be matched by transfusion of fresh frozen plasma and platelets, when available. Tranexamic acid (1 g IV over 10 minutes followed by an infusion of 1 g over 8 hours) reduces mortality in major haemorrhage.

4 Large-bore peripheral lines are preferred. Intraosseous access is an important alternative route in the shocked patient, and should be attempted promptly if normal peripheral access is difficult or impossible. Central venous access is time consuming, and a standard central venous catheter is unsuitable for rapid infusion of fluids. Insertion of a large-bore vascular device (e.g. a pulmonary artery catheter sheath) by a skilled operator may be considered. Alternatively, peripherally inserted large-bore venous devices are available.

5 Surgically correctible sources of blood loss should be sought and haemorrhage arrested. Some sources of haemorrhage may be controlled medically (e.g. oesophageal varices with infusion of IV octreotide).

6 The endpoint of fluid therapy is still the subject of debate. Normal parameters may be detrimental in patients with some conditions which require surgical control of a bleeding source (examples include ruptured abdominal aneurysm, ectopic pregnancy and truncal stab wounds). Inadequate fluid resuscitation is, however, still a cause of preventable death, particularly in younger shocked patients, and the aim of therapy in most patients is return of near-normal blood pressure. A sustained low pressure in bleeding patients is known to produce the triad of hypothermia, acidosis and

coagulopathy. Hypotension is also particularly detrimental in the setting of brain injury.

7 Ongoing blood loss may produce coagulopathy, requiring treatment with appropriate doses of cryoprecipitate, fresh frozen plasma, platelets and so on. New technologies such as rotational thromboelastometry (ROTEM) can guide factor replacement. Specialist haematological input is usually required where there is an ongoing need for blood products.

Cardiogenic shock

Cardiogenic shock results from cardiac dysfunction with de-creased cardiac output. With increasing ventricular dysfunction, florid pulmonary oedema may develop. There are often prominent clinical signs of right ventricular failure, such as jugular venous distension.

The most common initiating event for cardiogenic shock is acute ischaemic damage to the myocardium. Once more than 40% of the myocardium is affected, ejection fraction falls and cardio-genic shock results from the reduced cardiac output. Ischaemia can also trigger cardiogenic shock by producing papillary muscle dysfunction, septal defects, free-wall rupture or right ventricular infarction. Traditionally, tachy- and bradyarrhythmias are listed separately although both can cause shock.

Cardiogenic shock is a highly lethal condition with a mortality rate in excess of 80% if a non-invasive, supportive approach is used. Preventing cardiogenic shock from developing is the most effec-tive therapy, and every effort should be made to limit infarct size in patients with acute myocardial infarction (AMI). It seems clear that percutaneous transluminal coronary angioplasty (PTCA) or emergency coronary artery bypass is more effective than throm-bolytic therapy.

MANAGEMENT

1 Assess and treat ABCs.
2 Maintaining an adequate blood pressure can be difficult, particularly because the volumes of fluid used in normal resuscitation can have an adverse effect, causing further dilation of the compromised ventricle. The patient's condition does not always allow time for institution of sophisticated

monitoring (e.g. pulmonary artery catheter) and may force the clinician to administer empirical therapy. If the patient is already in pulmonary oedema, a fluid bolus should be avoided, but for other patients it is acceptable to try incremental small boluses of crystalloid as a first step (100–250 mL).

3 If there is no response to a fluid challenge, a vasopressor is required. Commonly used agents include dobutamine and dopamine.

4 Afterload reduction leads to improved cardiac function, but further reduction in blood pressure may compromise the function of other vital organs. Afterload reduction is therefore something to institute with caution to prevent exacerbation of hypotension.

5 Specific therapy includes aspirin, control of arrhythmias and reperfusion of the infarcted area.

6 Consider the use of intra-aortic balloon pump for patients who remain haemodynamically unstable.

Distributive shock

A number of pathological conditions cause distributive shock, the hallmarks of which are maldistribution of intravascular fluid through microvascular leak and/or vasodilation.

SEPTIC SHOCK

(See also Severe Sepsis in Chapter 23 Infectious Diseases.)

Septic shock results from a host response to infection with triggering of the innate immunological response. While the microbiological products are themselves harmful (e.g. endotoxin), a widespread and unregulated host response mediated by cytokines and chemokines and involving activation of leucocytes, complement and coagulation cascades, and neuroendocrine system which leads to widespread systemic inflammation and organ dysfunction/failure in the host.

Septic shock occurs in approximately 50% of those with gram-negative bacteraemia, and in about 20% of those with *Staphylococcus aureus* bacteraemia. The gram-negative organisms most often implicated are *Escherichia coli*, *Klebsiella*, *Pseudomonas*, *Enterobacter* and *Proteus* species.

Septic shock is marked clinically by signs of infection (although this may not be obvious in the immunocompromised or those at extremes of age) and vasodilation (classically warm peripheries despite hypotension). However, myocardial dysfunction can add to the instability caused by microvascular leak and vasodilation, and the patient may present with features of vasoconstriction (cool peripheries, skin mottling).

MANAGEMENT

1 Assess and treat ABCs. If intubation is required, the patient's haemodynamic status needs to be considered in terms of the precise timing and agents used. 'Lung protective' ventilation strategies should be employed (e.g. 5–7 mL/kg tidal volume initially).

2 Conventionally large volumes of IV fluid have been used to restore circulating volume and optimise stroke volume. The Surviving Sepsis Campaign recommends at least 30 mL/kg of IV fluid be administered in the first 3 hours in the patient with sepsis and hypoperfusion. Substantial reductions in sepsis mortality over the past two decades have coincided with the introduction of protocolised resuscitation in sepsis, including fluid boluses. However, emerging observational data show an association between fluid overload and increased mortality in sepsis, while randomised trial data from resource-poor settings in Africa have led to a reappraisal of the use of fluids. While the subject of ongoing clinical trials, a practical approach is to use 500–1000 mL fluid boluses judiciously titrated to clinically relevant endpoints, and not to delay commencing vasopressors by futile repeated attempts to improve perfusion with fluids where a sustained response cannot be achieved.

3 In addition to fluids, inotropes are likely to be necessary, and should be chosen to address the twin problems of decreased systemic vascular resistance and decreased myocardial function. Noradrenaline is an appropriate initial agent.

4 Invasive monitoring is usually required, including an arterial blood pressure monitor and central pressure monitoring. Recommended targets include:
   • central venous pressure (CVP) 8–12 mmHg
   • mean arterial pressure (MAP) > 65 mmHg
   • urine output > 0.5 mL/kg/h.

Central venous oxygen saturation monitoring and aggressive blood transfusion protocols are no longer recommended. Adjunctive haemodynamic support such as dobutamine, vasopressin and so on are guided by cardiac output monitoring in the ICU.

5 The source of sepsis should be aggressively and rapidly sought. It is appropriate to administer empirical antibiotic therapy unless a focus can be established. Other treatments may include surgical drainage, debridement or laparotomy.

6 Routine use of corticosteroids remains controversial in septic shock, and at the time of writing the results of a large multicentre clinical trial are awaited. However it is important to administer corticosteroids to those patients with shock who are likely to have adrenal insufficiency such as patients on long-term steroid therapy.

Anaphylactic shock
(See also anaphylaxis flow chart, Figure 5.1.)

Anaphylactic shock results from the release of chemical mediators from mast cells and basophils. These chemicals (including histamine, leukotrienes, tumour necrosis factor [TNF], various cytokines, etc.) cause vasodilation and capillary leakage, and subsequently hypotension. In addition, they can cause life-threatening compromise of the upper airway (angio-oedema) and ventilation (bronchospasm).

Clinically the syndrome is marked by a recent exposure to an allergen, the presence of urticaria/angio-oedema (90% of patients), bronchospasm, rhinitis, conjunctivitis and gastrointestinal cramping.

MANAGEMENT
1 Place the patient in the supine position (or left lateral position for vomiting patients).

2 Give IM adrenaline 1:1000, at a dose of 0.01 mg/kg bodyweight to a maximum dose of 0.5 mg (0.5 mL), injected into the lateral thigh. If no improvement after 5 minutes this may be repeated.

3 All patients will benefit from supplemental oxygen and IV fluids. Use normal saline.

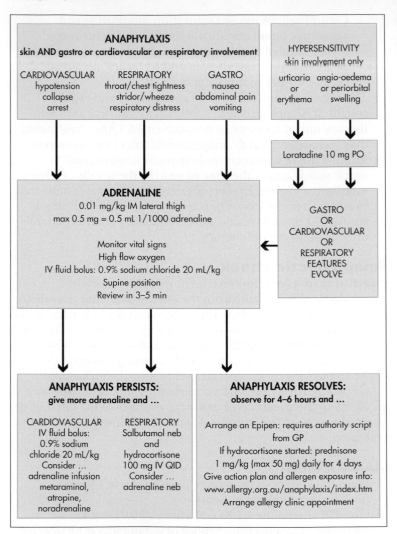

Figure 5.1 Allergic reactions: three-step management
Adapted from Amar SM, Dreskin SC. Urticaria. Prim Care Clin Office Pract 2008;35:141–57.

4 Support airway and ventilation. Be ready to deal with rapid progressive loss of airway. Be ready for resistant bronchospasm.

5 Remove the offending agent if possible.

6 Re-examine the patient frequently to assess progress. If resuscitation with IM adrenaline and IV normal saline is not effective, an infusion of IV adrenaline may be required: 1 mg of adrenaline added to 100 mL of normal saline can be run at 30–100 mL/h (5–15 microg/min) via a secure peripheral venous cannula.

7 Medications such as corticosteroids, antihistamines (H_1 and H_2) and antileukotrienes have no proven impact on the dangerous effects of anaphylaxis. They may have some benefit in treating mild allergic reactions involving skin. Promethazine can make vasodilation and hypotension worse.

Neurogenic shock

Neurogenic shock occurs when sympathetic tone is lost following spinal cord transection above the T6 level (T4–T8). Loss of sympathetic tone causes peripheral vasodilation and is classically associated with bradycardia.

MANAGEMENT

1 Assess and treat ABCs. If the level of injury is high enough (e.g. high cervical), there may be compromised ventilatory effort.

2 Engage in a thorough search for other causes of hypotension. Blood loss should be sought and confidently excluded before hypotension is attributed to neurogenic causes alone.

3 If neurogenic shock does need to be treated, it is relatively unresponsive to fluid resuscitation, and overhydration is to be discouraged. Patients may require treatment with inotropic/vasopressor agents to effectively raise blood pressure.

Obstructive shock

Obstructive shock is hypotension due to impeded venous return. Circulatory volume is normal, but blood flow through the heart is compromised.

Specific clinical signs are of impeded venous return (distended neck veins) and also of the cause.

Pericardial tamponade

Pericardial tamponade occurs when fluid accumulates in the pericardial space, compressing the heart and eventually impairing cardiac filling. Classically, patients manifest Beck's triad (hypotension, elevated JVP and muffled heart sounds), and may have marked pulsus paradoxus. However, clinical features can be unreliable and the diagnosis needs to be considered and actively excluded in shocked patients with risk factors (e.g. penetrating thoracic trauma, uraemia, malignancy). Clinical deterioration can be rapid. ECG may show electrical alternans, and the diagnosis can be established definitively with echocardiography.

MANAGEMENT

1 Assess and treat ABCs.
2 All patients benefit from IV fluids and oxygen.
3 Specific therapy is emergent pericardiocentesis (which ideally should be done with echo and ECG guidance) or open thoracotomy in the setting of acute trauma.
4 Other specific therapies depend on the cause of the effusion.

Tension pneumothorax

Obstructive shock results from a tension pneumothorax when raised intrathoracic pressure induces collapse of cardiac chambers and subsequent impaired cardiac filling. Specific signs include respiratory distress, with shift of the trachea from the midline and a hyperresonant, quiet chest on the side of the pneumothorax. The diagnosis is clinical and should be considered particularly in the settings of trauma, severe asthma or if the patient is receiving positive pressure ventilation. Treatment should not be delayed for a confirmatory chest X-ray.

MANAGEMENT

1 Assess and treat ABCs.
2 Specific therapy is to drain the pneumothorax, initially by finger thoracostomies, immediately followed by a formal intercostal catheter. Needle thoracostomy is often ineffective

and has been supplanted by finger thoracostomy in many health services.

3 Sucking chest wounds can cause a tension pneumothorax and should be covered with a non-permeable dressing stuck down on three sides, in addition to draining the pneumothorax.

4 A pneumothorax that resists drainage and continues to bubble vigorously may represent an injury to a major airway. Cardiothoracic help should be sought.

Pulmonary embolism

Massive pulmonary embolism can cause obstructive shock (see Chapter 16 Venous Thromboembolic Disease: Deep Venous Thrombosis and Pulmonary Embolism).

Summary

There are many causes of shock, but the initial general approach is always the same. Secure an airway, supplement ventilation if necessary, provide oxygen and resuscitate with IV fluids (except for cardiogenic shock). The cause of the shock should be sought, and specifically treated as appropriate.

Recommended readings

Harris D, Davenport R, Mak M et al. The Evolving Science of Trauma Resuscitation. Emerg Med Clin N Am 36 (2018) 85–106.

Loflen R, Winters ME Fluid Resuscitation in Severe Sepsis Emerg Med Clin N Am 35 (2017) 59–74.

Surviving Sepsis Campaign: International guidelines for Management of Sepsis and Septic Shock: 2016 Crit Care Med March (2017) 45:3.

Vincent JL, De Backer D. Circulatory Shock NEJM (2013) 369:18 Oct 31.

Chapter 6
Major haemorrhage
Marian Lee

'A 65-year-old man vomiting large amounts of bright blood. On warfarin for AF. GCS 15, SBP 60 and 80 after a litre of saline. ETA 3 mins.'

Haemorrhage refers to life-threatening bleeding, either evident or potential. The focus is to support the circulation and prevent multi-organ failure until source control is achieved. Strategies to support haemostasis are temporising measures while source control is definitive treatment that is context specific. Even so, they are crucial to the patient's outcome and need to be initiated from the outset. A good understanding of the principles behind the current practice of haemostatic resuscitation and permissive hypotension in the management of haemorrhage is indispensable to prioritisation and decision-making 'on the floor'.

Response to haemorrhage
HAEMODYNAMIC RESPONSE
The immediate loss of blood volume registers a fall in arterial pressure, triggering the baroreceptors to increase the sympathetic outflow. Tachycardia with vasoconstriction in the splanchnic and peripheral circulation follows. The outcome is preservation of the cerebral and coronary circulations. Hypotension may not be evident in the young healthy adult. This compensates for up to 15% of blood loss.

Beyond 15% blood loss, there is a further but limited rise in the heart rate and systemic vascular resistance. Hypotension is usually evident. At about 30–35% of blood loss, the sympathetic response is at its maximal. At haemorrhage greater than 40%, irreversible shock implying inevitable multiple organ failure is present.

RESTORATION OF BLOOD VOLUME

Apart from the haemodynamic response, transcapillary refill of the blood volume occurs. This mechanism refers to the movement of interstitial fluid into the capillaries. Normally, there is no net movement between these two extracellular fluid (ECF) compartments due to balanced hydrostatic and oncotic pressures (Starling forces). When intravascular volume loss occurs, vasoconstriction reduces the hydrostatic pressure driving fluid out of the capillaries, with no change in the capillary oncotic pressure. The result is movement of interstitial fluid into the capillaries until the Starling forces return to a new equilibrium. This mechanism is able to replace up to 75% of the plasma volume within 30 minutes.

Other compensatory mechanisms also promote a restoration of the volume and content of the haemorrhage. Activation of the renin-angiotensin-aldosterone system results in Na and water retention to replace the lost ECF compartment. The bone marrow releases reticulocytes and initiates haemopoiesis. Hepatic synthesis of albumin and coagulation factors occurs.

Clinical assessment

The clinical assessment is undertaken concurrently with the resuscitation. Information that is immediately relevant and essential are those that can provide a likely source of the haemorrhage, the estimated volume and the medications and co-morbidities that may impact on the management. A thorough examination is crucial in providing further data and must be done during the busy resuscitation process.

VOLUME

The volume is estimated from the history and evidence that might be available such as soaked clothing. The estimated amount may be compared with clinical findings to render more accuracy. In general, normal mental status, tachycardia and a blood pressure within the normal range are maintained up to 10–15% of haemorrhage in a young adult. Decompensation with altered mental status, hypotension with or without relative bradycardia occurs beyond a loss of 40%. The rise in respiratory rate and cool pale peripheries are less useful in volume estimation.

SOURCE
The source is often evident from the symptoms or signs. Bedside ultrasound is useful for identifying covert sources of haemorrhage.

MEDICATIONS
The medication list should be perused for drugs that impair haemostasis: anticoagulants and antiplatelet agents. Cardiac medications are important to note as they may impair the haemodynamic response to the haemorrhage.

Editorial Comment

Local pressure and/or tourniquet application is an essential early step in first aid and basic life support.

Management of haemorrhage
In the structured approach to haemorrhage, the priorities in resuscitation remain the same. The stabilisation of the airway and ventilation must take precedence over the circulation. However, shock will need to be accounted for in the interventions required to stabilise the airway and ventilation. The following will focus on the management of the circulation.

HAEMOSTATIC RESUSCITATION
Haemostatic resuscitation is directed primarily at optimising and promoting haemostasis. The aim is to prevent coagulopathy as a result of ongoing haemorrhage or due to treatment rendered. Apart from stopping the bleeding at the source, factors leading to coagulopathy are specifically targeted.

Causes of coagulopathy
There are three major factors that contribute to coagulopathy in haemorrhage. These are commonly present during the resuscitation.

1. Dilution of coagulation factors
Transcapillary refill of the intravascular compartment occurs shortly after blood loss. Giving crystalloids will further dilute the coagulation factors, compound the dilutional anaemia and cause

interstitial oedema from the proportional distribution of the fluid across the ECF compartment. Generalised oedema or pulmonary oedema are seen commonly in patients post-resuscitation.

2. Hypothermia

Large volumes of infused fluid at room temperature and exposure of the patient contribute to a fall in body temperature. Clotting activity falls with hypothermia, and at 33°C the activity is 50% of normal. Platelets are inactivated at low body temperatures and splenic sequestration may occur.

3. Acidosis

Acidosis is commonly from lactate production. Sources of lactate are multiple: anaerobic metabolism, endogenous and exogenous catecholamines and the use of normal saline.

Acidosis, coagulation factors and platelets

Acidosis impairs the coagulation factors, either directly or indirectly through the availability of ionised Ca. Thrombin production is impaired by acidosis with 50% of production occurring at a pH of 7.1.

Platelets do not tolerate acidosis. Below a pH of 7.4, they become spherical and lose their pseudopodia function.

Acidosis and the circulation

Acidosis causes a decrease in arterial vasomotor tone together with a reduced cardiac output. Pulmonary vasoconstriction is present. These adversities are compounded by the high risk of arrhythmia in the acidotic state. Additionally, acidosis reduces the response to endogenous and exogenous catecholamines.

Preventing coagulopathy: balanced transfusion of blood products

The early restoration of blood-like fluid in resuscitation in haemorrhagic shock prevents coagulopathy. Hence, crystalloids are kept to a minimum. A transfusion ratio of red blood cells, platelets and plasma of 1:1:1 is considered the optimal ratio. There is no universal consensus for this ratio but it is generally accepted to be beneficial.

Massive transfusion of blood products

A massive transfusion protocol (MTP) refers to the transfusion of a balanced solution of red blood cells, platelets and plasma. It is initiated when massive blood loss has occurred, defined as > 150 mL/min OR 50% of blood volume (approximately 2000 mL in a 70 kg patient) in 4 hours or an entire blood volume in 24 hours; alternatively, in a haemodynamically unstable patient, when a transfusion of > 4 units of packed red blood cell (PRBC) is anticipated.

The protocol has local adaptations. The commonality lies in the rapid and streamline response that accompanies its initiation AND the required monitoring of the outcome to defined endpoints. Initiation of the MTP occurs when the indication is met. The blood bank is notified and a standard pack composed of PRBC, platelets and fresh frozen plasma (FFP) are released. In general, the quantities are 4 units of PRBC, 4 units of FFP and 1 standard adult dose platelet. If a second box is required, the FFP may be replaced by cryoprecipitate if the fibrinogen level is < 1 g/L. Monitoring is required at intervals of 30–60-minutes. The titration points are as follows.

- FBC: Hb >70 g/L, platelet > 50×10^9/L (> 100×10^9/L for CNS injury)
- Coagulation profile: APTT/PT < 1.5 × normal, INR < 1.5
- Fibrinogen > 1 g/L

Tranexamic acid

Tranexamic acid is an antifibrinolytic agent. It acts by inactivating plasmin; hence, it cannot bind to fibrin and cause its degradation. It is used in trauma patients with haemorrhage as it has been shown to reduce mortality by 30% when used within 3 hours. In critically ill patients with upper gastrointestinal tract (GIT) haemorrhage in the ED, tranexamic use should be considered. Use in other causes of haemorrhage needs to be considered on a case-by-case basis. However, it is an old drug and is considered generally safe. It is given as a bolus dose of 1 g IV over 10 minutes and followed by 1 g over 8 hours.

PERMISSIVE HYPOTENSION

This is the delayed restoration of blood pressure to its normal range in haemorrhagic shock. The rationale is that a slowed flow would reduce the volume loss and facilitate thrombi formation at the sites of bleeding. The target is a mean arterial pressure (MAP) of 50 mmHg as this is thought to be the balance point between further blood loss and maintaining adequate organ perfusion pressure. It is generally accepted as beneficial in penetrating trauma but its application to other contexts has not been proven. It does make sense but there are situations where its use needs to be cautious. In particular, the MAP of 50 mmHg is too low for the elderly patient and those with associated traumatic brain injury.

ANTICOAGULANTS

Warfarin and direct-acting anticoagulants are both commonly encountered in clinical practice. Hence, their presence is to be expected. (See Table 6.1.)

Table 6.1 Anticoagulant actions and reversal

	Action	Characteristics	Half-life	Treatment in haemorrhage
Coumarin: warfarin	Acts on vitamin K and leads to reduced synthesis of vitamin K dependent coagulation factors II, VII, IX, X	Highly protein bound Hepatic metabolism Renal and faecal elimination Cannot be dialysed	40 hours	Vitamin K 5–10 mg IV Prothrombinex-VF at 50 units/kg IV If above is not available: FFP 15 mL/kg IV
Xarelto: rivaroxaban	Xa inhibitor	Protein bound Hepatic and renal metabolism	6–9 hours	Prothrombinex-VF use is not evidence based Refer to haematologist
Xaban: apixaban	Xa inhibitor	Protein bound. Hepatic and renal metabolism	12 hours	Prothrombinex-VF use is not evidence based Refer to haematologist

Continued

Table 6.1 Anticoagulant actions and reversal (cont.)

	Action	Characteristics	Half-life	Treatment in haemorrhage
Dabigatran	Direct thrombin inhibitor	Can be haemodialysed	12–15 hours	Idarucizumab: a monoclonal antibody fragment that binds to dabigatran 2.5 gram vials 2 vials IV over 5–10 mins No dose adjustment for renal impairment

Putting it together

A sequenced approach demonstrates the priorities required in the management of haemorrhage shock. The patient outcome is time critical and reliant on a well-rehearsed approach.

* Initial assessment and stabilisation of the airway and breathing must take into account the impact of the impending or evident circulatory collapse.
* Focused assessment needs to be directed towards the magnitude of the estimated blood loss, the likely cause AND significant co-morbidities including medications.
* Stop the bleeding: specific treatment of the source of bleeding. This is the definitive treatment.
* Begin haemostatic resuscitation.
  — Start blood products: initiate a massive transfusion protocol if indications are present, noting that the indications are inclusive of anticipated blood loss.
  — Minimise crystalloid use in the interim: use O negative PRBC if there is delay in the above or criteria not met.
  — Consider the use of tranexamic acid.
* Maintain body temperature within the normal range.
  — Warm the patient or prevent hypothermia.
* Invoke permissive hypotension in penetrating trauma and consider its use in other contexts.

- Monitor and adjust management to these endpoints.
  - Cause of haemorrhage has been rectified
  - Haemodynamic status: SBP 80–90 with MAP 50
  - Temperature $> 35°C$
  - pH > 7.3
  - Hb > 70 g/L, platelet $> 50 \times 10^9$/L
  - INR < 1.5; APTT < 40; fibrinogen > 1 g/L
  - Ionised Ca > 1.10 mmol/L

Summary

Haemorrhage is potentially life- or limb-threatening and needs to be viewed as such in the ED. Hence, a structured, prioritised team approach is mandated. The clear focuses in all aspects of the management are to: 1. source control; and 2. support the circulation until the source is controlled. The ultimate aim is to prevent multi-organ failure from irreversible shock.

- See also Chapter 5 Shock.
- See also Code Crimson in Chapter 4 Trauma.

Chapter 7
Burns

Ania Smialkowski

Overview

Burn injuries are common presentations to the ED. Most injuries occur around the household from accidental scald burns due to hot water or oil to contact thermal burns, particularly in the paediatric population. Other causes of burns include flash flame and explosions, particularly on work sites. Regardless of the cause of the burn, basic principles of first aid and burn management should be applied to decrease the zone of injury.

This chapter covers:
1 basic burn first aid
2 assessment of burn depth and injury
3 management of minor burns
4 emergency management of the severe burn
5 burn retrieval and referral guidelines.

Basic burn first aid

Appropriate basic first aid is effective within 3 hours of the burn injury. Effective first aid can reduce the zone of burn injury and result in a smaller, shallower burn.

1 Stop the burning (usually at the scene)
— Stop, drop, cover and roll
— Remove clothing
— If electrical burn, turn off power and remove patient from electrical circuit
— If chemical burn, irrigate with copious water
2 Cool the burn
— Use 20 minutes of continuous cool, clean water as soon as possible after the injury (effective up to 3 hours post)

— Any fluid between 8 and 25°C is acceptable; ideal temperature is 15°C

— Avoid hypothermia and do not use ice/iced water

Editorial Comment

Remember: a good history and examination of the whole patient analgesia tetanus status. Think of associated injuries: was it a faint, collapse, fit was it associated with drugs, alcohol, mental health issues, dementia, non-accidental injury.

Assessment of burn depth and injury

1 Burn depth assessment (Table 7.1)
  a Epidermal burn
    ○ Red, painful, dry, skin intact
    ○ Mild erythema not included in %TBSA
  b Superficial dermal burn
    ○ Blister, Redness, Moist, Painful, Oedema
    ○ Brisk capillary return
  c Mid–deep dermal burn
    ○ Sluggish capillary return to severely delayed or absent
    ○ Less painful or dull sensation
    ○ Dark pink to blotchy red or white
  d Full-thickness burn
    ○ No sensation
    ○ No capillary return
    ○ Leathery white/ black or yellow

Table 7.1 Burn depth

Depth	Partial thickness		Full thickness
	Superficial	Deep	
Colour	Pink	Pale	White
Blisters	Late	Early	–
Circulation	Present	±	Absent
Sensation	Painful	Decreased	Insensate
Healing	< 2–3 weeks	> 3 weeks	No

2 Electrical burns
   — Direct injury:
      ○ Low voltage < 1000 V
         • Localised to area of contact; no deep tissue damage
         • Can cause muscle spasm/tetany/immediate cardiac arrest
      ○ High voltage > 1000 V
         • Flashover burns or full-thickness entry/exit wounds and deep tissue damage
      ○ Lightning (extremely high voltage, high amps, DC)
         • Superficial or dermal flash burns, exit wounds on feet
         • Deep tissue damage (ear drum and corneal perforation)
         • Can cause immediate cardiorespiratory arrest requiring prolonged CPR
   — Indirect injury: flash, arc or thermal injury
   — Consequences of electrical burns
      ○ *Cardiac:* twenty-four hours of electrocardiogram (ECG) monitoring may be required for high-voltage injury, current passes through thorax, unconsciousness or abnormal ECG on arrival
   — Monitoring not essential if AC current, 220–260 V and asymptomatic
   — *Neurological:* LOC, seizures
   — *MSK:* compartment syndrome
      ○ Elevate limbs, monitor circulation
      ○ In patients with deep tissue damage, anticipate haemochromogenuria; insert a urinary catheter to both detect the earliest sign of urine discolouration and to monitor urine output; if pigments appear in urine, increase the fluid infusion rate

3 Chemical burns
   — Hand and upper limb most common site
   — Difficulty in assessing extent and depth
   — Can cause systemic toxicity, especially hydrofluoric acid
   — Chemical burns cause ongoing and progressive tissue damage until neutralisation or dilution

— *Hydrofluoric acid*
  ○ Severe injury, extremely painful
  ○ Burns to 2% of total body surface area (TBSA) may be fatal
  ○ Concentrations
    • < 20%: burn appears after 24 hours
    • 20–50%: burn apparent after several hours
    • 50%: immediately painful
  ○ Management:
    • Water irrigation
    • Topical calcium gluconate burn gel
    • Local injection subcutaneous Ca gluconate into burn wound (0.1–0.2 mL with 30-gauge needle, titrate to pain)
    • IV ischaemic retrograde infusion of Ca gluconate (Bier's block)
    • Early surgical debridement
    • Telemetry plus IV Ca^{++} plus Mg^{++} replacement
    • Promotion of F^- excretion: IV $NaHCO_3$, ± haemodialysis
    • Hand injury: digital fasciotomies plus intra-arterial Ca^{++}
    • Inhalation injury: respiratory support plus nebulised Ca^{++}
4 Assessing burn size
  — Large areas: use 'rule of nines' (Figure 7.1)
  ○ Body divided into areas of 9%
  ○ Paediatrics: for every year of life after 12 months take 1% from the head and add 0.5% to each leg
    • at 10 years of age, body proportions are the same as an adult
  — Small areas: use patient's palmar surface (fingers and palm of hand) which is equivalent to 1% TBSA

Management of minor burns

A minor burn is one which does not fit the transfer criteria and can be managed in a non-burn-unit hospital or clinic, including appropriate wound and pain management. Minor burns management is as follows.

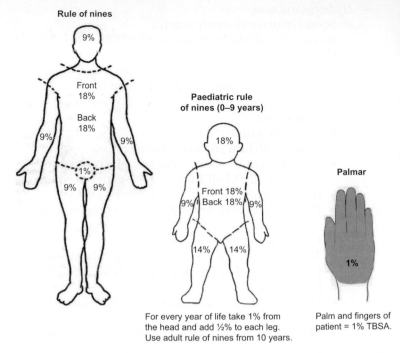

Figure 7.1 Rule of nines used to assess the percentage of body covered by burns

- Assess the burn wound.
- Deroof blisters (remove skin and fluid) after appropriate analgesia.
- Apply appropriate dressing.
- Arrange follow-up dressing and review.
- Prescribe pain relief as required.
- Contact a burn unit for any questions or for further review via emailed digital photograph or phone consultation.

Emergency management of the severe burn

The principles of the emergency management of severe burns are as follows.

1. PRIMARY SURVEY (ABCDE)

Airway and C-spine

- Clear the airway and secure if compromised.
- Protect C-spine if indicated by mechanism of injury.
- Large surface area burns > 35–40% TBSA should be intubated prior to transfer.

Clinical Pearl

A patient's airway may be adversely affected, particularly in flame burns/explosions in confined spaces and any burn involving the face and neck. If in doubt, intubate.

Breathing

- High-flow oxygen, pulse oximetry.
- Observe for stridor, hoarseness, oedema of face/neck, respiratory distress, presence of soot in nostrils or mouth, carbonaceous sputum.
- If in doubt, intubate.

Circulation

- Haemorrhage control.
- Monitor heart rate and blood pressure.
- If reduced perfusion of distal limbs, this may be due to hypovolaemia or tourniquet effect of limb burns and indication for escharotomy.

Disability

- Glasgow Coma Scale
- Pupils

Exposure

- Remove clothing and jewellery and any wet dressings or sheets.
- Keep patient warm.
- Log roll.

2. RESUSCITATE

- Fluid resuscitation
  — Two large IVCs
  — Modified Parkland formula
  — For burns > 15% TBSA adults or > 10% TBSA children
  — Area burnt (% TBSA) × weight (kg) × 3–4 mL = total mL in first 24 hours
  — Half given in first 8 hours since time of injury
  — Second half given next 16 hours
  — Use Hartmann's solution
  — Add maintenance plus glucose for children < 30 kg
  — Revise according to urine output (infusion rate guided by urine output, not formula)
    ○ Adult 0.5–1 mL/kg/hr
    ○ Children 1 mL/kg/hr if < 30 kg
- Analgesia
- Tests
  — Bloods, group and screen, ABG
  — ECG/cardiac monitoring, especially for electrical burns
- Tubes (lines, indwelling urinary catheter [IDC], nasogastric tube [NGT])

3. Secondary survey

- AMPLE history
  — Allergies, Medications, Past history, Last meal, Events/ environment leading to history
  — Information about burn: how hot, how long, closed space, clothing, first aid?
- Head to toe examination
  — Assess burn depth, size (% TBSA), site
- Tetanus
- Documentation and transfer
  — Document and discuss with statewide burns service
  — Prepare patient for transfer—early care of burn wound guidelines
    ○ Ensure first aid completed
    ○ Wash wounds with saline/sterile water
    ○ Deroof blisters

  ◦ Dressings
    • Glad wrap or non-adhesive dressing (Jelonet or Bactigras double layer) if being transferred immediately
    • Acticoat/silver dressing if delayed presentation to burns unit
    • Kerlix gauze or Velband/Webril and crepe bandage outer dressings
    • For facial burns apply paraffin ointment
  ◦ Elevate limbs
• Support—social worker etc.

Burns unit retrieval and referral guidelines

• Burns unit retrieval guidelines (time-critical transfer)
  — Intubated patient
  — Inhalation injuries
  — Head/neck burns
  — > 10% in children
  — > 20% in adults
  — Burns with significant comorbidities
  — Associated trauma
  — Significant preexisting medical disorder
  — Circumferential burn to limbs or chest that compromises circulation or respiration
  — Significant electrical including lightning injuries
  — Significant chemical (e.g. hydrofluoric acid)
• Burns unit referral/admission guidelines (not time critical)
  — Partial/full-thickness burns greater than 10% TBSA adults
  — Partial/full-thickness burns greater than 5% TBSA in children
  — Burns of special areas: face, hands, feet, genitalia, perineum, major joints and circumferential limb or chest burns
  — Electrical burns
  — Chemical burns
  — Burns with preexisting illness
  — Burns associated with major trauma
  — Burns at the extremes of age: young children and the elderly
  — Burn injury in pregnant women
  — Non-accidental burns

Indications to intubate are:
- Head/neck burns with increased swelling
- Stridor, hoarse voice, swollen lips
- Carbonaceous sputum/soot around nose/mouth
- Singed facial, nostrils, head hair
- Intra-oral oedema and erythema
- Possible inhalation injury

Intubate early if:
- the patient is unconscious
- head/neck burns are present with obvious/increasing swelling
- the patient is to be transported and may have potential airway compromise
- there are signs of respiratory dysfunction.

ESCHAROTOMY
- Eschar = thick, coagulated crust which develops following burn injury
- Full thickness/deep circumferential limb burns can have a tourniquet effect and cause vascular compromise
- Escharotomy = incision of the eschar to decompress the constrictive effects of the burn injury
- Generally done under sedation as a sterile procedure, can be done in resuscitation bay
- Full thickness incisions made into subcutaneous fat, extending into unburned skin. Incisions made on both sides of limbs/chest to adequately release constriction
- Haemostasis by diathermy or ligature
- Dress with Kaltostat, Jelonet and compressive bandages.

Online resources
Agency for Clinical Innovation (ACI) Statewide Burn Injury Service. clinical guidelines: burn patient management. 4th ed. 2019. Chatswood. Retrieved from: https://www.aci.health.nsw.gov.au/__data/assets/pdf_file/0009/250020/burn_patient_management_-_clinical_practice_guidelines.pdf

Australian & New Zealand Burn Association http://www.anzba.org.au/

Chapter 8
Patient transport, retrieval and pre-hospital care

Neil Ballard

Transferring critically ill or injured patients between hospitals is a potentially dangerous business. Although these transfers occur commonly, care needs to be taken to ensure that they are performed appropriately and safely. The Australasian critical care specialty colleges (Emergency Medicine, Anaesthesia, and Intensive Care Medicine) have issued a joint policy document specifying minimum standards of care required in these circumstances, and these are essential reading for staff involved (ACEM P03, *Guidelines for the Transport of Critically Ill Patients*, available on the website of the Australasian College of Emergency Medicine, www.acem.org.au).

Although intrahospital transport is often thought to be routine, or not thought about at all, the issues raised below with regard to interhospital transport must be considered.

Indications for retrieval

Patients need retrieval or transport to another facility when their needs are beyond the scope of the facility that they are in. They may require a higher level of critical care, specialist surgical or medical services (e.g. neurosurgery or interventional cardiology) or investigations such as an MRI.

Why the patient is being transferred always needs to be borne in mind, for this will guide the urgency of the transfer. Once it becomes apparent that the condition of the patient is beyond the scope of care of the referring hospital, initiation of the transfer process should commence. In some circumstances this will mean activating a retrieval team even before the patient arrives at hospital; for example, in the case of a multi-trauma patient and a small country hospital.

137

If the patient is being transferred for life-saving care (e.g. urgent neurosurgical decompression of an acute extradural haematoma), the patient needs to be packaged safely but quickly, taking time to do only procedures necessary for transfer. However, in other cases, such as a patient in septic shock being transferred for tertiary ICU care, time can be taken to optimise the patient's condition prior to transfer.

It is not unusual for critically ill patients to need transfer because no ICU beds are available. Time should be taken to ensure that this is the most appropriate course of action for a particular patient; if the patient is unstable or has a condition requiring urgent treatment and can be managed at the referring hospital, consideration should be given to moving another, more stable patient.

It is important to develop referral systems so that time is not wasted searching for a receiving hospital. These may be statewide or regional systems, or simply agreements between small hospitals and larger centres. An essential component of such systems is the ability of a practitioner in a small facility to be able to find a receiving hospital and get clinical advice with little difficulty, preferably via a single phone call.

The retrieval team

Interhospital patient transport should be performed by staff with the skills, experience and training to deal with potential problems that may arise during the course of the mission. Within Australasia, there are a number of specialised medical retrieval services which generally follow the staffing model of an experienced critical care doctor (emergency medicine, anaesthetics or ICU) plus either a paramedic or a flight nurse. As well as interhospital transfer of critically ill and injured patients, these services are also involved in pre-hospital care of critically injured patients.

If existing hospital staff are utilised in an interhospital transport, they need to be sufficiently experienced and skilled to make decisions and perform resuscitative measures in a potentially difficult environment, and they should be trained and familiar with the equipment that they use. The practice of sending an untrained junior doctor in the back of an ambulance with a critically ill patient can result in an adverse outcome for the patient, and a traumatic experience for the doctor involved.

Equipment

Monitors, syringe pumps and ventilators used in retrieval need to be light, robust and easy to use, with good battery life. Screens should be assessed for ability to be seen in variable light conditions (bright sunlight is particularly problematic) and at angles.

Airway, breathing and circulation equipment, plus appropriate medications and other necessary gear, should be kept in packs. These need to be checked regularly and staff involved in retrieval need to be familiar with the content and layout of these packs.

There should be redundancy of vital equipment (e.g. a spare laryngoscope and endotracheal tubes) in case of failure.

The retrieval environment

The hospital environment tends to be a familiar one: comfortable climate, controlled lighting, limited personal protection issues. However, interhospital transport of patients exposes both patient and staff to a number of different environments with various challenges.

Hot weather can result in dehydration and difficulty viewing monitors in bright sunlight. It can be difficult to assess a patient rugged up against the cold, or in the dark. Increasing altitude may result in hypoxia and cold. Interaction with unfamiliar staff of varying skills and experience at referring or receiving hospitals can present challenges, as can dealing with ambulance and other emergency services that one may come in contact with during interhospital patient transport. In such environments, the usual cues which alert one to deterioration in the patient's condition may be missed.

All of these elements impact on the patient, but also on the retrieval team. Lack of awareness of these hazards and precautions (e.g. food, fluids, good light sources) against them will result in fatigue and impaired decision-making.

Retrieval vehicles

The vehicles generally used for interhospital patient transport are road ambulances, helicopters and fixed-wing aircraft. They have some similarities in that they all offer cramped and noisy workplaces and are thus difficult places in which to perform assessments and procedures. Lighting will be worse than in hospital, power for equipment may or may not be available and motion sickness may affect the patient or attendants.

- Road ambulances are commonly used for short-distance interhospital transfers (less than 100 km), but care must be taken to secure equipment properly.
- Helicopters tend to be used for medium-distance transfers (100–300 km), and often have the advantage of flying direct from referring to receiving hospital, but are more susceptible to bad weather than other modes of transport. Because of noise and vibration, helicopters are a particularly difficult environment in which to perform clinical assessment or procedures.
- Fixed-wing aircraft have a greater range and fewer weight constraints than helicopters, but transfers involve road-ambulance legs and more patient movements to and from stretchers, all with the potential for mishap. Gravitational forces on take-off and landing may result in marked haemodynamic instability (including cardiac arrest), particularly with hypovolaemic patients.

Fixed-wing aircraft used as air ambulances tend to be pressurised, unlike helicopters where issues with hypoxia and gas expansion at altitude come into play. Gases expand by approximately 40% at an altitude of 8000 feet (2400 metres), and this may result in deleterious clinical effects if in a confined space. Pneumothoraces should be drained before transport.

An arterial partial pressure of oxygen (PaO_2) of 100 mmHg at sea level will fall to approximately 60 mmHg at 8000 feet if on the same fraction of inspired oxygen (FiO_2). This may make the difference between a patient being stable on high-flow oxygen via a non-rebreathing mask, and requiring intubation and ventilation. It may also result in medical attendants becoming hypoxic on minimal exertion during the mission, which may result in headaches, fatigue and impaired judgment.

The choice of retrieval vehicle should be made by a central tasking authority. This should take into account vehicle availability, weather, distance and clinical considerations.

Preparing a patient for retrieval

- The patient needs to be well packaged prior to interhospital transfer, always bearing in mind the clinical urgency of the case.

- It is difficult to do any procedures en route, so necessary procedures should be performed prior to departure, taking into account the likely or potential clinical course.
- If there is a concern about the airway, this should usually be secured by intubation prior to departure. The threshold for intubating a patient is lower than if they remain in a hospital environment.
- A minimum of two peripheral intravenous cannulas should be in place. Infusions should be rationalised to those necessary for transfer, and fluids should go through a pump set (blood-giving set) to ensure that they can run.
- Invasive blood pressure monitoring is more reliable than non-invasive readings, so an arterial line is preferable.
- Indwelling urinary catheters and gastric tubes are generally required. Awake patients should have an anti-emetic.
- Extreme care should be taken if moving an agitated or intoxicated patient. The risks of putting such patients in an aircraft are considerable, so transfer should either be deferred or involve sedation or even general anaesthesia.
- Sufficient medications and infusions for the mission should be immediately available.
- Copies of notes and imaging should go with the patient.
- Accurate determination of the patient's weight is essential, as the movement of obese patients can be logistically challenging and beyond the capacity of usual means. Patient weight beyond 130 kg will generally require specialised transfer methods, as will extreme height or width.
- Be sure to keep the patient's family aware of what is going on and where the patient is going. Give them an honest idea of the likely clinical course.

In transit

With a well-prepared patient, the time in transit is generally spent keeping a close eye on the patient and dealing with problems should they arise. Occasionally, however, significant resuscitation will be necessary which makes for an 'interesting' journey.

Particular care should be taken any time the patient is transferred between stretchers, and during loading and unloading vehicles. These are danger times for inadvertent disconnections

Table 8.1   ISBAR clinical hand-over tool

I	**Introduction** Identify yourself, your role and location. Identify the patient.
S	**Situation** State the patient's diagnosis/reason for admission and current problem.
B	**Background** What is the patient's history?
A	**Assessment** What are the most recent observations? What is your assessment?
R	**Recommendation** What do you want the person taking over care of the patient to do? When should this occur?

nswhealth.moodle.com.au/DOH/DETECT/content/00_worry/when_to_worry_06.htm

and even extubation, plus haemodynamically unstable patients can deteriorate with even minor stimuli.

A clear and detailed record of the transfer should be kept.

Hand-over

Good hand-over is vital to ensure appropriate ongoing care of the patient. Hand-over at the receiving hospital should be to the most senior medical officer, and must also include the nursing staff who will be looking after the patient. Hand-over should follow a structured framework such as the ISBAR tool (Table 8.1— introduction, situation, background, assessment, recommendation), addressing clinical course and the immediate needs of the patient. Ventilation, monitoring and infusions should be transferred from the retrieval to hospital equipment in a systematic manner, ensuring the patient is appropriately monitored at all times. Be sure to pass on contact details of the patient's family. This is a vulnerable time for the patient.

The retrieval team is responsible for directing the coordinated hand-over and transfer of care. A patient retrieval hand-over procedure is outlined in Table 8.2.

Table 8.2 Retrieval hand-over procedure

Hand-over: who, when, where, how	
Who	• The hand-over should be between the most senior hospital clinician responsible for the patient and the retrieval clinician.
When	• The hand-over should take place at a predictable time—an estimated time of arrival for the retrieval team should be provided, with the expectation that the relevant team is assembled at the designated time. • The hand-over should occur before the transfer of management begins (unless urgent resuscitation is required). This ensures that all staff listen to the hand-over and then focus on the systematic transfer of patient care.
What	• At hand-over the following information is exchanged, along with general ISBAR principles: — presenting problem and relevant past history; use MIST/AMPLE — initial and current management (including monitoring, infusions, ventilation) — response to management and current condition (including current vital signs) — a problem list of perceived issues that need addressing within the next 60 minutes.
How	1. Transfer to stretcher/bed • The hospital is responsible for ensuring that sufficient staff and equipment are available. The retrieval team is responsible for coordinating the move, as they are familiar with the retrieval equipment. 2. Transfer monitors • Monitoring should be transferred between the hospital monitors and retrieval bridge monitors one at a time. There should be no disruption to the continuity of monitoring. 3. Transfer therapies • Therapies should be transferred one at a time, at the direction of the retrieval team.

Continued

Table 8.2   Retrieval hand-over procedure (cont.)

Hand-over: who, when, where, how

Ventilation
— Hospital bed to retrieval stretcher = transfer ventilation last.
— Retrieval stretcher to hospital bed = transfer ventilation first; note that when transferring from retrieval to hospital equipment, the retrieval team will prescribe initial ventilation parameters.

Drug infusions
— One drug at a time, like-to-like, ensure no dead space.

Specific therapies
— That is, intercostal drainage systems, external ventricular drains (EVDs), Sengstaken–Blakemore tubes, IV fluids.

Routine therapies
— That is, nasogastric tubes, urinary catheters, etc.

Source: Modified from NSW Department of Health Retrieval Policy, 2011. Emergency medicine. https://acem.org.au/Documents/Policies/Guidelines-for-Transport-of-Critically-Ill-Patient

Pre-hospital care

Retrieval services are frequently tasked to the pre-hospital care of critically injured or difficult-to-access patents. Doctors in such services are generally specialists or advanced trainees in emergency medicine, anaesthetics or intensive care. Increasingly, pre-hospital and retrieval medicine is viewed as an area of subspecialty in these fields.

The role of the doctor in such teams is to utilise critical-care skills in the field; for example, rapid-sequence intubation, insertion of intercostal catheters or pre-hospital ultrasound scanning. The goal for medical pre-hospital teams is to provide these interventions in a safe and timely manner, accelerating rather than delaying the patient's journey to definitive care. Slightly more time spent in the field to intubate a patient may be time saved in the ED.

The challenges of working in difficult environments have led to the development of protocols for procedures such as rapid sequence intubation with the aim of improving performance and safety. These protocols may include challenge–response checklists, which are common in aviation. Increasingly, these protocols are finding their way into in-hospital care.

Editorial Comment

Every ED, especially those in smaller hospitals, must have an easily accessible document (e.g. on ED computers) that lists key phone numbers, checklists for doctors and nurses and how to organise transfers—the 'one phone call'—as well as who to call to have the matter escalated if the ED is overwhelmed or encountering a 'brick wall' at any receiving hospital. *Note*: Murphy's Law says—it will be at night, on the weekend and/or at holiday time!

Online resource
NSW Ambulance Protocols Version 2.0

Chapter 9
The seriously ill patient: tips and traps

Gordian WO Fulde

It is the purpose of every ED to assess, resuscitate, diagnose and treat, both definitively and symptomatically, the patients who walk or are wheeled in through the door.

The ultimate responsibility for this belongs to the medical officer. In order to cope when faced with a variable number of patients whose conditions vary in severity, an organised approach is essential.

There must be triage (sorting) and re-triage, especially if the department is busy. (See also Chapter 52 Nursing and Allied Health Advanced Practice and Adjunct Roles.)

The emergency doctor should use a priority problem-oriented approach and make clear decisions. As the leader of the team of medical officers, nurses, clerical staff, radiographers, porters and the many others who are often needed to attend to a sick patient, this approach is imperative. The doctor must assess, resuscitate and manage the patient and the patient's relatives. As a rule, decision-making is harder in the case of patients who are not critically ill. The majority of all admissions (60–70%) come from triage category 3. Such patients should be assessed and managed with emphasis on early symptomatic relief and reassurance.

A key to keeping control of a busy department is that the most senior medical and nursing staff must be aware of all patients (including those waiting in ambulances). This may involve, for example, after a resuscitation doing a 'flash' ward round to do a 'stocktake' and allocate priorities, make admission decisions, contact inpatient staff to come down or accept problems.

Emergency doctors must communicate well so that most parties, most of the time, have some idea what is happening or what they need to do. For example, with system problems, ensure you escalate 'up' early; that is, if beds are full and ambulances are waiting, ensure medical and nursing administration know (contacting them by mobile phone is best—they also want to know early).

Remember to ensure a safe and professional environment for patients and staff. Do not compromise this, as it is wrong and it will come back to bite you even though your motives were honourable.

Although it goes against human nature, ensure that difficulties are documented and submitted to the quality and risk system of your hospital. The system will respond, especially if serious or repeated problems are listed objectively. Emails to key people next working day also speed up action if critical issues are encountered. (See also Chapter 62 Administration and Governance in the ED.)

When attending to the many problems encountered in an ED, rely on good clinical common sense in order to avoid pitfalls. At all times, play it safe. Be suspicious of any complication. Never be afraid to ask or 'google'. The patient must be managed in as close to an 'ideal' fashion as possible. Distractions such as work pressure or the many other difficulties faced in EDs (e.g. bed shortages) should play no major role in individual management. Of course, good written documentation is essential as evidence of what was done and why.

Warning—red lights—beware

For all of us there are red warning lights that alert us to potential pitfalls.

- **Re-presentations to the ED.** Think it through again; do not just accept the last diagnosis.
- **Patient sent in by another healthcare professional** (e.g. GP, community nurse). They are asking for help from you and the hospital.
- **If pain is severe and unrelieved, worry!** You have probably missed something. Continuing out-of-character pain is a very common feature of misdiagnosis—so re-think! At the very least, observe and ask.
- **Repeated questions or protests** (e.g. the patient, the patient's mother, anybody who keeps telling you 'they are sick' or 'this is not normal for the patient') are a key indicator of pathology going on.
- **Triage categories 3 and 4** are often quite sick (especially if old).

- **Check vital signs frequently yourself** (BP, pulse, respiratory rate, temperature, blood glucose level, coma scale, oximetry). They change quickly.
- **Unpleasant patients (with or without difficult relatives).** Never vary your standard approach and management. Document all. This also applies to VIPs and friends. Always be polite, not rushed, try to sit down, get eye contact and listen. If not going well including mental health, excuse yourself and walk away, ask a colleague, preferably more senior, for help even to take over.
- **Hand-over patients.** Make sure you have the whole story and plan. In the United States this patient group features highly in court cases. Use the ISBAR tool (see Figure 8.1).
- **Poor history, poor examination.** History and examination are cornerstones of the diagnosis. If you are unable to get good facts, be very careful and conservative, and worry.
- **Investigations are never 100% accurate.** Even if a test is very expensive, do not worship it—it makes mistakes. Many tests confirm a diagnosis but do not fully exclude it. Look at the whole clinical picture. A multi-hundred-slice CT or multiple-tesla MRI or even an X-ray does not necessarily mean you are expert enough (even in spite of pretty reconstructions) to definitively report. CT MRIs are finding new lesions that were not seen before and that may not be pathological.
- **Urgent treatment** (see Law 1, below). Sometimes you must treat on suspicion, *now!* For example, tension pneumothorax, bacterial meningitis, narcotic overdose, hypoglycaemia. Early pain control may also be needed.
- **Pain.** Always listen to the patient; go through all details of the pain. (Avoid leading questions!) This way you will probably get the diagnosis. Treat pain very early.
- **Abnormal results.** With so many tests now available, learn to scan for pivotal ones (i.e. those associated with time-critical bad outcomes). Ideally the lab should let you know by phone until all results go back to the orderer by smartphone or such and alert you of an abnormal result via an alarm. An example of key abnormals is shown in Table 9.1.

Table 9.1   Critical results

Test (blood)	SI units	Low critical values (+ or <) Paediatric (> 1 month to 16 years)	Adult	High critical values (= or >) Neonate (up to 1 month)	Paediatric (> 1 month to 16 years)	Adult
General chemistry levels						
Sodium	mmol/L	130	125		150	160
Potassium	mmol/L	2.8	2.8		6.0	6.0
Bicarbonate	mmol/L	16	10		35	40
Glucose plasma	mmol/L	2.5	2.5		15	25
Phosphate	mmol/L	0.4	0.4		2.8	2.8
Magnesium	mmol/L	0.5	0.5		2.0	2.0
Calcium (total)	mmol/L	1.6	1.6		3.2	3.2
Calcium (ionised)	mmol/L	0.8	0.8		1.6	1.6
pH		7.2	7.2		7.5	7.5
pCO_2	mmHg	–	–		–	70
pO_2	mmHg	40	40		–	–
Lactate	mmol/L	–	–		4.0	3.4
COHb	%	–	–		10	10
MetHb	%	–	–		10	10
Bilirubin	micromol/L			280		
Uric acid	mmol/L			0.400		
Urea	mmol/L			20		
Creatinine	micromol/L			100		
Haematology						
Platelet count			$< 50 \times 10^9$/L			
Absolute neutrophil count			$< 1.0 \times 10^9$/L			
Hb			< 80 g/L			
WBC			$< 2.0 \times 10^9$/L or $> 30.0 \times 10^9$/L			

Decision-making tips

In the ED, we are all seeing older, sicker, more-complicated patients. You must focus on the following.

- What made the patient come to hospital? What do they hope for?

- Are all the vital signs okay?
- Do I need extra help, extra information (old notes, GP, specialist advice)?
- Problems → treatment, plan of management.

An important question is: 'Does the patient need admission to hospital?' This is better approached from the other perspective: 'Is it safe or appropriate to send the patient home?' If the answer is to be 'yes', refer to the discharge checklist in Box 9.1.

The patient must be able to cope alone. Is there anyone to help? Can the patient take necessary medications, prepare and eat meals and go to the toilet? Also, can the patient survive any likely complication of the medical condition? The fact that the ED was excessively busy at the time and the hospital was full will not be at all useful as an excuse in a legal inquiry or a court case relating to the management

---

Box 9.1   Discharge checklist—safe discharge, especially after-hours and for all elderly or disabled patients

1. Mobility: can the patient mobilise safely?
- Has the patient been observed to mobilise without assistance?
- If normally used, does the patient have a walking aid?
- Will the patient be able to sit in/get up from a chair?
- Will the patient be able to get into/up from bed?
- Will the patient be able to get from the transport vehicle into their residence (distance to front door, steps to negotiate)?

2. Social or family: is there adequate family or social support?
- Is someone available to take the patient home?
- Will someone be with the patient overnight if needed?

3. Nutrition, hygiene, comfort: can the patient attend to basic needs?
- Can the patient eat and swallow?
- Will the patient be able to shower/toilet without assistance (can they get clothes on and off)?
- Will the patient be able to prepare meals (can they open a can, is there food at home)?
- Is the patient pain free? Does the patient have medications to take?

4. Cognitive function: is the patient likely to place himself or herself in a dangerous position?
- Can the patient be expected to avoid unnecessary personal risk (is there a history of wandering, leaving gas outlets open, etc.)?
- Can the patient be expected to avoid self-harm, self-medicate?
- Can they understand and phone for help (e.g. have key phone numbers)?
- Need an emergency call system.

Box 9.1   Discharge checklist—safe discharge, especially after-hours and for all elderly or disabled patients (cont.)

5. Discharge instructions
- Letter
- Instructions understood
- Third party (GP, relative aware)

If NO has been answered for any of the above determine whether the problem/potential problem can be adequately addressed (e.g. if the patient cannot walk from the car into their place of residence, ambulance transport may be organised) and document strategies below.

_____

_____

_____

_____

If NO has been selected for any of the above and appropriate management strategies can be identified, the patient should not be discharged at this time.

Patients choosing to discharge against medical advice must be asked to sign themselves out.

---

of an individual who was inappropriately sent home. Always err on the side of safety and, if you are not sure what to do, get the most senior medical officer possible involved in the decision-making. Always write details in the notes of what was decided, by whom and why.

Usually some follow-up, either by a local doctor, specialist or outpatients department, is indicated. This must be organised and noted in the patient's record. This may need to be done later, in business hours.

Emergency department 'laws'
LAW 1: ALL PATIENTS ARE TRYING TO DIE BEFORE YOUR EYES

You must always think in terms of worst-case scenarios (e.g. cardiac infarcts, meningitis, subarachnoid haemorrhage, pulmonary embolism). This is even more vital where early specific treatment will cure and prevent death. It may seem dramatic, but if you treat or exclude these serious illnesses early, further management of the patient is often very straightforward. Remember, medicine is best geared to treat serious illnesses, and society expects us to get these right.

Once serious illness is excluded and explanations are given, the patient is often grateful and happy for follow-up by GP or specialist.

LAW 2: CALL FOR HELP EARLY!

The team approach for complicated emergencies, such as trauma and cardiac arrest, should be activated early (i.e. even before patients 'crash'). Early involvement of intensive specialists, those responsible for definitive care, is imperative. Never be reticent to ask for more help—a 'routine' case of acute pulmonary oedema is enough work for two doctors in the initial resuscitation phase. Always aim for the hypothetical optimum-care scenario (i.e. pretend that the patient is a loved relative).

If the patient is critical and unstable, call the arrest team or similar response team (e.g. medical emergency team) before it happens. The patient is much more likely to do better if you prevent the crash. See Table 9.2.

The patient who meets one or more of these criteria should be in a resuscitation area with adequate doctors and nurses. The 'drama' phase lasts only a few minutes and staff can return to their other patients as soon as you have control of ABCs.

Observation charts are now designed to highlight abnormal observations (e.g. Between the Flags). Do not ignore a deteriorating trend even if not abnormal yet.

LAW 3: BE FLEXIBLE

Many sick patients defy any discrete label or have a diagnosis backed up by clearly abnormal tests. Follow your clinical impression, keep looking and be prepared to be surprised and change your management direction. If in doubt, observe.

LAW 4: TREAT THE PATIENT, NOT JUST THE TESTS

Clinical impression (is this patient sick?) has been repeatedly shown to be highly accurate in picking up sick patients where scores, protocols, tests, and so on have not clearly 'ruled in' a diagnosis (e.g. acute coronary syndrome). If in doubt, watch, observe, ask.

Table 9.2 Calling for help criteria—now

Call for help for any patient who meets the following criteria

Change in	Physiology
	• Severe bleeding if from a limb? Tourniquet?
Airway	• Predicted difficult airway • Unable to obtain
Breathing	• All respiratory arrests • Respiratory rate < 5 breaths/min • Respiratory rate > 30 breaths/min • O₂ saturation < 90%
Circulation	• All cardiac arrests • Pulse rate < 40 beats/min • Pulse rate > 140 beats/min • Systolic blood pressure < 90 mmHg
Neurology	• Sudden fall in level of consciousness • Fall in GCS ≥ 2 points • Repeated or prolonged seizures • Not-intubated GCS < 9
Other—any patient you are seriously worried about who does not fit the above criteria	• For example: — Unable to obtain prompt assistance, resources — 'Difficulty speaking' — Agitation or delirium, violent — Any unexplained decrease in consciousness — Uncontrolled pain — Failure to respond to treatment

GCS = Glasgow Coma Scale score
Based on criteria set out in Parr MJ, Hadfield JH, Flabouris A et al. The medical emergency team: a twelve-month analysis for activation immediate outcome and not-for-resuscitation orders. Resuscitation 2001;50:39–44.

Do not feed the lawyers

• See above.
• Never openly criticise colleagues or management—you rarely have all the facts, let alone the other side's reasons. Clinical signs evolve and change.
• Respect the efforts of the healthcare workers. Do not talk shop (i.e. the imperfect world of healthcare and mistakes or problems) in public. It makes it worse for all. If there

are problems, use the system/process to improve it (i.e. be constructive)—there is always someone to discuss a problem with who can give advice on how to tackle it and achieve improvement. Also, positive feedback works well! Use it freely!

• Always find out early what the patient, relatives, GP, and so on expect or want, especially if it is not clear what the problem is or why they came. You will make a lot of people happy with your service, even if you can only give an explanation of why you cannot meet their immediate perceived need. You also will save a lot of time and expense.

• To have a really good work environment, where the patient and you will do well, see Table 9.3.

Table 9.3   Emergency department 10 commandments

1	IF IN DOUBT, ASK This includes asking medical, nursing, clerical and allied health staff
2	NO PATIENT IS TO BE DISCHARGED FROM THE EMERGENCY DEPARTMENT UNLESS THE EMERGENCY REGISTRAR/CONSULTANT KNOWS ABOUT IT Especially if sent in by a local medical officer (LMO)
3	BE SAFE: • universal protective measures • wash hands • safe shoes • safe sharps disposal • immunisations up-to-date • know 'needle-stick' protocol • know location of wall-mounted alarms • wear personal duress alarms • know hospital codes (see Figure 9.1)
4	IF YOU SUSPECT PROBLEMS, GET HELP EARLY
5	SEE PATIENTS IN THE TRIAGE ORDER THEY APPEAR ON THE EMERGENCY DEPARTMENT INFORMATION SYSTEM SCREEN and COMPLETE INFORMATION Print out discharge letter, instructions and results for the patient
6	ALWAYS CONSIDER ANALGESIA, GIVE ANALGESIA EARLY VIA THE MOST APPROPRIATE ROUTE (INTRAVENOUS UNLESS SPECIFICALLY CONTRAINDICATED)
7	WHILE ON DUTY IN THE DEPARTMENT, BEHAVE AS YOU WOULD EXPECT A DOCTOR TREATING YOUR FAMILY TO BEHAVE

Table 9.3   Emergency department 10 commandments (cont.)

8 TREAT EVERYBODY EQUALLY:
- socially
- medically
- be thorough and polite

9 WRITE NOTES GOOD ENOUGH TO USE IN A COURT APPEARANCE;
   DOCUMENT CLEARLY IN YOUR MEDICAL NOTES
   Include discharge instructions and whom notified

10 BE TIDY:
- appearance
- identification
- names—yours legible, patient's on history and medication charts
- do not leave X-rays out of packets and give back private
X-ray, etc.
- keep consultation rooms clean
- put used trays and sharps biohazard away appropriately
- doctors, keep your office tidy
- cot bedsides up when you leave the patient

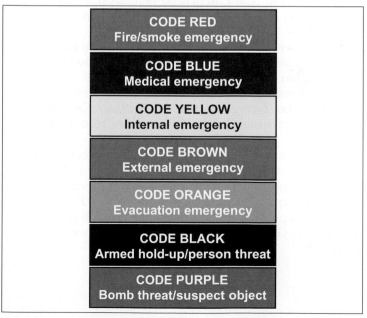

CODE RED
Fire/smoke emergency

CODE BLUE
Medical emergency

CODE YELLOW
Internal emergency

CODE BROWN
External emergency

CODE ORANGE
Evacuation emergency

CODE BLACK
Armed hold-up/person threat

CODE PURPLE
Bomb threat/suspect object

Figure 9.1 Hospital response codes

INTERACTION WITH POLICE, LEGAL PROFESSIONALS, THE MEDIA

In the first instance, *say nothing*—until you have checked with someone more senior who knows what you are allowed to say, what the normal protocol is (e.g. whether the responding person should be the treating consultant, hospital medicolegal officer, hospital public relation officer). An innocent comment taken out of context can cause no end of trouble.

The fun bits

Do these as much as you can.

- Teach students, nurses, allied health and community (CPR); use aids such as photos and handouts and involve the learners.
- Engage in research such as clinical audits and chart reviews (see the benchmark article by EH Gilbert, SR Lowenstein et al. Chart reviews in emergency medicine research: where are the methods? Ann Emerg Med 1996;27(3):305–9).
- Mentor medical students, trainees, nurses—join up with other centres.
- Simulation centres do course scenarios, and also have practice mannequins for anything from intubation to IVs (including intraosseous and LPs). Go and ask.
- Update yourself—ensure the department subscribes to journals, audio (*Emergency Medical Abstracts*, *Emergency Reports*, etc.), journal club, podcasts, online resources, and so on.
- Ensure that interesting articles are routinely circulated to staff; assist staff to attend conferences, courses, and so on.
- Socialise—support departmental social and sporting events; everybody should attend some of the activities. Ensure they are well publicised and preferably that each group is represented. Get to know your fellow workers better—make the effort!

Chapter 10
The approach to the patient with chest pain or dyspnoea

Patricia Saccasan and Anthony J Whelan

Chest pain, dyspnoea and haemoptysis are common and important symptoms which bring patients to the ED. The role of the emergency medical team is to rapidly identify high-risk patients, commence resuscitation if necessary, arrive at an accurate diagnosis, initiate appropriate therapies and arrange appropriate disposition. Some therapies are extremely time-dependent (e.g. reperfusion therapy for myocardial infarction) and good outcomes depend on early recognition of these seriously ill patients. However, the clinician must be aware of the tension between appropriate investigation and the costs associated with inappropriate admissions and tests.

Chest pain

The general public is increasingly aware of the importance of chest pain and the need for early presentation with this symptom. In American EDs, up to 7% of all presentations are for chest pain, prompting changes in the organisation of EDs so that many high-volume departments have specialised chest pain units where patients with this symptom are rapidly triaged and treated according to defined protocols. While there are many causes of chest pain, clinicians should be aware of disorders which are potentially life-threatening (Box 10.1). Before any chest pain patient is discharged, each of these diagnoses should at least be considered.

MYOCARDIAL ISCHAEMIA
(See also Chapter 11 Acute Coronary Syndromes.)

History
Recognition of the symptoms of myocardial ischaemia is crucial. Modern therapies significantly improve the outcome of patients

Box 10.1 Causes of chest pain	
Potentially life-threatening	**Not life-threatening**
Acute coronary syndromes	Chest wall pain/chest trauma
Pulmonary embolism	Gastro-oesophageal reflux
Aortic dissection	Oesophageal spasm
Tension pneumothorax	Pericarditis
Ruptured oesophagus	Mitral valve prolapse
Pneumonia	Herpes zoster
Pericardial tamponade	Myocarditis

with acute ischaemia and missing this diagnosis can be disastrous. In the United States, inappropriate discharge of patients who eventually are found to have acute coronary syndromes is the leading cause of litigation involving emergency physicians.

Take time to question the patient, using non-leading questions, to clarify the nature of the patient's pain.

- The pain of myocardial ischaemia is classically a deep visceral pain felt in the anterior chest but not localised to any part of the chest. Patients may describe heaviness, constriction, a sensation like a heavy weight or a dull ache.
- Pain usually comes on gradually, reaching a peak over a few minutes, and lasts at least a few minutes.
- Patients prefer to lie still and the pain is not exacerbated by the respiratory cycle, posture or food intake.
- Classical radiation patterns include spread to the neck, jaw or arms. Pain radiating to the left arm is more common than to the right. Heaviness (rather than pain) in both arms is also very suggestive.
- Autonomic accompaniments such as sweating, nausea, vomiting and anxiety are also of concern.

While the pain of myocardial ischaemia may be severe, the severity of the pain is not consistently related to the extent of ischaemia. Ischaemic pain often worsens with exertion. Angina usually lasts less than 20 minutes and there may be some benefit from oxygen and sublingual nitrates. The temporal pattern of angina is of prognostic significance (Table 10.1). Patients with a stable pattern of angina may not need admission but will need appropriate referral for follow-up.

Atypical presentations are common. Older patients, younger patients, women and diabetics are more likely to have presentations which are not immediately suggestive of myocardial ischaemia. Pain

Table 10.1   Braunwald classification of unstable angina

Class	Description	Risk of AMI/death in next year
I	New onset of exertional angina; angina with less effort; no rest pain	7%
II	Angina at rest within the last month but no pain in last 48 hours	10%
III	Angina at rest in the last 48 hours	11%

AMI = acute myocardial infarction

may be felt in the abdomen, jaw or arm (without chest pain), or an acute coronary syndrome may present only with dyspnoea, vomiting or syncope, and no chest pain at all. Women can often have atypical symptoms, such as fatigue, dyspnoea, nausea or abdominal symptoms. Thus a high index of suspicion is necessary and the diagnosis of myocardial ischaemia should be considered (and an ECG and biomarkers done) in all patients in whom this diagnosis is possible.

There may be overlap with other chest pain syndromes. Some patients describe burning pain suggestive of gastro-oesophageal reflux; and while sharp, stabbing or even pleuritic-type pain makes myocardial ischaemia unlikely, it does not exclude this diagnosis. Pope et al. (2000) found that up to 22% of patients with the principal complaint of sharp stabbing pain had an acute coronary syndrome.

A number of diagnostic decision tools using history and ECG findings to assist with diagnosis have been proposed (e.g. the acute cardiac ischaemia [ACI] predictive instrument, the thrombolysis in myocardial infarction [TIMI] score, GRACE score and HEART score) which probably increase the accuracy of diagnosis. Many of these are available online and as smartphone apps. However, a high index of suspicion is the most useful safeguard.

Risk factors
A previous diagnosis of myocardial infarction, stable angina or revascularisation procedures significantly increases the risk that a new presentation with chest pain is due to myocardial ischaemia. The presence of diabetes and increasing age are also important risks. A patient with diabetes presenting with chest pain should be assumed to have coronary artery disease until it has been proven otherwise. It is not clear whether a history of other risk factors for

atherosclerosis (smoking, hyperlipidaemia, family history) increases the risk that a new presentation with chest pain is due to myocardial ischaemia, these findings being very common in the general population. End-stage renal disease, amphetamine use and inflammatory states such as rheumatoid arthritis have been recently recognised as risk factors for coronary artery disease, as are acute infections such as influenza and community-acquired pneumonia.

OTHER POTENTIALLY LIFE-THREATENING CAUSES OF CHEST PAIN

Aortic dissection

(See also Chapter 28 Aortic and Vascular Emergencies.)

This is an important but rare disorder leading to severe chest pain associated with a significant mortality.

- Typically the pain is of abrupt onset and is of maximum intensity immediately, as opposed to the pain of myocardial ischaemia which builds up over minutes.
- The pain of aortic dissection often radiates through to the back, which is unusual in myocardial ischaemia.
- The pain may be described as 'tearing' and can be very severe, needing large doses of narcotics for control of pain.
- The appearance of a patient with severe pain and a non-specific ECG who appears shocked and diaphoretic, yet has a high blood pressure, is a strong clue to this disorder.
- A significant percentage of patients with thoracic aortic dissection will have experienced syncope or have neurological symptoms.

Risk factors for aortic dissection include Marfan's syndrome and other inherited disorders of connective tissue, hypertension, pregnancy, bicuspid aortic valve and previous invasive procedures involving the aorta. The addition of D-dimer measurements to clinical features may allow better risk stratification in suspected aortic dissection (the ADviSED risk score).

Pneumothorax

(See also Chapter 13 Respiratory Emergencies: The Acutely Breathless Patient.)

Pleuritic chest pain varies with the respiratory cycle and is usually worse on inspiration. Pneumothorax (air in the pleural space) is an important cause of pleuritic chest pain and is frequently associated with dyspnoea.

- Primary spontaneous pneumothorax occurs most frequently in younger males who are tall and thin but have no previous history of lung disease.
- Secondary spontaneous pneumothorax complicates chronic lung disease, especially COPD, asthma and cystic fibrosis.
- Iatrogenic causes such as recent insertion of central venous lines, biopsy procedures and commencement of assisted ventilation should be considered.

Pulmonary embolism
(See also Chapter 16 Venous Thromboembolic Disease: Deep Venous Thrombosis and Pulmonary Embolism.)
Pleuritic pain can also be caused by pulmonary embolism, where there is a complicating pulmonary infarction and pleural irritation; however, massive pulmonary embolism can also cause central chest discomfort suggestive of angina. This is life-threatening, associated with dyspnoea, syncope and haemodynamic collapse, and may reflect acute right ventricular dysfunction.

Pneumonia
(See also Chapter 13 Respiratory Emergencies: The Acutely Breathless Patient.)
Pleuritic chest pain is a common feature of respiratory tract infections which extend to the pleura. There should be other clinical features pointing to infection.

Ruptured oesophagus
Severe anterior chest pain following vomiting is characteristic of oesophageal perforation (Boerhaave's syndrome). While vomiting may occur in myocardial infarction, it usually follows the onset of chest pain rather than preceding it. Oesophageal perforation may also follow procedures, especially oesophageal dilation.

Cardiac tamponade
Chest pain may be a feature of cardiac tamponade which occurs when fluid accumulates within the pericardial space, compressing the heart and impeding diastolic filling. Often, however,

hypotension and shock are presenting problems. Causes of tamponade can include trauma, aortic dissection, invasive cardiac procedures, neoplastic disease, infection, hypothyroidism, drugs and inflammatory syndromes.

OTHER CAUSES OF CHEST PAIN
Pericarditis
Pain is usually felt in the anterior or left chest. The pain of pericarditis is sharp and severe and is not typically related to exertion. It is usually worse in the supine position and improves with sitting up and leaning forward. Acute pericarditis is diagnosed by the presence of at least two of four criteria: chest pain typical for pericarditis, a pericardial friction rub, new electrocardiographic changes or a new pericardial effusion.

Reflux
The pain of reflux is usually described as burning, commencing in the lower chest and 'rising' into the throat. There may be associated belching, waterbrash, dysphagia or odynophagia. Patients usually report relief with antacids but this response is not specific for reflux, and improvement with antacids or 'GI cocktails' may be seen in myocardial ischaemia. Thus, a response to antacids should not be used to rule out myocardial ischaemia.

Chest wall pain
This is the commonest cause of chest pain in outpatient practice. Pain is usually well-localised, jabbing or stabbing, lasting either for a fraction of a second or for hours or even days at a time. While a number of syndromes have been described, a precise diagnosis may not be possible. Generally pain that is described as coming from 'outside' the chest with a lancinating or knife-like quality is less likely to be due to myocardial ischaemia. Chest wall tenderness is common and pain that is reproduced by pressure on the chest wall is a non-specific finding. It should not be used to rule out myocardial ischaemia, and may co-exist with other more significant pathologies.

Anxiety
Chest pain may be associated with anxiety states and is an important component of the hyperventilation syndrome. This diagnosis

should only be reached after a thorough evaluation to exclude other, possibly life-threatening, possibilities.

Abdominal disease
(See also Chapter 26 Gastrointestinal Emergencies.)
Upper abdominal disorders such as cholecystitis, peptic ulcer disease, pancreatitis, hepatic and splenic disorders can be associated with chest pain which dominates the presentation and may appear out of proportion to the abdominal findings. Some of these disorders may be associated with ECG abnormalities, further confusing the diagnosis. Upper abdominal pain (without chest pain) may also represent an acute coronary syndrome. An ECG is important in all patients with epigastric and upper abdominal pain.

PHYSICAL EXAMINATION AND INITIAL MANAGEMENT

- Triage chest pain patients rapidly to urgent care. Important haemodynamic abnormalities should be recognised quickly.
- Commence oxygen treatment if the oxygen saturation is < 94%, and consider giving nitrates, taking care if it is the first dose for the patient or they are hypotensive. Recent use of sildenafil is a contraindication.
- Administer aspirin (300 mg PO stat unless there is a definite history of allergy) early, as this medication has been shown to considerably decrease the mortality rate in unstable coronary syndromes.
- Institute continuous cardiac monitoring and obtain IV access.
- Blood tests including troponins should be obtained.
- Take a focused history as all this is being implemented, as time is of the essence.
- An ECG should be done immediately.
  In addition look for the following.
 1 Impaired level of consciousness, presence of respiratory distress, diaphoresis, pallor and peripheral hypoperfusion.
 2 Raised jugular venous pressure, which may be indicative of acute heart failure, massive pulmonary embolism, tension pneumothorax or cardiac tamponade.
 3 Other signs of cardiac failure. Oedema is relatively non-specific but a 3rd heart sound is very suggestive of heart

failure. Signs of heart failure associated with an acute coronary syndrome place the patient in a high-risk group.

4 Peripheral pulses. Peripheral vascular disease is strongly associated with coronary artery disease. Compare pulses in both arms and measure the blood pressure in both arms if aortic dissection is possible. A difference of greater than 10 mmHg is significant but non-specific.

5 The praecordium. Clinical cardiomegaly is suggestive of left ventricular dysfunction. Similarly, a 3rd heart sound is usually abnormal. However, 4th heart sounds are common in the older population, particularly those with hypertension. Murmurs are frequently non-contributory, but features of severe aortic stenosis, mitral valve prolapse or hypertrophic cardiomyopathy may suggest a cause for chest pain. A mitral regurgitation murmur that coincides with the patient's pain and disappears with relief of pain is highly significant for high-risk ischaemia. A new systolic murmur may be indicative of an infarction of the papillary muscle, and the diastolic murmur of aortic regurgitation may suggest thoracic aortic dissection. A pericardial rub is an important sign but may be transient or only heard in certain postures.

6. The chest. Symmetry of breath sounds and deviation of the trachea should be sought. Look also for localised chest signs, particularly crackles, rubs, features of consolidation and evidence of pleural effusion. Chest wall tenderness is non-specific and is seen in many patients with and without important cardiorespiratory disorders.

7 Abdominal examination should be done routinely, particularly to look for a non-cardiac cause for the patient's symptoms.

8 Limbs. Look for oedema, pulses and signs of deep venous thrombosis (DVT).

INVESTIGATIONS
Electrocardiogram (ECG)
All patients complaining of chest pain should have an ECG, and previous ECGs should be obtained for comparison. An ECG may be transmitted by ambulance paramedics, or it should be taken immediately on arrival in the ED and interpreted within a maximum of 10 minutes. If the initial ECG is unhelpful and symptoms

continue, a repeat ECG in 15 minutes or with onset of new pain may be diagnostic. The ECG helps to triage patients into high, intermediate and low risk for myocardial ischaemia and is crucial in the selection of treatment.

A number of guidelines have evolved to standardise the process of assessment, early management and disposition of chest pain patients and these are often incorporated into local practice patterns.

ECG patterns are discussed in detail in Chapter 12 Clinical Electrocardiography and Arrhythmia Management.

Pathology tests

Troponins are the standard of care in this clinical setting. An elevated troponin strongly supports the diagnosis of an acute coronary syndrome and places the patient into a higher risk group. Two normal troponin values (on admission to the ED and 6 hours later) are very reassuring and may allow low-risk patients to be discharged safely from the ED, with appropriate follow-up.

Recent research indicates that 'accelerated diagnostic protocols' can allow more rapid assessment of chest pain patients, and safely distinguish between patients who may be safely discharged home and those who require further investigation. The ADAPT trial showed that low-risk patients could be safely identified with a two-hour protocol and discharged from the ED for outpatient follow-up.

Other causes for an elevated troponin include sepsis, acute pulmonary embolism, renal impairment and severe exacerbation of COPD. Some patients have persistent mild elevations of troponin, particularly if the high sensitivity tests are used. In this setting the clinician should look for the diagnostic rise and fall of an acute process superimposed on the baseline troponin elevation.

Remember that chest pain can still be of cardiac origin despite a negative troponin, although the risk of an adverse outcome in this setting is less. If clinical suspicion remains, the safe approach is to keep the patient for further observation and appropriate consultation.

D-dimer may be used as a screening test in patients with suspected pulmonary embolism, but should be combined with pre-test assessment of the risk of pulmonary embolism (Wells or Geneva score). Many other common disease processes cause an elevation in D-dimer (recent surgery, malignancy, infection, pregnancy) and the result of a D-dimer test needs to be placed in the clinical context before imaging tests are ordered, or a decision is made on patient disposition.

Other tests

A **chest X-ray** is a simple and important test in patients presenting with chest pain. As well as identifying pulmonary pathology, cardiomegaly and pulmonary venous congestion may also be found in patients with acute ischaemic syndromes.

Bedside **echocardiography** can be very helpful in the assessment of acute chest pain. Ultrasound machines are available in many EDs and many emergency doctors are now skilled in echocardiography. Detection of left ventricular wall motion abnormalities strongly suggests important ischaemia or previous infarction. Echocardiography may also detect pericardial effusion, aortic dilation or even dissection, although transoesophageal echocardiography (TOE) is far superior for aortic abnormalities.

Some EDs have access to facilities for **early stress testing**. Patients presenting with chest pain who have negative troponins and non-diagnostic ECGs may undergo an exercise stress test with or without nuclear medicine myocardial perfusion scanning. Negative results improve the probability that the cause of the chest pain is not ischaemic. The role of early stress testing is still being evaluated.

CT scanning is under investigation as a modality to assess chest pain patients, and its role in the ED is still evolving. Coronary artery calcification on CT does correlate with atherosclerosis, and recent advances in technology with rapid, multislice CT coronary angiograms can accurately demonstrate coronary lesions. Studies suggest that a negative CT coronary angiogram can be used to identify low-risk patients who can be safely discharged from the ED. CT pulmonary angiography is a very specific test which is widely used to confirm pulmonary embolism. A CT of the chest with contrast is indicated for suspected thoracic aortic dissection.

DISPOSITION

Figure 10.1 summarises an integrated approach to the work-up and disposition of the chest pain patient. A combination of symptoms, examination findings, ECG results and cardiac markers often allows a precise diagnosis in many patients. Perhaps even more importantly, the risk of adverse outcomes can be assessed. High-risk features

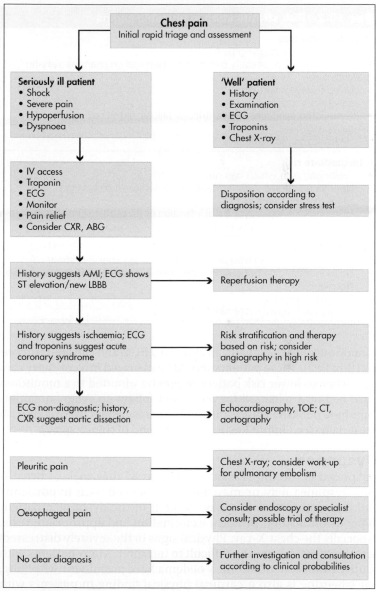

Figure 10.1 Chest pain algorithm

Box 10.2   Risk stratification in unstable angina

High-risk features
- Prolonged and ongoing pain
- ECG changes, especially dynamic ST depression changes varying with pain
- Deep T wave inversion
- Elevated troponin
- Associated syncope, left ventricular failure, mitral regurgitation or gallop rhythm
- Haemodynamic instability

Intermediate risk
- Prolonged pain which has now resolved
- New-onset angina with limitation of activities of daily living
- More than 65 years old
- History of previous myocardial infarction or revascularisation procedure
- ECG normal or old Q waves, or minor ST/T changes only

Low-risk features
- Angina of increased frequency, severity or at lower threshold
- New-onset angina beginning more than 2 weeks before presentation
- Normal ECG
- Negative troponin
- No high or intermediate risk features

---

include ongoing chest pain, an abnormal ECG and elevated troponins (Box 10.2). These patients should be managed in a coronary care unit, whereas lower risk patients might be admitted to a monitored ward bed or discharged for outpatient follow-up. Many organisations have published guidelines for the management of patients with chest pain (see Online Resources at the end of this chapter).

Dyspnoea

Dyspnoea is the unpleasant awareness of the work of breathing. Dyspnoea may or may not be associated with hypoxaemia and tachypnoea. Accurate assessment of the dyspnoeic patient depends on history, physical examination and appropriate tests, especially the chest X-ray. Physical signs in the severely distressed, breathless patient may be difficult to interpret. Many patients with acute cardiogenic pulmonary oedema have prominent wheezing, but wheezing is also a cardinal physical finding in patients with airflow obstruction.

HISTORY

Important points in the history include:

- previous cardiorespiratory disease, and previous best exercise capacity
- paroxysmal nocturnal dyspnoea—seen in both asthma and left ventricular failure (LVF)
- orthopnoea—more specific for LVF
- cough and sputum production, and features such as fever or upper respiratory tract infection
- peripheral oedema
- history of atopy
- medications, especially a history of use of cardiac medications or bronchodilators
- risk factors for DVT
- smoking.

PHYSICAL EXAMINATION

An immediate assessment is necessary to differentiate the critically ill patient from those who are less sick. Look for the following.

1 General appearance: diaphoresis, depressed level of consciousness, extreme respiratory distress and efficacy of ventilatory effort. Immediate ventilatory support may be necessary.

2 The presence of stridor, an important clue in the diagnosis of upper airway obstruction.

3 Vital signs including respiratory rate, heart rate and oximetry. Pulsus paradoxus may be present in severe airflow obstruction.

4 Cardiac examination. The presence of a 3rd heart sound (gallop rhythm) and a raised jugular venous pressure are very suggestive of heart failure.

5 Respiratory examination. Important points include symmetry of chest movement, the presence of subcutaneous emphysema and focal signs in the chest.

THE CHEST X-RAY (CXR)

Examination of a CXR is crucial in the assessment of the seriously ill patient with dyspnoea. Figure 10.2 summarises the interpretation of the CXR in the breathless patient. Recall that portable CXR

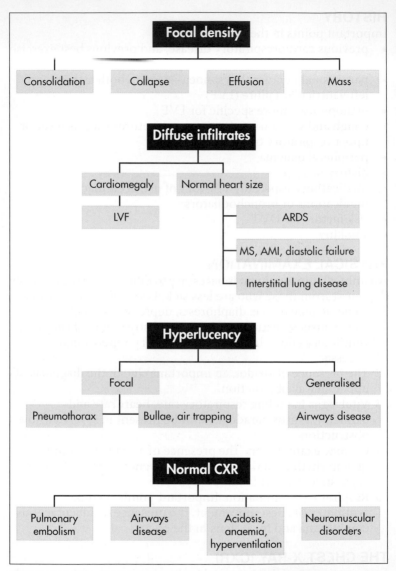

Figure 10.2 Chest X-ray interpretation in the breathless patient
AMI = acute myocardial infarction; ARDS = acute respiratory distress
syndrome; LVF = left ventricular failure; MS = mitral stenosis

machines have inherent technical limitations, in particular making assessment of heart size difficult.

OTHER TESTS

1 Arterial blood gases (ABGs). Indicated in all dyspnoeic patients to quantify the degree of hypoxaemia and demonstrate the presence of hypercarbia and acid–base abnormalities. A widened alveolar–arterial gradient may be a clue to subtle disorders such as pulmonary embolism; however, blood gas patterns are not specific for any disorder but do reflect the severity of the disease process.

2 ECG.

3 Spirometry. In patients who can cooperate, spirometry can diagnose and quantify airflow obstruction. Most modern electronic spirometers can display a flow–volume loop which can be helpful in the diagnosis of upper airway obstruction.

4 D-dimer. When combined with a clinical assessment of pre-test probability (e.g. using the Wells criteria), D-dimer can be helpful in the assessment of possible pulmonary embolism. A negative test in a patient with low pre-test probability makes pulmonary embolism unlikely. A positive test is non-specific.

5 Imaging tests for pulmonary embolism. **CT pulmonary angiography** is a very specific test which is used to confirm pulmonary embolism. A significant dose of iodine-containing IV contrast is necessary and thus the test may be contraindicated in some patients, particularly those with significant renal impairment. **Nuclear medicine ventilation–perfusion lung scanning** is also valuable in the diagnosis of suspected pulmonary embolism. Local availability may dictate which of these tests is used. Both tests are associated with significant radiation exposure. Many EDs use protocols to select patients, based on pre-test probability and D-dimer, to limit inappropriate use of these expensive scans. **Doppler ultrasound** is useful in the diagnosis of a deep venous thrombosis where pulmonary embolism is suspected, and other forms of imaging may not be appropriate.

6 Echocardiography. This can be very helpful in the acutely breathless patient; important information about left and right ventricular size and function, the presence of a pericardial

effusion and important valvular disease can be quickly assessed.

7 Other blood tests may be helpful in selected patients. A full blood count provides crucial information which can rule out anaemia as a cause for dyspnoea, and an elevated white cell count supports an inflammatory or infective basis for the patient's presentation.

DISPOSITION AND MANAGEMENT

Disposition and management depend on the underlying cause. Hypoxaemia should be treated with appropriate oxygen therapy, aiming to achieve adequate oxygen saturation as measured with pulse oximetry. Carbon dioxide narcosis should be suspected in the seriously ill dyspnoeic patient with a depressed level of consciousness, and careful titration of oxygen therapy based on serial arterial blood gases may be necessary. Target ranges for oxygen saturation may need to be modified in these patients (88–92%). Non-invasive ventilation should be considered early in the distressed patient with impaired gas exchange.

Haemoptysis

(See also Chapter 14 Haemoptysis.)

Haemoptysis is defined as the coughing of blood from the respiratory tract. Usually it is clear that the blood is coming from the respiratory tract, as the patient describes an associated cough. Sometimes differentiation from haematemesis is difficult, and blood loss from the upper airway, particularly the nose, may be difficult to exclude.

Most haemoptysis is **minor**, and should prompt a search for the cause, usually starting with a CXR. In a stable patient with minor haemoptysis, investigations may be commenced in the ED and continued as an outpatient.

Large-volume haemoptysis is life-threatening and frightening. It is often difficult for the patient to estimate the volume of blood loss. Guidelines suggest that 300–600 mL of blood expectorated in 24 hours constitutes massive haemoptysis. The immediate threat is not hypovolaemia, but hypoxaemia related to blood in the airways and lung parenchyma (the estimated volume of the airways is 100–200 mL).

CAUSES OF HAEMOPTYSIS

- Cancer. This should always be suspected in a patient with a history of smoking. A clear CXR does not rule out cancer but makes the diagnosis less likely; bronchoscopy is indicated in this setting. Massive haemoptysis is unusual in malignancy.
- Bronchiectasis. Massive bleeding can occur from abnormally dilated bronchial arteries in patients with longstanding bronchiectasis.
- Infections, particularly tuberculosis and other cavitary lung diseases. Old cavitary lung disease may be complicated by fungal colonisation (mycetoma), which is frequently associated with haemoptysis. Simple bronchitis may be associated with minor haemoptysis.
- Vascular disorders. Pulmonary embolism, mitral stenosis, arteriovenous malformations and aneurysms are all associated with haemoptysis of varying severity.
- Vasculitis. Systemic lupus erythematosus, Goodpasture's syndrome, granulomatosis with polyangiitis (formerly known as Wegener's granulomatosis) and other pulmonary vasculitides are associated with repeated haemoptysis, pulmonary parenchymal haemorrhage and an aggressive course. Often there is associated renal disease.
- Previous aortic surgery for coarctation can be associated with aorto-bronchial fistulas which can produce massive haemoptysis.
- Other causes include anticoagulant therapy, coagulopathy and trauma.

In Australia the commoner causes of massive haemoptysis are old cavitary lung disease, bronchiectasis and pulmonary vasculitis.

MANAGEMENT OF MASSIVE HAEMOPTYSIS

Massive haemoptysis is a serious emergency which usually requires a multidisciplinary team. Important early steps include the following.

1 Assess oxygenation and the airway—urgent intubation may be necessary.
2 Arterial blood gases and appropriate oxygen therapy.
3 IV access and appropriate volume replacement.
4 Full blood count, cross-match and coagulation screen.

5 Urgent chest X-ray.
6 If there is unilateral disease and the affected side is known, nurse with the diseased lung down, to protect the healthy lung.
7 Bronchoscopy. This should be done with appropriate anaesthetic support; sometimes rigid bronchoscopy is necessary to provide better suction and maintenance of airway patency.
8 CT scan.
9 Urgent consultation with a thoracic surgeon and an interventional radiologist.

Definitive management depends on the cause. Options include bronchoscopic techniques to control bleeding, angiography with embolisation of feeding arteries and thoracotomy with resection.

LESSER DEGREES OF HAEMOPTYSIS

Management depends on the cause, based on history, risk of malignancy and CXR. If admission is not indicated, appropriate follow-up, perhaps for bronchoscopy, should be arranged.

Recommended readings

Backus BE, Six AJ, Kelder JC. Chest pain in the emergency room: a multicentre validation of the HEART score. Crit Pathw Cardiol 2010;9(3):164–169.

Chew DP, Scott IA, Cullen L et al. National Heart Foundation of Australia and Cardiac Society of Australia and New Zealand: Australian clinical guidelines for the management of acute coronary syndromes (2016). Med J Aust 2016;205(3):128–133.

Chunilal SD, et al. (2003). Does this patient have pulmonary embolism? JAMA 2003;290:2849–2858.

Cullen L, Greenslade JH, Hawkins T et al. (2017). Improved assessment of Chest pain Trial (IMPACT): assessing patients with possible acute coronary syndromes. Med J Aust 2017;207(5):195–200.

Mehta, L. et al. Acute Myocardial Infarction in Women: A Scientific Statement from the American Heart Association. Circulation 2016, March;133(9):916.

Nazenian P, Mueller C, de Matos Soeiro A et al. (2017). Diagnostic accuracy of the Aortic Dissection Risk score plus D-dimer for acute aortic syndromes (the ADviSED Prospective Multicentre Study). Circulation 2017 doi:10.1161/CIRCULATIONAHA.117.029457

Parsonage WA, Milburn T, Ashover S et al. (2017). Implementing change: evaluating the Accelerated Chest pain Risk Evaluation (ACRE) project. Med J Aust 2017;207(5):201–205.

Pope JH, Aufderheide TP, Ruthauser R et al. Missed diagnosis of acute cardiac ischemia in the emergency department. N Engl Med 2000; 342:1163–70.

Sakr L, Dutau H. Massive haemoptysis: an update on the role of bronchoscopy in diagnosis and management. Respiration 2010;80:30–58.

Than M, Cullen L, Aldous et al. 2-hour accelerated diagnostic protocol to assess patients with chest pain symptoms using the contemporary troponins as the only biomarker (ADAPT). J Am Coll Cardiol 2012;59:2091–2098.

Wells PS, Anderson DR, Rodger M et al. Excluding pulmonary embolism at the bedside without imaging: management of patients with suspected pulmonary embolism presenting to the emergency department by using a simple clinical model and D-dimer. Ann Intern Med 2001;135:98–107.

Chapter 11
Acute coronary syndromes

Kevin Maruno

Acknowledgment

The author wishes to acknowledge the content used from the previous edition of *Emergency Medicine* which was provided by Paul Preisz.

Assessing patients who may have an acute coronary syndrome (ACS) is a frequent and important part of the work performed in an ED. Patients most often present with 'typical' chest pain, dyspnoea, palpitations, syncope or pre-syncope. Some patients (particularly the elderly, diabetic or renal failure patients) may have atypical pain, or no pain, or just vague non-specific symptoms such as lethargy or deterioration in daily function. It is important to consider all presentations of an ACS, while also taking into consideration other life-threatening conditions.

Although many units now use a protocol approach, important alternative conditions need to be rapidly diagnosed. Some of these conditions may be immediately life-threatening, such as pulmonary embolism, aortic dissection, pneumothorax or severe pancreatitis, while others may be investigated and managed over time as an inpatient (e.g. pneumonia, cholelithiasis) or outpatient (e.g. musculoskeletal pain, gastro-oesophageal reflux disease). Alternative cardiac diagnoses (e.g. pericarditis) and non-cardiac diagnoses (e.g. peptic ulcer disease) as well as cardiac injury secondary to other illness (e.g. sepsis) should all be considered.

The acute coronary syndromes typically seen in the ED consist of the ST-elevation myocardial infarctions (STEMIs) and the second and larger group, non-ST-elevation acute coronary syndromes (NSTEACSs). NSTEACSs are then risk-stratified based on short-term prognosis as *high-risk*, *intermediate-risk* and *low-risk ACS* (Box 11.1).

Box 11.1	**Initial patient assessment and stratification**
STEACS ST-elevation acute coronary syndrome usually referred to as STEMI (ST-elevation myocardial injury)	**NSTEACS** Non-ST-elevation acute coronary syndrome Stratify: • high risk • intermediate risk • low risk

Editorial Comment

STEACS and NSTEACS are equal terms for STEMI and non-STEMI in this chapter.

Safe assessment

The patient should be assessed in a safe environment. Symptoms and signs which may indicate an ACS need to be identified as soon as possible so that treatment can be initiated to avoid or minimise myocardial damage and to avert the risk of life-threatening complications. A defibrillator must be immediately available with staff trained in its use.

• Assign a high priority at triage to patients who may have an ACS.
• Provide ECG monitoring and supplemental oxygen (if SaO_2 is less than 93% on room air) and insert an IV cannula as soon as possible.
• Send blood samples for testing and provide analgesia (nitrates and/or morphine) and, unless contraindicated, give oral aspirin (300 mg).
• An ECG should be performed and reviewed on presentation (within 10 minutes of arrival) to look for arrhythmias and for diagnostic changes related to acute coronary artery occlusion, most importantly **STEMI**. If no STEMI is present, then **NSTEAC** and alternative diagnoses are considered.

A patient presenting with acute chest pain or other symptoms suggestive of an ACS should receive care guided by an evidence-based Suspected ACS Assessment Protocol or pathway (see Figure 11.1).

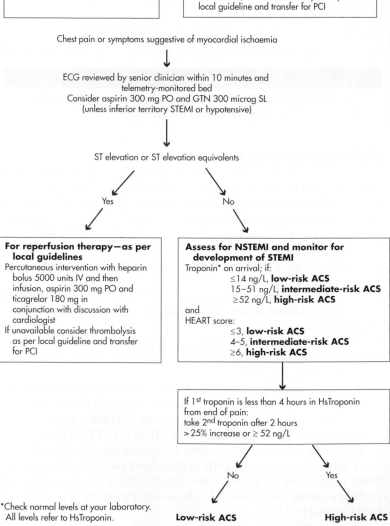

Key questions to ask yourself are:
Does this patient have a STEMI?
Does this patient have a NSTEMI?
Does this patient have an intermediate or high risk of MACE in 30 days?

For reperfusion therapy: as per local guidelines
Percutaneous injection with heparin bolus 5000 units IV and then infusion, aspirin 300 mg PO and ticagrelor 180 mg in conjunction with discussion with cardiologist
If unavailable, consider thrombolysis as per local guideline and transfer for PCI

Chest pain or symptoms suggestive of myocardial ischaemia

ECG reviewed by senior clinician within 10 minutes and telemetry-monitored bed
Consider aspirin 300 mg PO and GTN 300 microg SL (unless inferior territory STEMI or hypotensive)

ST elevation or ST elevation equivalents

Yes

No

For reperfusion therapy—as per local guidelines
Percutaneous intervention with heparin bolus 5000 units IV and then infusion, aspirin 300 mg PO and ticagrelor 180 mg in conjunction with discussion with cardiologist
If unavailable consider thrombolysis as per local guideline and transfer for PCI

Assess for NSTEMI and monitor for development of STEMI
Troponin* on arrival; if:
  ≤14 ng/L, **low-risk ACS**
  15–51 ng/L, **intermediate-risk ACS**
  ≥52 ng/L, **high-risk ACS**
and
HEART score:
  ≤3, **low-risk ACS**
  4–5, **intermediate-risk ACS**
  ≥6, **high-risk ACS**

If 1st troponin is less than 4 hours in HsTroponin from end of pain:
take 2nd troponin after 2 hours
> 25% increase or ≥ 52 ng/L

No

Yes

*Check normal levels at your laboratory.
All levels refer to HsTroponin.

Low-risk ACS

High-risk ACS

Figure 11.1 Chest pain pathway

DIAGNOSING ACUTE CORONARY SYNDROMES
History and examination
Typical presentations of ACS involve chest discomfort at rest or for prolonged periods (prolonged is defined as > 10 minutes, not relieved by sublingual nitrates) or recurrent chest discomfort or discomfort associated with syncope or acute heart failure.

Some important points of immediate history include the time of onset of pain, the character or quality of the pain, exertion-related pain and associated symptoms such as diaphoresis, nausea and sweating. Radiation of pain to arms, jaw and shoulder is particularly suggestive.

Risk factors and comorbidities, allergies and contraindications to treatments should also be documented. The main cardiac risk factors include diabetes, hypertension, hyperlipidaemia, smoking, chronic renal disease and family history of premature heart disease. Note that although cardiac risk factors increase the likelihood of disease (particularly in those under 40 years of age), their absence does not exclude the diagnoses. Patients of Aboriginal descent are particularly at risk.

Physical examination is directed towards identifying signs of complications and comorbidities of ACS and finding alternative diagnoses. There may be tachycardia or bradycardia, hyper- or hypotension, sweating, nausea or evidence of heart failure (dyspnoea, basal crepitations, 3rd heart sound, poor peripheral perfusion). **Importantly, there may be no specific physical findings in many patients with ACS.**

Cardiac myonecrosis is demonstrated by increased levels of cardiac biomarkers (such as troponins), and can occur in ACS with or without ECG changes. The testing interval to 'rule out' myocardial infarction may be reduced using an accelerated diagnostic strategy such as the ADAPT or HEART protocols. This combines a risk score, negative ECGs and serial troponins to exclude major short-term cardiac events to enable outpatient care.

The indication for initial urgent reperfusion therapy is clinical presentation consistent with ACS and acute ECG change. This is defined as persistent ST-segment elevation of ≥ 1 mm in two contiguous limb leads, ST-segment elevation of ≥ 2 mm in two contiguous chest leads or new left bundle branch block (LBBB) pattern.

Investigation

Initial investigation

When STEMI is diagnosed on clinical and ECG criteria, revascularisation therapy is time-critical so there should be no delays waiting for investigations prior to revascularisation. In other circumstances, the tests shown in Table 11.1 should be obtained.

Table 11.1   Tests to aid in the diagnosis and stratification of patients with ACS*

Test	Comment
Full blood count	• Anaemia or polycythaemia may need treatment, baseline platelet count (particularly if heparin is to be used)
Coagulation PT and APTT	• Guides anticoagulant therapy
Serum chemistry	• Hypokalaemia increases the risk of arrhythmia • Hypomagnesaemia may be present if patient taking some diuretics or has liver/renal disease
Renal function	• Creatinine (and eGFR calculation); kidney disease is a risk factor for high- and intermediate-risk ACS • Drug dosage may require adjustment if renal impairment present (e.g. heparin, sotalol)
Troponin I or T**	• May take hours to rise, two or more measurements over time may be required (delta change); remains elevated 5–14 days • Some high-sensitivity assays may be interpreted in as little as 4 hours from the onset of pain
Serum lipids	• Initiating treatment of hyperlipidaemia within the first few days (e.g. with statins) may be required

Table 11.1   Tests to aid in the diagnosis and stratification of patients with ACS (cont.)

Test	Comment
Blood glucose	• Diabetes may be undiagnosed (especially mild NIDDM); control of high blood glucose levels may improve outcomes
Chest X-ray (CXR)	• May show heart failure, cardiomegaly • Do not delay urgent treatment to obtain a CXR • Do not send potentially unstable patient out of resuscitation monitoring area for CXR

APTT = activated partial thromboplastin time; eGFR = estimated glomerular filtration rate; NIDDM, non-insulin-dependent diabetes mellitus; PT = prothrombin time.
*Additional tests such as high-sensitivity C-reactive protein (CRP) and B-type natriuretic protein (BNP) or Pro-BNP are still being evaluated. In some settings bedside cardiac echocardiography can be valuable as it may be able to provide information on wall motion (myocardial ischaemia or infarction), ejection fraction (heart failure, systolic or diastolic dysfunction), valvular disease (aortic stenosis, acute mitral valve chordae disruption), free wall rupture, aortic or pericardial disease. An alternative diagnosis of pulmonary embolism can sometimes be made when significant right heart abnormality is seen on echo. Drug screening (cocaine, amphetamines) may be relevant.
**Elevated or rising troponin T and I measurements indicate myocardial damage and are predictors of increased risk of cardiac mortality. It may take several hours for troponin levels to rise and a series of tests may be required. Troponin may sometimes also be elevated in patients with heart failure, tachycardia, myocarditis, pericarditis, renal failure or other non-ischaemic cardiac injury.

Management of STEMI

1 **Patients presenting within 12 hours with STEMI should have urgent time-critical reperfusion** (PCI or fibrinolysis)
   — When percutaneous coronary intervention (PCI) can be commenced without undue delay, this is the treatment of choice based on current evidence. The maximum acceptable delay is 90 minutes from first medical contact with symptom onset < 120 minutes, or 60 minutes if within 1 hour of symptom onset.
   — The benefits of PCI over thrombolysis are still present up to 12 hours after the onset of symptoms if PCI can be performed within 2 hours. Late presentation after symptom onset (> 4 hours), primary PCI is preferred due to lower efficacy with fibrinolytic therapy.

— PCI is also the preferred treatment for *unstable patients* or those with *ongoing symptoms* or evidence of *failed fibrinolytic therapy* on ECG (i.e. 'rescue PCI'). This is seen as persistent (> 50% of initial) ST elevation 90 minutes after administration of the agent. Fibrinolysis can be repeated if PCI is not available; however, benefit may be gained from early routine PCI regardless of success of pharmacological reperfusion.

— Early coronary artery bypass graft (CABG) surgery may also be considered for some patients, especially if they have anatomy that is unsuitable for stenting or have associated cardiogenic shock, valve injury or other structural complications.

— Patients who decline PCI or have contrast allergy or other contraindications to PCI should be considered for fibrinolysis. Fibrin-specific bolus agents such as tenecteplase or reteplase are now the usual choices, although streptokinase can be used unless the patient is an Indigenous Australian or Torres Strait Islander or has received streptokinase before.

— Contraindications to fibrinolysis are given below.

2 **Give anti-platelet drugs + antithrombotic drug**
Anti-platelet drugs

— Give aspirin and a second antiplatelet drug such as clopidogrel.

— The use of a potent oral antiplatelet agent (e.g. prasugrel or ticagrelor) should be considered as an alternative to clopidogrel for subgroups at high risk of recurrent ischaemic events (e.g. those with diabetes, stent thrombosis, recurrent events on clopidogrel or a high burden of disease on angiography). This may be less appropriate in patients at increased risk of bleeding (e.g. those aged > 75, those with prior stroke or transient ischaemic attack [TIA] and those with low bodyweight).

— Glycoprotein IIb/IIIa inhibitors (e.g. abciximab) are of most benefit in patients undergoing PCI, and can be considered during PCI in those with high-risk angiographic features, or ongoing ischaemia with standard medical treatment and undue delay to PCI.

— *Note*: Patients who have been given clopidogrel can still have urgent CABG surgery although this is not ideal.

3 **Antithrombotic drugs**

— Give heparin as unfractionated IV heparin or subcutaneous enoxaparin (but avoid changing from one to the other).

— Patients having fibrinolysis should also receive antithrombotics (this is optional if the fibrinolytic used is streptokinase).

— Among patients with STEMI undergoing primary PCI, the use of bivalirudin can be considered as an alternative to heparin and glycoprotein IIb/IIIa inhibitors.

Additional treatment in STEMI are shown in Table 11.2.

Table 11.2   Additional treatment in STEMI

Therapy	Dose	Comments
Oxygen	6 L (non-rebreather)	• All patients when SaO_2 < 94% (room air) • Issues (uncommon) with patients retaining CO_2
Aspirin	300 mg PO (soluble or rapidly absorbable)	• True allergy may contraindicate
Nitrates	Sublingual or spray or titrated IV	• Headache, flushing, hypotension may occur with higher doses
Morphine	2.5–5.0 mg IV increments	• Nausea, decreased LOC and ventilation, hypotension
Metoprolol	25 mg PO	• Asthma, bradycardia, heart block, other side effects and contraindications
Clopidogrel or Ticagrelor	600 mg PO loading 180 mg PO	• Increased bleeding risk • Increased risk of bleeding, dyspnoea, bradycardia
Heparin	Low-molecular-weight or unfractionated protocols	• Bleeding risk, HITS

Continued

Table 11.2   Additional treatment in STEMI (cont.)

Therapy	Dose	Comments
Tencotoplase	Single dose based on body weight; 5 mg = 1000 IU < 60 kg: 30 mg 60–69 kg: 35 mg 70–79 kg: 40 mg 80–89 kg: 45 mg ≥ 90 kg: 50 mg	• Bolus dosing over 5 seconds
Abciximab	IV protocol	• Not with fibrinolytics (or at least reduce dose), in select cases only
Frusemide	40–80 mg IV	• Used when LVF present • Higher doses needed if renal impairment present

HITS = heparin-induced thrombocytopenia syndrome; LVF = left ventricular failure; LOC = level of consciousness

CONTRAINDICATIONS TO FIBRINOLYSIS

• **Absolute**: acute haemorrhage is likely to cause death or severe disability
   — *Current*:
      ○ Significant uncontrollable bleeding or major bleeding diathesis
      ○ Suspected aortic dissection
   — *Past history*:
      ○ Any past proven intracranial haemorrhage
      ○ Known structural cerebral vascular lesion
      ○ Intracranial neoplasm
      ○ Major head injury within the past 3 months
      ○ Ischaemic stroke within the past 3 months
• **Relative**: clinical judgment is required to gauge the relative risk, particularly if the alternative of PCI may be possible, even with some delay
   — *Current*:
      ○ Pregnancy
      ○ Anticoagulant therapy

- ○ Non-compressible vessel puncture
- ○ Prolonged traumatic CPR
- ○ Active peptic ulcer
- ○ Uncontrollable hypertension (systolic pressure > 180 mmHg or diastolic pressure > 110 mmHg)
- ○ Major surgery within the past 3 weeks
- ○ Significant internal bleeding within the past 4 weeks
— *Past history*:
  - ○ Ischaemic stroke more than 3 months ago, dementia, other intracranial abnormality that is not an absolute contraindication
  - ○ Long-term poorly controlled hypertension

Editorial Comment

In general, after initial high-flow oxygen therapy further oxygen is dictated to maintain the oxygenation (SaO_2 > 90%) while avoiding further hyperoxia exposure.

ADJUNCTIVE TREATMENTS IN ACS

Reperfusion confers outcome benefit, particularly the combination of aspirin and PCI or fibrinolysis. Additional therapies also convey incremental improvement, although this is not as marked and will add to the risk of adverse events. Consider methods to reduce bleeding risk (e.g. titrate antithrombotic agents to optimal dose for weight and renal function).

Stratifying ACS without diagnostic STEMI ECG changes: NSTEACS patients

Risk stratification is essential to guide investigations and subsequent management in NSTEACS. History, examination and investigation features direct stratification, and management based on risk group should proceed rapidly with early involvement of senior staff. Use of an evidence-based accelerated diagnostic pathway can assist in estimating both ACS-related morbidity and mortality while reducing unnecessary investigations and therapies in low-risk patients.

Management of NSTEACS
FOR ALL PATIENTS WITH NSTEACS

- Risk should be stratified as HIGH-, INTERMEDIATE- or LOW-risk ACS.
- Initially give aspirin unless contraindicated.
- All patients are treated with analgesia (nitrates, morphine) as required and oxygen to keep $SaO_2 \geq 94\%$.

HIGH-RISK ACS PATIENTS

1 Dual anti-platelet drugs (e.g. aspirin plus clopidogrel).
2 Antithrombotic drugs (e.g. unfractionated heparin or subcutaneous enoxaparin).
3 Beta-blockers should be given unless contraindicated.
4 Arrangements should be made for admission and coronary angiography except in those with severe comorbidities.

INTERMEDIATE-RISK ACS PATIENTS

1 Anti-platelet drugs (e.g. aspirin alone).
2 Accelerated diagnostic evaluation either as an inpatient or, if considered medically safe and logistically possible, as an outpatient within 72 hours. Diagnostic and provocation tests include CTCA (CT coronary angiography), stress echo, nuclear perfusion scans (sestamibi) and exercise stress tests.

LOW-RISK ACS PATIENTS

After an appropriate period of observation and assessment, may be discharged for outpatient follow up if negative biomarkers, no high-risk ECG changes and resolved pain.

Additional management (STEMI and NSTEACS)

- Optimise the heart rate. Significant bradycardia or tachycardia—associated with poor cardiac output (e.g. hypotension, syncope/pre-syncope heart failure or oliguria)—requires treatment with appropriate antiarrhythmics or pacing.
- Analgesia with nitrates and/or morphine should be provided as needed.

- Hypotension may require careful IV fluid volume optimisation, titration of therapeutic drugs and, in some patients, inotropes. Hypertension may resolve with analgesia or beta-blockers when appropriate but, rarely, if unresponsive consider potent agents (diazoxide, sodium nitroprusside) with close monitoring.
- Treat heart failure, if present, with nitrates and other standard therapy (BiPAP) +/− diuretics.
- Medical therapy (usually a statin) is now recommended for most patients with ischaemic heart disease unless contraindicated.
- If being discharged, ensure patients diagnosed with ACS have begun an appropriate medication regimen, including aspirin (with clopidogrel in some patients), a beta-blocker, ACE inhibitor, statin and/or other treatment as required.
- Provide patients with support and advice to address the risk factors at a suitable time. A chest pain management plan is often appropriate. For all patients and their families, consider the level of social support and provide assistance for those at risk through referral to cardiac, rehabilitation and other services (e.g. social work, drug and alcohol misuse clinic). Consider patient support groups.

Cocaine-induced chest pain

Although only a minority of patients (less than 6%) with chest pain associated with cocaine use will have proven cardiac myonecrosis, cocaine (a vasoconstrictor) has multiple effects that can contribute to the development of myocardial ischaemia hours or days after ingestion. Even small doses have been associated with vasoconstriction of coronary arteries, which may be more accentuated in patients with pre-existing coronary artery disease. Cocaine users have been shown to have accelerated atherosclerosis as well as elevated levels of CRP, von Willebrand factor and fibrinogen. Anterior and inferior infarctions are equally likely and most are non-Q wave. Initial typical ischaemic ECG changes are relatively uncommon. In general, beta-blockers should be avoided in these patients and benzodiazepines are often used. Mortality overall is relatively low.

Patient transfer

Patients in a facility without specialist cardiology services and PCI facilities who have been diagnosed with STEMI and treated with fibrinolysis should be transferred to an appropriate tertiary cardiology unit. Those with a large area of at-risk myocardium, poor left ventricular function or renal failure should be transferred urgently. Adjunctive reperfusion therapies should be commenced before transfer.

Chapter 12
Clinical electrocardiography and arrhythmia management

Kevin Maruno

Acknowledgment

The authors wish to acknowledge the content used from the previous edition of *Emergency Medicine* which was provided by Allen Yuen, Carmel Crock and Paul Preisz.

This chapter examines the clinical use of the ECG, one of the most important diagnostic tools in an ED. It must be stressed, however, that the ECG may appear normal, even in the presence of severe cardiac disease.

The reader should have knowledge of basic cardiac electrophysiology and anatomy, which will help in diagnosing and localising lesions from the ECG.

Indications

ECGs are indicated:
- early, to assist in diagnosis and treatment of potentially life-threatening disorders
- routinely, as part of cardiac assessment.

They should be performed in all cases of chest pain, upper abdominal pain, dyspnoea, collapse, post-arrest, palpitations, syncope, dizziness, loss of consciousness and shock; also in any patient with a history of hypertension, fluid or electrolyte imbalance, drug overdose or other conditions that may affect the heart.

ECG interpretation

This is most usefully done in the context of the presenting symptoms and signs, which fall into three main groups:

1 chest and upper abdominal pain, dyspnoea, shock
2 collapse, palpitations, syncope, dizziness, altered consciousness

3 electrolyte disturbances, drug overdose, environmental emergencies.

The ECG should be examined for rate, rhythm, axis, P wave, PR interval, QRS morphology, ST–T segment, T wave and QT interval.

With chest pain, particular attention is paid to the ST–T segment and Q waves. The underlying lesions may be determined by ECG pattern recognition. It is useful to have a previous ECG for comparison, since any changes will have more significance.

1 CHEST AND UPPER ABDOMINAL PAIN, DYSPNOEA, SHOCK

History and examination are the mainstays of assessment, with the ECG playing a complementary role. The main conditions requiring early diagnosis are acute myocardial infarction (AMI), unstable angina, aortic dissection and pulmonary embolism (PE).

Myocardial infarction

Note that the initial ECG may be normal in about half of patients with AMI.

The earliest change is ST elevation, which may occur within 30 minutes of onset of pain, and is the basis upon which a decision regarding thrombolysis or angioplasty is made.

ST elevation

- ST elevation $\geq$ 1 mm in I and aVL suggests a lateral AMI (Figure 12.1), usually due to occlusion of branches of the circumflex or left axis deviation (LAD) arteries.
- ST elevation $\geq$ 1 mm in II, III and aVF suggests inferior AMI, usually due to occlusion of the right coronary artery; in some cases, the left coronary system may be the site of occlusion, if the left coronary artery (LCA) is 'dominant'.
- ST elevation $\geq$ 2 mm in chest leads suggests anterior or anteroseptal (if only in V_1–V_3) AMI, which occurs with occlusion of the left main coronary or its branches.

If a coronary thrombus is treated early with thrombolysis or angioplasty, the ST elevation can regress and further myocardial damage may be prevented. It is therefore vital that the diagnosis is made rapidly so that reperfusion can occur urgently with

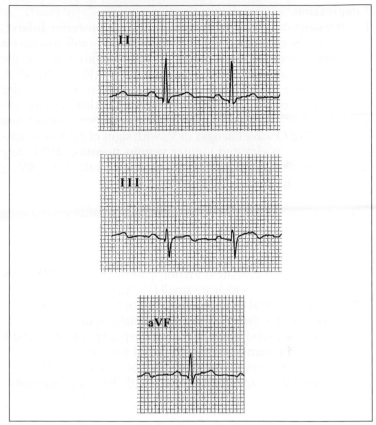

Figure 12.1 Inferior AMI, earliest changes: minimal ST elevation in leads II, III, aVF

cardiology involvement early. The diagnosis should be made on the basis of a concerning ischaemic history and the ST elevation in two concurrent leads prior to any blood results.

Normal 'high ST-take-off' in anterior chest leads can confuse the diagnosis when the chest pain is atypical, but it is better to err in suspecting an acute cardiac event than to clear the patient when in doubt. Consult with an emergency doctor, cardiologist or registrar.

ST depression

ST depression > 2 mm in V_1 may indicate a posterior infarct, and this may be confirmed in ECG leads $V_{7,8,9}$. $V_{1,2}$ will also have a prominent R wave and tall T waves. Posterior infarcts are usually caused by occlusion of the right coronary artery (RCA). The RCA also supplies the sinoatrial (SA) and atrioventricular (AV) nodes and the bundle of His. Occlusion of the RCA is therefore associated with potentially serious bradyarrhythmias.

Minor ST or Q wave changes in V_1 with signs of right ventricular failure, such as elevated jugular venous pressure (JVP), may point to a right ventricular infarct: right ventricular leads $RV_{3,4,5}$ may show characteristic ST elevation.

Q waves

- Q waves > 2 mm, > 40 ms follow in those leads showing ST elevation, if the infarct evolves (Table 12.1). They may appear within the first hour or, more commonly, within 2–6 hours (Figure 12.2). Differentiate from non-pathological septal Q waves in I, II, aVF or V_5, V_6, which are small (< 2 mm) and narrow.
- A non-pathological Q wave can occur in III; it is narrow, < 2 mm and less than one-third the height of the QRS complex, and may disappear during deep inspiration. A small Q wave in III is significant if associated with one in II.
- Sometimes Q waves do not develop, but AMI can still be suspected if there are small R waves with 'lack of progression

Table 12.1 Infarct localisation—the ECG pattern distribution (early ST elevation, later Q waves)—will help to localise the site of infarction, and the usual coronary artery occluded

ECG pattern distribution	Site	Infarct-related artery
I, aVL	Lateral	Circumflex
II, III, aVF	Inferior	Right coronary, circumflex
V_2–V_4	Anterior	Left anterior descending (LAD)
V_1, V_2 (large R, ↓ ST)	Posterior	Right coronary

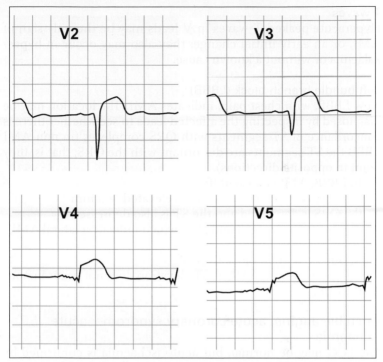

Figure 12.2 Anterior AMI, later changes: Q waves, prominent coved ST elevation V_2–V_5

of R waves' across the anterior leads (normally the R wave increases in amplitude from V_2 to V_4). These infarcts are often associated with inverted T waves.

- NSTEMIs refers to AMIs without any ST elevation. Blood should be sent for troponins on arrival of the patient with chest pain so that, where there is no ECG evidence of AMI, the diagnosis is not missed.

R wave

A prominent R wave in V_1, and often V_2, suggests a posterior infarct, as well as incomplete right bundle branch block (RBBB), right ventricular hypertrophy (RVH) or left accessory pathway.

T waves

Hyperacute peaked T waves in V leads may be the only sign of AMI, or an early initial change; they also may occur in hyperkalaemia or without a known cause.

Left bundle branch block (LBBB)

New LBBB, with chest pain, indicates AMI. The location may be diagnosed by inspecting the affected leads to see whether there is concordance of ST segments with QRS complexes (in non-AMI LBBB the ST segments are discordant with the QRS; that is, they point in opposite directions).

In LBBB, AMI is present if:

- the QRS is upright and the ST is elevated > 5 mm
- the QRS is depressed and the ST is also depressed
- there are Q waves in I and aVL, which indicate a lateral AMI.

Right bundle branch block (RBBB)

RBBB does not mask AMI, as ST elevation does not occur in non-AMI RBBB.

Unstable angina, acute coronary syndrome, acute ischaemia

The ECG may be normal, but acute ischaemia is confirmed by 2 mm or more ST depression in anterior or standard leads. This may be induced by exercise. If angina is prolonged greater than 20 minutes, then this can be regarded as pre-infarctional.

Left ventricular hypertrophy

- Left axis deviation
- S in V_2 + R in V_5 > 35 mm
- ST depression anterior chest leads (LV strain)

Pericarditis

- Extensive ST elevation, concave upwards
- PR depression

Myocarditis

Non-specific ST–T changes.

Aortic dissection

The ECG is non-specific, with associated hypertensive changes in the majority.

If the dissection involves the coronary ostia, resultant myocardial ischaemia or infarction may be seen, especially in the inferior leads. The cardiac surgeon should be notified urgently.

Pulmonary embolus (PE)

Over 40% of patients show no significant change; therefore, a normal ECG does *NOT* rule out a pulmonary embolus. ECG findings include:

- sinus tachycardia
- RBBB, usually partial
- R axis deviation
- $S_1Q_3T_3$ (acute cor pulmonale)
- ST elevation in aVR
- anterior T wave inversion V_1–V_4 (Figure 12.3); differentiate from the normal T-wave inversion found in some youths, athletes and African-American people in V_1–V_3.

Anticoagulation is indicated (see Chapter 16 Venous Thromboembolic Disease: Deep Venous Thrombosis and Pulmonary Embolism). Consult urgently for compromised patients following massive PE as they may need urgent thrombolysis or embolectomy.

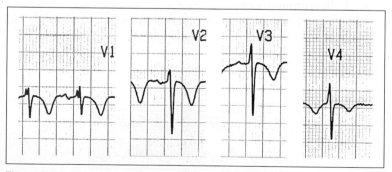

Figure 12.3 Acute pulmonary embolism: partial RBBB, inverted T waves V_1–V_4

2 COLLAPSE, PALPITATIONS, SYNCOPE, DIZZINESS, ALTERED CONSCIOUSNESS

The ECG can help to determine a cardiac cause.

AMI, acute ischaemia, unstable angina or acute coronary syndrome

These can cause syncope or coma as a result of vasovagal reaction, cardiogenic shock, tamponade or any of the following arrhythmias.

Ventricular asystole

Absence of any electrical activity with a 'flat' ECG is asystole requiring CPR and the use of adrenaline as part of advanced life support (ALS) guidelines.

Ensure that leads are attached and recording amplitude is correct, as low-voltage VF may be misinterpreted as asystole. Defibrillation should be tried, if there is any doubt.

Ventricular fibrillation (VF)

This grossly irregular and variable amplitude arrhythmia is easy to recognise (Figure 12.4), unless it is low in amplitude (fine VF), when it can be mistaken for asystole (if in doubt, treat as VF). It requires:

- immediate defibrillation beginning with 200 J biphasic or 360 J monophasic, with
  - CPR commencement
- adrenaline 1 mg IV, repeated every 3 minutes as required, and
- amiodarone 5 mg/kg or 300 mg bolus IV as the mainstays of drug therapy
- treatment of any of the causes.

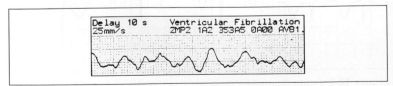

Figure 12.4 Ventricular fibrillation

Ventricular tachycardia (VT)

A wide-complex tachycardia represents VT (Figure 12.5) in over 90% of cases, approaching 100% in patients with prior AMI. If in doubt, treat as VT.

Most VT occurs in the setting of structural heart disease, usually ischaemic.

- Pulseless VT is treated as for VF with immediate (unsynchronised) defibrillation (200 J biphasic) with CPR and ALS.
- If the patient is unstable (chest pain, hypotension or acute pulmonary oedema), prompt synchronised electrical cardioversion at 150–200 J biphasic should be performed (once sedated).
- If the patient is not haemodynamically compromised, electrical or chemical cardioversion is warranted, often with cardiology advice. Drugs used may be lignocaine 1–1.5 mg/kg, procainamide 1 mg/kg or amiodarone 300 mg over 1 hour.

VT can occur in the absence of structural heart disease, and this type of VT may last for seconds to weeks and generally has a benign prognosis. Cardiology consultation regarding medical management is advised.

Diagnostic difficulty occurs in cases of supraventricular tachycardia (SVT) with aberrancy/intraventricular conduction defect, which can mimic the ECG appearances of VT. Look for signs of AV dissociation, which would be diagnostic of VT. There should be typical LBBB or RBBB changes; otherwise regard as VT, especially in the older patient where VT is much more likely.

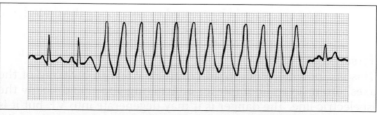

Figure 12.5 Ventricular tachycardia: onset from sinus rhythm

Table 12.2 Causes of prolonged QT interval and torsades de pointes

Cause	Specific drugs, conditions
Antiarrhythmics	Quinidine, procainamide, disopyramide, amiodarone, sotalol
Antipsychotics	Risperidone, fluphenazine, droperidol, pimozide, clozapine, olanzapine, thioridazine, haloperidol, chlorpromazine
Antidepressants	Tricyclics: amitriptyline, imipramine, clomipramine, dothiepin, doxepin
Anti-infective	Macrolides: erythromycin, clarithromycin, azithromycin, roxithromycin Quinolones: ciprofloxacin, moxifloxacin, norfloxacin Antifungals: fluconazole, ketoconazole Antimalarials: hydroxychloroquine, mefloquine, quinine
Miscellaneous drugs	Cisapride, cocaine, methadone, lithium, sumatriptan, organophosphates
Cardiac disease	Ischaemia, complete heart block
Electrolyte disturbances	Hypomagnesaemia, hypocalcaemia, hypokalaemia
Hypothyroidism	
Congenital long QT syndrome	

Prolonged QTc interval

A QTc (corrected for the rate) of over 0.44 s predisposes to VT and torsades, and should be corrected as soon as possible. Table 12.2 lists the causes of a prolonged QTc, which may progress to torsades de pointes.

Prolonged QTc should be treated by correcting the underlying cause, usually by withdrawing the offending agent.

Torsades de pointes

This is a polymorphic broad-complex VT with 'twisting of the axes', often several complexes alternating above and below the isoelectric line. The danger is it may degenerate into VF, but it is more often self-limiting. Causes include drugs which prolong the QT interval, electrolyte disturbances and ischaemia.

- Treatment involves drug withdrawal, IV magnesium sulfate 2 g bolus over 1 minute, followed by an infusion, and correction of electrolytes and ischaemia.
- An isoprenaline infusion or transcutaneous overdrive pacing may be used to accelerate the heart rate and terminate the arrhythmia.
- Unsynchronised cardioversion 200 J biphasic is recommended for haemodynamic instability; however, torsades may be resistant to electrical therapy.

Brugada syndrome

This is a disorder which causes VF and polymorphic VT, and which can be inherited in an autosomal dominant pattern. It is more common in South-East Asians and males, and there may be a family history of sudden cardiac death. There is an abnormality in the cardiac sodium (Na^+) channel. It should be considered in any young male presenting with syncope, seizures, chest pain, sudden cardiac arrest, a family history of unexplained death or the incidental finding of a Brugada pattern on routine ECG.

The ECG features of Brugada are ST elevation and T wave inversion in leads V_1–V_3, mimicking a RBBB. Figure 12.6 shows a type 1. These changes may be transient. The rarer types 2 and 3 have 'saddleback' ST segments with upright T waves.

Treatment is insertion of an implantable cardiac defibrillator (ICD).

Heart block

High-degree heart block, particularly if associated with AMI, may deteriorate to complete heart block requiring urgent pacing. Incomplete occlusions can cause intermittent blocks.

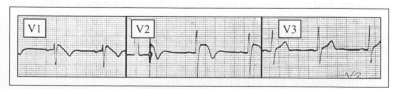

Figure 12.6 Brugada syndrome type 1
Courtesy of Dr Jitu Vohra, Cardiologist, Epworth and Royal Melbourne Hospitals, Victoria.

First-degree AV block
The PR interval is > 0.2 s.

Second-degree, Möbitz type I, Wenckebach
The PR interval increases progressively until a 'dropped beat', with no QRS/ventricular response, occurs. The subsequent PR interval is shorter than the PR before the dropped beat.

Second-degree, Möbitz type II
The PR interval is constant, in association with frequent dropped beats, often regular (e.g. 1 in 3). Deterioration results in a high rate of progression to complete heart block.

No treatment is indicated for first- and second-degree blocks unless there is ischaemia or poor cardiac output, when atropine 0.3–0.6 mg IV may be given with supplementary oxygen.

Third-degree, complete AV/heart block (CHB)
There is no P to QRS relationship; all of the atrial impulses are blocked at the AV node, so that regular P waves (rate > 50) are seen with an independent, idioventricular, QRS with a rate of around 30–40. If the QRS complex arises just below the AV node, the QRS may be narrow and normal in appearance (junctional AV block). More-distal rhythms are relatively wide (> 0.12 s). In general, the broader escape rhythms are more unstable, and more likely to progress to ventricular standstill.

Patients with complete heart block (CHB) may decompensate with poor cardiac output, hypotension or loss of consciousness (Stokes–Adams attack).
- Urgent treatment with atropine 0.3–0.6 mg IV, isoprenaline infusion and/or pacing are indicated.
- Atropine appears to be more effective for narrow-complex CHB, and may worsen the block in broad-complex CHB.

Bundle branch block (BBB)
BBB generally indicates disease in the main conducting system, and syncope can result from an associated AMI with decompensation, progression to CHB and asystole.
- **LBBB** (Figure 12.7), due to functional or anatomical block of the LBB and delayed depolarisation of the left ventricle,

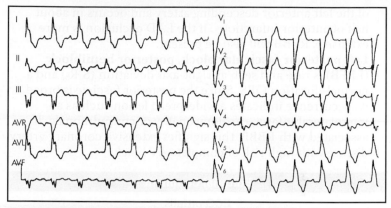

Figure 12.7 Left bundle branch block

is seen as an rS in V_1 and a broad RR^1 in V_5, V_6 with a wide QRS (> 0.12 s). It can be benign, but it is more commonly associated with ischaemic heart disease (IHD) and hypertension. It is important to note that evidence of AMI may still be seen on the ECG (see earlier section Myocardial Infarction).

- **RBBB** (Figure 12.8), due to functional or anatomical block of the RBB and delayed depolarisation of the right ventricle, is seen as an RSR^1 pattern in V_1, V_2 with a wide QRS (> 0.12 s) and is often benign, but can also be a sign of acute right heart strain, such as acute pulmonary embolism. AMI is not disguised by an RBBB.

- **Left anterior fascicular block, anterior hemiblock (LAFB)** is seen as left-axis deviation ($q_1R_1S_3$) and a normal-duration QRS. In patients with chest pain, it signifies partial occlusion

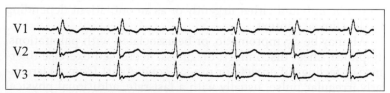

Figure 12.8 Right bundle branch block

of the left anterior descending artery and occurs in about half of anterior infarctions. If the LAD occlusion is more extensive, RBBB will also be present.

♦ **Left posterior fascicular block, posterior hemiblock (LPFB)** is rare and seen as right-axis deviation (S_1R_3) and a normal-duration QRS. Since the posterior fascicle is broad, its occurrence indicates a widespread lesion such as an inferolateral infarct, cardiomyopathy or cor pulmonale. If associated with RBBB, this signifies extensive coronary artery disease with high risk of complete AV block.

Editorial Comment

ECG pitfalls

- Posteroinferior STEMI
- STEMI in aVR
- Hyperacute T waves
- New upright T waves in V_1
- Arrhythmogenic right ventricular dysplasia
- Brugada syndrome
- Wellens syndrome
- Sgarbossa criteria in LBBB and pacemaker patients

Remember: if the ECG is not normal, especially if something 'does not look right' or looks complicated, ask, scan and send, fax for advice.

These pitfalls can be hard but the ECG is not normal.

Atrial fibrillation (AF)

The commonest clinically significant cardiac arrhythmia seen in EDs is AF (Figure 12.9). This may be a first episode or recurrent, which is then subclassified as *paroxysmal* (self-terminating, < 24 hours), *persistent* (sustained > 7 days) or *permanent*. There are many causes and clinical settings for AF, and investigation should be initiated either urgently or as an outpatient depending on the clinical context.

AF may be asymptomatic, or be associated with palpitations, dyspnoea, chest discomfort, dizziness, decreased exercise tolerance or feelings of anxiety or pre-syncope. Apart from an irregularly irregular pulse, usually with a fast rate, additional physical findings vary. Heart failure may be present. Signs of associated

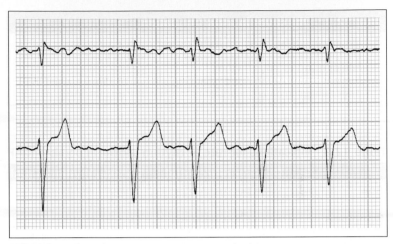

Figure 12.9 Atrial fibrillation

cardiovascular disease (e.g. mitral valve disease, ischaemic heart disease or hypertension) may be present. Signs of the underlying cause (e.g. anaemia, sepsis or thyrotoxicosis) may be present. AF with a very rapid ventricular rate (> 200 bpm) suggests the possibility of an underlying accessory pathway.

Acute AF may be associated with alcohol (and some other drugs), surgery, electrocution, myocardial infarction, myoperi-carditis, pulmonary embolism, lung diseases, hyperthyroidism, metabolic conditions and many other causes. Treatment of these may lead to resolution.

Up to two-thirds of new or recurrent episodic AF may resolve without treatment within the first 24 hours. When associated with another illness, treatment of the primary problem may lead to reversion to sinus rhythm. Investigation for both cardiac disease, particularly structural or ischaemic disease, and underlying causes should be undertaken. Echocardiography, particularly transoesophageal echocardiography (TOE), is very useful. The risk of stroke should be considered in each patient.

Management objectives (see Box 12.1) to give symptomatic relief and to prevent tachycardia-induced cardiomyopathy is either by rate control or by rhythm control (Table 12.3).

Box 12.1 Objectives in atrial fibrillation

1 Identify and treat causative factor.
2 Decide on rate or rhythm control, and implement treatment to slow rate or revert to sinus rhythm.
3 Prevent thromboembolism, balancing the risk of stroke against the risk of bleeding on anticoagulants.

Table 12.3 Indications for rate or rhythm control in persistent AF

	Consider rate control	Consider rhythm control
Age	Older people (> 65 years)	Younger people (< 65 years)
Symptoms	Few or no symptoms	Severe symptoms
AF type	Permanent	Lone AF or new-onset
Complications	People without congestive heart failure	People with congestive heart failure
Contraindications	People with contraindications to antiarrhythmic drugs or cardioversion	People eligible for antiarrhythmic drugs or cardioversion
Comorbidities	People with coronary artery disease	AF secondary to treated/corrected precipitant

Adapted from NHMRC Clinical Practice Guideline.

- Rate control can be best achieved with drugs such as beta-blockers, verapamil or diltiazem. Digoxin, while no longer considered first choice, may be useful in those with heart failure due to its inotropic effects. Drugs that slow atrioventricular conduction are contraindicated in those with accessory pathway.
- Rhythm control can be achieved by either electrical cardioversion or pharmacotherapy. Pharmacological restoration to sinus rhythm may be achieved by agents such as flecainide or amiodarone; however, careful assessment of safety and likely efficacy of the chosen agent is required for each patient. Flecainide is contraindicated in those with structural heart disease.

Electrical cardioversion in the ED requires most importantly a safe environment (see Figure 12.10). A resuscitation area and staff trained in airway and resuscitation equipment is essential.

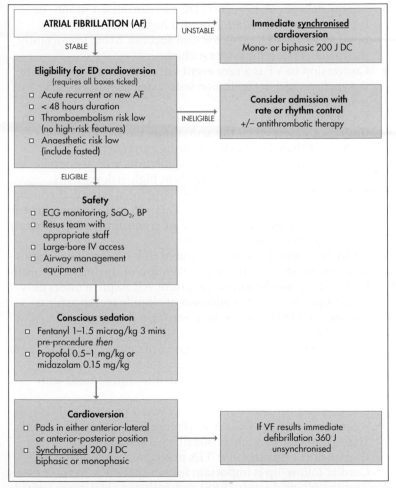

ATRIAL FIBRILLATION (AF)

UNSTABLE →

Immediate <u>synchronised</u> cardioversion
Mono- or biphasic 200 J DC

STABLE ↓

Eligibility for ED cardioversion
(requires all boxes ticked)
☐ Acute recurrent or new AF
☐ < 48 hours duration
☐ Thromboembolism risk low (no high-risk features)
☐ Anaesthetic risk low (include fasted)

INELIGIBLE →

Consider admission with rate or rhythm control
+/− antithrombotic therapy

ELIGIBLE ↓

Safety
☐ ECG monitoring, SaO₂, BP
☐ Resus team with appropriate staff
☐ Large-bore IV access
☐ Airway management equipment

Conscious sedation
☐ Fentanyl 1–1.5 microg/kg 3 mins pre-procedure *then*
☐ Propofol 0.5–1 mg/kg or midazolam 0.15 mg/kg

Cardioversion
☐ Pads in either anterior-lateral or anterior-posterior position
☐ <u>Synchronised</u> 200 J DC biphasic or monophasic

→ If VF results immediate defibrillation 360 J unsynchronised

Figure 12.10 Pathway for electrical defibrillation of atrial fibrillation
Adapted from American College of Cardiology/American Heart Association/European Society for Cardiology Guidelines for the management of patients with atrial fibrillation, 2006.

- The need for cardioversion may be immediate (e.g. hypotension, worsening heart failure) or semi-elective.
- Patients require procedural sedation (e.g. propofol, midazolam or other agents) with airway management and monitoring.
- Energy delivery at 150–200 J DC (synchronised mono- or biphasic) is usually adequate, with higher energy levels possibly increasing cardioversion success. Most importantly, the cardioversion must be synched.
- Conversion to VF is a rare event but necessitates immediate unsynchronised defibrillation with usual advanced ALS management.
- Cardioversion also carries a risk of thromboembolism, with this risk greatest when the arrhythmia has been present for greater than 48 hours. Following cardioversion, atrial 'stunning' may occur, and anticoagulation may need to be continued for 4 weeks afterwards in high-risk patients.

Independent of rate or rhythm control strategy, thromboembolism risk requires addressing. This will include the intrinsic risk of thromboembolism, choice of treatment, risk of major haemorrhage and patient preference.

- Multiple studies have demonstrated that oral anticoagulation with warfarin is effective for prevention of thromboembolism in patients with chronic or recurrent AF. Aspirin offers only modest protection. The addition of clopidogrel to aspirin may be used in those in whom warfarin is contraindicated or unreliable.
- Other agents, particularly the direct thrombin inhibitors such as dabigatran, are currently under evaluation.
- When anticoagulation is indicated, initial treatment with enoxaparin is often used.
- The decision for anticoagulation is based on risk, and risk scores such as $CHADS_2VASC$ (Figure 12.14) may be helpful. High-risk features such as metallic valves, rheumatic heart disease or recent stroke or TIA needs to be assessed.

Cardiac follow-up is important for new patients. In some cases electrophysiological study (EPS) and catheter ablation is considered. Atrial appendage closure, pulmonary vein isolation, treatment for valvular heart disease and other surgical management may also be appropriate in selected patients. All patients put on either rhythm or rate control drugs will need to be monitored for adverse effects.

Atrial flutter

Generally, atrial flutter has an atrial rate of 300 bpm with variable block (commonly 2:1 or 3:1). It has the same causes as AF, and may be treated similarly. Despite its regular rate, it may still result in atrial thrombus.

Flutter waves may be most obvious in the inferior leads or V_1, and are described as having a sawtooth appearance. Rate control is as for AF. The most effective treatment is synchronised cardioversion, beginning with 50–100 J biphasic. Pharmacological agents are less effective in reverting atrial flutter than atrial fibrillation. The same precautions regarding anticoagulation apply for atrial flutter. Cardiology follow-up is necessary as it responds well to ablation.

Paroxysmal supraventricular tachycardia (PSVT)

PSVT has a regular rate, usually 150–200 bpm (range 100–280 bpm; see Figure 12.11). It is a junctional tachycardia, where the AV node is an integral part of the arrhythmia circuit.

AV nodal re-entry tachycardia (AVNRT) is where the circuit is within the AV node itself, while AV re-entry tachycardia (AVRT) is where an additional (accessory) pathway is involved.

- Vagal manoeuvres such as Valsalva with leg raise (REVERT manoeuvre) may terminate PSVT.
- Adenosine is effective and relatively safe to use for chemical reversion, given as IV boluses through a wide-bore (e.g. 18-gauge in cubital fossa) IV cannula of incrementally

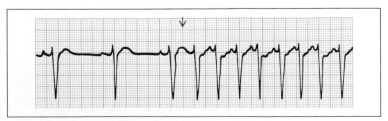

Figure 12.11 Paroxysmal supraventricular tachycardia

increasing doses of 6 mg, 12 mg or up to 18 mg if needed. In some patients, it causes a feeling of impending doom.

- Verapamil 5 mg IV slowly at 1 mg/minute may be used with care, but it can cause intractable hypotension, CHB and asystole, especially if the patient is also on a beta-blocker or digoxin.
- Radiofrequency ablation (RA) may be needed if adenosine is unsuccessful.

SVT with intraventricular conduction defect (aberrant conduction), such as when there is a concurrent BBB or WPW syndrome causing a broad QRS complex, is difficult to differentiate from VT. Adenosine is safe for SVT with BBB, but in WPW it may cause hypotension and an unstable ventricular arrythmia.

Wolff-Parkinson-White syndrome (WPW)

WPW is due to pre-excitation of the ventricles by an accessory pathway, bypassing the AV node, resulting in a short PR interval and a slurred upstroke or 'delta wave' on the R wave, best seen in V_2-V_6 (see Figure 12.12).

If associated with a dominant R in V_1 and inverted T waves in V_1-V_4, this is due to a left accessory path (type A WPW); otherwise the accessory path is on the right (type B WPW). The ECG of type A WPW can be mistaken for a posterior AMI.

Serious paroxysmal tachyarrhythmias can occur by retrograde re-entry mechanisms or by rapid conduction of superimposed AF/atrial flutter, such as when digoxin is used for treating AF when WPW is unrecognised. Impulses may be rapidly conducted down

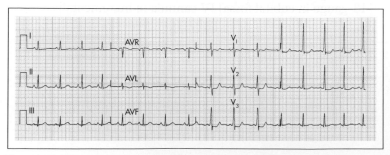

Figure 12.12 Wolff-Parkinson-White type A with typical delta waves

the accessory path and cause a bizarre ECG with variable-width QRS tachycardia, hypotension and eventual VF arrest.

• Treat WPW tachyarrhythmias with cardioversion if unstable.
• Medical or electrical reversion may be tried if stable: IV procainamide 100 mg over 2 5 minutes, up to a total dose of 1 g (watch for and suspend if hypotension or QRS widening).
• AV blocking drugs are contraindicated.
• Radiofrequency ablation or surgery may be needed.

Editorial Comment

Cardiac monitoring of ECG leads by apps on a patient's own computer, iPad, smartphone and smart watch is becoming more widespread and useful.

Holter monitoring

Despite a history suggestive of palpitations, no arrythmia may be detected during ED assessment. The patient should be considered for admission for cardiac monitoring or have Holter monitoring as an outpatient.

Holter monitoring involves attaching a patient to a portable personal ECG monitor, which records usually two ECG channels on tape or computer for 24 hours. A technician then scans the recordings by computer and identifies periods of arrhythmia, which are then presented to the cardiologist for review to see if episodes of palpitations, syncope, angina, and so on can be explained.

• Sinus bradycardia < 35 bpm, sinus pauses < 3 s, Wenckebach, brief runs of AF, multiple atrial ectopics and isolated ventricular ectopic beats may all be found in otherwise normal persons, and do not warrant treatment.
• Sustained arrhythmias are more significant, particularly in symptomatic patients.
• Holter monitoring is also useful in checking response to antiarrhythmics.

3. ELECTROLYTE IMBALANCE, DRUG OVERDOSE, ENVIRONMENTAL EMERGENCIES

Arrhythmias can arise as a result of any of these conditions.

Potassium or magnesium imbalance

Potassium or magnesium imbalance cause similar effects and are important to recognise early, as each may progress to serious arrhythmias if uncorrected.

Hyperkalaemia or hypermagnesaemia

Hyperkalaemia or hypermagnesaemia may cause tall, peaked T waves, flat P waves, wide QRS and undefined ST–T changes. Higher levels will cause various tachyarrhythmias including VT, sine wave patterns and, eventually, asystole.

Hypokalaemia or hypomagnesaemia

Hypokalaemia or hypomagnesaemia may result in a prolonged QT, flattened T waves and small U waves; note that U waves may occur in healthy people in V_2–V_4, but the T waves are normal. ST depression and first- or second-degree heart block may also be seen. Lower levels can cause atrial and ventricular arrhythmias, notably torsades de pointes.

Calcium imbalance

Hypercalcaemia

Hypercalcaemia shortens the ST and the Q–T intervals, but widens the T wave. Bradycardias, BBB, second-degree heart block and CHB can deteriorate to asystole if levels are markedly elevated.

Hypocalcaemia

Hypocalcaemia lengthens the ST and therefore the Q–T interval, with risk of VT and torsades. A prolonged QTc may be caused by any drug which causes hypocalcaemia, hypokalaemia and hypomagnesaemia.

Environmental emergencies

Hypothermia and electrocution are examples causing cardiac effects.

Hypothermia

With severe hypothermia, cardiac effects can be related to the temperature. The initial response is a sinus tachycardia for temperatures down to 32°C, then bradycardia for temperatures down to about 30°C. Osborn waves, which are deflections at the end of the QRS complex and in the same direction as the QRS, appear at around 30°C and increase in height as the temperature falls. Various arrhythmias occur down to 27°C, when VF may occur and cause death. In some patients, VF does not occur, and the temperature can fall as low as 22°C, culminating in fatal asystole. Gradual rewarming and ALS should be instituted early to avoid this.

See also Chapter 43 Drowning and Chapter 46 Hypothermia and Hyperthermia.

Electrocution
Cardiac effects can vary from nil to ST changes, transient arrhythmias, BBB, heart block, myocardial necrosis and cardiac asystole. If the route from entry to exit points traverses the torso, cardiac damage is more likely.
- A low current of 10–100 microamps, resulting from stray currents or earthing faults in household equipment, can cause a microshock, which can result in VF arrest.
- If the skin resistance is lowered by moisture, a 0.24 milliamp (mA) current from a 240 volt source can be increased to a current of 240 mA and cause a macroshock, with resultant VF.
- Contact with high-tension power lines (> 1000 A) or a lightning strike (> 12 000 A) can cause cardiorespiratory arrest from asystole (more commonly) or VF. Early ALS may save these patients, but the severity of their burns will determine their fate.
See also Chapter 45 Electrical Injuries.

Axis (electrical pathway mapping)
Axis generally refers to the QRS axis and the direction of depolarisation in the ventricles as reflected in the frontal plane (the anterior chest wall). It is best illustrated by a clock face with each numerical division representing 30° (see Figure 12.13).
- The horizontal direction can be determined by inspecting Lead I, to see whether the QRS deflection is mainly *up* (positive impulse moving from right to left) or *down* (negative impulse from left to right).
- The vertical direction is reflected in aVF (the vertical axis). If the QRS deflection is mainly up, the impulse is travelling

towards the foot, and if the QRS is down, the impulse is towards the head.

Combining this information, the quadrant in which the QRS vector lies can be determined.

- QRS in LI up, in aVF up—vector in left lower quadrant (normal axis)
- QRS in LI up, in aVF down—vector in left upper quadrant (left axis deviation)
- QRS in LI down, in aVF up—vector in right lower quadrant (right axis deviation—RAD)
- QRS in LI down, in aVF down—vector in right upper quadrant (indeterminate or extreme RAD).

To determine the axis more accurately (within 30°), note which limb or standard lead has the most isoelectric QRS (equally up and down); the axis is at 90° to this in the predetermined quadrant (use Figure 12.13). The range of normal axis can extend from −30° to +90°, as patients who are obese can have a more horizontal heart (vector in left upper quadrant), while those who are asthenic have a more vertical heart (90° axis). Thus, if the QRS is isoelectric in lead aVR, and the above criteria point to the left upper quadrant (LAD), then a perpendicular (90°) to the aVR axis gives an axis of −60° in the left upper quadrant. The QRS axis is then −60° in the frontal plane.

Significance

- **Left axis deviation.** LAD should raise the suspicion of anterior hemiblock (left anterior fascicular block—LAFB), often as a result of occlusive disease of the left anterior descending artery or cardiomyopathy.
- **Right axis deviation.** RAD suggests posterior hemiblock (right posterior fascicular block—RPFB) and usually right (occasionally, left) coronary artery disease, right ventricular hypertrophy, acute cor pulmonale (as in massive pulmonary embolus) or cardiomyopathy.

In general, the vector moves towards hypertrophy, and away from infarction.

The CHA_2DS_2-VASc calculator for atrial fibrillation (Figure 12.14) evaluates ischaemic stroke risk in patients with atrial fibrillation.

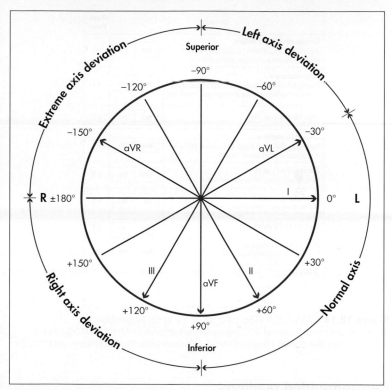

Figure 12.13 The QRS frontal plane cardiac axial reference system
Yuen Derek, after Fisch C, Mirvis D, Goldberg A. Electrocardiography. In: Libby P, Bonow R et al. (eds). Braunwald's Heart disease. 8th edn. Philadelphia: WB Saunders; 2007 https://www.chadsvasc.org/ CHADssVASC https://chadsvasc.org/

Criteria			Poss. Point
Congestive heart failure Signs/symptoms of heart failure confirmed with objective evidence of cardiac dysfunction	Yes	No	+1
Hypertension Resting BP >140/90 mmHg on at least 2 occasions or current antihypertensive pharmacologic treatment	Yes	No	+1
Age 75 years or older	Yes	No	+2
Diabetes mellitus Fasting glucose >125 mg/dL or treatment with oral hypoglycemic agent and/or insulin	Yes	No	+1
Stroke, TIA ( ), or TE ( ) Includes any history of cerebral ischemia	Yes	No	+2
Vascular disease Prior MI ( ) peripheral arterial disease, or aortic plaque	Yes	No	+1
Age 65 to 74 years	Yes	No	+1
Sex Category (female) Female gender confers higher risk	Yes	No	+1
SCORE Risk of stroke 0 - Low-risk 1 - Moderate 2 - High-risk			

Figure 12.14 CHA_2DS_2-VASc calculator for atrial fibrillation
Modified from Van den Ham et al. Comparative Performance of ATRIA, CHADS$_2$, and CHA$_2$DS$_2$-VASc Risk Scores Predicting Stroke in Patients With Atrial Fibrillation. JACC. 2015.

Recommended readings

Pisters R, Lane DA, Nieuwlaat R, de Vos CB, Crijns HJ, Lip GY. A novel user-friendly score (HAS-BLED) to assess one-year risk of major bleeding in atrial fibrillation patients: The Euro Heart Survey. Chest 2010;138(5):1093–100.

EHRA / EACT / ESC Committee for Practice Guidelines. Guidelines for the management of atrial fibrillation: the Task Force for the Management of Atrial Fibrillation of the European Society of Cardiology (ESC). Europace. 2010 Oct;12(10):1360–1420. doi: 10.1093/europace/euq350.

Lip GY, Frison L, Halperin JL, Lane DA. Identifying patients at high risk for stroke despite anticoagulation: a comparison of contemporary stroke risk stratification schemes in an anticoagulated atrial fibrillation cohort. Stroke. 2010 Dec;41(12):2731–2738. doi: 10.1161/STROKEAHA.110.590257. Epub 2010 Oct 21.

Lip GY, Nieuwlaat R, Pisters R, Lane DA, Crijns HJ. Refining clinical risk stratification for predicting stroke and thromboembolism in atrial fibrillation using a novel risk factor-based approach: the euro heart survey on atrial fibrillation. Chest. 2010;137:263-272.

Management of antithrombotic therapy in atrial fibrillation patients presenting with acute coronary syndrome and/or undergoing percutaneous coronary or valve interventions: a joint consensus document of the European Society of Cardiology Working Group on Thrombosis, European Heart Rhythm Association (EHRA), European Association of Percutaneous Cardiovascular Interventions (EAPCI) and European Association of Acute Cardiac Care (ACCA) endorsed by the Heart Rhythm Society (HRS) and Asia-Pacific Heart Rhythm Society (APHRS). Eur Heart J. 2014 Aug 25. pii: ehu298.

Van den Ham et al. Comparative Performance of ATRIA, CHADS2, and CHA2DS2-VASc Risk Scores Predicting Stroke in Patients With Atrial Fibrillation. JACC. 2015.

Chapter 13
Respiratory emergencies: the acutely breathless patient

Bronwyn Orr and John Roberts

Acknowledgment

The authors wish to acknowledge the content used from the previous edition of *Emergency Medicine* which was provided by Craig Hore.

General principles

Exclude airway compromise, which may be subtle, as the cause of acute breathlessness. Management of airway problems always comes first. Dyspnoea is a sensation which has multiple aetiologies and can be difficult to assess.

There may be several reasons why the patient with comorbidities experiences dyspnoea. This patient may require comprehensive treatment strategies to optimise their condition and thus relieve their symptoms.

Initial goals in assessment and management are to:

1 identify and treat life-threatening abnormalities of gas exchange, acute onset or deterioration of hypoxia and hypercarbia
2 commence non-invasive ventilation in the form of bi-level positive airway pressure (BiPAP) or continuous positive airway pressure (CPAP) where indicated
3 identify when intubation and ventilation is required and initiate this therapy
4 identify and commence specific treatment to relieve respiratory distress based on initial history and examination
5 formulate a plan of investigation and management of cases where the exact cause of respiratory distress is unknown or uncertain.

Triage all patients presenting with a respiratory system emergency to a monitored acute bed. Obtain IV access. Arterial blood gases (ABGs), chest X-ray and BiPAP services should be available.

Oxygen therapy

Delivery of oxygen is one of the most common therapies in the ED and an important component of resuscitation. Acute hypoxaemia is immediately life-threatening, and the 'first-line drug' for hypoxaemia is oxygen! It is a safe drug: the complications of oxygen therapy are concentration- and time-dependent, uncommon and take time to develop. Other aspects of oxygen delivery may also need to be improved in the hypoxaemic patient, especially cardiac output, haemoglobin, tissue perfusion and reducing tissue O_2 requirements (see Table 13.1).

Essentially, oxygen should be delivered to all patients who have acute respiratory failure to maintain a partial arterial pressure (PaO_2) of 60–80 mmHg (or a $PaO_2 > 55$ mmHg in chronic respiratory failure). The lowest fraction of inspired oxygen (FiO_2) that provides an acceptable PaO_2 should be chosen. Choosing the right mode of delivery is also important.

OXYGEN DELIVERY SYSTEMS
Simple delivery systems
These are variable performance systems—the FiO_2 delivered not only depends upon the oxygen flow rate, but also on the rate and depth of respiration. The FiO_2 delivered by various systems can be estimated (Table 13.2).

Table 13.1 O_2 therapy

SaO$_2$ (%)	PaO$_2$ (mmHg)	Level
98	100	Arterial blood
90	60	
75	40	Venous blood
50	26	
~33	~20	Tissue

SaO_2 = oxygen saturation; PaO_2 = partial pressure of oxygen in arterial or venous blood or tissue
Note: When $SaO_2 \approx$ 60–90%, there is a linear relationship between SaO_2 and PaO_2.

Table 13.2 **Estimation of the fraction of inspired oxygen (FiO_2)
achieved by simple delivery systems**

Flow rate (L/min)	FiO_2
2 (nasal prongs)	0.25
3 (nasal prongs)	0.28
4 (nasal prongs)	0.30
6	0.40
8	0.45
15	0.65
15 (reservoir mask)*	0.70

*If a double wall supply is used, a flow rate of 30 L/min and FiO_2 up to 0.90 can be achieved.

- **Nasal prongs.** These are easy to use and usually well tolerated by the patient, allowing them to eat, drink and talk without interrupting oxygen delivery. They are ineffective if the patient has blocked nasal passages or is an obligate mouth breather. Flow rates > 4 L/min can lead to mucosal drying and are less well tolerated.
- **Hudson mask.** A simple and easy way to deliver oxygen but delivery is variable (see Table 13.2). Flow rates < 4 L/min are not recommended as rebreathing can occur.

Entrainment systems
- **Venturi masks.** This system uses the Bernoulli effect to entrain a fixed amount of air to mix with oxygen. This is an example of a fixed performance system—the FiO_2 delivered is more independent of patient factors. Nonetheless, it may vary in patients with very high peak inspiratory flow rates. One commonly used system delivers the following options: 24/28/35/40/50/60% oxygen. The lower concentrations are especially useful for patients with chronic obstructive pulmonary disease (COPD) and CO_2 retention.

Partial rebreathing systems
- **Reservoir masks.** These can achieve a higher FiO_2 than simple masks, but it is essential to keep the reservoir inflated with O_2.

This can require high flow rates. This is a good initial choice for most conscious, unwell, hypoxaemic patients in the ED.

• **Anaesthetic circuits.** Mentioned for completeness; rarely used in the ED setting.

Non-rebreathing systems

• **Resuscitation bags** (e.g. Laerdal, Baxter). The commonly used bags are self-inflating, and have a series of one-way valves and a reservoir bag. The aim is to keep the reservoir bag at least 75% inflated with O_2. An FiO_2 of close to 100% can be delivered if 15 L/min O_2 is used and the reservoir bag is inflated (50% without a reservoir bag). There is a growing trend to use disposable, single-use bags to help overcome the problem of incorrect assembly and sterilisation. The ability to use a bag–mask system is a vital skill that should be learned and mastered early!

• Gas-driven inflating valves (e.g. Oxy-viva).

Others

• Positive-pressure ventilators
• Non-invasive positive-pressure ventilation (e.g. CPAP, BiPAP)
• High-flow nasal oxygen using humidification units and specialised delivery circuits are being used more frequently, especially in paediatrics; FiO_2 up to 1.0 can be delivered along with small amounts of PEEP
• Hyperbaric oxygen (HBO) therapy

Other delivery systems are dealt with in more detail in other chapters of this text.

Investigations in respiratory emergencies
ARTERIAL BLOOD GASES (ABGs): OXYGENATION AND VENTILATION

ABGs reflect oxygenation (PaO_2), ventilation ($PaCO_2$) and acid–base status. The last is dealt with in more detail in Chapter 21 Acid–base and Electrolyte Disorders.

It should be noted that venous blood gases are increasingly performed in the ED. They are less painful and faster to perform than ABGs and provide most of the necessary information required in the ED.

Oxygenation

Remember that, even for 'normal' lungs, the PaO_2 varies with the following parameters.

- **The inspired O_2 concentration (FiO$_2$).** Never take ABGs, or try to interpret ABGs, without noting the FiO$_2$. If room air, this is 21% (i.e. FiO$_2$ = 0.21).

- **Age.** PaO_2 falls with age. As a rough guide to what to expect at a given age, use the following estimation:

$$PaO_2 \approx 105 - \left(\frac{1}{3} \times age \right)$$

- **Altitude.** PaO_2 falls by ~3 mmHg for each 1000 feet (~300 m) above sea level.

- **Temperature.** For each degree Celsius rise (or fall) in temperature, the PaO_2 will rise (or fall) by ~5%.

- **pH.** For each 0.1 decrease (or increase) in pH, the PaO_2 will increase (or decrease) by ~10%.

Do not take oxygen off a hypoxic patient to perform ABGs. Perform the ABGs with the patient on oxygen and note the FiO$_2$. The A–a gradient (the difference between alveolar and arterial oxygen pressure, $P_{A-a}O_2$) is calculated from the alveolar gas equation:

$$PAO_2 = PiO_2 - (PaCO_2/R)$$

PAO_2 is the alveolar oxygen tension and R is the respiratory quotient (usually 0.8). The partial pressure of inspired oxygen (PiO_2) is determined by the atmospheric pressure, which varies with altitude. Usually, it is assumed that the patient is breathing at sea level, that atmospheric pressure is 760 mmHg and that the water vapour pressure is 47 mmHg. There is usually a small difference between the PAO_2 and the PaO_2—the A–a gradient or $P_{A-a}O_2$.

- $P_{A-a}O_2 < 15$ mmHg is normal.
- $P_{A-a}O_2 = 20$–30 mmHg reflects mild pulmonary dysfunction.
- $P_{A-a}O_2 > 50$ mmHg reflects severe pulmonary dysfunction. Note that pulmonary embolism is only one of many causes of an increased $P_{A-a}O_2$.

The gradient varies with age: add three for each decade over the age of 30 years.

The PAO_2 can also be quickly estimated using one of the following rules of thumb:

- If breathing room air

$$PAO_2 \approx 145 - PaCO_2$$

- If breathing supplemental O_2

$$PAO_2 \approx 6 \times \%O_2 \quad or$$

$$PAO_2 \approx (7 \times \%O_2) - PaCO_2$$

The causes of hypoxia

There are four main types of hypoxia:

1 **stagnant hypoxia** resulting from decreased cardiac output
2 **anaemic hypoxia** resulting from decreased haemoglobin
3 **histotoxic hypoxia** resulting from decreased oxygen-binding capacity
4 **hypoxaemic hypoxia** resulting from decreased O_2 saturation.

The take-home message from this list is that the patient can be 'hypoxic' with a normal O_2 saturation. Perhaps the most obvious example is histotoxic hypoxia resulting from CO poisoning.

Acute respiratory failure is generally associated with hypoxaemic hypoxia. The problem is getting the oxygen from the lungs into the capillaries. **Ventilation/perfusion (V/Q) mismatch** is the commonest cause.

- At one extreme of V/Q mismatching, there is normal ventilation but *abnormal perfusion* (**dead space ventilation**). This mismatching affects the exchange of O_2, resulting in hypoxaemia. Hypercarbia occurs to a lesser extent, as CO_2 diffuses more easily than O_2. The classic example is pulmonary embolism.
- At the other extreme, there is normal blood flow but *abnormal ventilation* (**shunt**). This is most commonly a result of **venous admixture** where capillary blood and alveolar gas do not equilibrate, such as when blood is flowing through a consolidated lung. The larger the shunt, the less responsive it is to supplemental O_2.

Ventilation

Hypercarbia (↑ $PaCO_2$)

The commonest cause of hypercarbia is alveolar hypoventilation. This can be due to a variety of problems, such as airway obstruction, narcotics, CNS disorders, peripheral nervous system (PNS) disorders, chest wall disorders. Remember there are other uncommon causes of hypercarbia, including V/Q inequality (e.g. COPD, emphysema); increased CO_2 production (e.g. hyperpyrexia, hypercatabolism, thyrotoxicosis, inappropriate carbohydrate load); and increased dead space (e.g. physiological—V/Q mismatch or 'dead space ventilation', equipment—long ventilator tubing and circuitry).

The clinical effects of hypercarbia

- Respiratory drive will typically be increased, unless it is suppressed due to the underlying cause of the hypercarbia (e.g. CNS disorders, narcotics).
- There is a rise in endogenous catecholamines leading to tachycardia, hypertension, increased CO, increased cerebral blood flow and raised intracranial pressure (ICP).
- Peripheral vasodilation typically occurs.
- The patient initially becomes anxious and restless, followed by a decreased level of consciousness and eventually coma if it remains uncorrected.

The 'chronic CO_2 retainer'

Some patients with chronic respiratory disorders (e.g. COPD) have a chronically elevated $PaCO_2$. The chemoreceptors adjust to this elevated level and essentially become less 'sensitive' to fluctuations in $PaCO_2$, relying more on changes in PaO_2—the so-called 'hypoxic drive'. A high FiO_2 could depress ventilation by decreasing this hypoxic stimulus. This is the theory, but clinically it actually rarely occurs in patients with acute respiratory failure.

Hypoxia can kill quickly, so give oxygen to the hypoxaemic patient. If the patient may have chronic CO_2 retention, still give oxygen, accepting a PaO_2 of 50–60 mmHg or even less.

OTHER INVESTIGATIONS IN RESPIRATORY EMERGENCIES

The chest X-ray (CXR)

The CXR is one of the most useful investigations in the patient with respiratory failure. In order to interpret the film correctly, and to avoid missing important findings, a good routine for assessing the CXR is a must. The principles of chest radiography, and other chest imaging modalities, are dealt with in more detail in Chapter 48 Diagnostic Imaging in Emergency Patients.

The lung can react in a similar fashion to a variety of insults. Therefore, there are no absolute rules in terms of radiological patterns that allow us to distinguish between these insults with 100% accuracy. *It is important to always interpret the CXR in the light of your clinical history and examination findings!* There will be times when an acutely short-of-breath patient presents to the ED and is found to be hypoxaemic without any significant changes seen on CXR. The differential here includes pulmonary vascular disease (e.g. emboli), respiratory problems (e.g. asthma, early COPD, early chronic lung disease, early pneumonia) and non-respiratory problems (e.g. compromised airway, high oxygen consumption, hyperthermia, intracardiac shunt).

Tests of forced expiration

These tests are effort- and technique-dependent and may not be able to be properly performed when the patient is acutely breathless. As such, they are rarely performed in the ED and are often more appropriate in the ward setting.

- **Peak expiratory flow rate (PEFR)** is measurable using a simple, portable flow meter. It is reproducible by most patients after several practice efforts. PEFR may be reduced in COPD, asthma and respiratory muscle weakness. PEFR may be normal or increased in restrictive lung diseases such as fibrosis. It is perhaps most useful as a monitor for asthmatic patients in the outpatient/home setting. It may also be helpful in the ED as one of the means to assess discharge suitability of asthmatic patients (e.g. PEFR should be at least 75% of predicted or best).
- **Forced vital capacity (FVC)** is the volume of air that can be exhaled with maximum force following a full inspiration. It varies with age, sex, height and general physique.

- **Forced expiratory volume in 1 second (FEV_1)** is the maximum amount of air that can be forcibly exhaled in 1 second following a full inspiration. FEV_1 is reduced in disease that affects airflow, lung elasticity and/or the state of the chest wall, including respiratory musculature. If FEV_1 improves by $> 15-20\%$ following bronchodilator therapy, there is said to be reversible airway obstruction. FEV_1 normally accounts for $> 75\%$ of the FVC. In obstructive airway disease, FEV_1/FVC is classically $< 70\%$. In restrictive lung disease, FEV_1/FVC is classically normal or increased.

Microbiological methods

Treatment of suspected severe respiratory infections should not be delayed while awaiting the results of laboratory tests. A causal pathogen is found in less than 50% of cases of community-acquired pneumonia. This percentage decreases even further if the cultures are taken after antimicrobials have been given.

Blood cultures can often be collected in the ED before antimicrobial therapy is commenced. Ideally, two sets should be taken at least 1 hour apart from separate sites. The second set may not be possible when rapid empirical therapy is indicated.

The value of **sputum culture** is limited but may be improved if the sputum is purulent, properly collected—not contaminated by the upper respiratory tract (e.g. saliva, epithelial cells) and, where possible, taken before antibiotics are given—and transported to the lab within 2 hours of collection. Where bacterial infection is not likely (e.g. many upper respiratory tract infections), cultures are usually not indicated. Respiratory syncytial virus (RSV) immunofluorescent-labelled antibody examination of exfoliated cells in nasopharyngeal secretions may be undertaken in paediatric acute bronchiolitis; however, this rarely changes management.

The **nature of the sputum** may be helpful: copious, pink frothy sputum is characteristic of acute left ventricular failure; copious, purulent, pungent sputum of lung abscess; clear, watery sputum of alveolar cell carcinoma; and rusty, mucoid sputum of pneumococcal pneumonia.

Invasive respiratory investigations

Invasive techniques such as percutaneous needle biopsy, diagnostic bronchoscopy, transbronchial biopsy and bronchoalveolar lavage are rarely undertaken in Australasian EDs. An exception is diagnostic and/or therapeutic **thoracentesis**.

Pleural fluid is normally a pale yellow colour. It is turbid in the setting of empyema or parapneumonic effusion. Blood in pleural fluid may be due to trauma, malignancy or pulmonary infarction. Other common analyses of pleural fluid include:

- protein (pleural fluid protein < 30 g/L represents a transudate; > 30 g/L represents an exudate)
- lactate dehydrogenase (LDH) (pleural fluid : serum LDH ratio < 0.6 represents a transudate; > 0.6 represents an exudate)
- white cell count (leukocytes may be due to a parapneumonic effusion, pulmonary embolus or empyema; lymphocytes may be due to tuberculosis, malignancy or a vasculitis)
- glucose (pleural fluid glucose may be < 50% serum glucose levels in bacterial infections, malignancy, rheumatoid arthritis and systemic lupus erythematosus [SLE])
- cytology (malignant cells, mesothelial cells), and
- culture.

Life-threatening conditions presenting with breathlessness

ACUTE ASTHMA

Initial management

1. Give oxygen and salbutamol 2 × 5 mg ampoules nebulised immediately, if not already commenced, after taking a brief history and physical examination.
2. Focus on delivering oxygen, reversing the bronchospasm and relieving symptoms as soon as possible in a high-acuity, well-supervised, monitored area with IV access.

Assess severity

Assess severity as mild, moderate or severe and life-threatening using signs of physical exhaustion, cyanosis, speech, PEFR, oxygen saturation, heart rate, respiratory rate and pulsus paradoxus (abnormal decrease in blood pressure on inspiration). Refer to Table 13.3.

Table 13.3 Initial assessment of acute asthma in adults

Findings	Mild	Moderate	Severe and life-threatening*
Physical exhaustion	No	No	Yes Paradoxical chest wall movement
Talks in:	Sentences	Phrases	Words
Pulse rate	< 100/min	100–120/min	> 120/min[†]
Pulsus paradoxus	Not palpable	May be palpable	Palpable[‡]
Central cyanosis	Absent	May be present	Likely to be present
Wheeze intensity	Variable	Moderate to loud	Often quiet
PEFR	More than 75% of predicted (or best if known)	50–70% of predicted (or best if known)	Less than 50% of predicted (or best if known) or less than 100 L/min[#]
FEV$_1$	More than 75% of predicted	50–75% of predicted	Less than 50% of predicted or less than 1 L
Oximetry on presentation			Less than 90% Cyanosis may be present**
Arterial blood gases (assay)	Not necessary	Necessary if initial response poor	Necessary[††]
Other investigations	Not required	May be required	Check for hypokalaemia Chest X-ray to exclude other pathology (e.g. infection, pneumothorax)

*Any of these features indicates that the episode is severe. The absence of any feature does not exclude a severe attack.
[†]Bradycardia may be seen when respiratory arrest is imminent.
[‡]Paradoxical pulse is more reliable in severe obstruction. Its presence (especially if > 12 mmHg) can identify patients whc need admission. Its absence in those with severe exacerbations suggests respiratory muscle fatigue.
[#]Patient may be incapable of performing test.
**Measurement of oxygen saturation is required: many patients look well clinically and may not appear cyanosed despite desaturation. PaO$_2$ < 60 mmHg indicates respiratory failure.
[††]PaCO$_2$ > 50 mmHg indicates respiratory failure.
Reproduced with permission from 'Initial Assessment of Acute Asthma In Adults', page 50 of *The Asthma Management Handbook* 2006 published by The National Asthma Council Australia. www.nationalasthma.org.au/handbook

Spirometry is the most accurate marker of severity, but is usually not clinically appropriate in the ED.

Features of severe and life-threatening asthma include paradoxical chest wall movement, exhaustion, sweating, vomiting, panic, speaking in short phases or words only, pulse rate $> 120/min$, pulsus paradoxus > 12 mmHg, central cyanosis, quiet, *NOT* wheezy chest, PEFR $< 50\%$ of predicted or < 100 L/min, $FEV_1 < 50\%$ of predicted or 1 L, pulse oximetry $< 90\%$.

Difficult-to-treat patients are usually those who have delayed presentation and/or deteriorated despite outpatient steroid treatment.

Also observe carefully the patient who has childhood onset of asthma, is steroid-dependent, has previously been intubated or has a history of severe episodes, especially requiring ICU admission, as they are at increased risk.

Further treatment

1 Ipratropium bromide 2 mL (500 microg) with salbutamol q 20 mins for the first hour (optional in moderate severity, not required in mild cases, followed by 500 microg nebs 4–6 hourly if required).

2 Magnesium 10 mmol IV in 100 mL NaCl over 20 minutes if severe and not initially responding to salbutamol and ipratropium.

3 Hydrocortisone 100 mg IV or equivalent (maximum adult dose) in severe and life-threatening cases, within an hour of presentation; repeat 6-hourly and review at 24 hours.

4 Oral steroids for moderate severity (e.g. prednisolone at 2.0 mg/kg (maximum 50 mg) daily).

5 Salbutamol continuously nebulised until dyspnoea improves, then reduce frequency slowly.

IV salbutamol, 250 microg (0.5 mL of 500 microg/mL solution) IV bolus over 1 minute, then IV infusion at 5–10 microg/kg/hour may be used in critical care areas or if continuous nebulised salbutamol is unable to be effectively delivered, which is very rare. IV salbutamol frequently causes a lactic acidosis.

Adrenaline 0.5 mg IM or slowly IV in severe, prearrest cases, if anaphylaxis may be present. In these circumstances, adrenaline is best administered in 0.1 mg boluses (1 mL of 1:10 000 solution) or 1 mg in 100 mL burette titrated slowly. Subsequent adrenaline infusions should be prepared and titrated based on local hospital protocols.

Intubation and ventilation, while often seen as a last resort, are required for respiratory arrest or exhaustion leading to an immediate prearrest state. Asthmatic patients who are intubated are at risk of barotrauma and are ventilated using permissive hypercapnia. Senior assistance should be sought for intubation and adjustment of ventilation parameters in asthmatic patients.

Assess response to therapy

- Use the same criteria used to assess severity.
- Severe and life-threatening cases require ABGs, CXR and electrolytes.
- Observed deteriorations in oxygen saturation monitoring require prompt treatment.
- Continuous metered-dose inhaler (MDI) or nebulised salbutamol can result in blood levels equivalent to therapeutic salbutamol infusions. Patients who are hypoventilating, have mucus-obstructed airways or are not responding to nebulised salbutamol may require parenteral therapy.
- Patients with COPD may begin to deteriorate due to hypercarbia associated with high oxygen flow and reduced hypoxic drive, signalling the need for reduced FiO_2 and/or BiPAP support.

Admission, discharge, follow-up

Observe until the patient is clearly fit for discharge. Longer periods of observation may be required if the patient presents at night or if review, follow-up and compliance with therapy may be compromised.

Every patient discharged following an acute asthma episode should have a clear follow-up plan, including a review of medications, precipitating factors and need for an asthma action plan.

ACUTE EXACERBATION OF COPD

Patients with COPD, because of their marginal lung function at diagnosis, are prone to significant symptoms with minor precipitants. The precipitant may include acute infection (most commonly), small pneumothoraces, deteriorations in cardiac performance and arrhythmias and may be complicated by acute anxiety and increasing O_2 consumption.

Smoking is the commonest cause of COPD and acute interventional counselling is as effective as any other measure in reducing smoking in all ED patients.

Indigenous Australians continue to lose significantly more quality life years because of smoking and COPD.

Initial stabilisation

1 Give oxygen initially, titrated to O_2 saturation > 90%. Monitor carefully for hypercarbia and intervene before significant decrease in LOC or loss of hypoxic drive.
2 Commence nebulised bronchodilator therapy with salbutamol and ipratropium bromide.
3 Give IV hydrocortisone 200 mg.
4 Monitor respiratory rate, ECG, pulse oximetry.
5 Obtain IV access.
6 Assess sputum volume, colour, ABGs, spirometry (if patient is able to perform) and CXR.
7 If patient febrile or appears septic, sputum and blood cultures.

Further treatment

1 Regular nebulised salbutamol 5 mg q4h and ipratropium bromide 500 microg q6h.
2 Antibiotics per *Therapeutic Guidelines* if evidence of infection. If IV antibiotics are required due to severity, inability to safely swallow, use guidelines for community-acquired pneumonia, usually Class III or IV.
3 Hydrocortisone IV maximum 400 mg/day. Long-term steroid therapy is only indicated where reversible bronchospasm has been identified. If the patient is able to swallow, oral steroids (prednisolone 50 mg daily then tapered) are appropriate.
4 Consider additional treatment with nitrates and diuretics if pulmonary oedema is also a factor. Crackles on auscultation may be preexisting due to pulmonary fibrosis rather than pulmonary oedema; check old records.
5 BiPAP is highly effective in acute symptom relief, treatment of hypercarbia and exhaustion. Many intubations have

been prevented by early institution of BiPAP. BiPAP should be initialised with care and with consideration of the fact that many of these patients become acutely claustrophobic and take time to adjust to their face being covered and the sensation of the pressure changes.

Patients who have reported good quality of life despite home O_2 therapy may request intubation in the event of respiratory arrest or BiPAP failure, if there is a reversible precipitating factor.

Advance directives should be checked and respected.

Admission, discharge, follow-up

All but the most minor exacerbations presenting to hospital will require admission.

GP liaison, multidisciplinary community care, pulmonary rehabilitation programs, influenza vaccination and establishment of advance directives continue to improve patient outcomes and reduce length of stay and readmission rates.

ACUTE PULMONARY OEDEMA

This topic is covered in Chapter 15 Acute Pulmonary Oedema.

PNEUMONIA

- Initially, presentation may be subtle, with fever and malaise.
- Pleuritic chest pain, sputum and dyspnoea may not occur until more advanced, unless there is a significant preexisting respiratory comorbidity.
- Pneumonia presenting with respiratory distress generally represents a severe case likely to require ICU monitoring and management.
- CXR may not be helpful until later in the course of the illness and after rehydration.
- The immediate threats to life are hypoxaemia and systemic sepsis.

Management

1 Initiate high-flow oxygen.
2 Obtain IV access.
3 Initiate sepsis management if examination reveals signs of sepsis.

4 Blood culture from a minimum of two sites, nose and throat swabs, urinary antigens for pneumococcus and *Legionella* and sputum culture are helpful to potentially rationalise and target antibiotic therapy.

5 Commence antibiotic therapy as soon as cultures taken in high parenteral doses using antibiotic guidelines.

6 CURB65 score is useful in outpatient setting to predict mortality and need for admission.

7 The Pneumonia Severity Index is more accurate in predicting short term mortality, but requires ABGs (see Figure 13.1).

8 SMART-COP is a score which requires ABGs and serum albumin, but more accurately predicts need for intensive respiratory or vasopressor support (IRVS).

Consider that respiratory symptoms may be secondary to severe sepsis from another source.

Be aware of the aggressive therapy required for the immuno-suppressed patient or hospital-acquired pneumonia and the unique challenges of pneumonia in residents of high-level-care nursing homes.

Consider severe acute respiratory syndrome (SARS) and *Legionella* as potential causes, particularly in rapidly deteriorating cases associated with respiratory failure.

SPONTANEOUS PNEUMOTHORAX

Traumatic pneumothoraces are treated more aggressively and are covered in Chapter 3 Resuscitation Procedures.

The classic presentation of spontaneous pneumothorax is that of the thin, tall young man with pleuritic chest pain and dyspnoea. Spontaneous pneumothoraces occur in families and can be recurrent.

Illness such as COPD and asthma may be associated with spontaneous pneumothorax, especially in association with acute exacerbations where the pneumothorax may have precipitated the presentation.

Initial stabilisation

The immediate threat to life is the tension pneumothorax which, if untreated, will lead to circulatory collapse. Circulatory collapse is preceded by extreme and rapidly deteriorating respiratory distress.

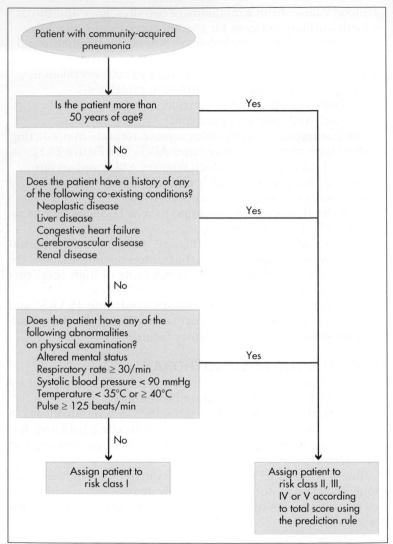

Figure 13.1 The Pneumonia Severity Index, used to determine a patient's risk of death. The total score is obtained by adding to the patient's age—in years for men or in (years – 10) for women—the points assigned for each additional applicable characteristic. *Based on Fine MJ, Auble TE, Yealy DM et al. A prediction rule to identify low-risk patients with community-acquired pneumonia.*

Continued

CHARACTERISTIC	NO. OF POINTS ASSIGNED
Demographic factors	
Age	
Men	Age (in years)
Women	Age (in years) − 10
Nursing home resident	+10
Coexisting illnesses	
Neoplastic disease	+30
Liver disease	+20
Congestive heart failure	+10
Cerebrovascular disease	+10
Renal disease	+10
Findings on physical examination	
Altered mental status	+20
Respiratory rate ≥ 30/min	+20
Systolic blood pressure < 90 mmHg	+20
Temperature < 35°C or ≥ 40°C	+15
Pulse ≥ 125 beats/min	+10
Laboratory and radiographic findings	
Arterial pH < 7.35	+30
Blood urea nitrogen ≥ 30 mg/dL	
(11 mmol/litre)	+20
Sodium < 130 mmol/litre	+20
Glucose ≥ 250 mg/dL (14 mmol/litre)	+10
Haematocrit < 30%	+10
Partial pressure of	
arterial oxygen < 60 mmHg	
or oxygen saturation < 90%	+10
Pleural effusion	+10

Stratification of risk score			
RISK	RISK CLASS	SCORE	MORTALITY
Low	I	Based on algorithm	0.1%
Low	II	≤ 70	0.6%
Low	III	71–90	0.9%
Moderate	IV	91–130	9.3%
High	V	>130	27.0%

Figure 13.1, cont'd *N Engl J Med 1997; 336:243–50, as presented in Halm EA, Teirstein AS. Management of community-acquired pneumonia. N Engl J Med 2002; 347(25):2039–44. http://www.asthmahandbook.org.au/*

Tension pneumothorax leading to significant compromise will be obvious clinically.

The presence of tension is independent of the size of the pneumothorax, although it will progressively enlarge unless there is marked gas trapping in the affected lung. The patient may be agitated and confused and appear restless with dyspnoea, tachypnoea and cyanosis. The affected hemithorax will appear hyperinflated, neck veins distended.

The patient will be tachycardic and hypotensive. Tracheal shift, if palpable, will be away from the side of the pneumothorax. Auscultation reveals reduced or absent breath sounds on the affected side. The affected hemithorax is hyperresonant to percussion. Subcutaneous emphysema, if present, may become suddenly worse.

- Identify the affected hemithorax and place a 12-gauge IV cannula in the 2nd intercostal space, midclavicular line. Attach it to a flutter valve or leave it open to air. (Alternatively, needle decompression can be performed in the same location as a tube thoracostomy, 4th–5th intercostal space, just anterior to the mid axillary line.)
- Needle thoracostomies with IV cannulas are prone to block or kink and may be too short to drain reliably unless a longer than standard cannula is used.
- Placement of the cannula commits to a formal tube thoracostomy.
- Experienced practitioners adept at rapid insertion of tube thoracostomy will be less likely to need needle thoracostomy. Nonetheless, the patient must not be allowed to deteriorate or remain untreated if a slow process of tube thoracostomy is anticipated.
- Initiate high-flow oxygen.
- Obtain IV access for sedation and analgesia in the case of tube thoracostomy.

Specific treatment
Treatment options are available, depending on the patient's underlying condition and the response of the pneumothorax.

1 **Conservative management as an outpatient**
- Suitable for patients with a small pneumothorax, no preexisting lung disease, mild symptoms and no hypoxia. The pneumothorax is treated with high-flow oxygen while being assessed, but is not drained. The patient is discharged after remaining stable for 4–6 hours of observation.
- The patient is advised to seek follow-up X-rays (12–48 hours, shorter if a repeat X-ray is not taken prior to discharge), and full resolution and clearance is required before flying or diving. Discharge is not advised if any doubts exist as to the patient's ability to return promptly to hospital.

2 **Aspiration of pneumothorax**
- Suitable for patients with moderate symptoms and a 20–40% pneumothorax with no underlying lung disease (secondary spontaneous pneumothorax).
- An IV cannula and three-way tap or other catheters designed for the purpose may be used.
- A pigtail catheter inserted using Seldinger technique may be safer and also effective if continuous drainage is required.
- The pneumothorax is aspirated using a three-way tap and then X-rays are repeated.
- If the pneumothorax has recurred on repeat CXR, a formal tube thoracostomy should be performed or, if a suitable catheter was used initially, it may be connected to an underwater drain and low suction.

3 **Tube thoracostomy**
- The best choice for those with a large pneumothorax or significant underlying lung disease.
- Use as much local infiltration of 1% lignocaine as can be safely administered to the site of insertion, especially the parietal pleura and liberal IV analgesia and sedation.
- Place the tube in the 4th–5th intercostal space and directed superiorly.
- Avoid placing the tube where lung adhesions may be present as seen on CXR. Use the 2nd intercostal

space midclavicular line if necessary. Connect to low suction.

Large pneumothoraces are regarded as $> 2–3$ cm of collapse; however, treatment decisions regarding 'smaller' pneumothoraces should be based on the patient's stability, as determinations of pneumothorax size from CXR are notoriously inaccurate.

Male smokers have a 20-fold increased risk of primary spontaneous pneumothorax.

COPD and cystic fibrosis patients have increased risk and associated mortality.

Recurrent spontaneous pneumothoraces (i.e. same hemithorax) should be referred to a thoracic surgeon for possible thoracoscopic treatment.

PULMONARY EMBOLISM

This topic is covered in Chapter 16 Venous Thromboembolic Disease: Deep Venous Thrombosis and Pulmonary Embolism.

ACUTE LUNG INJURY (NON-CARDIOGENIC PULMONARY OEDEMA)

- This represents a range of conditions characterised by inflammation or injury causing increased permeability of lung tissue and exudation of fluid into the alveoli.
- Wet, stiff lungs make gas exchange and ventilation difficult.
- The condition may not become apparent until the patient starts to decompensate and tire, hours after the initial insult. Further decompensation is likely and should be anticipated.
- Respiratory dysfunction may become apparent as late as 48 hours or longer after the initial insult and may take weeks or months to resolve.
- Causes include pulmonary contusion, aspiration, chemical pneumonitis, narcotic overdose, near drowning, transfusion of blood products, SARS, avian influenza and severe sepsis.
- When invasive ventilation is required, care should be taken to avoid further ventilator-associated lung injury, as these patients are particularly at risk, especially from barotrauma.

ANAPHYLAXIS WITH BRONCHOSPASM

(See also Chapter 5 Shock, Figure 5.1.)

- Anaphylaxis may present with respiratory distress with or without shock as a result of the type 1 hypersensitivity reaction.
- Initial management is with adrenaline 0.5 mg intramuscular injection (IMI). These patients may require repeat doses and/or intravenous adrenaline infusions as well as treatment with bronchodilators and steroids.
- They can be identified by known history of allergy and precipitants, airway involvement with signs of oedema and voice changes, urticaria and pruritus. Suspect also when 'asthma' is of sudden onset without obvious precipitant.
- Following this initial therapy the patient should also receive oral prednisone (1 mg/kg maximum 50 mg) or IV hydrocortisone (5 mg/kg maximum 200 mg).
- Observe the patient for at least 4 hours from last adrenaline injection and longer if late at night or living far from hospital.

HYPERVENTILATION

- Organic causes of hyperpnoea and hypocapnia must be considered and excluded initially.
- A CXR will be normal and ABGs will show respiratory alkalosis.
- Patients may present with non-exertional chest pain, blurred vision, palpitations, paraesthesia, carpopedal spasm, fear, panic and hysteria.
- Treatment is with patient education and relaxation techniques, the goal being to achieve self-control.
- Antidepressants possibly have a role in recurrent cases but should not be initiated in the ED.
- A short course of benzodiazepines may be of limited use, for some patients.
- Mitral valve prolapse may present with atypical chest pain, palpitations, dyspnoea, anxiety and panic attacks—so, if a typical click is heard and associated ECG changes seen, an outpatient echocardiogram should be arranged.
- 'Paper bag breathing' is not recommended.

Editorial Comment

ABC (airway, breathing, circulation)—beware of breathing, as deterioration can be subtle; look for trends in observations and tests.

Respiratory rates are very good measures of the degree of respiratory compromise.

Pulse oximetry—respond if low or drops.

For ventilated patients with high and increasing oxygen requirements and reversible conditions, early consultation with retrieval ECMO (extracorporeal membrane oxygenation) services, where available, is advised.

Chapter 14
Haemoptysis

Rahul Santram

Haemoptysis is defined as the expectoration of blood or blood-stained sputum derived from below the level of the glottis.

The lung has a dual arterial blood supply.

1 Pulmonary arteries
  — Low pressure system (20/10 mmHg)
  — Responsible for 99% of the arterial blood supply
  — Take part in gas exchange
2 Bronchial arteries
  — High pressure system
  — Nourish the supporting structures of the airways including the blood vessels
  — Source of bleeding in 95% of cases

Life-threatening disease may be causing haemoptysis, hence warranting urgent investigation.

Haemoptysis can be classified as minor and massive depending on the volume of blood loss.

Massive haemoptysis is where excessive bleeding disrupts breathing; this can be 600 mL/24 hours or 50 mL following a coughing episode. It is not the loss of blood that is usually the danger; rather, it is the hypoxia due to blood obstructing the larger airways and gas exchange surfaces. Mortality from massive haemoptysis is approximately 30% and this is contributed to by underlying malignancy or coagulopathy.

The majority of haemoptysis (95% of cases) is of a minor nature and after an initial set of investigations (CXR, FBC, EUC [electrolytes, urea and creatinine]) in the ED can be followed in an outpatient setting.

• Aetiology: broad differential

- Infection: bacterial or viral bronchitis or pneumonia. Cavitatory lung diseases like TB. Old cavitatory lung lesions may become infected with fungi resulting in a mycetoma.
- Neoplastic: small cell lung cancer, squamous cell lung cancer, carcinoid, bronchial cancer and lung metastases. A clear CXR does not exclude cancer especially if there is a history of smoking. Consider high-resolution CT chest +/− bronchoscopy.
- Bronchiectasis: long-standing bronchiectasis results in abnormally dilated bronchial arteries which are prone to erosion and thus massive bleeding.
- Vascular: PE, arteriovenous malformation (AVM), pulmonary hypertension, aortobronchial fistula.
- Vasculitis: granulomatosis with polyangiitis, SLE, Goodpasture's syndrome and other autoimmune vasculitides.
- Cardiac: mitral stenosis, tricuspid endocarditis and heart failure.
- Haematologic: coagulopathy (idiopathic and iatrogenic), DIC, platelet dysfunction and thrombocytopenia.
- Traumatic: pulmonary contusion, lung laceration and tracheobronchial rupture.
- Others: iatrogenic (biopsy, aspirate, instrumentation), pulmonary endometriosis, FB aspiration, amyloid and 20% cases are idiopathic.
- Spurious: haematemesis, epistaxis, sinusitis and pharyngeal tumour.

Overall, the most common cause of haemoptysis is bronchitis.

In Australia, the common causes of massive haemoptysis are previous cavitatory lung disease and bronchiectasis pulmonary vasculitis.

Pertinent history is:

- frank blood, streaks of blood or blood mixed with purulent sputum
- amount of blood loss (a patient's ability to estimate volume is limited)
- smoking history—nicotine, THC, other drugs
- known lung, renal or heart disease
- anticoagulant or antiplatelet use
- coughing or vomiting.

Previous episodes would suggest a chronic condition.
Management of massive haemoptysis:

- resus bay, comprehensive monitoring.
- assess need for urgent airway security.
- oxygen to correct hypoxaemia.
- large-bore IV.
- replace volume with crystalloid and blood products.
- CXR, FBC, EUC, coagulation testing and urgent crossmatch plus group and hold
- tranexamic acid 1 g IV
- patient to be nursed in a sitting up position
- reverse coagulopathy if present—use antidotes if required
- early involvement of anaesthetics, thoracic medicine, cardiothoracic surgery and interventional radiology
- may need selective bronchial intubation to protect the good lung or endobronchial tamponade of the bleeding lung
- therapies available will depend on the nature of pathology: bronchoscopy, bronchial artery embolisation (98% success, 20% rebleed rate), surgical resection (lobectomy, pneumonectomy).

Chapter 15
Acute pulmonary oedema

Anthony FT Brown

Overview

Acute pulmonary oedema (APO) is one of the acute heart failure (AHF) syndromes that include the spectrum from acute decompensated (chronic) heart failure (ADHF), hypertensive AHF, high-output heart failure and right-heart failure, to the more dramatic APO and cardiogenic shock.

APO accounts for up to 1% of ED visits, with a 7.4–15% in-hospital mortality and up to as high as a 40% 1-year mortality.

Although the classical gasping, frail, elderly patient may dominate the doctor's perspective, APO presents to the ED in a diverse population, from those with an underlying acute coronary syndrome (ACS), whether an ST-elevation myocardial infarct (STEMI) or non-ST-elevation myocardial infarct (NSTEMI), those with an acute hypertensive event, to those with chronic decompensated heart failure, or a non-cardiogenic cause.

All have subtly different historical, examination and investigation findings, and may require a wide array of urgent treatment modalities.

Pathophysiology

APO may be divided into cardiogenic and non-cardiogenic causes.

ACUTE CARDIOGENIC PULMONARY OEDEMA

Acute cardiogenic pulmonary oedema is the most severe manifestation of congestive heart failure, and is associated with an increase in lung fluid secondary to hydrostatic leakage from pulmonary capillaries into the alveoli and interstitium of the lungs. Underlying this is an abrupt rise in left-ventricular end-diastolic pressure and left atrial pressure related to left-ventricular dysfunction.

The causative heart disease leading to left-ventricular failure may be predominantly systolic failure with impaired cardiac contractility; that is, with an ejection fraction (EF) under 40%, diastolic failure with impaired myocardial relaxation and distensibility (but with a normal or even supranormal EF), or with a combination of both.

APO may develop out of the blue, or be precipitated in patients with existing heart disease as a result of an acute cause such as ischaemia, an arrhythmia or medication change.

Box 15.1 lists the potential causes of cardiogenic pulmonary oedema, whether related to predominant systolic or to diastolic dysfunction, with common precipitating factors.

Box 15.1   Causes of cardiogenic pulmonary oedema
Precipitating factors
• Myocardial ischaemia
• Cardiac arrhythmia:
— tachycardia, including atrial fibrillation
— bradycardia, conduction abnormality
• Volume overload, including blood transfusion
• Hypertensive crisis
• Cardiac infection: myocarditis, endocarditis
• Renovascular disease, including renal artery stenosis
• Systemic infection, including septic shock
• Medication-related:
— inappropriate reduction of therapy
— drug non-compliance
— cardiac depressant (beta-blocker)
— salt-retaining (non-steroidal anti-inflammatory drug [NSAID])
• High-output state: anaemia, thyrotoxicosis, beriberi
Predominant systolic heart failure
• Acute coronary syndrome
• Hypertension
• Valvular disease, particularly acute aortic or mitral regurgitation
• Myocarditis, such as Coxsackie B or echovirus
• Cardiomyopathy
Predominant diastolic heart failure (up to 50% of all patients)
• Hypertension, including renovascular disease
• Aortic stenosis (indicates critical disease)
• Acute coronary syndrome
• Cardiomyopathy—hypertrophic (HCM) or restrictive

NON-CARDIOGENIC PULMONARY OEDEMA

Non-cardiogenic pulmonary oedema occurs without a rise in pulmonary capillary wedge pressure > 18 mmHg, and may result from a wide variety of mechanisms that include:

- increased capillary permeability in acute respiratory distress syndrome (ARDS), septicaemia, aspiration of gastric contents, inhaled toxins, pancreatitis, uraemia or near-drowning
- mixed or unknown causes such as neurogenic pulmonary oedema, high-altitude pulmonary oedema (HAPE), transfusion-related acute lung injury (TRALI), heroin overdose, smoking freebase cocaine, eclampsia, pulmonary embolism and post lung re-expansion
- decreased oncotic pressure such as in hypoalbuminaemia, usually in combination with another cause above.

NEUROGENIC PULMONARY OEDEMA

This is a rare cause of APO developing within a few hours of an acute neurological insult associated with sympathetic over-reactivity and intracranial hypertension. Typical causes include prolonged seizures, head injury or a subarachnoid or intracerebral haemorrhage.

It usually resolves over 48–72 hours, determined by the management and course of the underlying primary neurological insult.

Clinical features
HISTORY

Patients may be too distressed to give a history until after aggressive medical management, but may report chest pain, palpitations, a change in medication or recent fever (see Box 15.1) as a precipitating cause, or remember previous flash episodes of 'fluid on the lung'.

Acute breathlessness is universal, and may occur precipitately, or be progressive on a background of cough, exertional dyspnoea, orthopnoea, paroxysmal nocturnal dyspnoea (PND) and dyspnoea at rest.

Other non-specific features such as fatigue and nocturia may occur in those with previously compensated heart failure. Finally, confusion, coma and respiratory arrest can ensue.

EXAMINATION

- Patients with APO are frightened, sweaty, restless, unwilling to lie down, and may wheeze or froth pink sputum in extreme cases.
- Tachypnoea, tachycardia, reduced oxygen saturation, hyper- or hypotension and cyanosis all occur.
- Inspiratory basal crackles, bilateral pleural effusions, a raised jugular venous pressure (JVP) from secondary right-heart failure and a 3rd heart sound S_3 gallop are typical.
- Conversely in non-cardiogenic pulmonary oedema, patients may have a warm periphery, bounding pulse and usually absence of an S_3 gallop or jugular venous distension.
- A new systolic murmur can indicate an acute mechanical complication such as papillary muscle rupture or an acquired ventricular septal defect (VSD) in the setting of an acute myocardial infarction (AMI).

Differential diagnosis

Pulmonary embolism (PE) and acute pneumonia must be considered, as PE is predisposed to in heart failure, and severe pneumonia may of itself lead to non-cardiogenic pulmonary oedema.

Investigations
ELECTROCARDIOGRAM (ECG)

This is essential to diagnose an AMI, arrhythmia or heart block, and may determine the need for time-critical reperfusion therapy in the presence of chest pain particularly with STEMI. See Chapter 11 Acute Coronary Syndromes.

It may also indicate underlying heart disease with left-ventricular strain or hypertrophy, pre-existing coronary artery disease or even an electrolyte disturbance such as tall peaked T waves in acute hyperkalaemia.

CHEST X-RAY (CXR)

CXR can confirm the presence of APO, but due to its relatively poor sensitivity, it should not be used to rule out the diagnosis when oedema fluid is not visible, or in the presence of technical issues particularly with a portable film that is 'poorly penetrated.'

The CXR may help to differentiate APO from an exacerbation of chronic obstructive pulmonary disease (COPD) or asthma.

1 Typical CXR features of cardiogenic pulmonary oedema include cardiomegaly, pulmonary venous congestion with upper lobe diversion, perihilar 'bat's wing' infiltrates, Kerley B engorged subpleural lymphatics, interstitial oedema and small pleural effusions.

2 A normal heart size may occur in acute valvular rupture, diastolic dysfunction, myocarditis or non-cardiogenic causes of pulmonary oedema.

3 Non-cardiogenic pulmonary oedema will also show patchy or peripheral oedema, rather than even and central. Kerley B-lines and pleural effusions are usually not present.

BEDSIDE ULTRASOUND
Lung ultrasound
Bedside lung ultrasound demonstrates a bilateral alveolar interstitial syndrome (AIS) pattern, typically with multiple B-lines less than 3 mm apart, associated with hypoechoic (i.e. dark) basal effusions. Severe pulmonary oedema may lead to confluent B-lines appearing like a 'snowstorm'.

Echocardiography
Bedside transthoracic echo can rapidly evaluate for ventricular size, global or regional systolic dysfunction, diastolic dysfunction, a valvular disorder and for pericardial disease. It is of particular early value to demonstrate a suspected complication of ACS including acute valvular rupture.

LABORATORY TESTS
A full blood count, electrolyte and liver function tests, troponin, coagulation profile and thyroid function test should be sent, but usually add little to the immediate management.

Biomarkers
Troponin
An elevated troponin may indicate myocardial damage from an ACS, particularly in the presence of new ECG changes, but also

occurs in the absence of ACS, for instance in severe sepsis or from a PE.

B-type natriuretic polypeptide (BNP)

Other biomarkers such as BNP and *N*-terminal (NT) pro-BNP are of most value when the diagnosis is uncertain, such as the patient with acute dyspnoea possibly due to exacerbation of an underlying respiratory disorder such as COPD rather than a cardiac cause. A BNP level under 100 pg/mL makes heart failure unlikely (approximate negative likelihood ratio [LR] = 0.1), and above 400 pg/mL makes heart failure likely (approximate positive LR = 6).

However, between 100 and 400 pg/mL is an 'indiscriminate zone' that necessitates clinical judgment with further testing. In addition, both markers may be raised in the presence of renal disease, PE and cor pulmonale, and conversely both may be low in 'flash' APO, acute papillary muscle rupture and the obese.

Thus BNP use in the ED is uncommon, and in the ICU can be problematic; it may be better suited to assessing progress in response to therapy.

Blood gases

A bedside venous blood gas (VBG) will rapidly demonstrate underlying anaemia, hyper- or hypokalaemia and acidosis. Conversely, as with other laboratory tests, doing an ABG adds nothing to the immediate management and serves only to delay therapy. It may be useful to monitor hypercapnia in the non-responding patient, possibly following insertion of an invasive arterial line.

Management of APO

1 Sit the patient upright, apply high-flow oxygen via a non-rebreathing mask if there is hypoxia with oxygen saturations below 93% or shock, and prepare for non-invasive ventilation in a resuscitation area.
2 Commence vasodilator therapy with nitrates to reduce preload, particularly in patients with systolic blood pressure (SBP) above 140 mmHg.
   a Give glyceryl trinitrate (GTN) 150–300 microg sublingually. This dose may be repeated. Remove the tablet or cease if hypotension (SBP below 100 mmHg) occurs.

   b Change to a GTN infusion in resistant cases, particularly those associated with ischaemic chest pain. Add 200 mg GTN to 500 mL 5% dextrose (i.e. 400 microg/mL) in a glass bottle with low-absorption polyethylene infusion set. Commence at 1 mL/h (6.66 microg/min) and gradually increase to 20 mL/h or more, taking care to maintain SBP above 100 mmHg.

3 Give frusemide 40 mg IV or twice the usual oral daily dose if already taking frusemide tablets, which may be repeated after 20–30 minutes.

   a No randomised controlled trial has shown a mortality benefit with the use of frusemide alone in acute decompensated heart failure, whether as a bolus or as an infusion, but it is logical particularly with fluid overload.

   b Avoid overdiuresis, as this may activate neurohormonal systems with a deterioration in renal function and a worsened outcome, particularly in those presenting hypertensive with predominant diastolic dysfunction.

4 Give small increments of morphine *only* when there is chest pain with dyspnoea that is resistant to nitrates, starting at 0.5 mg morphine IV in the elderly up to 2.5 mg in younger patients.

   a Do not use morphine routinely, particularly if non-invasive ventilation is planned, or the patient is becoming tired or even obtunded with a rising arterial partial pressure of CO_2 ($PaCO_2$). Morphine is also contraindicated in suspected underlying COPD or asthma.

   b Morphine also does not reduce mortality and may worsen acidosis.

5 Commence non-invasive ventilation (NIV) in those who do not respond to the above standard pharmacological therapy.

   a Use continuous positive airway pressure (CPAP) via a tight-fitting face mask, high-flow gas circuit and starting with 10–15 cmH_2O.

   b CPAP improves lung mechanics and enhances left-ventricular performance, reducing the need for endotracheal intubation (relative risk [RR] 0.44) and the in-hospital mortality (RR 0.64).

c   Bi-level positive airway pressure (BiPAP) non-invasive positive-pressure ventilation (NIPPV) is an alternative, starting at 10/5 cmH$_2$O (inspiratory/expiratory positive airway pressures). However, it is more complex to set up and costly, and although it reduces the need for intubation in cardiogenic pulmonary oedema (RR 0.54), there is contradictory evidence as regards reduction of the in-hospital mortality.

Disposal

1   The majority of patients respond to standard pharmacological therapy plus NIV.
   a   Arrange admission to a coronary care or telemetry unit if there are ongoing cardiac issues such as pain, ischaemia, arrhythmias or an electrolyte disturbance and close monitoring or respiratory support are necessary.
   b   Otherwise, particularly in the elderly patient with brief decompensation of chronic heart failure, admit the patient to a non-monitored medical bed.
2   Patients who present hypotensive with SBP < 90 mmHg in cardiogenic shock, or who deteriorate and/or do not tolerate pharmacological vasodilation, have a poor prognosis with a mortality up to 80%.
   a   Call for senior help if you have not already done so. Manage the patient as for cardiogenic shock with endotracheal intubation and mechanical ventilation, applying 5–10 cmH$_2$O positive end-expiratory pressure (PEEP).
   b   Support the circulation with an inotrope such as dobutamine 2–30 microg/kg/min. This invariably requires adding a vasopressor such as noradrenaline or adrenaline for worsened hypotension, but the higher myocardial oxygen demand may ultimately be deleterious.
   c   Organise reperfusion therapy—such as acute angioplasty or coronary revascularisation— in the setting of a STEMI.
   d   Look for a treatable mechanical cause with bedside transthoracic echocardiogram, such as an acute valvular rupture or VSD, and arrange immediate cardiac surgical referral if one of these is found.

   e Admit the patient to intensive care. An intra-aortic balloon pump may be used as a temporising measure while valvular or VSD repair is organised (see above), or even a left-ventricular assist device in suitable, usually younger patients with a potentially reversible cause, or pending cardiac transplantation.

3 Non-cardiogenic pulmonary oedema is managed according to the underlying primary cause (e.g. antibiotics for infection), and with non-invasive or invasive respiratory support as necessary.

Clinical Pearls

- Up to half of all cases of acute decompensated heart failure may include diastolic dysfunction with a preserved ejection fraction.
- Make sure to look out for potentially reversible causes such as a STEMI (arrange urgent reperfusion therapy), or acute valvular rupture (arrange urgent surgery).
- Bedside lung ultrasound has similar if not better sensitivity (normal rules out) and specificity (abnormal rules in) for acute pulmonary oedema compared with CXR.
- Avoid giving morphine, and start NIV early in the management.

Online resources

National Institute for Health and Care Excellence (NICE). Acute heart failure: diagnosis and management. Clinical Guideline [CG187]. October 2014. Retrieved from: www.nice.org.uk/guidance/cg187

Purvey M, Allen G. Managing acute pulmonary oedema. Aust Prescr. 2017;40:59–63. doi:10.18773/austprescr.2017.013

UpToDate: multiple topics including 'Pathophysiology of cardiogenic pulmonary edema'; 'Approach to acute decompensated heart failure in adults'; 'Treatment of acute decompensated heart failure: General considerations'; 'Treatment of acute decompensated heart failure in acute coronary syndromes'; 'Noncardiogenic pulmonary edema'. See www.uptodate.com/

Chapter 16
Venous thromboembolic disease: deep venous thrombosis and pulmonary embolism

Tim Green

Acknowledgment

The author wishes to acknowledge George Jelinek and Martin Duffy who contributed previous versions of this chapter.

Introduction

Venous thromboembolism (VTE) has a significant untreated mortality of up to 30%. Mortality within a month of diagnosis is 6% for DVT and 12% for PE. While hospitalisation or recent hospitalisation itself is the major risk factor for developing VTE, up to 43% of cases are acquired in the community and commonly present to EDs.

While both DVT and PE have a number of characteristic clinical features, these are neither sensitive nor specific and clinical diagnosis is difficult. ED evaluation involves a structured approach of risk stratification, screening investigations, a search for alternative diagnoses and selection of an appropriate imaging strategy. The approach taken in an individual ED will depend on its case-mix and the availability of key modalities of investigation, and a balance must be struck between the harms of undiagnosed disease and the adverse events associated with both invasive investigations and anticoagulation.

While VTE is increasingly safely treated in the community, often in a hospital in the home (HITH) setting, it is important to identify patients who may need invasive therapies such as thrombolysis or surgery. While parenteral and oral anticoagulation effectively decrease morbidity and mortality from VTE, they pose a not inconsiderable cost, inconvenience and risk of harm, so it is critical that a firm diagnosis of VTE is made before committing a patient to long-term therapy.

Pathophysiology

Predisposition to VTE is best understood by analysis of Virchow's triad of *venous stasis*, *vessel wall injury* and *hypercoagulable states* and forms the basis of most clinical decision rules for VTE.

- Stasis may result from immobility (particularly in hospital), external compression by pelvic tumours or lower limb plaster splints.
- Vessel wall injury may be the result of trauma, surgery or intravascular device.
- Hypercoagulability is a feature of pregnancy, oral contraceptive pill or hormone replacement therapy (HRT) use, cancer and a number of thrombophilic disorders (see Box 16.1).

Age is an important risk factor for VTE, via a number of mechanisms: increasing venous valve incompetence, acquired thrombophilia such as malignancy, increased risk of comorbid diseases such as cardiac failure, renal disease or the need for surgery, particularly joint replacement.

Venous thrombi, particularly when fresh, may dislodge and embolise centrally to the right ventricle and pulmonary arterial circulation or paradoxically via a patent foramen ovale or atrial septal defect into the systemic circulation. Patients with proximal leg or pelvic vein DVT will develop PE in approximately 50% of cases. Calf vein DVT are much less likely to embolise to the lungs but are the most common source of paradoxical emboli.

Pulmonary emboli lead to hypoxaemia by increasing both anatomical and physiological dead space. Multiple or large emboli

---

Box 16.1 Thrombophilic disorders associated with VTE

Antithrombin III deficiency
Protein C deficiency
Protein S deficiency
Factor V Leiden
Prothrombin G20210A
Homocysteinaemia
Antiphospholipid syndrome
Elevated factor VIII
Elevated factor IX
Elevated factor XI
Elevated fibrinogen

---

will lead to an increase in pulmonary vascular resistance, which in turn leads to increasing right ventricular wall tension and may lead to right ventricular dysfunction. Increased right ventricular wall pressure may compress the right coronary artery as well as impairing subendocardial blood flow, and precipitate myocardial ischaemia. This may be accompanied by micro-infarction and elevation of cardiac biomarkers such as troponin. Massive PE will eventually cause paradoxical interventricular septal motion, left ventricular diastolic dysfunction and impaired cardiac output. Death is the result of circulatory shock and myocardial ischaemia.

Therapeutic anticoagulation inhibits formation of new clot. Fresh clot is more friable and prone to embolise. In time, existing clot ages and becomes more stable, decreasing the risk of embolism. With therapeutic anticoagulation the fibrinolytic pathway is able to partially or completely remove preexisting clot. The success of this process will be measured in the incidence of post-phlebitic complications such as oedema and venous ulcers in the lower limb following DVT or chronic pulmonary hypertension and cor pulmonale complicating PE.

Clinical features

DVT may cause calf and/or thigh pain and lower limb swelling but is frequently asymptomatic. Typical signs of DVT, including unilateral swelling, oedema, erythema, local warmth and tenderness along the distribution of deep veins, are variable in frequency and examination may be entirely normal. Extensive pelvic or proximal DVT may present with a grossly swollen, painful limb of pale or dusky blue appearance (phlegmasia alba dolens and phlegmasia cerulea dolens, respectively). These presentations represent an acute limb threat and mandate aggressive inpatient therapy, frequently with catheter-delivered thrombolysis or thrombectomy.

Patients with **PE** may or may not have clinical evidence of concomitant DVT. Common but non-specific symptoms of PE include dyspnoea, pleuritic chest pain, apprehension and cough (> 50%). Haemoptysis, sweats, syncope and non-pleuritic pain are less common (15–30%). Apart from tachycardia and tachypnoea, physical signs of PE such as pleural rubs, loud P2 or gallop rhythm are relatively rarely found. Massive PE should be considered in patients who present with sudden cardiovascular decompensation, syncope, unexplained hypoxia, shock or pulseless electrical activity (PEA) cardiac arrest.

DIFFERENTIAL DIAGNOSES
DVT
- Ruptured Baker's cyst, cellulitis, muscle strain/haematoma, superficial venous thrombophlebitis, chronic venous insufficiency

PE
- Pulmonary: pneumonia, asthma, COPD, pneumothorax, pleurisy
- Cardiovascular: ACS, pericarditis, CCF, aortic dissection
- Musculoskeletal: chest wall strain, rib fracture
- Anxiety

Diagnostic approach and clinical decision rules

ED assessment for patients presenting with symptoms of possible VTE is focused on searching for and ruling out alternative diagnoses, establishing the clinical likelihood for VTE and determining whether diagnostic imaging is required. Clinical impression, or pre-test probability (PTP), is best guided by one of many validated clinical decision rules that have been produced for both DVT and PE. Such risk stratification combined with the measurement of D-dimer can either rule out significant risk of VTE or mandate specific imaging.

DVT
Wells et al. have published clinical decision rules for both DVT and PE. Wells' criteria for DVT are listed in Table 16.1.
- Low risk: score = 0, DVT risk is 5%. With negative D-dimer, risk is < 1% and VTE is effectively ruled out.
- Intermediate risk: score 1 or 2, DVT risk is 17%.
- High risk: score 3 or greater, DVT risk is 53%.
- Intermediate and high-risk patients require further assessment with ultrasonography. If ultrasonography is negative but D-dimer is positive, repeat ultrasound in 1 week should be recommended.

Table 16.1 Clinical model for predicting the pre-test probability of DVT

Clinical characteristic	Score
Active cancer (patient receiving treatment for cancer within the previous 6 months or currently receiving palliative treatment)	1
Paralysis, paresis or recent plaster immobilisation of the lower extremities	1
Recently bedridden for 3 days or more, or major surgery within the previous 12 weeks requiring general or regional anaesthesia	1
Localised tenderness along the distribution of the deep venous system	1
Entire leg swollen	1
Calf swelling at least 3 cm larger than that on the asymptomatic side (measured 10 cm below tibial tuberosity)	1
Pitting oedema confined to the symptomatic leg	1
Collateral superficial veins (non-varicose)	1
Previously documented DVT	1
Alternative diagnosis at least as likely as DVT	−2

Scoring method indicates high probability if score is 3 or more; moderate if score is 1 or 2; and low if score is 0 or less. In patients with symptoms in both legs, the more symptomatic leg was used.
Reproduced from Wells PS, Owen C, Doucette S, et al. Does this patient have deep venous thrombosis? JAMA. Jan 11 2006;295;20:199–207 with permission.

Pregnant and postpartum women should not be assessed with these criteria and should generally all have ultrasonography if DVT is suspected.

If a patient presents out of hours and ultrasound is not available, the risks of treatment without formal diagnosis must be assessed against the risk of bleeding. Bleeding into a calf muscle tear leading to compartment syndrome is an increasingly recognised complication. While individual risk assessment should apply, generally intermediate risk patients should not be anticoagulated while awaiting ultrasound, while high-risk patients usually should.

PE

For patients in whom the clinical 'gestalt' for PE is low (< 15%), the PE Rule-out Criteria (PERC Rule) can be applied prior to ordering D-dimer or imaging. The mnemonic HADCLOTS represents

8 clinical criteria which if all met can effectively rule out PE without further investigation.

H Hormone: no oestrogen use/pregnancy
A Age < 50 years
D DVT/PE: no previous history
C Coughing blood: no haemoptysis
L Leg swelling: absence of unilateral limb swelling
O Oxygen: $SaO_2 > 95\%$
T Tachycardia (absence): HR < 100 bpm
S Surgery: nil recent (< 28 days)

A myriad of clinical decision rules have been described for evaluation of PE. The Wells PE Score remains the most commonly used (Table 16.2).

- Low pre-test probability as judged by a Wells score ≤ 4 combined with a negative D-dimer effectively rules out PE without requiring imaging.
- Patients with positive D-dimer or a Wells score > 4 may have PE diagnosed or ruled out with CT pulmonary angiography.
- V/Q scanning can be considered in patients with a normal chest X-ray when contrast and radiation exposure need to be avoided/minimised. An alternative strategy is to perform

Table 16.2   Wells PE score

Clinical feature	Points
Suspected DVT	3
Alternative diagnosis less likely than PE	3
Heart rate > 100 bpm	1.5
Prior VTE	1.5
Immobilisation within prior 4 weeks	1.5
Active malignancy	1
Haemoptysis	1
Score < 2: low risk (3.4%) Score 2–6: moderate risk (27.8%) Score > 6: high risk (78.4%)	

Adapted from Wells PS, Anderson DR, Rodger M et al. Excluding pulmonary embolism at the bedside without diagnostic imaging: management of patients with suspected pulmonary embolism presenting to the emergency department by using a simple clinical model and D-dimer. Ann Intern Med 2001;135:98–107.

lower limb ultrasound first, with a positive diagnosis of DVT obviating the need for further investigation.

Investigations

- **ECG:** mainly performed to exclude acute myocardial ischaemia or pericarditis, ECG may reveal signs of right ventricular strain. Sinus tachycardia is common, as is anterior T wave inversion. The classical S_1, Q_3, T_3 pattern is relatively specific for PE but quite rarely seen.
- **Chest X-ray:** the main purpose of chest radiography is to establish alternative diagnoses such as pneumonia or pneumothorax. In cases of PE, chest X-ray is often normal or near-normal. Signs of focal oligaemia (focal decrease in vascular markings) or pulmonary infarction (such as the Hampton's hump, a peripheral wedge-shaped density above the diaphragm) are not common. Atelectasis and small pleural effusions are often non-specific markers of PE.
- **Blood gases:** although blood gas analysis may provide useful information of acidosis in moderate to severe PE, the diagnostic utility of identifying hypoxaemia, hypocarbia or elevated A–a gradient is not great and is not helpful in determining whether imaging is necessary. Evidence of hypoxaemia is easily diagnosed using non-invasive pulse oximetry.
- **D-dimer:** D-dimer is produced during the breakdown of fibrin by plasmin and is a marker of the presence of clot and in vivo thrombolysis. A good-quality quantitative D-dimer enzyme-linked immunosorbent assay (ELISA) has a sensitivity of about 80% for DVT and 95% for PE and is subsequently a useful test to rule out VTE, particularly if the assessment of clinical likelihood is low. Unfortunately, the specificity of D-dimer is low, and it is frequently elevated in patients with acute illness (such as ACS, cancer or sepsis), in the postoperative period and during and after pregnancy.
- **Troponin:** elevation in cardiac biomarkers such as troponin, while not diagnostic of VTE, is a marker of severity of PE and may predict complications and mortality.
- **Ultrasound:** Doppler ultrasound has almost completely replaced contrast venography in the diagnosis of DVT.

DVT is manifest by lack of vein compressibility, direct visualisation of thrombus and abnormal Doppler flow response to compression. Whole-leg colour-flow Doppler ultrasound is performed by radiology departments and vascular laboratories and has a sensitivity of 91–96% and a specificity of 98–100%. Bedside ultrasound in the ED, using a limited technique of 2-point compression of the femoral and popliteal veins, is being increasingly used to exclude proximal vein DVT and is a skill that can be readily acquired by competent ED sonographers.

- **CT pulmonary angiography (CTPA):** modern multi-detector spiral CT scanners are able to obtain images with a resolution of less than 1 mm and are able to diagnose very small peripheral emboli. CTPA has now completely replaced conventional pulmonary angiography. In addition to diagnosing or ruling out PE, CT may establish an alternative diagnosis by imaging pathology in the lung or aorta. Modern CTPA has a sensitivity of 83% and a specificity of 96%. CTPA may not be readily available in smaller centres or after hours. Contrast allergy and renal impairment limit its safety in some groups, and the cumulative radiation burden of modern medicine remains a concern.
- **Ventilation–perfusion scan:** V/Q scanning is now a second-line test for PE, but still has a role in patients intolerant to iodine-containing contrast and by virtue of its lower radiation dose in pregnant patients. V/Q scanning is of most utility in patients without underlying acute or chronic lung disease. High-probability V/Q scans and normal V/Q scans are able to diagnose or exclude PE. Intermediate-probability scans are common and necessitate another diagnostic approach.
- **Other imaging:**
  — CT contrast venography may be performed immediately after CTPA without requiring further IV contrast to diagnose proximal DVT.
  — DVT may also be diagnosed as an incidental finding during abdominal/pelvic contrast CT.
  — Gadolinium-enhanced contrast magnetic resonance angiography (MRA) may be used in cases where ultrasound is not diagnostic.

— Bedside echocardiography is of particular use in evaluating critically ill patients in the ED resuscitation room with right ventricular dilation, hypokinesis, and rarely direct clot visualisation may diagnose massive PE or one of its mimics (AMI, pericardial tamponade, aortic dissection).

• **Tests for underlying thrombophilia in confirmed cases of VTE:** while testing for underlying thrombophilic disorders has traditionally been advocated, some now question the cost–benefit of this. Idiopathic (versus provoked) VTE is associated with a similar risk of recurrence as VTE associated with a thrombophilic disorder, and it is argued that a decision about the duration of anticoagulation can be made for all idiopathic VTE without extensive testing. An exception is the antiphospholipid syndrome, which if diagnosed in a patient with VTE mandates lifelong anticoagulation.

Treatment
ANTICOAGULATION

Traditional anticoagulation for all VTE has been with heparin and warfarin, with heparin being discontinued when the international normalised ration (INR) is therapeutic. With the exceptions of submassive/massive PE, pregnancy and cancer-associated VTE, non-vitamin K oral anticoagulants (NOACs) are being commonly used as single agents to treat both DVT and PE, and this is supported by high-quality evidence.

• NOACs can be started without bridging heparin and do not require monitoring. Apixaban 10 mg BD for 7 days, continuing with 5 mg BD or rivaroxaban 15 mg BD for 3 weeks followed by 20 mg daily are commonly used regimens but caution is required in patients with renal impairment.

• Low-molecular-weight heparin (LMWH) such as enoxaparin is usually preferred to unfractionated heparin. LMWH allows outpatient treatment in selected patients in a typical dosage of enoxaparin 1.0 mg/kg BD or 1.5 mg/kg daily.

• Caution should be exercised in obese patients and in patients with renal impairment. Patients weighing > 100 kg should have LMWH dose calculated for 100 kg.

- Unfractionated heparin remains the treatment of choice for hospitalised patients at high risk of bleeding, requiring invasive procedures or with renal failure.
- Oral anticoagulation with warfarin may be started concurrently with heparin with a target INR in the range of 2–3.
- Warfarin or NOAC is usually continued for 3–6 months but may be recommended as lifelong treatment in patients with a high risk of recurrence.

GRADUATED COMPRESSION STOCKINGS

Use of stockings reduces the risk of post-phlebitic syndrome following DVT and is recommended for all unless preexisting leg ulceration or extensive varicosities contraindicate it.

VENA CAVAL FILTERS

These may be considered in cases where anticoagulation is contraindicated or where PE has recurred despite therapeutic anticoagulation.

THROMBOLYSIS/SURGERY/ECMO

Treatments for haemodynamically unstable PE include thrombolysis (with alteplase or tenecteplase), catheter-directed thrombolysis, thrombus aspiration, surgical thrombectomy and the use of venoarterial extracorporeal membrane oxygenation.

Limb-threatening proximal DVT may be treated with local thrombolytic therapy using urokinase infused into a distal cannula.

Disposition

Most patients with DVT can be managed as outpatients. Exceptions include extensive proximal DVT, limited cardiorespiratory reserve, high risk of bleeding, risk of poor compliance with therapy and inadequate social supports. Patients with confirmed PE are usually admitted to hospital. Recent studies argue that carefully selected patients with PE may be safely discharged from the ED or after a short period of in-hospital observation.

Editorial comment

The literature and clinical practice are allowing for increasing treatment of patients at home with follow-up after discharge. The management of this important clinical group will change markedly with newer anticoagulant therapy and refinement of at-risk groups.

Pearls and pitfalls in venous thromboembolic disease are given opposite.

Chapter 17
Neurological emergencies

Gonzalo Aguirrebarrena

Acknowledgment

The author wishes to acknowledge the contribution to this chapter that was provided by Raymond Garrick AM.

Altered mental status

- A change in mental state can be expressed as an acute memory impairment and disorientation, confusion, behaviour disturbance, confabulation, delusions, hallucinations or agitation. Patients with psychiatric conditions have preserved attention and cognition but impaired thought process. The Glasgow Coma Scale (GCS) gives a standard way of recording and monitoring the level of consciousness (see Chapter 27 Neurosurgical Emergencies).
- Coma signifies diffuse disturbance of the central nervous system (CNS) function (e.g. trauma, epilepsy, drugs, hypoxia, hypoglycaemia or metabolic abnormality) or it can be due to a brainstem lesion or compression.

HISTORY

History should be taken from patient's contacts including family, workplace, police, ambulance officers, family doctor, and so on. Past medical history, medications, recent trauma, substance abuse and recent illness can guide to the diagnosis of the aetiology of the current mental state.

EXAMINATION

Look for signs of:

- changes in thought process including delusion and non-auditory hallucinations (more likely to be due to non-psychiatric medical disorders)

- head injury
- raised intracranial pressure (hypertension, bradycardia with dilated and non-reactive pupil is classical; see Chapter 27 Neurosurgical Emergencies)
- alcohol (acute intoxication, Wernicke's, delirium tremens)
- narcotics (needle track marks, pinpoint pupils) and anxiolytics
- psychostimulants (agitation, dilated pupils, tachycardia, hypertension)
- tricyclic antidepressants (TCA) (tachycardia, hypotension +/− seizures)
- hypoxia (tachypnoea, cyanosis and abnormal pulse oximetry)
- hypercapnia (history of chronic airway limitation, inappropriate O_2 treatment given in patient with CO_2 retention)
- metabolic cause (hypo/hyperthyroid, hypo/hyperglycaemia, hepatic or renal failure)
- infections (hyperthermia/hypothermia, tachycardia, hypotension)
  - measure temperature rectally; axillary or tympanic measurement is inaccurate in severe hypothermia
  - systemic infection—pneumonia, urine infection, septicaemia
  - cerebral infection—meningitis, encephalitis, acquired immunodeficiency syndrome (AIDS dementia complex)
- seizures (postictal, complex partial or absence status)
- CNS pathology (brain mass, haemorrhagic or ischaemia stroke)
- deficiency states (thiamine, vitamin B_{12}).
  Look for specific CNS signs.
- Pupils: dilated pupil with impaired response to light may signify a 3rd nerve lesion due to transtentorial herniation. When bilateral, it may suggest brainstem injury or psychoactive drugs. Small pupils occur with pontine lesions, opiates, clonidine or cholinergic effect.
- Eye movements: test by following a target or reflex with head turning (oculocephalic reflex). Failure of **conjugate** gaze to the side of the hemiplegia is common with a hemisphere lesion. When severe, the head and eyes stay deviated away

from the hemiplegic side. **Dysconjugate** gaze is indicative of lesions of the 3rd, 4th and 6th cranial nerves or their nuclei or connections in the brain stem.

- Fundoscopy: look for papillo-oedema which usually indicates raised intracranial pressure. Pre-retinal haemorrhage (Terson's syndrome) suggests subarachnoid haemorrhage (SAH).
- Motor signs: look at posture and for absence of spontaneous movements.
- Tone: classically increased in serotoninergic syndrome but, with acute CNS damage, decreased tone is usual.
- Tendon reflexes: classically increased but may be absent or reduced with an acute lesion.
- Plantar responses: classically extensor but may be absent with an acute lesion.

INVESTIGATIONS

- Blood count, blood sugar level (BSL), electrolytes, urea and creatinine, liver (LFTs) and thyroid (TFTs) function tests and calcium
- Serum paracetamol and alcohol level
- Venous blood gases (pH and pCO_2 level)
- Urine analysis: for microscopy, drug screening, glucose and ketones
- If sepsis is suspected: blood and urine culture; lumbar puncture should only be performed if there are no contraindications (see the section on Lumbar Puncture below)
- ECG (bradycardia: clonidine, cholinergic or gamma hydroxy butyrate [GHB] overdose; wide QRS: tricyclic antidepressant [TCA] overdose)
- Cerebral CT scans (first-line)
- Chest X-ray (CXR)

Management

1 Ensure a patent airway and adequate oxygenation.
2 Establish venous access.
3 Treat hypo/hyperglycaemia and symptomatic severe hyponatraemia.

4 Give naloxone 0.4 mg IV/IM, up to 2 mg over 10 minutes for signs of narcotics overdose.

5 Give thiamine 100–200 mg IV for unknown cause of coma or signs of alcoholism/neglect.

6 Treat underlying conditions and follow sepsis guidelines.

7 Monitor neurological signs and GCS half-hourly.

8 Maintain normal pulse, BP, temperature, hydration, monitor urine output and perform pressure care.

9 Raised intracranial pressure requires immediate neurosurgical consultation. Treatment to gain time for definitive surgery may include:

   a passive hyperventilation to a PCO_2 of 30–35 mmHg

   b mannitol 20% (0.5–1.0 g/kg) by IV infusion over 20 minutes

   c in proven cerebral tumours, dexamethasone 8 mg IV.

Seizures

Fits are usually self-limiting, and no urgent drug treatment is needed. However, prolonged or multiple fits require urgent treatment.

HISTORY

Obtain history of:

- epilepsy, antiepileptic drug and compliance
- fever (meningitis, encephalitis, HIV, malaria)
- alcohol intake or illicit drug use (amphetamines, TCA, benzodiazepines withdrawal)
- medications which may cause hyponatraemia or trigger seizures
- previous pseudo-seizures
- malignancy and its treatment (metastasis, hypercalcaemia)
- eclampsia in women of childbearing age.

During fits:

1 Minimise injury from burns, cuts or falls, protect the head, and roll into decubitus to avoid aspiration.

2 Determine if the seizure was partial simple or complex, and generalised tonic/clonic or absence will guide management.

3 Clear airway as soon as tonic-clonic movements cease.

4 Do not put anything between the teeth during a fit.

5 Exclude hypoglycaemia at bedside.

6 Insert IV cannula and take blood sample.

INVESTIGATIONS

- Blood count, electrolytes, renal function, glucose and calcium
- Assay for antiepileptic drugs and alcohol level
- Consider other tests for less-common causes: HIV, syphilis
- Brain CT scan if first episode or change in characteristics of seizure
- Imaging may be deferred for an outpatient MRI and EEG if: age < 40 with first isolated seizure, normal physical exam, no history of fever, head injury, malignancy or immunosuppression.

Prolonged or frequent fitting (status epilepticus)

Major generalised seizures lasting more than 20 minutes, or recurring rapidly without regaining consciousness in between, is a life-threatening neurological emergency.

TREATMENT

Treatment should be commenced after 5 minutes of continuous generalised seizure. This situation demands prompt airway management, high-flow oxygen, IV drug therapy, monitoring and support.

1 Arrange transfer to a resuscitation area while establishing IV access and commencing drug treatment.
2 Give midazolam 2.5–5 mg IV with repeated boluses up to 15 mg (child, 0.15–0.2 mg/kg bolus). IM administration can be used if venous access is delayed. Alternatives to midazolam are:
  — lorazepam 2–4 mg bolus IV (child, 0.1 mg/kg bolus)
  — diazepam 5–10 mg IV, (child, 0.1–0.2 mg/kg bolus).
3 Add phenytoin 18 mg/kg IV at no more than 50 mg/minute if patient is not already taking phenytoin (child, administer 18 mg/kg IV at no more than 25 mg/minute). Monitor ECG and vital signs.
  OR
  Sodium valproate 20 mg/kg IV (maximum 80 mg/kg) slow IV injection
  OR
  Levetiracetam 1000 mg IV (commonly used but with no definitive evidence).

4 If seizures persist despite treatment, anaesthetise with thiopentone or propofol and muscle relaxant, provide ventilatory support and admit to intensive care unit.

5 Monitor temperature, oxygenation, acidosis, lactate, hydration, urine output, serum electrolytes and EEG.

6 Re-establish or adjust long-term oral anticonvulsants.

Cerebrovascular disease

Stroke is either cerebral infarction or haemorrhage. CT scans show haemorrhage immediately, but the signs of infarction are usually delayed for several hours. Transient ischaemic attack (TIA) is a focal ischaemic neurological deficit which usually clinically resolves in less than 1 hour and no signs of infarction in neuroimaging.

COMMON PATTERNS OF NEUROLOGICAL IMPAIRMENT

- Hemisphere (likely embolic): hemiplegia with dysphasia or sensory inattention
- Lacunar infarct (likely hypertensive): internal capsule/pons (pure motor hemiplegia), thalamus (pure sensory)
- Brainstem (vertebrobasilar system disease embolic or dissection): bilateral motor signs, sensory decline (Pontine), diplopia, ataxia, vertigo/nystagmus, cranial nerve signs

Ischaemic stroke

- **Medical emergency. Door to Physician** < 10 minutes, door to CT interpretation < 45 minutes, door to treatment < 1 hour
- Ischaemic strokes account for 85% of strokes.
- Ensure a clear airway, adequate oxygenation and circulation.
- Exclude stroke mimics (e.g. seizure, hypoglycaemia, sepsis, hypoxia, hyponatraemia, drug overdose [usually alcohol], Bell's palsy, hemiplegic migraine, syncope, conversion disorder).
- Document neurological deficits and level of consciousness.
- Identify any cardiovascular abnormalities (e.g. atrial fibrillation [AF], prosthetic valve, signs of endocarditis or recent AMI [cardiac embolus], and carotid bruit/dissection [neck vessel disease]).

- Perform urgent cerebral CT scans to exclude haemorrhage or space-occupying lesions.
- Nil by mouth (NBM) until bedside swallow screen is performed.
- Aspirin as soon as haemorrhage is excluded and thrombolysis is not indicated.
- Perform regular monitoring of neurological status, blood glucose, blood pressure and hydration status.

INVESTIGATIONS

- Perform full blood count (FBC), electrolytes, creatinine, blood glucose level, coagulation studies, urinalysis, ECG and chest X-ray.
- Initial CT and computed tomography angiography (CTA) scans can be normal for ischaemic stroke, as infarction can be visible hours to days after the onset. Urgent CT and CTA are used to exclude haemorrhage or brain mass, rule out dissection, localise thrombus/vasculature abnormalities to allow the commencement of antiplatelet, thrombolytic agents or mechanical thrombectomy.
- Magnetic resonance imaging (MRI) and magnetic resonance angiography (MRA) shows infarction immediately after a stroke and can distinguish a new from an old infarct. Small lesions and brainstem lesions invisible in CT scans can be seen with MRI.
- Perform transthoracic echocardiography and carotid Doppler ultrasound studies. Transoesophageal echocardiography (TOE) may be needed to exclude cardiac embolism.

THROMBOLYTIC THERAPY IN STROKE

- Thrombolysis is indicated for ischaemic stroke if the hospital is set up for this. The NIHSS is > 6 and < 20, thrombolysis can commence within 4.5 hours of symptom onset and there are no known contraindications. Contraindications are listed in Chapter 11 Acute Coronary Syndromes.
- Alteplase 0.9 mg/kg up to a maximum dose of 90 mg; 10% of alteplase is given stat and 90% is given as IV infusion over 60 minutes. No antiplatelet or anticoagulation agents for 24 hours.

MECHANICAL CLOT RETRIEVAL

- Endovascular clot retrieval has shown significant neurological and survival benefit up to 24 hours after onset of symptoms, with or without previous thrombolytic therapy.
- Patients should be immediately retrieved to a Stroke Centre as soon as a proximal anterior circulation clot has been detected in the CTA.
- Patients with a proximal posterior circulation clot may also benefit from early mechanical thrombectomy, but this must be up to the discretion of the Stroke Centre.
- Candidates for mechanical clot retrieval that require transportation should start thrombolysis prior to departure if within 4.5 hours of symptom onset.

STROKE MANAGEMENT CHECKLIST

- Oxygenation: maintain oxygen saturation at > 95%.
- Neurological status: hourly GCS and neurological observation for first 4 hours or until stabilised.
- Body temperature: control fever at < 37.5°C with paracetamol.
- Blood glucose: correct BSL if < 3 or > 11 mmol/L.
- Blood pressure: if not a tPA candidate, reduction of no more than 15% is indicated if systolic blood pressure (SBP) is > 220 mmHg or diastolic blood pressure (DBP) is > 120 mmHg (use PO labetalol). If a tPA candidate, BP goal is SBP < 180 mmHg / DBP < 110 mmHg (use IV labetalol).
- NBM and IV fluid to maintain hydration until swallow screen is performed.
- Urine output: bladder catheterisation may be needed if urinary retention or decreased GCS.
- Deep-vein thrombosis (DVT) prophylaxis: subcutaneous low-molecular-weight heparin (LMWH) if not contraindicated.
- Antiplatelet therapy: start aspirin 300 mg stat then 150 mg daily.
- Anticoagulation: heparin infusion is only indicated in cases of carotid or vertebral artery dissection. Anticoagulation is protective in the long term in patients with AF or other cardiac disease causing embolism.
- Positioning: support for hemiparetic limbs, prevention of injury to the neglected side and general pressure care.

- Stroke unit: admission to a specialised stroke unit has proven benefits in reducing secondary complications and mortality.

Transient ischaemic attack (TIA)

TIA is a neurological dysfunction due to thrombotic or embolic arterial occlusion that results from focal brain or retinal ischaemia, usually lasts less than 1 hour and often resolves by the time of ED presentation. To be considered a TIA, the episode must have complete clinical resolution (NIHSS 0), have no signs of acute infarction in the initial neuroimaging and have all relevant differential diagnosis ruled out.

The diagnosis of TIA is intended to identify patients that would benefit from preventive therapy.

Transient monocular visual loss is very suggestive of carotid artery stenosis.

The initial ED investigations for TIA should be the same as those given for stroke, as above. Antiplatelet therapy can be commenced after cerebral haemorrhage is excluded by CT scan.

Depending on each medical centre risk stratification protocol, admission or specialised clinic referral may be needed to avoid delays in TIA assessment (LDL level, carotid doppler, echo and Holter monitor) and stroke prevention measures (antiplatelet therapy, anticoagulation, blood pressure control, statins or carotid revascularisation).

The ABCD^2 score (Box 17.1) is used as a risk prediction tool at 7 days after the TIA event. A score < 4 has a stroke risk of around 2%. Equal or above 4 represents a risk of around 10%.

Spontaneous intracerebral haemorrhage

- Haemorrhage accounts for 15% of all strokes.
- Associated with high mortality—a 12-month survival rate of 30%.
- Bleeding due to anticoagulant therapy is common.
- Haemorrhage may be due to rupture of small vessels damaged by hypertension.
- With older age, amyloid angiopathy is common.
- Bleeding can be from arteriovenous malformation or aneurysm.

Box 17.1 ABCD² score (maximum 7 points)	
Age	
> 60 years	1 point
< 60 years	0 points
Blood pressure when first assessed after TIA	
SBP > 140 mmHg or DBP > 90 mmHg	1 point
SBP < 140 mmHg or DBP < 90 mmHg	0 points
Clinical features	
Unilateral weakness	2 points
Isolated speech disturbance	1 pint
Other	0 points
Duration of TIA symptoms	
> 60 minutes	2 points
10 to 59 minutes	1 point
< 10 minutes	0 points
Diabetes	
Present	1 point
Absent	0 points

- Initial assessment and management are similar to ischaemic stroke, as listed above.
- Hypertensive intracerebral haemorrhage will usually be in the internal capsule/striatum, pons or cerebellum. Intracerebral haematoma from a berry aneurysm will arise from near the circle of Willis, and peripheral haematomas suggest amyloid angiopathy.
- MRI and contrast cerebral angiography may be needed to define suspected aneurysm or arteriovenous malformation (AVM).

TREATMENT

Treatment is as per the stroke management checklist given above, with the following modifications.

1 Cease all antiplatelet or warfarin therapy and if needed reverse anticoagulation.
2 Gradually decrease SBP to < 180 mmHg and DBP < 120 with labetalol or esmolol.
3 Hydration: fluid restriction may be needed, as syndrome of inappropriate antidiuretic hormone secretion (SIADH) is common.

4 Consult neurosurgeon for possible surgical interventions. Surgical drainage may improve the outcome for cerebellar haematoma.

5 Surgery may also be considered for the presence of hydrocephalus, posterior fossa bleeding, marked mass effect or haematoma associated with AVM or aneurysm.

Subarachnoid haemorrhage (SAH)
CLINICAL FEATURES

- SAH accounts for 50% of all haemorrhagic strokes.
- SAH should be considered in patients presenting with sudden onset of severe headache (> 95% of cases of SAH), sometimes described as the 'worst ever' 'thunderclap' headache with or without neurological findings. Syncopal episodes occur in around 15% of cases and vomiting is common. Although less frequent, SAH can present with sudden-onset unilateral headache, corresponding to the side of the aneurysm.
- Up to 50% of patients experience a 'warning bleed' associated with headache which settles spontaneously or with simple analgesia 1–3 weeks before. Re-presentation with second bleed is usually catastrophic and associated with poor outcome. It is often due to a ruptured berry aneurysm and sometimes due to a vascular malformation.
- Hypertension, polycystic disease and aortic coarctation are associated with berry aneurysms. Monoamine oxidase therapy or illicit drugs such as cocaine and amphetamines may result in acute hypertension complicated with SAH.
- On examination, look for meningism, altered level of consciousness, confusion or focal neurological signs (such as hemiparesis or dysphasia). Papillo-oedema may be present. Pre-retinal haemorrhage (Terson's syndrome) is virtually diagnostic and is associated with a higher Hunt and Hess score. A cranial bruit may indicate an arteriovenous malformation. Absence of physical signs cannot exclude SAH.

Note: Migraine is not a likely diagnosis in a first-time severe headache.

INVESTIGATIONS

- Non-contrast brain CT scans have sensitivity over 99% when performed in the first 6 hours of the onset of the pain. In the first 24 hours will demonstrate subarachnoid blood in 90–95% of cases. Sensitivity of CT scans decreases with time: 80% positive at 3 days and 50% at 1 week. Increasing evidence supports the use of high-quality CT scan reported by an experienced radiologist performed in the first 6 hours of onset of headache to definitively rule out SAH. In these cases, a lumbar puncture (LP) or CTA would only be indicated in high-risk patients (classic clinical presentation, positive family history).
- LP is necessary if there is high clinical suspicion of SAH and the CT scan does not provide a diagnosis. The diagnosis of SAH is dependent on the finding of red cells or xanthochromia in the CSF. Xanthochromia is due to breakdown products of haemoglobin in the CSF and is usually present within 6–12 hours and lasts up to 2 weeks of the haemorrhage. Hence, LP should be delayed for 12 hours from the onset of symptoms to minimise false-negative findings. Spectrophotometry detects products of blood breakdown from oxyhaemoglobin to bilirubin. They can be detected up to a month from the symptoms.
- CT angiography has evolved as the preferred imaging modality for the cause of the haemorrhage. MRI can be used as the next tier of investigation modality, particularly in subacute presentations (> 3 days of bleed).
- SIADH, temporary hyperglycaemia and cardiac tachyarrhythmias may complicate the bleed.

GRADING SYSTEMS

The **Hunt and Hess score** (Table 17.1) is used to assess the clinical severity of the presentation based on examination.

The **Fisher score** (Table 17.2) predicts likelihood of vasospasm based on CT scan.

TREATMENT

1 General supportive with airway protection, adequate oxygenation and blood pressure control.

Table 17.1   Hunt and Hess score

Grade	Neurological status
1	Mild headache
2	Severe headache, neck stiffness, no neurological deficit
3	Drowsy, confused, mild neurological deficit
4	Stuporous, hemiparesis
5	Coma, decerebrate posturing

Table 17.2   Fisher score

Grade	Characteristics of blood in CT
1	No blood seen
2	Diffuse deposition or thin layers < 1 mm thick
3	Localised clot or layers 1 mm or thicker
4	Intracerebral or intraventricular clot extension

2 Relieve headache and restlessness. Use narcotic analgesia for headache and antiemetics.

3 Maintain blood pressure in normal range by analgesia and sedation. Antihypertensive therapy should be used with caution.

4 Restrict fluids to 1200–1500 mL per day.

5 Anti-spasm drug treatment (nimodipine 60 mg every 4 hours) should be commenced within 48 hours of haemorrhage to reduce delayed cerebral ischaemia.

6 Regularly monitor neurological signs.

7 Bed rest with head up by 30° in a dark, quiet room.

8 Urgent surgical clipping or coiling of the aneurysm or excision or embolisation of an arteriovenous malformation remain the definitive treatments.

Headache

Headache represents 2–4% of all ED visits and over 95% are benign and self-limiting. The goal is to exclude potentially serious conditions and to relieve pain. Important diagnoses to be considered are:

- subarachnoid haemorrhage (see earlier this chapter)
- meningitis/encephalitis

- migraine
- giant cell (temporal) arteritis
- trigeminal neuralgia
- acute narrow-angle glaucoma (see Chapter 38 Ophthalmic Emergencies)
- hypertensive encephalopathy
- space-occupying lesions (see Chapter 27 Neurosurgical Emergencies).

Meningitis
CLINICAL FEATURES

- Headache with fever suggests meningitis, and there may be vomiting, photophobia, neck pain or stiffness, confusion, irritability, coma or fitting.
- Examine for neck stiffness and also purpura or sepsis in meningococcaemia; sources of infection (e.g. middle ear, sinusitis, cerebrospinal fluid [CSF] leak); or viral infection such as mumps or mononucleosis. Kernig's and Brudzinski's signs are poorly sensitive but highly specific examination manoeuvres to identify meningitis.
- Elderly patients rarely have the classic clinical presentation, have higher rate of complications and mortality.
- Usual bacteria involved in adults and children are *Streptococcus pneumoniae*, *Neisseria meningitidis* (less common after vaccination was introduced) and gram-negative bacilli (in < 3 years of age).
- In elderlies, alcoholic, transplant or dialysis patients consider Listeria. In neonates, consider group B Streptococcus, *Escherichia coli* and Listeria.

INVESTIGATIONS

- FBC, C-reactive protein (CRP), electrolytes, creatinine, blood glucose and CXR.
- Blood cultures (positive in over 50% of bacterial meningitis).
- Nose, throat and ear swabs.
- Viral cultures, viral antibody titres.
- Brain CT scans must be obtained before an LP is performed if there is focal neurological signs, altered conscious state, papillo-oedema, recent seizures, immune-deficiency or HIV-positive.

- An LP is needed to confirm the diagnosis and to identify and culture the organism. It should be delayed if there is risk of herniation, abnormal coagulation (anticoagulation or severe thrombocytopenia), epidural abscess or haemodynamic instability (see Table 17.3).

TREATMENT

1 Give IV antibiotics as soon as the possibility of bacterial meningitis is realised. Do not wait for CT scans or LP. (Blood cultures or CSF polymerase chain reaction (PCR) may assist when antibiotic treatment has rendered the CSF negative to Gram stain and culture.)

2 Ceftriaxone 2 g IV every 12 hours (children 50 mg/kg/day).

3 Appropriate antibiotic for known organism/sensitivity (e.g. benzylpenicillin 1.2–1.8 g every 4 hours [children 350 mg/kg/day] IV for *Meningococcus* or *Pneumococcus*).

4 Steroid therapy (IV dexamethasone 10 mg 6-hourly or 0.15 mg/kg) is believed to reduce neurological sequelae in *H. influenzae* or pneumococcal meningitis (evidence not conclusive). Initial dose should be given prior to antibiotic therapy.

5 Treat sepsis, disseminated intravascular coagulation, adrenal failure, SIADH and other complications.

6 Prophylaxis: it is recommended that household contacts of confirmed meningococcal and *Haemophilus influenzae* type b

Table 17.3 Laboratory findings for CSF in meningitis

	Normal	Bacterial	Viral	Tuberculosis or fungal
White cell count/mL	< 5, and < 1 polymorphs	> 1000 Polymorphs predominant	< 500 Monocytes predominant	< 500 Monocytes predominant
Glucose (mmol/L)	2.5–3.5	Low (< 40% of BSL)	Normal	Low
Protein (g/L)	0.15–0.45	High	Normal	High
Gram stain and culture	−ve	+ve in 80%	−ve	−ve
Antigen	−ve	+ve in 80%	−ve	−ve

meningitis be given prophylactic antibiotics. Healthcare workers are not at increased risk for the disease and do not require prophylaxis unless they have had direct mucosal contact with the patient's secretions, as might occur during mouth-to-mouth resuscitation, endotracheal intubation or nasotracheal suctioning. The choices of prophylaxis can be rifampicin, ciprofloxacin or ceftriaxone.

Lumbar puncture (LP)
INDICATIONS
The major role for LP in the ED is the diagnosis of infection or bleeding within the central nervous system.

PREPARATION
Discuss with the patient or carer indications, procedure and possible complications of the procedure, and obtain verbal or written consent.

COMPLICATIONS
- Post-LP headache (15–20%). Patients present with worsening frontal or occipital headache 12–72 hours after the procedure. The incidence of headache can be reduced by using a small-sized LP needle (22-gauge) or pencil-point tip with a side hole (Sprotte needle) rather than sharp cutting tips. Bed rest has not been shown to improve the incidence of headache. Treatment in the first 24 hours of pain includes simple oral analgesia and caffeine. If severe headache persists for longer than 24 hours, an epidural blood patch is indicated.
- Other complications include:
  - epidural haematoma (more likely if post procedure anticoagulation is given)
  - local trauma to spinal cord or nerve roots
  - infection such as discitis or epidural abscess.

INTERPRETATION OF CSF FINDINGS
- Although certain CSF characteristics may be highly suggestive of viral or bacterial infection, ED doctors should not be falsely reassured by viral 'like' CSF.

- Normal CSF pressure is 5–20 cmH$_2$O when the patient is horizontal. High pressure may indicate the presence of space-occupying lesions, specific infections such as *Cryptococcus* or CSF outflow obstruction. Low pressure is associated with severe dehydration or CSF leak.
- Macroscopic appearance:
  — normal—clear and colourless
  — infection—cloudy
  — blood—pink or frank blood
  — old blood (> 12 hours)—yellow (xanthochromia).
- CSF laboratory testing:
  — microscopy for cell count, differential, Gram stain and culture
  — biochemistry: glucose, protein and lactate (elevated in bacterial meningitis)
  — xanthochromia and spectrophotometry if SAH is suspected
  — acid-fast bacillus and India ink stains if tuberculosis or *Cryptococcus* is suspected
  — antigen and PCR testing, mainly if antibiotic therapy was given prior to LP.

Additional considerations

Pre-treatment with antibiotics will diminish the yield of Gram stains and cultures but will not affect the CSF cell count or lactate level.

- The initial CSF cell counts may show lymphocytosis in bacterial meningitis.
- The presence of a clot in one of the tubes or the clearing of CSF blood-staining from tubes 1–3 suggests traumatic LP.

Encephalitis
CLINICAL FEATURES

- Headache and fever with focal neurological signs, altered cognition or fits suggest encephalitis.
- Impaired level of consciousness and delirium are common.
- There is overlap between meningitis and encephalitis.
- Encephalitis is mostly viral. Sometimes the specific virus can be identified from associated clinical features (e.g. mumps,

rabies) or from laboratory tests, cultures and antibody titres, or from the epidemiology (e.g. Murray Valley encephalitis).

- Herpes simplex encephalitis demands early diagnosis as treatment is life-saving.
- Immunocompromised patients can present with parasitic or fungal as well as viral infections (e.g. toxoplasmosis, cytomegalovirus, progressive multifocal leuco-encephalopathy).

Investigations
- FBC, CRP, EUC, BSL and CXR
- Viral cultures and antibody titres
- Cerebral CT scans often show subtle changes, hypoattenuation in a temporal lobe and mass effect may be present
- Lumbar puncture—WCC 50–500/mL, mild elevation in protein, normal glucose; CSF sent for viral cultures, antibody titres and PCR for HSV and other viruses
- MRI is more sensitive and more specific than CT scans

Treatment
- Specific treatment is not available except for herpes simplex encephalitis which responds to aciclovir 10 mg/kg in IV infusions every 8 hours for 10 days. Each dose must be infused over not less than 1 hour.
- This drug should be commenced urgently on suspicion of herpes simplex encephalitis (i.e. clinical encephalitis with cells in the CSF).

Migraine
CLINICAL FEATURES
- The pathophysiology of migraine is complex and poorly understood. It is defined as idiopathic recurring severe headache disorder with attacks that last 4–72 hours.
- There is often presence of a family history and sometimes triggers such as food or menstruation.
- The headache may be preceded or accompanied by a prodrome or aura of visual, auditory, motor or other neurological symptoms (25% of patients). Aura with

no headache has been well described as representing a diagnostic challenge, because it can be mistaken for a transient ischaemic attack.

- Typical characteristics include gradual onset, throbbing quality, unilateral location, nausea, vomiting, photophobia and prostration. Major but temporary neurological signs may result from migraine, causing diagnostic problems (e.g. aphasia, hemiplegia).
- Investigations will be normal and should be directed towards excluding other serious diseases as suggested by the clinical features—SAH, meningitis and so on.
- Although not life-threatening, migraine causes great suffering. When the diagnosis is secure, the goal is to relieve pain and other associated symptoms. Possible triggers should be identified in order to prevent further episodes (alcohol, flashing lights, stress, change in sleeping pattern, menstruation).

TREATMENT

Patients presenting with migraine should be fast tracked as effectiveness of treatment increases when started soon after the onset of symptoms.

1 Soluble aspirin 600–900 mg and paracetamol 1–1.5 g 4-hourly, up to 4 g/day.

2 Metoclopramide (10 mg orally, IM or IV) has both antiemetic and direct analgesic effect.

3 Non-steroidal anti-inflammatory drugs (NSAIDs): ibuprofen 400–800 mg orally or indomethacin 100 mg rectally.
   If previous experience with these measures has failed:

4 Chlorpromazine: very effective treatment in 80% of patients who are unresponsive to oral analgesics. Give chlorpromazine 12.5 mg in 1 L of normal saline over 30 minutes. Further 12.5 mg, up to 37.5 mg can be administered if headache persists. Hypotension should be treated with 500 mL boluses of normal saline and acute dystonia is treated with 2 mg of IV benztropine.

5 Serotonin agonists are effective in 60–75% of cases, specially associated with NSAIDs. Sumatriptan recommended dose is 50–100 mg orally, 10–20 mg intranasally or 6 mg SC. Other

triptans may be used: eletriptan 40–80 mg orally, naratriptan 2.5 mg orally, rizatriptan 10 mg wafer or zolmitriptan 2.5–5 mg orally.

6 Dexamethasone 8 mg IV is recommended as a preventive measure in patients with recurrent presentations.

If treatment with the above measures has also failed, consider:

7 Dihydroergotamine, a potent vasoconstrictor. The recommended dose is 0.5–1 mg SC or IM or IV with metoclopramide to minimise the gastrointestinal side effects. Note that ergot compounds are contraindicated with concomitant triptans.

Note: Narcotics are not advised.

Giant cell arteritis (temporal arteritis)
ASSESSMENT
This disorder needs urgent diagnosis and steroid treatment, as delay may result in loss of vision. It often occurs in females over the age of 50 (mean 75 years of age), and gradual-onset severe headache may be the only symptom. Amaurosis fugax can be an early manifestation. Jaw claudication, tenderness and swelling over the temporal artery may be present.

The diagnosis is confirmed by a high ESR and CRP, temporal artery biopsy and response to steroids.

TREATMENT
- If the clinical diagnosis is likely, commence steroid therapy immediately.
- Prednisone 1 mg/kg PO for giant cell arteritis with no visual loss.
- Methylprednisolone 1 g/day IV for 3 days for giant cell arteritis with visual loss.
- Response within hours to the first dose of steroids can be diagnostic. Temporal artery biopsy and ESR help plan long-term treatment.

Trigeminal neuralgia
Recurrent unilateral sharp and short-lived episodes of pain localised in any or all the 5th cranial nerve branches distribution, usually caused by a nerve root compression by a vein or artery,

that can have simple triggers such as shaving, light touch, face washing or chewing.

The pain can be associated with facial muscles spasm (tic douloureux).

INVESTIGATIONS

High-resolution MRI is the most appropriate diagnostic test to rule out vascular compression of the nerve as well as the rarer multiple sclerosis or structural lesions such as cerebellopontine angle tumours.

TREATMENT

- First-line treatment is pharmacological. Carbamazepine 100 mg twice daily, incrementing by 200 mg daily, up to 1200 mg. Other options are baclofen, gabapentin or lamotrigine.
- Second-line treatment includes invasive approach with botulinum toxin injection and microvascular surgical decompression.

Other causes of headache

Many other diseases of ears, eyes, nose, sinuses, teeth and tempo-romandibular joints may cause head pain.

BELL'S PALSY

Assessment

This is a rapid-onset unilateral peripheral facial nerve palsy of unknown cause, with reduced forehead and eyelid move-ments and sagging of the corner of the mouth. Other features include ear pain, decreased tearing, hyperacusis and taste disturbance.

Examination

- Conduct a neurological examination and look for vesicles or scabbing at or in the external ear canal (herpes zoster Ramsay Hunt syndrome) or a mass in the parotid gland.
- Sparing of the forehead and eyelid muscles is suggestive of an upper motor neuron lesion because of bilateral innervation to this area.

Treatment

- Start treatment within 3 days of symptom onset with oral prednisone 60–80 mg daily for 5–7 days.
- Eye care with artificial tears and eye patch while sleeping to prevent drying and abrasion of the cornea.
- Antiviral agents have not been shown to have benefit over placebo in the absence of signs to suggest herpes zoster.

Neuro-muscular disorders
GUILLAIN-BARRÉ SYNDROME

- Post infectious rapidly progressing symmetric bilateral ascending weakness (7 days to 4 weeks), associated with decreased tendon reflexes in the affected limbs, muscle pain, autonomic dysfunction and paraesthesia to distal limbs.
- Miller Fisher syndrome is a variant with cranial nerve involvement, resulting in facial, oculomotor or bulbar weakness, which may extend later on to limb weakness.
- Twenty per cent will develop respiratory failure requiring respiratory support.
- Diagnosis is based on the clinical features supported by protein level elevation with normal white cell count in CSF (cytoalbuminological dissociation), and acute demyelinating polyneuropathy or acute motor axonal neuropathy in nerve conduction studies.
- Respiratory function tests and severity of muscle weakness will guide the need for ICU admission.
- Treatment is with intravenous immunoglobulin (IVIg) 0.4 g/kg/day for 5 days or plasma exchange.

MYASTHENIA GRAVIS

- Autoimmune disease that presents with generalised proximal skeletal muscle weakness (upper more than lower limbs) that often affects the ocular muscles with diplopia and ptosis.
- The Lambert-Eaton myasthenic syndrome is a variant usually associated with cancer that presents with skeletal muscle weakness affecting lower more than upper limbs and rarely involves ocular muscles.
- Diagnosis is based on clinical features and the presence of antibodies against acetylcholine receptors.

- Treatment is based on acetylcholinesterase inhibitors (pyridostigmine or neostigmine), prednisone with azathioprine, or rituximab. IVIg or plasma exchange might be indicated in severe exacerbations.

Periodic paralysis

- Primary periodic paralysis is a group of disorders that include hypokalaemia paralysis (hypoPP), hyperkalaemic paralysis (hyperPP) and Andersen-Tawil syndrome (A-TS which can present with hyper-, normo- or hyperkalaemia), characterised by mutation of sodium, calcium and potassium channel genes.
- Young patients present with self-limited flaccid muscle weakness usually triggered by diet or exercise.
- Diagnosis is confirmed by genetic testing.
- Andersen-Tawil syndrome is a potentially lethal disorder associated with prolonged QT/QU syndrome in the absence of hypokalaemia that can lead to polymorphic ventricular tachyarrhythmia.
- Treatment is based on carbonic anhydrase inhibitors such as acetazolamide or dichlorphenamide, plus gentle potassium supplementation in hypoPP and A-TS with hypokalaemia, or inhaled beta-2 agonists in hyperPP and A-TS with hyperkalaemia.
- In hypokalaemic attacks there is elevated serum but normal total body potassium. Therefore, large potassium doses or slow-release formulations should be avoided to avoid rebound hyperkalaemia.
- Prevention of new attacks is based on acetazolamide or dichlorphenamide in the three variants of primary PP, plus high-carbohydrate diet and hydrochlorothiazide in hyperPP, low-carbohydrate diet and potassium supplements in hypoPP.
- Management of secondary hypokalaemic periodic paralysis associated with hyperthyroidism, hyperaldosteronism or renal tubular acidosis is based on treatment of the underlying condition.

Chapter 18
Poisoning and overdose

Kate Sellors

Acknowledgment

The author wishes to acknowledge the content used from the previous edition of *Emergency Medicine* which was provided by Dr Fiona Chow.

Poisons Information Centre
Telephone 13 11 26
The NSW Poisons Information Centre (PIC) provides the latest poisons information to the public, as well as toxicology advice to health professionals on the management of poisoned and envenomed patients. Telephone advice is available 24 hours a day from anywhere in Australia.

Overview

- Poisoning and overdoses are common presentations to the ED, comprising 1–2% of all ED visits.
- Most overdoses are by deliberate attempts to self-harm, although accidental poisonings frequently occur, especially in the paediatric and elderly populations.
- Poisonings can also occur as a result of non-accidental injury, negligence and through environmental exposures. Most exposures occur through ingestion; however, other routes include insufflation (snorting), inhalation, mucous membrane or cutaneous exposure, and by parenteral injection.
- The role of the emergency doctor is to rapidly assess the poisoned patient, provide resuscitation and stabilisation, followed by specific treatments if necessary.

- Also important is the knowledge of when to declare the poisoned patient medically fit for discharge from hospital, and to arrange appropriate disposition and follow-up.
- Patients presenting after a deliberate overdose are often at the peak of a psycho-social crisis. They should be treated with empathy and referred for psychological assessment once medically fit.
- This chapter will outline the assessment and approach to the poisoned patient, followed by detailed information on specific common and serious presentations. Further information can be obtained from the Poisons Information Centre (see above), or from the online eTG resource: Toxicology and Wilderness.

Resuscitation

The initial management of any poisoned patient is an evaluation of early life-threats to the airway, breathing and circulation, and resuscitation as necessary. Good resuscitation and supportive care ensure survival in the majority of patients.

CARDIAC ARREST

- Cardiac arrest is treated according to standard advanced life support (ALS) principles, with the addition of specific interventions for toxin-induced cardiac arrest (Table 18.1).
- Patients with cardiac arrest following poisoning are frequently younger and have fewer comorbidities than those suffering cardiac arrest from other causes. Recovery with good neurological outcome has been reported in patients with cardiac arrest following poisoning, even

Table 18.1 Potential interventions in toxic cardiac arrest

Toxin	Intervention
Calcium-channel blocker or beta-blocker	High-dose insulin euglycaemia therapy
Sodium-channel blocker	Sodium bicarbonate
Local anaesthetic	Intravenous lipid emulsion
Digoxin	Digoxin antibody fragments
Organophosphates	Atropine

after many hours of CPR. For this reason, prolonged resuscitative efforts should be made, along with urgent consultation with a toxicologist or the Poisons Information Centre for advice.

• Consider the early use of cardiopulmonary bypass (ECMO) to facilitate prolonged resuscitation.

Pearls and Pitfalls
Prolonged resuscitation efforts are warranted in patients suffering toxin-induced cardiac arrest.

AIRWAY, BREATHING AND CIRCULATION

• Attention to the ABCs are paramount in the poisoned patient, as many will present with a depressed level of consciousness and can deteriorate quite quickly.

• Direct airway injury can occur following the ingestion of corrosive substances and early endotracheal intubation is indicated in patients with signs of airway compromise including stridor, drooling or dysphagia.

• Compromised airway patency and inadequate respiratory drive can lead to hypoventilation; intubation and ventilation is indicated in these cases. Note that the hypoventilation of opiate toxicity may be reversed with the use of naloxone which may obviate the need for intubation and ventilation.

• Hypotension should be treated initially with boluses of IV fluids.

• Refractory hypotension in the poisoned patient has various causes. Seek expert advice. Treatment may include inotropes, vasopressors and/or high-dose insulin.

• Several drugs can cause cardiac arrhythmias in overdose— most notably sodium-channel blockers causing widening of the QRS, and a variety of drugs that prolong the QT and may cause torsades de pointes.

Pearls and Pitfalls
Oxygen administration may mask hypoventilation in the poisoned patient. Monitor respiratory rate closely.

COMA

- Reduced GCS is a common toxic effect of many drugs and poisons.
- Look for reversible causes and treat urgently—hypoglycaemia, hypercapnia, opiate intoxication.
- The priority is focused on establishing a patent and protected airway.
- If coma is not a predicted outcome of the overdose, then investigate for other causes. This may include a CT of the brain.
- Comatose patients require attention to pressure areas and adequate fluid hydration.

SEIZURES

- Toxic seizures are generalised.
- The most common agents that cause toxic seizures are tramadol, amphetamines, tricyclic antidepressants, venlafaxine and bupropion.
- Other causes of drug-related seizures include hypoxic seizures from opiate toxicity and alcohol or benzodiazepine withdrawal.
- Detect and correct hypoglycaemia if present.
- First-line treatment of toxic seizures is benzodiazepines.
- Second-line treatment is barbiturates.
- Pyridoxine is the antidote for seizures caused by overdoses of isoniazid.
- Focal or partial seizures indicate a non-toxicological cause, or a complication of a toxicological cause, and should prompt further investigation.

Pearls and Pitfalls

Phenytoin is contraindicated in toxic seizures as it is less effective than benzodiazepines and may itself exacerbate cardiac conduction abnormalities in the setting of overdose.

HYPERTHERMIA

- Hyperthermia is seen in the setting of the sympathomimetic syndrome, serotonin syndrome and neuroleptic malignant syndrome.

- Temperatures of $> 39°C$ are life-threatening due to multi-organ failure and require aggressive treatment.
- Cooled fluids, ice packs, cooling mats, sedation and paralysis can be used to lower body temperature.

AGITATION

- Agitation is a common feature of patients who overdose.
- This may be due to drug or alcohol intoxication, or emotional crisis, or may be a feature of the overdose taken (e.g. anticholinergics, sympathomimetics).
- Manage agitation initially with verbal reassurance and de-escalation.
- If this fails, the first-line treatment of agitation should be with benzodiazepines, either given orally or by the IM or IV route as necessary.
- Other options include sedative antipsychotics (e.g. droperidol).
- Parenteral sedation must occur in an area where the patient can be closely monitored.

Risk assessment

The risk assessment is the cornerstone of decision-making in managing the poisoned patient. It informs the treating clinician to the likelihood of serious outcomes, and the need for intervention or specific therapies. The risk assessment is based on the following key pieces of information (Box 18.1).

Box 18.1   Risk assessment of the poisoned patient

- Agent
  — Drug name or type
  — Dose
  — Route of exposure
- Time since ingestion
- Patient factors
  — Age
  — Weight
  — Comorbidities
  — Co-ingestions
- Actions or events since exposure
- Clinical signs and symptoms
- Investigation results

FURTHER HISTORY

- Corroborative history is frequently required to make an assessment and should be sought from the patient's family, friends and treating GP.
- Ambulance officers can provide key information regarding medications, empty pill packets or drug paraphernalia found at the scene.
- A 'worst-case' scenario is often valuable, based on calculating the maximal amount of drug the patient had access to.

EXAMINATION

A thorough physical exam of the poisoned patient is an essential component of the risk assessment. Assess each overdose patient for signs of toxicity, or features of a toxidrome (see Table 18.3). Assess closely for signs of associated injuries.

Findings from examination may include the following.

- Skin: track marks, signs of injury or compartment syndrome, hot/dry skin versus sweaty/clammy skin.
- Eyes: miosis, mydriasis, nystagmus, icterus.
- Respiratory: respiratory rate, bronchorrhoea, signs of aspiration.
- CVS: blood pressure, pulse.
- Abdomen: presence of bowel sounds, tenderness.
- Neurological: GCS, tone, reflexes, nystagmus, presence of clonus.

INVESTIGATIONS

The investigations that are required will vary with different presentations.

Pearls and Pitfalls
Routine screening with an ECG and a paracetamol level are recommended for all overdose presentations.

Other investigations that may be of use include:
- full blood count (FBC)
- electrolytes and creatinine (EUC)
- blood sugar level (BSL)

- liver function tests (LFTs)
- venous blood gas (VBG)
- coagulation studies (anticoagulant overdoses, certain paracetamol overdoses)
- creatinine kinase (rhabdomyolysis)
- troponin (sympathomimetics)
- specific drug levels (e.g. digoxin, lithium, phenytoin, salicylate, carbamazepine, ethanol)
- abdominal X-ray (to confirm radio-opaque ingestions or ileus)
- CT brain (to exclude other causes of presentation, or complications of overdose)
- beta-hCG if the patient is a female of child-bearing age.

Pearls and Pitfalls

Qualitative urine drug screens are expensive and rarely alter the management of the acutely poisoned patient. False negatives and false positives can occur and not all drugs of abuse are screened for. For this reason they are not recommended for routine screening.

Decontamination

Decontamination is not essential for all poisoned patients. The decision about whether or not to decontaminate a patient must weigh up the risk of toxicity versus the benefit and risk of decontamination.

SKIN DECONTAMINATION

- Some toxins are absorbed via dermal, mucosal and inhalational routes. In these cases the patient's clothes should be removed and bagged, and the body washed with soapy water.
- The classic example is exposure to organophosphates.
- Resuscitation should occur concurrently and must not be delayed by decontamination efforts as the risk to staff is often overstated.

Box 18.2 **Complications of gastrointestinal decontamination**
Vomiting
Aspiration pneumonitis
Bowel obstruction or perforation
Distraction of staff from resuscitation and other supportive care priorities

GASTROINTESTINAL (GI) DECONTAMINATION

- GI decontamination is associated with complications (see Box 18.2). Therefore, its use depends on assessing the risk of toxicity and hence the need for decontamination.
- If the overdose is associated with significant risk of toxicity and supportive care or antidotal therapy alone is insufficient to ensure a good outcome, then GI decontamination should be considered.
- It is unlikely to be of benefit if more than 2 hours have elapsed from the time of overdose. Exceptions to this are overdoses of slow-release medications, drugs that have anticholinergic properties and drugs that undergo entero-hepatic circulation.

SINGLE-DOSE ACTIVATED CHARCOAL

- The efficacy of activated charcoal is time-dependent and therefore should be considered in those presenting within 1 hour when the poisoning is assessed to be high risk.
- The main complication of charcoal is pulmonary aspiration, especially in the obtunded patient.
- Toxins not well absorbed by charcoal are listed in Table 18.2.
- The dose is 50 g for an adult or 1 g/kg in children. Patients must have a protected airway.

Table 18.2 Toxins not well absorbed by activated charcoal

Toxin	Examples
Alcohols	Ethanol, isopropyl alcohol, methanol, ethylene glycol
Metals	Lithium, iron, mercury, potassium, lead, arsenic
Corrosives	Acids, alkalis
Hydrocarbons	Turpentine, kerosene, eucalyptus oil, benzene

- Mixing activated charcoal with ice-cream makes it more palatable for children.

WHOLE BOWEL IRRIGATION

- Decontamination with bowel prep (e.g. polyethylene glycol) hastens the elimination of poorly absorbed or slow-release medications before they can be absorbed.
- Complications include vomiting, aspiration and GI trauma. It is also very messy and requires intensive nursing support.
- Occasions where it may be of use include life-threatening ingestions of iron, potassium, lithium, slow-release verapamil or diltiazem and 'body packers'. Discuss potential cases with a clinical toxicologist.

SYRUP OF IPECAC

- In the past ipecac was used to induce emesis, and traditionally was recommended for paediatric toxic ingestions. It is no longer routinely recommended nor available.
- The amount of toxin removed is unreliable, it does not alter patient outcomes and its use can result in complications such as aspiration pneumonitis.

GASTRIC LAVAGE

- Lavage has not been shown to be beneficial in the general management of the acutely poisoned patient. Complications include aspiration and GI perforation.
- Toxicologists may recommend it for life-threatening overdoses, where the agent is thought to be within the stomach, and when the airway is protected.

Enhanced elimination

- Enhanced elimination refers to techniques employed to increase the rate of removal of a toxin from the body.
- The most common methods include multi-dose activated charcoal, urinary alkalinisation and dialysis.
- Once again, the decision about whether to attempt enhanced elimination is based on balancing the risk and severity of toxicity against the benefit and complications of the elimination technique.

MULTI-DOSE ACTIVATED CHARCOAL (MDAC)

- MDAC may decrease drug absorption in some cases (Box 18.3). This method of drug elimination works best when the drug involved has a small molecular weight, has a prolonged elimination time and a small volume of distribution.
- The dose is 1 g/kg up to 50 g given every 4–6 hours.
- It is contraindicated in the presence of an ileus or bowel obstruction, and in the patient without a protected airway. Charcoal itself can cause an ileus.
- Always check for the presence of bowel sounds before administering the next dose.

URINARY ALKALINISATION

- Urinary alkalinisation increases the urinary elimination of certain acids by promoting the ionisation and preventing reabsorption in the renal tubules. This can be achieved by the intravenous administration of sodium bicarbonate.
- The main indication is in symptomatic salicylate overdose.
- In adults, the dose is a bolus of 1 mmol/kg sodium bicarbonate followed by an infusion of 100 mmol in 1 L 5% dextrose over 4 hours. Target urinary pH is > 7.5.
- The main complication is of hypokalaemia, and IV K^+ supplementation is invariably required.

HAEMODIALYSIS

- Haemodialysis can enhance the elimination of various toxins (Box 18.4)
- Indications for dialysis would include failure to clinically improve despite maximal supportive care, inability to excrete

Box 18.3	Toxins for which multiple-dose activated charcoal may be useful	
Carbamazepine	Phenobarbitone
Colchicine	Theophylline
Dapsone	Quinine
Phenytoin	

Box 18.4	**Drugs amenable to enhanced elimination by dialysis**
Carbamazepine	Potassium
Lithium	Toxic alcohols
Salicylates	Sodium valproate
Theophylline	Phenobarbitone
Metformin	

or metabolise the drug due to hepatic or renal failure, associated metabolic abnormalities (e.g. hyperkalaemia or metformin-induced lactic acidosis) or a potentially lethal plasma concentration of a drug.

Toxidromes

The clinical presentation of some poisonings may be predictable based on the pharmacology of the drug or substance involved. Some classic toxidromes are listed in Table 18.3.

Table 18.3 Features of selected toxidromes

Toxidrome	Agents associated with the toxidrome	Clinical features
Anticholinergic	Antihistamines Tricyclic antidepressants Antipsychotics Atropine Carbamazepine Anticholinergic plants (e.g. *Datura*)	Agitated delirium Sedation Mydriasis Tachycardia Dry mouth and skin Hyperthermia Ileus Urinary retention
Cholinergic	Organophosphate pesticides Carbamate insecticides Chemical warfare nerve agents Dementia drugs (e.g. donepezil) Myasthenia drugs (e.g. neostigmine)	Agitation, coma, seizures Muscle fasciculation, weakness, paralysis Salivation, lacrimation, diaphoresis, bronchorrhoea, vomiting, diarrhoea Miosis Bradycardia or tachycardia

Continued

Table 18.3   Features of selected toxidromes (cont.)

Toxidrome	Agents associated with the toxidrome	Clinical features
Serotonin Syndrome	SSRIs SNRIs MAOIs St John's wort Tramadol TCAs Amphetamines	Mental status changes: anxiety, agitation, confusion Autonomic stimulation: hyperthermia, tachycardia, hypertension, mydriasis Neuromuscular excitation: increased tone (lower limbs > upper limbs), hyperreflexia, clonus, tremor, rigidity
Sympathomimetic toxidrome	Catecholamines Amphetamines Cocaine Xanthines (e.g. theophylline, caffeine) MAOIs Noradrenaline reuptake inhibitors (e.g. venlafaxine)	Tachycardia Hypertension Hypotension (severe cases) Hyperthermia Agitation, delirium Seizures Coma Mydriasis Metabolic acidosis

Editorial Comment

Beware mixed overdoses including with alcohol (never assume just 'dead' drunk) are very common:
- observe closely
- assume unknown cocktail of drugs
- assume worst-case scenario, late at night or early morning.

Specific toxins
BENZODIAZEPINES

- Overdoses of benzodiazepines are common and have a good prognosis with supportive treatment.
- CNS and respiratory depression are the main toxic effects.
- The toxic dose of benzodiazepines varies widely, due to differences between patients in tolerance and dependence. The elderly and those with respiratory comorbidities (e.g. COPD) are at greater risk of complications.

- The clinical features of benzodiazepine overdose include drowsiness, respiratory depression and coma. Bradycardia and hypotension can be seen in large overdoses.
- The majority of benzodiazepine overdoses do not require intubation and can be safely managed with supportive care and close monitoring.
- Charcoal decontamination is not indicated.
- Flumazenil (a competitive benzodiazepine antagonist) may confirm the diagnosis but is generally not used for treatment, unless reversing iatrogenic conscious sedation or if advanced airway management is unavailable, due to the risk of precipitating a withdrawal syndrome and seizures.

OPIOIDS

- This group of drugs includes those derived from opium as well as those that have opiate-like activity.
- Opioid-related overdoses and deaths have risen sharply in Australia over the last decade, with the majority now due to prescription painkillers such as oxycodone and fentanyl. It is the leading cause of death by poisoning in children.
- The classic features of opiate overdose are CNS depression, respiratory depression and miosis.
- Several drugs in this group have atypical toxic effects (Table 18.4).
- Patients should be closely observed and monitored for CNS and respiratory depression.
- Complications of opioid overdose include pulmonary aspiration, hypoxic brain injury, compartment syndrome, renal failure and rhabdomyolysis.

Table 18.4 Atypical opioids

Opioids	Atypical effect of clinical significance
Tramadol	Serotonin syndrome, seizures
Dextropropoxyphene	Seizures, wide QRS arrhythmias (sodium-channel blockade), hypotension
Methadone	Prolonged QT interval, torsades de pointes
Pethidine	Seizures, serotonin syndrome
Fentanyl	Chest wall rigidity

- Check the duration of action of the opioid involved. Some are as short as several hours (fentanyl, heroin) and others as long as 24 hours (methadone and controlled-release forms of morphine and oxycodone). This may help to predict the duration or symptoms and the likelihood of requiring a naloxone infusion or intensive care.
- Be mindful of more unusual routes of opioid overdose such as ingestion of transdermal fentanyl patches.

Pearls and Pitfalls
Do not provide oxygen in the absence of ventilatory support as respiratory depression may be masked.

NALOXONE

- Indications for naloxone (an opioid antagonist) include significant respiratory depression (RR < 8) or CNS depression (GCS < 12).
- Give an initial bolus dose of 100 microg IV (400 microg IM) repeated every minute until an adequate response has been achieved.
- Give smaller incremental doses (e.g. 50 micrograms IV) in the opioid-dependent patient to prevent withdrawal.
- Large doses of naloxone may be required to reverse buprenorphine overdoses (a partial mu agonist).
- The duration of action of naloxone is short (0.5–1 hour). This may be adequate in a short-acting opioid overdose (e.g. heroin), but repeat boluses may be required with longer-acting opioid overdoses.
- A naloxone infusion may be necessary if repeated boluses are required, or if a controlled-release opioid has been taken.

Pearls and Pitfalls
Naloxone can be given with impunity to accidental paediatric opioid overdoses. Give a 400 microg bolus IV to confirm or exclude the diagnosis.

PARACETAMOL

Introduction

- Paracetamol is the most readily available simple analgesic in the world and is responsible for a large proportion of deliberate self-poisonings and accidental paediatric exposures. It is also the leading pharmaceutical agent responsible for calls to the Poisons Information Centre in Australia.

- While hepatic failure and death are uncommon, paracetamol remains the most common cause of fulminant hepatitis in the western world. Thankfully, the early administration of N-acetylcysteine (NAC) is almost universally life-saving. See Table 18.5.

- There are many clinical scenarios in which paracetamol toxicity is encountered, each with a unique approach to risk assessment and management. Care must be taken in ensuring the correct aspect of the guideline is being applied to each individual patient.

- Accidental toxicity is frequently seen in patients taking repeated supratherapeutic doses of paracetamol for painful conditions (e.g. dental pain). Paracetamol is also found in many over-the-counter cold and flu and migraine preparations. Remember to take a careful medication history, particularly quantities of paracetamol ingested in patients presenting with painful conditions.

Guidelines and treatment nomogram

The nomogram for the management of paracetamol poisoning remains unchanged from previous guidelines; however, updated recommendations have been made to the management of massive paracetamol overdose and paediatric paracetamol ingestions.

Table 18.5 **Three-stage N-acetylcysteine infusion—adults**

Initial infusion	150 mg/kg of N-acetylcysteine diluted in 200 mL 5% glucose infused over 1 hour
Second infusion	50 mg/kg of N-acetylcysteine in 500 mL 5% glucose infused over 4 hours
Third infusion	100 mg/kg of N-acetylcysteine in 1 L 5% glucose infused over 16 hours

Resuscitation

- Resuscitation is rarely required for isolated paracetamol overdoses.
- The exception is massive paracetamol ingestions, which can cause early decreased level of consciousness and lactic acidosis.
- Supportive management and the use of NAC are the mainstays of treatment.

Risk assessment

Potentially hepatotoxic doses of paracetamol are outlined in Box 18.5.

Decontamination

- In awake, cooperative patients, offer 50 g (1 g/kg in children) of activated charcoal within 2 hours of ingestion (up to 4 hours for modified-release preparations).
- This reduces the absorbed paracetamol dose and may obviate the subsequent need for NAC.
- Activated charcoal should not be forced on uncooperative adults or children.

Commencing NAC immediately

NAC should be commenced immediately if:

- presentation is 8–24 hours after a known time of ingestion; the infusion can be ceased or continued once

Box 18.5	Paracetamol dosing that may be associated with hepatic injury
Acute single ingestions	• 200 mg/kg or 10 g (whichever is lower) over a period of < 8 hours
Repeated supratherapeutic ingestions	• > 200 mg/kg or 10 g (whichever is less) over a single 24-hour period • > 150 mg/kg or 6 g (whichever is lower) per 24-hour period over the preceding 48 hours • > 100 mg/kg/day or 4 g/day (whichever is lower) for more than 48 hours, in those who also have symptoms indicating possible liver injury (e.g. abdominal pain, nausea or vomiting)

the paracetamol level and results of transaminases are analysed
- time of ingestion is unknown and serum paracetamol is detectable
- there are signs of hepatic injury after any paracetamol overdose.

Acute single ingestions

Paracetamol levels measured > 4 hours post-ingestion are plotted on the nomogram to determine the risk of hepatotoxicity and the requirement for NAC therapy. See Figure 18.1.

Presentation within 8 hours of an acute ingestion

- Measure the serum paracetamol level (at 4–8 hours) and plot it on the nomogram. If there is a delay in obtaining a paracetamol level beyond 8 hours from ingestion, then commence NAC while awaiting the result.

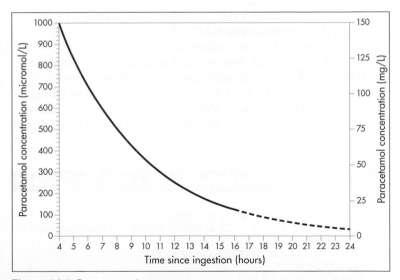

Figure 18.1 Paracetamol nomogram
Note: Ensure the correct units are used when utilising the paracetamol nomogram.

- If the level is plotted below the treatment line, no further medical treatment is required.
- If the level is plotted above the treatment line, then commence NAC therapy. No further investigations are required.
- Those patients with very high paracetamol levels (double the treatment line) may benefit from an increased NAC dose—see the section on massive paracetamol ingestions.

Presentation between 8 and 24 hours after an acute ingestion

- NAC should be commenced immediately.
- Measure the serum paracetamol level and an alanine aminotransferase (ALT) test.
- If the paracetamol level plots above the treatment line, then continue the NAC.
- If the level plots under the treatment line and the ALT is < 50 U/L, then cease the NAC infusion. No further investigations are required.
- If the level plots under the treatment line, but the ALT is raised, then continue the NAC infusion.
- Measure the ALT at the end of the NAC infusion.
- If the ALT is normal, then no further treatment is required.
- If the ALT is abnormal, continue NAC (100 mg/kg over 16 hours) and recheck ALT every 12–24 hours until falling.
- If ALT > 1000 U/L check INR, renal function and platelet count every 12–24 hours. See Box 18.6 for criteria for referral to a liver transplant unit.

Box 18.6   Indications for discussion with a liver transplant unit

- INR > 3.0 at 48 hours post-ingestion, or > 4.5 at any time
- Oliguria or creatinine > 200 micromol/L
- Persistent acidosis (pH < 7.3) or arterial lactate > 3 mmol/L, despite resuscitation
- Systolic hypotension with BP < 80 mmHg
- Hypoglycaemia
- Severe thrombocytopenia
- Encephalopathy of any degree, or alteration of consciousness (GCS < 15), not associated with sedative co-ingestions.

Acute paracetamol ingestion with unknown time of ingestion

+ Treat the patient as if it is a delayed presentation.
+ Commence NAC immediately and measure a paracetamol level and an ALT.
+ Treat the patient as per the > 8 hours scenario above.

Massive paracetamol ingestions

+ Patients who have ingested > 30 g paracetamol should be offered activated charcoal up to 4 hours post-overdose.
+ Patients who have paracetamol levels above double the nomogram line are considered high risk. They may develop hepatotoxicity despite being treated within 8 hours with NAC.
+ Consult the PIC for the most current advice on these patients. Many toxicologists will recommend doubling the concentration of NAC in the third bag from 100 mg/kg to 200 mg/kg over 16 hours.
+ Measure paracetamol levels and ALT at the end of the NAC infusion. Continue NAC at a rate of 100 mg/kg over 16 hours if the ALT > 50 U/L or if the paracetamol level is > 10 mg/L (66 micromol/L).

Management of 'staggered' ingestions

+ A staggered overdose is one of multiple doses taken over a 24-hour period.
+ If it has been less than 8 hours since the first dose, the patient can be treated as per the < 8 hours section above.
+ If it has been more than 8 hours since the first dose was ingested, then treat the patient as per the > 8 hours scenario above.
+ In both cases, plot the paracetamol level on the nomogram assuming that the entire dose was taken at the *earliest* possible time.

Repeated supratherapeutic ingestions

+ This scenario occurs in the setting of patients taking repeated supratherapeutic doses of paracetamol over several days, often for self-medication for painful conditions (e.g. dental pain).

- In children it is often a dosing error.
- Patients who have possible repeated supratherapeutic ingestions should have a paracetamol level and an ALT measured.
- If the ALT < 50 U/L and the serum paracetamol concentration is < 20 mg/L (132 micromol/L), then no further treatment is required.
- If there is any other result, then commence NAC and repeat the paracetamol level and ALT at 8 hours.
- If ALT is normal or static and paracetamol level is < 10 mg/L (66 micromol/L), cease the NAC. No further treatment required.
- If ALT is abnormal or worsening, continue NAC and check ALT and other bloods at 12-hourly intervals.

Management of modified-release paracetamol ingestions

- Some formulations of paracetamol available in Australia are modified-release (e.g. Panadol osteo), which has the potential for delayed peak serum paracetamol levels when taken in overdose.
- Patients should be offered activated charcoal up to 4 hours post-overdose.
- If more than 200 mg/kg or 10 g (whichever is lower) has been ingested, then NAC should be started immediately.
- Paracetamol levels should be taken at 4 (or more) hours post-ingestion and repeated 4 hours later. If both levels are below the treatment line, then NAC can be stopped.
- If either level is above the line, then continue NAC as per the 'single ingestion' section above.

N-acetylcysteine (NAC)

- NAC given within 8 hours of a paracetamol overdose is almost completely protective of subsequent hepatotoxicity.
- It is given as a three-stage infusion over 21 hours.
- Doses should be calculated for actual weight, with a ceiling of 110 kg. See Table 18.5.
- Anaphylactoid reactions occur in 10–50% of patients receiving NAC, manifested by rash, wheeze and mild hypotension.

- Management includes temporary halting or slowing of the infusion, administration of antihistamine or bronchodilators, and then recommencing the infusion.
- Severe and life-threatening reactions are unusual. Rarely adrenaline is required for severe allergic reactions to NAC.

STIMULANTS

- Stimulants refer to a diverse group of chemicals (Table 18.6) that share clinical features of increasing alertness and energy.
- They are commonly referred to as 'uppers'.
- Stimulants act on a variety of neurotransmitters, including noradrenaline, dopamine and serotonin.
- There is huge variability in the chemical constituents of street drugs.
- In overdose, they can cause the sympathomimetic toxidrome (Table 18.7) and are potentially lethal.

Cocaine

- Cocaine is a powerful sympathomimetic and also has vasospastic and sodium-channel blocking effects.
- Cocaine intoxication is rapid, with features occurring within the first hour and lasting several hours.

Table 18.6 Stimulants

Drug name	Common street names
Cocaine	Coke, crack, Charlie, blow
3,4-Methylenedioxy-N-methamphetamine	Ecstasy, E, eccy, pills, MDMA
Methamphetamine	Ice, speed, meth, crystal meth
Para-methoxyamphetamine (PMA), para-methoxy-N-methylamphetamine (PMMA)	Red Mitsubishi, Dr Death, pink ecstasy
Synthetic cathinones (e.g. methylenedioxypyrovalerone 4-methylmethcathinone)	Bath salts, MDPV, mephedrone, miaow-miaow
Novel phenethylamines	NBOMes, N-Bomb, 25-I-NBOMe
Methylphenidate, dexamphetamine	

Table 18.7 **Clinical features and complications of stimulant overdoses**

System	Clinical effect
CNS	Euphoria Anxiety, agitation Hallucinations, psychosis Seizures, coma
Cardiovascular	Tachycardia, hypertension Arrhythmias Acute coronary syndromes Vascular dissections
Other	Hyperthermia Mydriasis Rhabdomyolysis, renal failure Subarachnoid haemorrhage Pneumothorax, pneumomediastinum Hyponatraemia (MDMA)

- Co-ingestion with alcohol increases the toxic effect of cocaine.
- Cocaine is more likely than the other amphetamines to cause seizures, arrhythmias and myocardial ischaemia.
- Patients presenting with chest pain must be worked up for cardiac ischaemia.

Amphetamines

- Patients may present with acute intoxication, with complications of abuse or in an acute psychosis.
- Amphetamines are more hallucinogenic due to greater dopaminergic effects.
- MDMA can sometimes induce the syndrome of SIADH and can lead to hyponatraemia, coma and seizures.
- The most common presentation of methamphetamine intoxication is of profound agitation and psychosis. These patients often require parenteral sedation.
- PMA and PMMA are stimulants with hallucinogenic effects similar to MDMA. They have been linked to deaths in patients thinking they were taking MDMA. They cause a severe serotonin syndrome and multi-organ failure.

- Synthetic cathinones or bath salts are potent stimulants that can cause an excited delirium. They can cause a severe sympathomimetic toxidrome and multi-organ failure.

Management of stimulant overdose

- Benzodiazepines are the treatment of choice for stimulant-induced agitation, seizures, tachycardia and hypertension.
- Second-line therapies for hypertension include glyceryl trinitrate (GTN) or sodium nitroprusside infusions.
- Beta-blockers are contraindicated because of the potential for unopposed alpha stimulation. This can result in increased blood pressure, reduced coronary blood flow and reduced left ventricular function.
- Cocaine-induced broad-complex tachycardia is treated with boluses of sodium bicarbonate.
- Acute coronary syndromes are treated with standard therapies including aspirin and GTN. Beta-blockers should be avoided. Thrombolysis is contraindicated if there is uncontrolled hypertension.
- Hyperthermia requires rapid cooling to prevent multiple organ failure. This may require intubation, sedation and paralysis.
- Manage rhabdomyolysis with aggressive IV fluid hydration.
- Severe hyponatraemia ($Na^+ < 120$ mmol/L) with altered mental status or seizures is treated with hypertonic saline.

GAMMA-HYDROXYBUTYRATE (GHB) AND ANALOGUES

- This group of drugs consists of GHB, gamma-butyrolactone and 1,4-butanediol. They are structural analogues of the inhibitory neurotransmitter GABA.
- They are clear, colourless and reasonably tasteless drugs with minimal hangover effects which makes them palatable to the user and sometime implicated as a date-rape drug.
- Street names include GBH (grievous bodily harm), liquid ecstasy, fantasy and 'G'.
- The most prominent clinical feature of toxicity is a rapid onset of coma, often to a GCS score as low as 3. Varying GCS over a short period of time can also occur. For example, a

patient can oscillate from GCS 6 to 10 and then back to 6 in a period of minutes.

- Other clinical features of GHB intoxication include mild bradycardia and hypotension, mild respiratory depression, sweatiness, vomiting and, rarely, myoclonic jerks.
- Due to the rapid onset and short duration of action, there is no role for decontamination.
- Patients have a good outcome with supportive care including close observation in a resuscitation bay, placing the patient in the left lateral (recovery) position, and intubation and ventilation if there is not prompt recovery of GCS.
- The drug has a short duration of action, with most patients recovering within 1–4 hours.
- Mild hypotension and bradycardia are common features, but rarely require intervention.
- GHB has a cumulative effect with repeated dosing and an additive effect with other CNS depressants such as alcohol and benzodiazepines. In these settings, recovery may be slower.
- Patients who are not improving or who have an atypical presentation should be further investigated (e.g. CT brain).

KETAMINE

- Ketamine is a dissociative general anaesthetic agent. It is usually snorted but can also be ingested or injected.
- Street names include 'K', special K or vitamin K. Users feel detached from their immediate surroundings, feel euphoric, have 'out-of-body' experiences (flying, floating) and hallucinate. They do not respond to stimuli in their external surroundings.
- It is generally short-acting and fatalities are rare.
- Effects can vary from appearing inebriated to being calm or agitated or violent. With larger doses, incoordination, confusion and coma can occur.
- The clinical signs of ketamine intoxication include hypertension, tachycardia, hypersalivation, pain insensitivity and a blank stare ('the K-hole').
- Treatment options, depending on the clinical setting, include supportive care, sedation with benzodiazepines and advanced airway management.

- Chronic ketamine abuse can lead to painful haemorrhagic cystitis of the bladder.

CANNABINOIDS
(For more information on cannabis see Chapter 19 Drugs and Alcohol.)

- Cannabinoids are the active substances from *Cannabis sativa* and include cannabinol, cannabidiol and tetrahydrocannabinol (THC). The principal psychoactive cannabinoid is delta-9-THC.
- Marijuana is the name for a mixture of dried leaves and flowers of the plant. Hashish is the pressed resin. Hashish oil is the oil from hashish.
- These substances may be smoked or ingested. Effects are apparent within minutes of smoking, and from 1–3 hours after ingestion.
- Clinical effects are relatively mild and include sedation, euphoria and disinhibition. Large doses can cause tachycardia, orthostatic hypotension, CNS depression, anxiety and rarely psychosis. Overdoses in children have caused coma.
- Serious toxicity is rare. The mainstay of treatment is supportive, with reassurance and benzodiazepines and/ or occasionally antipsychotics for gentle sedation in the agitated, paranoid or psychotic patient. Psychiatric symptoms are often due to underlying disorders.
- A syndrome of cyclical nausea, vomiting and abdominal pain, the 'cannabis hyperemesis syndrome', is seen occasionally in chronic cannabis users. Sufferers often find relief from hot showers. The best cure is cessation of cannabis use, but symptomatic relief can be achieved in the ED with topical capsaicin cream, antiemetics and low doses of antipsychotics with antiemetic effects (e.g. droperidol).

LSD
- Lysergic acid diethylamide (LSD) is a synthetic hallucinogen which is able to alter and distort perception, thought and mood.
- It is sold as capsules, tablets, liquid or on liquid-impregnated paper which is ingested.

- The onset of effects after ingestion occur within 30–60 minutes and last approximately 10–12 hours.
- Auditory and visual hallucinations occur, along with distortion of size, shape and colour. Synaesthesia—a crossing-over of the senses—is often described as 'seeing sounds' or 'hearing colour'.
- The common presentation to an ED is in those suffering a 'bad trip' (i.e. dysphoric and scary hallucinations). Treatment involves providing a quiet room with minimal stimuli, reassurance and, if necessary, benzodiazepine sedation.
- Potentially life-threatening complications include cardiovascular collapse, hyperthermia and the serotonin syndrome. These are seen only in the setting of massive overdose.

AMYL NITRITE

- Amyl nitrite is a volatile nitrite and vasodilator.
- Vials of amyl nitrite are known by their street name 'poppers'. They are most commonly inhaled.
- Clinical effects include facial flushing and light-headedness (the 'rush'), euphoria, muscle relaxation, disinhibition and increased libido.
- It can cause methaemoglobinaemia, especially if accidentally ingested.
- Clinical effects of methaemoglobinaemia are consistent with those of hypoxia (Table 18.8).
- Pulse oximetry typically reads around 85% and fails to improve with supplemental oxygen.
- Diagnosis relies on detection of methaemoglobinaemia on co-oximetry.
- Treat symptomatic patients and those with levels > 20% with methylene blue. The dose is 1–2 mg/kg IV over 5 minutes.

Table 18.8   Clinical effects of methaemoglobinaemia

Methaemoglobin (%)	Clinical effects
10–20%	Cyanosis
20–50%	Dizziness, fatigue, headache, tachycardia, anxiety
> 50%	Tachypnoea, lethargy, coma, seizures, death

- Response should be apparent within 1 hour. If not, methylene blue dosing may be repeated.
- Monitor response with serial methaemoglobin level checks.

BETA-BLOCKERS

- Sotalol and propranolol are the most toxic of all the beta-blockers in overdose.
- The other beta-blockers are less toxic in overdose, unless co-ingested with other agents that have cardiovascular effects.
- Other predictors of severity include advancing age and preexisting cardiac disease.
- Clinical manifestations are usually apparent by 4 hours post-ingestion (Table 18.9) unless slow-release preparations are taken.
- Patients should be managed in an area where they can receive continuous cardiac monitoring and resuscitation if necessary.
- Propranolol overdoses are managed as a tricyclic antidepressant overdose with intubation, ventilation and administration of sodium bicarbonate (see section on TCA overdose).
- Bradycardia and hypotension can be managed with initial IV fluid boluses, atropine and high-dose insulin (Box 18.7). Adrenaline and/or isoprenaline infusions can be used as a

Table 18.9 Clinical effects of beta-blocker overdose

System	Clinical features
Cardiovascular	Bradycardia
	Hypotension
	Bradyarrhythmias—1st- to 3rd-degree heart block
	QRS widening (propranolol)
	QT prolongation (sotalol)
CNS	Delirium
	Coma
	Seizures (propranolol)
Metabolic	Hypo/hyperglycaemia
	Hyperkalaemia
Respiratory	Bronchospasm
	Pulmonary oedema

Box 18.7 **High-dose insulin euglycaemic therapy (HIET) for use in beta-blocker or calcium-channel blocker toxicity**

Indications
- Calcium-channel blocker or beta-blocker poisoning with cardiovascular collapse

Steps
- Correct hypoglycaemia if present with a bolus of 50 mL 50% glucose IV.
- Give short-acting insulin 1 unit/kg IV bolus.
- Commence insulin infusion 1 unit/kg/hr.
- Maintain euglycaemia with a glucose infusion titrated to BSLs.

Notes
- HIET takes 30–60 minutes to exert its inotropic effect.
- Hypokalaemia is an expected complication and serum potassium should be monitored and replaced as necessary.
- Insulin infusions may need to be titrated up to 10 units/kg/hr. Discuss severe cases with a clinical toxicologist.

---

temporising measure until the insulin exerts its inotropic effects.
- Temporary cardiac pacing is also an option for refractory bradycardia and hypotension, although capture may be difficult.
- Torsades de pointes due to QT prolongation is a feature of sotalol overdose. It is managed with magnesium and isoprenaline or overdrive pacing.
- Glucagon is no longer recommended for beta-blocker overdoses. Although effective, it has a short half-life and hospital stocks are often quickly exhausted.

Calcium-channel blockers
- The centrally acting calcium-channel blockers verapamil and diltiazem are potentially lethal in overdose. Death is due to profound cardiovascular collapse. The peripherally acting calcium-channel blockers (Box 18.8) are relatively less toxic in overdose.
- Children, the elderly, those with cardiovascular disease and those who co-ingest other cardiac toxins are most susceptible to severe effects.
- Clinical features of calcium-channel blocker overdose are outlined in Table 18.10.

Box 18.8   Types of calcium-channel blockers

Centrally acting:
- verapamil
- diltiazem

Peripherally acting:
- amlodipine
- felodipine
- lercanidipine
- nifedipine

Table 18.10   Clinical features of calcium-channel blocker overdose

System	Clinical features
Cardiovascular	Hypotension Bradycardia and arrhythmogenic shock Myocardial ischaemia Cardiac arrest
Neurological	Confusion, drowsiness (due to hypotension)
Metabolic	Hyperglycaemia Lactic acidosis Hypocalcaemia

Decontamination

- Activated charcoal should be offered to all patients who have overdosed within 1 hour of standard release and 4 hours of sustained-release preparations.
- Whole bowel irrigation can be considered in patients with large verapamil or diltiazem overdose who present within 4 hours and before toxicity is established.

Management of calcium-channel blocker (CCB) overdose

- Patients need to be closely observed for features of toxicity with continuous cardiac monitoring and frequent ECG analysis. Consider early invasive blood pressure monitoring in symptomatic patients.
- Atropine boluses can be given initially for symptomatic bradycardia or conduction disturbances.
- Hypotension needs to be treated aggressively in a step-wise manner with IV fluids, IV calcium, high-dose insulin and inotropes.

- Calcium can reverse some of the toxic effects of CCB poisoning. Calcium gluconate is preferable to calcium chloride as it is less irritating when given through peripheral veins. The dose is calcium gluconate 10% 30 mL (1 mL/kg in children) given over 10 minutes, repeated as necessary to maintain serum ionised calcium above 2.0 mEq/L.
- The choice of inotrope is guided by whether the hypotension is mainly due to myocardial depression, bradycardia or peripheral vasodilation. An echocardiogram can help guide therapy. Noradrenaline and adrenaline are both recommended, with noradrenaline favoured in the presence of vasodilatory shock.
- Temporary cardiac pacing can be attempted; however, electrical capture may be difficult to achieve and may not be associated with improved haemodynamics.
- VA-ECMO should be considered in centres where it is available for cases of refractory cardiogenic shock.
- In the case of cardiac arrest, prolonged attempts at resuscitation are warranted. Seek urgent expert help while maintaining good-quality CPR.

TRICYCLIC ANTIDEPRESSANTS (TCAs)

- Examples of TCAs include amitriptyline, clomipramine, dothiepin, doxepin, imipramine and nortriptyline.
- TCAs inhibit the reuptake of noradrenaline and serotonin, and also have anticholinergic and antihistaminergic properties.
- Overdoses can be life-threatening, particularly at doses > 10 mg/kg.
- Signs of toxicity (Table 18.11) manifest early, and rapid deterioration can occur.
- Charcoal is contraindicated with an unprotected airway, due to the risk of rapid coma.
- Early intervention with management of coma, seizures and cardiac arrhythmias is life-saving.
- All patients must be closely monitored and observed for a minimum of 6 hours post-ingestion.
- ECGs are essential to monitor for toxicity and guide therapy. Key ECG abnormalities include QRS widening, PR prolongation, a tall R wave in aVR and QT prolongation.

Table 18.11   Clinical signs of TCA toxicity

System	Clinical signs
CNS	Sedation
	Coma
	Seizures
Cardiovascular	Sinus tachycardia
	Hypotension
	Broad-complex tachyarrhythmias
	Broad-complex bradyarrhythmias (pre-arrest)
	Cardiac arrest
Anticholinergic effects	Delirium
	Mydriasis
	Urinary retention
	Ileus

- The degree of QRS widening can be used to predict complications; a QRS of > 100 ms is predictive of seizures, > 160 ms is predictive of ventricular arrhythmias.

Management of TCA overdose

- At the first sign of CNS depression, the patient should be intubated and hyperventilated. The target is a pH of 7.5.
- Seizures are often brief and self-limiting. They can be treated with benzodiazepines if necessary.
- Hypotension is treated with IV fluids and inotropes.
- If progressive QRS widening is associated with any sign of decreased GCS or cardiovascular instability, then boluses of sodium bicarbonate should be given titrated to a narrowing of the QRS. Give 1–2 mmol/kg IV every 3–5 minutes. Intubation and hyperventilation should occur concurrently, targeting a pH of 7.5.
- In the event of cardiac arrest, give repeated boluses of sodium bicarbonate (100 mmol or 2 mmol/kg IV, repeated every 1–2 minutes), along with standard advanced cardiac life support (ACLS) protocols, until a perfusing rhythm is restored.
- Antiarrhythmics such as amiodarone and beta-blockers are contraindicated.
- Defibrillation tends to be unsuccessful.

- Patients who are clinically well at 6 hours post-overdose with a normal ECG may be medically fit for discharge.

Editorial Comment

Beware: intentional or accidental–recreation overdose can be fatal if different classes of antidepressants (even 1–2 tabs) are taken, due to different mechanisms of action multiplying toxicity.

SELECTIVE SEROTONIN REUPTAKE INHIBITORS (SSRIs)

- SSRIs are widely prescribed for anxiety and major depression. Examples include citalopram, escitalopram, fluoxetine, fluvoxamine, paroxetine and sertraline.
- When taken as a single agent in overdose, the clinical course is usually benign regardless of the dose taken. Patients will often be asymptomatic or display only mild serotonergic features.
- Co-ingestion of other serotonergic agents (e.g. MAOIs, SNRIs, tramadol) greatly increases the risk of developing the serotonin syndrome.
- Features of serotonin syndrome are outlined in Table 18.3.
- Citalopram and escitalopram can cause QT prolongation.
- Treatment of mild serotonin syndrome includes reassurance and benzodiazepine sedation if required.
- More severe features (e.g. rigidity, hyperthermia, seizures) require aggressive therapy with intubation, sedation and active cooling.
- Patients who are asymptomatic at 6 hours post-overdose of most SSRIs may be medically cleared.
- Overdoses of citalopram > 600 mg and escitalopram > 300 mg require longer observation (13 hours) due to the risk of delayed QT prolongation.

SELECTIVE SEROTONIN AND NORADRENALINE REUPTAKE INHIBITORS (SNRIs)

- Examples of SNRI antidepressants include venlafaxine and desvenlafaxine.

- SNRIs, particularly venlafaxine, are potentially life-threatening in overdose.
- Common early symptoms are of a mild serotonin syndrome (see SSRIs above).
- There is a risk of seizures that increases with the dose ingested. A seizure is almost guaranteed with ingestions > 4.5 g.
- Cardiovascular toxicity is seen with large ingestions, including hypotension, QRS and QT prolongation and occasionally tachyarrhythmias.
- Treatment is supportive, with benzodiazepines for seizures and mild serotonergic features.
- Due to the risk of delayed toxicity, patients must be observed for a minimum of 16 hours.

QUETIAPINE

- Quetiapine is an atypical antipsychotic that is widely prescribed for both bipolar affective disorder and schizophrenia.
- In overdose it causes dose-dependent CNS depression ranging from mild sedation to deep coma. Greater toxicity can be expected with overdoses > 3 g.
- Tachycardia and mild anticholinergic side effects are frequently seen.
- Hypotension can complicate large overdoses, due to peripheral alpha blockade.
- Paradoxically, adrenaline can worsen the hypotension, and noradrenaline is the inotrope of choice.
- Minor QT prolongation has been reported, but quetiapine does not cause torsades de pointes and routine ECG monitoring is not required.
- Single-dose activated charcoal should be offered to quetiapine overdoses > 2 g presenting within 2 hours of ingestion (if GCS 15), or to those who have been intubated. It may lessen the requirement for intubation and the duration of symptoms.
- Patients with significant sedation or coma should be intubated.
- Treat hypotension with IV fluids +/- noradrenaline.

- Agitation should be treated cautiously with benzodiazepines, knowing that this may worsen the CNS depression.
- There is good prognosis with supportive and intensive care.
- Patients who are clinically well at 6 hours following overdose can be medically cleared.

Pearls and Pitfalls

Check for urinary retention in patients presenting with quetiapine overdose. It is a frequent cause of agitation in these patients.

LITHIUM

- Lithium is a mood stabiliser that has a narrow therapeutic index. It is entirely excreted by the kidneys.
- Lithium toxicity is encountered in two different scenarios: acute overdose and chronic toxicity.
- Acute lithium overdose is frequently benign, and causes gastrointestinal symptoms of nausea, vomiting, abdominal pain and diarrhoea. The treatment is supportive with IV fluid rehydration and monitoring of electrolytes and renal function.
- Chronic lithium toxicity is the more common and serious entity.
- It frequently occurs in older patients whose lithium excretion is reduced by renal impairment.
- Clinical features of chronic lithium toxicity are outlined in Table 18.12.
- Risk factors for the development of chronic toxicity include dehydration, renal impairment, drug interactions (e.g. NSAIDs, ACE inhibitors, SSRIs and diuretics) and older age.
- Nephrogenic diabetes insipidus is associated with chronic lithium use and can contribute to toxicity.
- Lithium levels do not correlate well with severity of toxicity; however, levels of > 2 mmol/L are associated with severe toxicity. The normal therapeutic index is 0.4–0.8 mmol/L.
- Management of chronic lithium toxicity includes ceasing lithium and any other medications that may contribute to renal impairment. Renal function and electrolytes are closely

Table 18.12   Features of chronic lithium toxicity

System	Features
Neurological	Tremor
	Hyperreflexia
	Ataxia
	Rigidity
	Hypertonia
	Myoclonus
	Seizures
	Coma
Cardiovascular	Hypotension
	QT prolongation

monitored, and IV normal saline is given both to rehydrate the patient and to enhance renal lithium excretion.

• The role of haemodialysis should be discussed with a clinical toxicologist. It is generally recommended for patients with severe clinical symptoms or those with levels > 2.5 mmol/L and renal impairment.

• All patients with chronic toxicity will require admission as resolution often takes days to weeks.

Pearls and Pitfalls

Always consider lithium toxicity in patients who take lithium and present with neurological symptoms or signs.

Chapter 19
Drugs and alcohol
Kate Sellors

Acknowledgment
The author wishes to acknowledge the content used from the previous edition of *Emergency Medicine* which was provided by Fiona Chow, Alex Wodak and Gordian Fulde.

Introduction
- People use alcohol and drugs for many reasons: for enjoyment, to relax, out of curiosity, to be part of a group, as a coping mechanism or to minimise physical and/or psychological pain and trauma.
- Substances that fall in this category can be either licit (e.g. alcohol, nicotine, prescribed drugs) or illicit (e.g. heroin, cocaine).

Issues related to the use of drugs and alcohol include the following.
- Acute intoxication or overdose.
- Chronic organ damage.
- Physical dependence and subsequent withdrawal syndromes.
- Psychiatric illness.
- Social problems (e.g. homelessness, criminality).
- A drug and alcohol history should be taken as part of a routine history on patients presenting to the ED. Direct but non-judgmental language should be used when questioning patients (e.g. 'Have you ever injected drugs?', rather than 'Are you a drug user?'). When one drug problem is identified, enquire about other substance use, as poly-drug use is common.
- Patients presenting to the ED with an alcohol or drug-related problem present an ideal opportunity for the treating doctor to make an assessment of the magnitude of the problem, provide a brief intervention and refer for longer-term support.

Box 19.1   Helpful links

Alcohol and Drug Foundation: https://adf.org.au, 1300 85 85 84
Alcohol Drug Information Service: 1800 422 599
Alcoholics Anonymous: http://aa.org.au, 1300 222 222
Narcotics Anonymous: https://www.na.org.au, 1300 652 820
SMART Recovery Australia: https://smartrecoveryaustralia.com.au

---

- Brief interventions can be as simple as emphasising the harms related to their drug or alcohol use and encouraging a patient to cut down or abstain.
- Patients can be directed to seek further information and assistance from their GPs, specialised drug and alcohol centres, or from numerous not-for-profit self-help organisations—see Box 19.1.

Editorial Comment

Emergency departments must have a ZERO tolerance of verbal abuse and physical violence. Ensure policies and practices are known and used for the safety of patients and staff. De-escalation, retreat, call for help (duress alarms for all staff).

Alcohol
EPIDEMIOLOGY

- About 1 in 13 adults drink alcohol every day.
- A quarter of all adults drink at levels that place their long-term health at risk.
- The risk of hazardous drinking is equal across all socioeconomic groups.
- The sex differences in hazardous drinking patterns has narrowed in the younger population, with the prevalence of problematic drinking among young women now matching their male counterparts.

IMPACT ON THE EMERGENCY DEPARTMENT

- Alcohol is the second leading cause of drug-related hospital admissions and deaths after tobacco.
- One in eight ED presentations is related to alcohol.

- Patients may present with a spectrum of alcohol-related problems, including acute intoxication, trauma associated with alcohol use, alcohol withdrawal or a complication of long-term alcohol abuse.

SAFE DRINKING LEVELS

The NHMRC have published guidelines to reduce health risks from drinking alcohol. They suggest the following.

- More than 2 standard drinks a day for healthy men and women will increase the lifetime risk of harm from alcohol-related disease or injury.
- More than 4 standard drinks on a single occasion for healthy men and women will increase the risk of alcohol-related injury.
- Not drinking alcohol is the safest option for children and young people < 18 years of age.
- There is no safe drinking level for women who are pregnant or who are breastfeeding.

Significant dependence is associated with the regular consumption of more than 8 standard drinks per day.

STANDARD DRINKS

- One Australian standard drink contains 10 g ethanol.
- This equates to 1 can (375 mL) of mid-strength beer, 1 nip (30 mL) of spirits (40%) or 100 mL of wine (10–13%).

COMPLICATIONS OF ACUTE INTOXICATION

- Increased risk of accidental injury including motor vehicle accidents (MVAs), falls, drownings and violent assaults
- Risky sexual behaviours including sexually transmitted infections (STIs) and unintended pregnancy
- Increased risk of self-harm and suicidality

COMPLICATIONS OF CHRONIC ALCOHOL ABUSE

- Cardiovascular disease: atrial fibrillation, cardiomyopathy, hypertension
- Malignancy: oropharynx, oesophagus, liver, colorectum and female breast
- Malnutrition conditions: Wernicke-Korsakoff syndrome, folate deficiency, vitamin A deficiency, niacin deficiency

- Gastrointestinal: cirrhosis, hepatitis, gastritis, pancreatitis, GI haemorrhage
- Psychiatric: depression, anxiety, self-harm
- Neurological: dementia, cerebellar degeneration, peripheral neuropathy
- Metabolic: hypokalaemia, hypomagnesaemia, hypocalcaemia
- Haematological: anaemia, thrombocytopenia, leucopenia

ACUTE INTOXICATION

- Clinical features of acute alcohol intoxication are initially of euphoria and decreased inhibitions, following by progressively worsening slurred speech, ataxia and CNS depression. See Table 19.1.
- Severity of clinical effects correlates with the ethanol level; however, there is a high degree of inter-individual variability due to individual tolerance.
- Co-ingestion of other CNS depressants (e.g. benzodiazepines) increases the risk of CNS and respiratory depression.
- Alcohol poisoning can be lethal.

Table 19.1 **Clinical effects of alcohol at different concentrations**

Blood alcohol concentration (BAC) (%)	Clinical effects
Up to 0.05%	Talkative Relaxed
0.05–0.08%	Reduced inhibitions Impaired judgment and movement
0.08–0.15%	Slurred speech Slowed reflexes Impaired balance and coordination
0.15–0.3%	Decreased level of consciousness Nausea and vomiting Memory blackouts Loss of bladder control
0.3–0.4%	Coma Respiratory depression
> 0.4%	Lethal dose (with notable exceptions)

- Many EDs have access to alcohol breathalysers which can provide rapid and non-invasive estimates of blood alcohol concentration.
- In most patients, the serum ethanol concentration decreases by approximately 0.02%/hr. This may be useful in estimating time to sobriety.

TREATMENT OF ACUTE ALCOHOL INTOXICATION

- Alcohol intoxication on its own is usually a benign entity and requires only supportive care with careful monitoring of the patient's airway and level of consciousness.
- Consider differential diagnoses for the patient's condition—a missed diagnosis of a head injury or ketoacidosis could be fatal.
- Provide a safe environment for the patient to prevent injuries to themselves and to staff.
- IV fluids and antiemetics are often prescribed, but have no evidence of benefit to the intoxicated patient.
- Monitor for signs of withdrawal.
- Once the patient has sobered up, take an accurate and non-judgmental drug and alcohol history, and provide opportunistic intervention and referral as necessary.

Editorial Comment

Use alcohol withdrawal scale but beware dual diagnosis (e.g. pneumonia can be a fatal mis-diagnosis).

ALCOHOL WITHDRAWAL SYNDROME

- Alcohol withdrawal syndrome usually starts within 6–24 hours of abrupt cessation or decreased consumption of alcohol, and typically persists for up to 72 hours.
- In patients who are tolerant to high BACs, withdrawal symptoms develop before the BAC drops to zero.
- Characteristic symptoms include sweating, anxiety, tachycardia, tremor, agitation and hyperthermia.
- Hallucinations (tactile and visual) occasionally occur.
- Delirium tremens (the DTs) is a rare and severe form of alcohol withdrawal and is characterised by confusion,

hallucinations, severe tremor and autonomic hyperactivity. It is a medical emergency that requires prompt identification and treatment with benzodiazepines and supportive care. Symptoms can last days to weeks.

♦ Interestingly, alcohol withdrawal is rarely a problem in the setting of advanced chronic liver disease. In these patients, hepatic encephalopathy can mimic the alcohol withdrawal syndrome.

ALCOHOL WITHDRAWAL SCALE

The alcohol withdrawal scale (AWS) is a commonly used and easy way of assessing and documenting the severity of withdrawal symptoms and response to treatment. It is important to note that the AWS is not a diagnostic tool, but one of measurement.

♦ AWS score ≤ 4 = mild withdrawal
♦ AWS score 5–7 = moderate withdrawal
♦ AWS score ≥ 8 = severe withdrawal

Table 19.2   Alcohol withdrawal scale

Perspiration	0—Nil 1—Moist skin 2—Beads of sweat 3—Whole body perspiring 4—Maximal sweating, wet clothes
Tremor	0—Nil 1—Slight tremor 2—Constant slight tremor 3—Constant marked tremor
Anxiety	0—Nil 1—Slight apprehension 2—Understandable fear 3—Anxiety with intermittent panic 4—Constant panic
Agitation	0—Nil 1—Slight restlessness 2—Moving constantly but obeys requests to stay in bed 3—Constantly restless, gets out of bed for no reason 4—Maximally restless; aggressive

Continued

Table 19.2   Alcohol withdrawal scale (cont.)

Temperature	0—Temperature of < 37.0°C 1—Temperature of 37.1–37.5°C 2—Temperature of 37.6–38.0°C 3—Temperature of 38.1–38.5°C 4—Temperature of > 38.5°C
Hallucinations	0—No evidence of hallucinations 1—Distortion of real objects, aware these are not real if pointed out 2—Appearance of new objects or perceptions, aware these are not real if pointed out 3—Believes the hallucinations are real but still oriented 4—Hallucinating, preoccupied and cannot be diverted
Orientation	0—Fully oriented 1—Fully oriented in person but unsure of place or time 2—Fully oriented in person but disoriented in place and time 3—Disoriented with short periods of lucidity 4—Completely disoriented, no meaningful contact can be obtained

MANAGEMENT OF ALCOHOL WITHDRAWAL

- Manage the patient in a calm and quiet environment (often difficult in the ED).
- Patients suffering only mild symptoms can be managed in an outpatient environment with reassurance and follow-up.
- Patients with more severe symptoms, or those at risk of severe withdrawal (see Box 19.2), require inpatient management.
- Diazepam, a long-acting benzodiazepine, is the most frequently used sedative for the management of withdrawal symptoms.

Box 19.2   Predictors of severe alcohol withdrawal

Older age
Medical or surgical co-morbidities
Past history of DTs or alcohol withdrawal seizures
Severe withdrawal symptoms in the presence of an elevated BAC
Biochemical derangement (e.g. hypokalaemia or hyponatraemia)
Deranged LFTs

- Dosing regimens vary—but commonly patients are loaded with repeated doses of oral diazepam (e.g. 20 mg given PO every 2 hours) until their symptoms diminish. A cumulative dose of 60–80 mg is often adequate and should not be exceeded without senior review. Generally no further doses of diazepam will be required.
- Patients with milder symptoms who are being discharged home can be given small doses of diazepam (e.g. 5–10 mg every 6–8 hours prn) for 24–48 hours.
- Oxazepam is used in the patient with liver failure or respiratory failure as it is shorter-acting and has no active metabolites; 15 mg of oxazepam is roughly equivalent to 5 mg of diazepam.
- As alcohol-dependent patients are often thiamine deficient, give thiamine 300 mg IV daily for 3–5 days, followed by 300 mg orally daily for 5–7 days.

ALCOHOL-RELATED SEIZURES

- Seizures occur in 1–5% of episodes of alcohol withdrawal.
- They usually occur early, 6–48 hours after the last drink is consumed.
- The seizures are typically generalised (tonic-clonic) and occur as a single event.
- Intravenous diazepam (5–10 mg) is the first-line anticonvulsant of choice.
- A patient presenting with their first seizure should be investigated. Subsequent seizures are only investigated if they are prolonged, unusual (e.g. focal) or occur more than 48 hours after alcohol cessation.
- Patients with evidence of head trauma, those who do not regain full consciousness and those with focal neurological signs should undergo a CT brain to exclude an intracranial haemorrhage. Subdural haematomas occur more commonly in patients who drink large quantities of alcohol because of frequent falls, coagulopathy and cerebral atrophy.

WERNICKE'S ENCEPHALOPATHY

- Wernicke's Encephalopathy is a life-threatening complication of thiamine deficiency.

- Classic triad of ophthalmoplegia or nystagmus, ataxia and global memory impairment. However, patients only rarely present with all three signs.
- Untreated, it can progress to the irreversible Wernicke-Korsakoff syndrome of permanent cognitive impairment.
- Thiamine is cheap and safe and should be given in high doses to those suspected of having the syndrome. Start with thiamine 500 mg IV tds.

Pearls and Pitfalls

Thiamine should be given before any carbohydrate load (e.g. IV glucose) as giving glucose in the setting of thiamine deficiency may precipitate Wernicke's encephalopathy.

ASSESSMENT AND MANAGEMENT OF HAZARDOUS ALCOHOL USE

- Remember to ask every patient in a non-judgmental manner about alcohol consumption. Do not ask 'Do you drink a lot?', but rather 'Do you drink alcohol?'
- Then ask for details regarding the number of days per week that alcohol is consumed, and the quantity and type of drink on each occasion.
- Assess the severity of alcohol dependence by asking about early-morning alcohol withdrawal symptoms, and the timing of the first drink of the day.
- Enquire about alcohol-related problems, including marital, employment, legal and financial complications.
- The 'CAGE' questions (Box 19.3) are helpful to detect alcohol abuse and dependence. Two or more positive responses identify patients with lifetime risk of alcohol problems.

Box 19.3 'CAGE' questions

Cut down: Have you ever tried to cut down your drinking?
Annoyed: Have you ever been annoyed by criticism of your drinking?
Guilty: Do you feel guilty about your drinking?
Eye-opener: Do you need an eye-opener when you get up in the morning?

Box 19.4   Brief intervention using the 'FRAMES' acronym

Feedback: Provide the patient with a risk assessment of their drinking patterns.

Responsibility: Emphasise that the decision to change behaviours lies with the patient.

Advice: Give clear advice about reducing or stopping alcohol intake entirely.

Menu: Provide options and ideas to help a patient change their behaviour.

Empathy: Ensure a warm, empathetic and collaborative approach.

Self-efficacy: Give the patient optimism that they can change their behaviour.

- Even brief interventions by clinicians can be very effective in reducing alcohol consumption in patients with hazardous (but non-dependent) drinking patterns.
- Establish rapport with the patient, advise them of the hazards of their current levels of consumption and establish a goal of either reducing intake or abstaining from alcohol altogether.
- The FRAMES acronym (Box 19.4) is a useful framework for providing advice to the patient.

Patients should finally be referred for long-term follow-up to their GP or local drug and alcohol treatment centre.

Nicotine

- The prevalence of smokers in Australia continues to fall, with a current rate of 15% of adults smoking tobacco daily.
- Smoking rates are higher in certain groups, such as those with mental illness, Aboriginal and Torres Strait Islander people, prisoners, people with alcohol or other substance abuse problems and those from culturally diverse backgrounds, including refugees.
- Even very brief interventions (as little as 1 minute!) are associated with a reduction in smoking prevalence.
- Most hospitals are now smoke-free environments, which reduces smoking-related risks to patients, staff and visitors, and reduces the community's exposure to second-hand smoke.

- Admitted patients who smoke may require support to manage their nicotine dependence while in hospital.
- This includes offering nicotine-replacement therapy (NRT) to all smokers with evidence of dependence (smoking within 30 minutes of waking and/or > 10 cigarettes per day).
- Smokers should be encouraged to speak to their GP and access the Quitline (www.quitnow.gov.au).

Cannabis

- Cannabis is the most commonly used illicit drug in Australia, with a lifetime prevalence of 35%.
- Ten per cent of Australians aged 14 reporting having used cannabis in the last 12 months.
- People aged in their 20s are most likely to use cannabis.
- Long-term effects of cannabis use include an increased risk of respiratory disease (including cancer), decreased memory and learning and decreased motivation.
- Cannabis may trigger schizophrenia in those who are already at risk of developing it, and can hasten the age of onset of first psychosis.
- Dependence can develop with frequent and regular use of cannabis and a withdrawal syndrome is described with symptoms of mood and sleep disturbance.
- There are no pharmacotherapy treatments for cannabis withdrawal or relapse prevention. Cognitive behavioural therapy and other psychosocial interventions are the mainstay of treatment.
- See Chapter 18 Poisoning and Overdose for information regarding cannabis overdose and the cannabis hyperemesis syndrome.

Injecting drug users
EPIDEMIOLOGY

- Injecting drug use is associated with considerable morbidity and mortality, including risk of death from overdose and transmission of blood-borne viruses.
- Approximately 0.6% of Australians aged between 15 and 64 are estimated to be injecting drug users.

- Men inject drugs more frequently than women, and the most common age group is 35–44.
- Intravenous poly-drug use is common among injecting drug users.

COMPLICATIONS OF INTRAVENOUS DRUG USE

- Vascular complications: phlebitis, sclerosis, arterial thrombosis, DVTs
- Bacterial infections: abscesses, cellulitis, right-sided endocarditis, septicaemia, botulism, tetanus
- Viral infections: hepatitis C, hepatitis B, HIV; the rate of hepatitis C in intravenous drug users in Australia is high (57%), while HIV is low (1%)
- Intoxication: aspiration pneumonia, hypoxic organ damage, compartment syndrome, rhabdomyolysis
- Overdose

Opioids
See the Opioid section in Chapter 18 Poisoning and Overdose.

OPIOID WITHDRAWAL SYNDROME

- The features of opioid withdrawal include intense craving, anxiety, insomnia, mydriasis, nausea, vomiting, diarrhoea and abdominal pain.
- While unpleasant, opioid withdrawal syndrome is not dangerous.
- Opioid withdrawal is not associated with seizures, delirium or high fever. These features should prompt the consideration of associated alcohol or benzodiazepine withdrawal, or a complication such as sepsis or head injury.
- The onset of withdrawal symptoms typically occurs within 12 hours after the last dose of morphine or heroin, peaks at day 2 and resolves within a week. Methadone withdrawal occurs later and can last for 2 weeks.
- Symptoms can be managed symptomatically with paracetamol and NSAIDs for pain relief, metoclopramide for nausea and loperamide for control of diarrhoea.

- Oral diazepam can be used to treat agitation and anxiety in the ED. Exercise caution in prescribing benzodiazepines in the outpatient setting as concurrent benzodiazepine use with opiates increases the risk of fatal overdose.
- Opioid-dependent patients who are admitted to hospital with an intercurrent illness may require the administration of an opioid during admission to prevent withdrawal symptoms. In this setting, buprenorphine is recommended.

LONG-TERM TREATMENT OF OPIOID DEPENDENCE

- Patients should be counselled that help is readily available.
- The risks of sharing needles should be discussed, and patients should be offered testing for blood-borne diseases (hepatitis B and C, and HIV).
- Long-term treatment includes both psychosocial support (e.g. cognitive behavioural therapy, counselling and social supports) and pharmacological substitutes.
- Methadone (an opiate agonist) and buprenorphine (a partial agonist) are both commonly prescribed as maintenance treatment.
- They prevent withdrawal symptoms, reduce craving and reduce the rates of recidivism among drug users.
- Clinicians are required to be authorised to prescribe methadone for addiction. These patients require referral to a specialised drug and alcohol service.

Pearls and Pitfalls

Methadone can cause prolongation of the QT interval, and deaths due to cardiac arrhythmias have been reported. Be careful when prescribing drugs that can prolong the QT interval to methadone users.

Benzodiazepines

See the Benzodiazepines section in Chapter 18 Poisoning and Overdose.

- Dependence and tolerance develop rapidly in people who use benzodiazepines.

- Long-term users of even low doses of benzodiazepines can develop tolerance and features of withdrawal on cessation.
- The elderly are a particularly vulnerable group for benzodiazepine use and complications (e.g. falls, cognitive impairment).
- Benzodiazepine use is common in poly-drug users, who will frequently seek prescriptions from ED doctors to fuel their habits.
- Requests for benzodiazepine should be treated with caution and prescriptions should not be issued to patients without good justification.

WITHDRAWAL

- The timing of the withdrawal syndrome depends on the pharmacokinetics of the particular benzodiazepine that is being taken.
- In general, withdrawal symptoms occur 2–5 days after cessation, reach a maximum on day 7–10 and can take 2–3 weeks to fully abate.
- The symptoms of withdrawal are of rebound anxiety, insomnia, restlessness and poor concentration. Perceptual disturbance can occur.
- The major complications are of delirium and seizures.

MANAGEMENT

- Generally, benzodiazepine dependence should be managed by the patient's GP.
- The patient should be stabilised on divided daily doses of diazepam, which is then gradually reduced over the course of weeks. The rate of reduction can be titrated against symptoms.
- Inpatient management is not usually required.
- Patients who are admitted to hospital for other reasons may undergo withdrawal from even low doses of long-term benzodiazepines. This is a particular problem in the elderly who may develop a delirium. For these patients, it is safest to continue the patient's preadmission benzodiazepine dosing, with recommendations to gradually wean the dose once the patient has recovered from medical illness.

Box 19.5   Indicators of drug-seeking behaviour

Asking for specific drugs by name
Claiming multiple allergies to alternative drugs
Irritability when asked about specific symptoms
Refusal of investigation, examination or alternative therapies
Presenting out of hours, or when usual prescriber is away
Claiming medications or prescriptions were lost or stolen

- The poly-drug user may report very high daily doses of benzodiazepine use. In the event of these patients being admitted to hospital, prescribe no more than 40% of their regular intake, or 80 mg diazepam/day (whichever is lower). Remember that the goal is safety (prevention of seizures) rather than sedation.

Drug-seeking behaviour

- See Box 19.5 for indicators of drug-seeking behaviour.
- People who misuse prescription drugs will often present to the ED requesting prescriptions for medications of abuse.
- Be cautious of the patients requesting scripts for opiates, benzodiazepines and psychotropics including quetiapine, olanzapine, dexamphetamine and methylphenidate.
- There is no typical demographic of the drug-seeking patient. Drug dependencies occur in patients of all ages, both men and women, and across all ethnic and socioeconomic classes.
- Clinicians must weigh up the risks of not treating a patient's pain, versus the risk of prescribing drugs of abuse to a dependent patient.
- When asked to provide a prescription for a drug of abuse, a risk-limiting approach is to prescribe only a day or two's worth of medication and recommend the patient follow-up with their usual prescriber.

Pearls and Pitfalls

The Prescription Shopping Programme (phone 1800 631 181) helps clinicians identify patients who may be drug seeking by keeping track of the number of different prescribers and prescriptions filled for each patient.

Chapter 20
Endocrine emergencies

Glenn Arendts

Emergencies in patients with diabetes

Diabetes mellitus (commonly called 'diabetes') is a disorder of glucose metabolism due to a relative (type 2) or absolute (type 1) insulin deficiency. With the rising rate of obesity in the community, diabetes is becoming increasingly common, and type 2 rather than type 1 diabetes is now often seen in young patients.

Diabetic patients may present to the ED with acute life-threatening derangements of glucose metabolism, with complications related to long-standing diabetes, or with unrelated health problems which require concurrent management of their diabetes.

DIABETIC KETOACIDOSIS (DKA)
Overview

DKA is due to insulin deficiency resulting in acidosis with ketosis, hyperglycaemia and fluid and electrolyte losses. It may be the presenting problem in patients with previously undiagnosed diabetes. The principles in assessment and management of DKA are identifying and treating the precipitating cause, assessing the severity of the illness, correcting fluid and electrolyte disturbances and administering insulin.

Assessment

Patients with DKA commonly present with vomiting, polydipsia, polyuria, shortness of breath and abdominal pain. History and examination should be directed at identifying the precipitating event and assessing the degree of dehydration. Most commonly, DKA is precipitated in patients with type 1 diabetes by intercurrent infection, although other causes should be considered (see Box 20.1). It almost always occurs in patients with type 1 (insulin-dependent)

Box 20.1 Precipitants of DKA

- First presentation of insulin-dependent diabetes
- Non-compliance/errors with insulin therapy
- Infection
  — Urinary tract
  — Respiratory tract
  — Gastrointestinal
  — Skin
- Other
  — Steroid medication
  — Myocardial infarction
  — Pancreatitis
  — Thyroid disease/surgery/pregnancy/trauma
  — Alcohol abuse

---

diabetes, but occasionally is seen in patients with non-insulin-dependent diabetes.

A bedside venous blood sample will confirm the diagnosis by the presence of plasma ketones with acidosis (pH < 7.3 or bicarbonate < 15 mmol/L). An elevated blood sugar level (BSL > 12 mmol/L) occurs in more than 90% of cases, but rarely DKA can occur with a normal range BSL in patients with a history of diabetes. Urinary ketones will also be present but with the widespread availability of blood ketone testing in the ED makes urine testing less useful.

Other important investigations include the following.

- Urea, electrolytes and creatinine (UEC): potassium (K^+) abnormalities are common and creatinine may be elevated
- Full blood count (FBC): elevated white cell count (WCC) suggests infection
- Midstream urine for microscopy and culture
- Blood culture if febrile
- Liver function tests; amylase and lipase if abdominal pain
- HbA_{1c} level: this indicates the level of blood sugar control over the past 3 months in long-standing diabetics
- ECG for silent myocardial infarction or arrhythmias

Management

Patients with DKA are often extremely ill and should be initially managed in an area of the ED with continuous ECG and oximetry monitoring, and regular blood pressure measurements. Ongoing regular measurement of BSL and serum K1 should continue throughout treatment.

Fluid and electrolyte therapy

All patients with DKA are volume-depleted and require rehydration with intravenous fluids.

- Hypotension (systolic BP < 100 mmHg) should be treated with boluses of normal saline up to 2000 mL until BP has improved.
- In the normotensive adult patient, 1 L of normal saline should be given over the first hour, followed by another 1 L over the next 2 hours.
- Subsequent fluid therapy will be guided by clinical assessment of pulse rate and hydration status, but some patients will require 5–8 L of fluid over the first 24 hours.
- A dextrose-containing solution should be commenced once the BSL falls below 15 mmol/L, in addition to ongoing sodium requirements.

Potassium depletion is a feature of DKA, even in the presence of an initial elevated serum K^+. Serum potassium should be measured as soon as possible and is often available on the initial blood gas results. The administration of intravenous fluids and insulin will rapidly lower the measured K^+. If the initial K^+ is > 5.5 mmol/L, the level should be rechecked every 30–60 minutes as it will inevitably fall as a consequence of rehydration (and insulin treatment). Table 20.1 outlines the rate of potassium replacement. Monitoring of K^+ levels every 1–2 hours is essential during the initial phase of treatment.

Phosphate and magnesium levels are commonly low in DKA; however, there is no evidence to support the routine replacement of these electrolytes. Intravenous bicarbonate is of no proven benefit in patients with DKA, as the acidosis usually improves with

Table 20.1 Guide to potassium replacement in DKA

Serum K^+ (mmol/L)	Replacement therapy
> 5.5	Nil—repeat test in 1 hour
3.5–5.5	KCl 5–10 mmol/h
< 3.5	KCl 20 mmol/h, cardiac monitoring

rehydration and insulin therapy. Bicarbonate should not be given without consulting a critical-care specialist or endocrinologist.

The measured sodium level should be corrected for the elevated glucose, as the high BSL will artefactually dilute the sodium. The equation is:

$$\text{true sodium} = \frac{(\text{measured sodium} + [\text{BSL} - 10])}{3}$$

Insulin therapy

Rehydration increases insulin sensitivity, and therefore insulin therapy should not precede fluid therapy.

In the initial phase, insulin should be delivered via continuous IV infusion. A second IV line is usually required for this purpose. A common regimen is 50 units of Actrapid in 50 mL of normal saline via a syringe pump. The insulin infusion should commence at 0.05–0.1 units/kg/h (2–8 units/h), aiming for a fall in BSL of 3–4 mmol/h. The BSL should be measured hourly initially, and the insulin infusion adjusted according to the rate of fall.

The insulin infusion should continue until the serum bicarbonate is greater than 20 mmol/L, regardless of the BSL. Once the BSL falls below 15 mmol/L, rehydration should continue with a dextrose-containing solution. Subcutaneous insulin can be commenced once the patient has adequate oral intake and is no longer acidotic. The first SC dose is given before the insulin infusion is ceased.

Other therapy

- Treatment of associated infection with appropriate antibiotics
- Thromboembolic (DVT) prophylaxis
- An indwelling catheter is occasionally needed in the critically ill to monitor urine output

Ongoing management

The aim of treatment is to correct fluid and electrolyte disturbances, lower the BSL to normal and control ketosis over 12–24 hours.

- Strict monitoring of BSL and serum K^+ every 1–2 hours initially is vital.

- Other electrolytes, especially sodium, should be checked at least twice daily.
- Regular reassessment of the patient's hydration status and acidosis is necessary to determine ongoing fluid management.
- The patient needs to remain closely monitored with hourly observations while the insulin infusion continues.

Cerebral oedema is a rare but life-threatening complication of DKA that is more common in children and usually occurs in the first 12 hours of therapy. Symptoms such as a falling level of consciousness, progressive headache, bradycardia and a rising blood pressure may indicate cerebral oedema and patients with any of these symptoms require urgent senior medical review.

HYPEROSMOLAR HYPERGLYCAEMIC STATE (HHS)
Overview
This condition occurs primarily in older patients with non-insulin-dependent diabetes, although it has several clinical features in common with DKA. It is characterised by relative, rather than absolute, insulin deficiency leading to hyperglycaemia, hyperosmolarity and dehydration, with little or no acidosis or ketosis.

The goals of therapy are identification and treatment of the precipitating event, controlled correction of fluid and electrolyte abnormalities and correction of hyperglycaemia.

Assessment
HHS often presents with non-specific signs such as confusion, vomiting and weight loss, developing over days to weeks in elderly patients with undiagnosed or poorly controlled diabetes. Polyuria and polydipsia are not universally present. There are many possible precipitating events, which are summarised in Box 20.2. These patients often have multiple comorbidities and may be on multiple medications.

Physical examination is focused on assessing the degree of dehydration and looking for evidence of a precipitating cause. The diagnosis is suggested by the presence of severe hyperglycaemia (often > 30 mmol/L) and serum hyperosmolarity (> 320 mOsm/L), with minimal acidosis (pH > 7.3).

Box 20.2 Precipitants of HHS

- Poor compliance
- Newly diagnosed diabetes
- Infection
  - Urinary tract
  - Respiratory
  - CNS
  - Skin
- Cardiovascular events
  - Acute myocardial infarction
  - Cerebrovascular accident/intracranial haemorrhage
  - Mesenteric ischaemia
- Other
  - Gastrointestinal haemorrhage
  - Pancreatitis
  - Renal failure
  - Diuretic therapy

Important early investigations include the following.

- UEC: severe dehydration may be associated with hypernatraemia. The sodium level should be corrected for the BSL as mentioned earlier. Potassium depletion and renal impairment are common.
- Septic screen: urine, blood, skin swabs +/− CSF for culture.
- Chest X-ray: for evidence of infection and to evaluate heart size and presence of cardiac failure.
- ECG: for evidence of myocardial infarction or atrial fibrillation.
- CT of head: for cerebrovascular accident (CVA) or intracranial haemorrhage in patients with an altered level of consciousness.

Management

These patients often have an altered level of consciousness and may have multiple comorbidities including heart and renal disease. Therefore they must be closely observed with full cardiorespiratory monitoring.

Fluid and electrolyte therapy

In the presence of shock (hypotension or poor tissue perfusion), fluid therapy should begin with 500 mL boluses of normal saline until blood pressure and tissue perfusion are restored. After correction of shock, fluid replacement should be performed carefully. Although these patients are often profoundly dehydrated, this has usually occurred over a period of days and overly rapid replacement of fluid may lead to pulmonary oedema.

- Most patients will have a fluid deficit of 8–12 L and this should be replaced over a 24–48 hour period.
- Fluid therapy should begin with 1 L of normal saline every 2–4 hours.
- If, after correction of shock with normal saline, the corrected sodium is > 155 mmol/L or the osmolality is rising, normal saline can be replaced by ½ saline/2.5% dextrose solution. The patient should be regularly assessed for clinical evidence of fluid overload.

Potassium levels will fall rapidly once the patient is rehydrated and receiving insulin. Potassium replacement at 5–10 mmol/h should commence if the K^+ is < 5.0 mmol/L and urine output has been established. In the presence of oliguria and renal failure, K^+ replacement should be more cautious.

Insulin therapy

As for DKA, an IV insulin infusion should be commenced only after initiating fluid therapy. Patients with HHS are often insulin-sensitive and usually require 0.05 units/kg/h to achieve a fall in BSL of 3–5 mmol/h. As hyperglycaemia has developed over a long time period, it is appropriate to correct the BSL slowly, aiming for normalisation over 24 hours. Most guidelines recommend ceasing IV insulin in HHS once the BSL decreases to 13–16 mmol/L.

Other therapy

Precipitating illnesses should be actively sought and treated. Serious diagnoses such as mesenteric ischaemia must be considered. Thromboembolic prophylaxis is particularly important in HHS due to the thrombogenic effect of profound dehydration, and the presence of serious comorbidities.

HYPOGLYCAEMIA
Causes
Hypoglycaemia most commonly occurs in diabetic patients on insulin or oral hypoglycaemic therapy. It can also occur in

non-diabetics secondary to diseases such as sepsis, alcohol, hepatic failure, renal failure and insulin-producing tumours.

In diabetics, hypoglycaemia may be due to excess insulin or oral hypoglycaemic treatment, missed meals, physical exertion and alcohol. It may be the first presentation of renal impairment in patients on sulfonylureas.

Clinical features

Hypoglycaemia predominantly affects the brain and the autonomic nervous system.

- Neurological signs can vary widely and include agitation, aggressive or bizarre behaviour, coma, seizures, confusion, dysarthria and focal deficits such as hemiparesis (mimicking stroke).
- Autonomic features include sweating, tremor, blurred vision, vomiting and anxiety.
- The diagnosis is confirmed on finger-prick sampling.

The diagnosis should be considered in all patients presenting with confusion, seizures or an altered level of consciousness.

Therapy

Hypoglycaemia is easily reversed with oral or intravenous glucose. Prolonged, untreated hypoglycaemia can lead to permanent brain dysfunction, so early diagnosis and treatment is essential.

- If the patient is still awake, oral glucose in the form of a sweet drink, biscuit or other sugary substance may be enough to restore BSL. If the patient is unable to swallow, 20 mL of 50% dextrose (adult dose) is given as an intravenous push through an IV cannula, followed by a 20 mL saline flush (to prevent phlebitis). If the patient does not recover within 2–3 minutes, or the BSL remains < 3 mmol/L, the dose can be repeated.
- If intravenous access is not possible, 1 mg of IM glucagon may temporarily reverse hypoglycaemia if the patient has normal hepatic function. This should be followed by oral or IV glucose.

Hypoglycaemia secondary to oral hypoglycaemic agents may be recurrent and prolonged, particularly in the presence of renal impairment. These patients can require a dextrose infusion and observation in hospital until the BSL is stable.

Once the BSL is restored, assessment and treatment of the precipitating cause is essential.

THE 'HIGH-RISK' DIABETIC PATIENT

As well as the acute derangements of glucose metabolism outlined, diabetic patients are at risk of other acute pathologies due to the long-term complications of their illness.

Infection

Diabetics are functionally immunocompromised and thus are more prone to infection and at greater risk of systemic sepsis than the general community. They may have significant infection in the absence of the usual clinical signs such as fever or elevated WCC. Therefore, diabetic patients with actual or potential infection warrant more extensive work-up than other patients, with a lower threshold for tissue and blood cultures, soft-tissue imaging and hospital admission. In particular, soft-tissue infections are often polymicrobial and may invade into deeper structures such as muscle and bone.

Infarction

Macro- and microvascular disease seen in diabetic patients makes them more prone to acute vascular compromise in many organ systems, including the heart, brain, kidneys, gut, eyes and peripheral vasculature. Acute myocardial ischaemia may present atypically with minimal or absent chest pain, unexplained acute heart failure or non-specific vomiting. Abdominal pain in a diabetic patient has many potentially serious causes, including mesenteric ischaemia, myocardial infarction, leaking aortic aneurysm or renal infarction. Therefore these patients require thorough investigation.

Other

Most patients with long-standing diabetes will have some impairment of renal function and are at relatively high risk of acute renal impairment, which may be precipitated by any illness that leads to dehydration. Serum creatinine should be measured in any diabetic patient who presents with systemic illness.

Long-standing retinopathy may be acutely complicated by retinal haemorrhage, infarction or detachment, and any diabetic patient with acute eye symptoms should have urgent ophthalmology review.

THE DIABETIC PATIENT WITH UNRELATED ILLNESS

In addition to the specific conditions for which they are at higher risk, diabetics are subject to the same spectrum of illness and injury as the general population. Admission to hospital requires concurrent management of their diabetes as well as their acute illness, and this should begin in the ED. Poor glycaemic control in hospitalised diabetics increases the risk of death and infection and prolongs hospital stay. Acute illness will usually increase an individual's basal insulin requirements and most diabetics will require upward adjustment of insulin therapy in the early part of their hospital admission.

The BSL should optimally be maintained in the region of 5–8 mmol/L and there are several methods available to achieve this. Most hospitals have well-developed local protocols for managing diabetes, and these should be followed closely. For critically ill patients, particularly those with acute stroke, myocardial infarction and sepsis, blood sugar control is best achieved by continuous insulin infusion with close monitoring of finger-prick BSLs.

All patients with type 1 (insulin-deficient) diabetes who are not critically ill should continue to receive regular SC therapy with intermediate- and short-acting insulin, but will usually require higher doses. This is preferable to 'sliding-scale' insulin therapy, as it provides more-stable glucose control. Additionally, some type 2 diabetics will require a period of insulin therapy during hospitalisation, even if they are not usually managed with insulin. Apply the same insulin dosing principles for type 1 patients in these circumstances.

Adrenal emergencies
HYPOADRENAL CRISIS (ACUTE ADRENOCORTICAL INSUFFICIENCY)
Presentation and clinical features

Hypoadrenal crisis develops in two clinical settings. Occasionally, the patient presents with acute haemorrhagic destruction of the adrenal glands due to sepsis, burns, trauma or anticoagulant therapy. More commonly, the crisis develops as an acute deterioration in patients with Addison's disease or other causes of chronic adrenal failure. This can be due to increased steroid requirements (e.g. infection), drug interactions that increase steroid metabolism, or non-compliance with maintenance steroid therapy.

The presenting symptoms are often non-specific and include lethargy, dizziness, nausea, diarrhoea and abdominal pain. However, in severe cases the patient presents with haemodynamic collapse—hypoadrenalism needs to be considered in any patient with unexplained shock.

Differential diagnosis
The differential diagnosis is very broad due to the non-specific presentations seen. Ascribing hypoadrenal symptoms to gastro-enteritis or other intra-abdominal conditions is the most common mis-diagnosis made.

Investigations
If acute hypoadrenalism is suspected, the following initial investigations may be helpful. Ideally these are done prior to starting treatment with steroids, unless the patient has frank shock and it is unsafe to delay treatment.

- UEC: the combination of a low bicarbonate level, hyponatraemia and hyperkalaemia is highly suggestive of hypoadrenal crisis. Renal failure may occur.
- BSL: hypoglycaemia.
- Blood gases: non-anion-gap metabolic acidosis.
- Ca^{2+}: hypercalcaemia (mild only).
- Random plasma cortisol level: a low level in the setting of acute stress is highly suggestive of adrenocortical insufficiency.
- Short corticotrophin test: this requires a baseline cortisol level, the administration of IV corticotrophin and then a repeat cortisol level 30–60 minutes later. This must occur prior to the administration of hydrocortisone (but not dexamethasone). In most cases of suspected insufficiency testing is possible, but if the patient is moribund and treatment cannot be delayed, omit this test.

Management
1 Fluids. The patient may present with haemodynamic collapse and require immediate resuscitation.
 — Hypotension should be treated initially with 1000 mL boluses of normal saline.

— Hypoglycaemia, if present, should be treated initially with 20 mL of 50% dextrose IV.

— Shock may be refractory to fluid resuscitation until hydrocortisone therapy is commenced. Even with adjuvant steroids, the patient may need vasopressor support in decompensated shock.

— After resuscitation, further fluid requirements should be determined by assessment of the patient's hydration status. Normal saline should be used to replace any fluid deficit over the next 24–48 hours. If the patient has associated persistent hypoglycaemia, adding 50 g dextrose to each bag of normal saline given is preferable to using a dextrose-containing solution with a low sodium concentration.

— Blood glucose, Na^+ and K^+ levels should be measured every 2–3 hours initially.

2 IV hydrocortisone (100 mg every 6 hours) should be given promptly.

3 Other important acute management issues include the treatment of any underlying precipitants, such as infection.

The majority of patients improve within 24 hours of commencing this treatment regimen. Oral combined glucocorticoid and mineralocorticoid therapy may then be commenced. Patient education after the acute treatment phase is over, concerning increasing their maintenance steroid requirements at times of stress or illness, is a vital part of management.

Thyroid emergencies
THYROTOXIC CRISIS ('THYROID STORM')
Presentation and clinical features

Patients at risk of thyrotoxic crisis usually have either undiagnosed or poorly treated hyperthyroidism. The precipitants of thyrotoxic crisis that should be looked for are shown in Box 20.3, although the cause can be elusive.

Thyrotoxic crisis represents the extreme of hyperthyroidism, and the diagnosis is a clinical one. Three signs in particular help distinguish thyrotoxic crisis from uncomplicated hyperthyroidism:

• hyperpyrexia (temperature > 39°C)
• extreme tachycardia (heart rate usually 130–200 beats/min, may be in AF)

Box 20.3   Precipitants of thyrotoxic crisis

- Intercurrent illness or stress: infection, labour, major vascular events such as CVA
- Drugs: thyroxine overdose, amiodarone, iodinated dyes, salicylates, cessation of anti-thyroid drug therapy
- Trauma: multi-trauma, thyroid gland surgery, vigorous palpation of thyroid gland

---

- CNS disturbance, ranging from restlessness to agitation, confusion and coma.

    Vomiting and diarrhoea are common. Potentially life-threatening cardiac complications (arrhythmias, cardiac failure) occur in more than 50% of patients.

Differential diagnosis
- Sepsis/meningitis
- Heat stroke
- Toxicological:
  — anticholinergic poisoning
  — sympathomimetic poisoning (e.g. amphetamines)
  — neuroleptic malignant syndrome
  — serotonin syndrome
  — alcohol withdrawal

Investigations
No single test confirms the diagnosis of thyrotoxic crisis. Thyroid function tests (TFTs) confirm hyperthyroidism, but the levels of T_3 and T_4 in thyrotoxic crisis are usually no different from those in uncomplicated hyperthyroidism, and treatment should not be delayed for the TFT results. Hyperglycaemia, hypokalaemia, hypercalcaemia, abnormal liver function and leucocytosis occur. CXR and ECG looking for specific cardiac complications should be performed.

Management
1 Supportive care. Patients with thyrotoxic crisis are usually extremely unwell and require continuous ECG, BP and temperature monitoring. Unstable arrhythmias and cardiac

failure may be evident at presentation and require urgent treatment.

These patients are hypermetabolic and have markedly increased oxygen, fluid, electrolyte and glucose requirements. High-flow oxygen by mask should be started. The patient may require 4–6 L of IV fluid in the first 24 hours, although less-aggressive fluid resuscitation is often necessary in the elderly or those with heart failure. Hyperpyrexia should be treated with external cooling methods, for example axillary and groin cold packs.

2 Beta-adrenergic blockers. These antagonise the peripheral end-organ effects of thyroid hormones and are the mainstay of emergency therapy. Oral (or nasogastric (NG)) propranolol commenced at 40 mg every 6 hours is the treatment of choice, although higher doses may be required.

Intravenous propranolol is not currently commercially available in Australia and, if the patient requires intravenous beta-blockade, esmolol is an option due to its very short half-life. All beta-blockers can worsen cardiac failure and hypotension.

3 Anti-thyroid treatment. Oral or NG propylthiouracil reduces the further synthesis of thyroid hormones and prevents the peripheral conversion of T_4 to the more active T_3. A loading dose of 400 mg followed by 200 mg every 6 hours is a typical regimen. Note that propylthiouracil can cause severe hepatic injury and is not recommended for long-term use after the crisis is over.

4 Corticosteroids improve survival in thyrotoxic crisis. Hydrocortisone 100 mg IV every 6 hours is an appropriate choice.

Cholestyramine or similar gut resins have been used to bind T_4 in the gut, but is not routine ED care.

HYPOTHYROID CRISIS ('MYXOEDEMA COMA')
Presentation and clinical features
Myxoedema coma occurs most commonly following some pre-cipitating event in a patient with unrecognised hypothyroidism (Box 20.4). The diagnosis is clinical and a high index of suspicion is required.

Box 20.4	Precipitants of hypothyroid crisis

- Intercurrent illness
  - Infection
  - GI tract bleed
  - CVA
- Drugs
  - CNS depressants
  - Beta-blockers
  - Cessation of thyroxine therapy
- Environmental
  - Extreme cold exposure

Myxoedema coma is the clinical extreme of hypothyroidism and is characterised by multi-organ failure due to reduced cellular metabolism. The cardinal features are:

- decreased conscious state
- hypoventilation progressing to respiratory failure
- bradycardia and hypotension
- hypothermia.

Increased total body water is common, leading to oedema, pleural and pericardial effusions and hyponatraemia. Paralytic ileus and urinary retention may occur.

Differential diagnosis
- Environmental hypothermia
- Encephalopathies (e.g. hepatic, uraemic)
- Cardiogenic shock
- Sepsis

Investigations
The diagnosis of myxoedema coma is clinical, although TFTs confirm hypothyroidism. A rapid free T_4 assay is often available and, if normal, excludes the diagnosis. Other important investigation abnormalities include:

- UEC—hyponatraemia, renal failure
- BSL—hypoglycaemia
- blood gases—elevated CO_2, hypoxia
- FBC—anaemia, low WCC
- ECG—bradycardia, prolonged QT interval
- CXR—pleural and pericardial effusions.

Hypothyroid crisis patients are commonly septic without exhibiting any of the usual clinical features of sepsis, and should have a septic screen as part of their initial work-up.

Management

1 Supportive care. These patients are profoundly unwell and require management in an area with full monitoring and resuscitation equipment.

Intubation and ventilation is often needed but requires special precautions due to hypothermia and gastric stasis.

Though oedematous, patients may have reduced intravascular volume; hypotension should initially be treated with 500 mL boluses of warmed IV normal saline.

Hypoglycaemia, if present, should be immediately corrected with 20 mL of 50% dextrose IV. Do not use hypotonic fluids; add dextrose to normal saline for maintenance if required.

Re-warming with warm blankets or a Bair Hugger is recommended provided it does not cause worsening hypotension from vasodilation.

2 Thyroid hormones. These are the mainstay of therapy in myxoedema coma. Controversy exists regarding the optimal dose, route and rate of thyroid hormone replacement. T_4 alone, T_3 alone or a combination of the two are all described.

As hypothyroid crisis usually develops slowly, rapid replacement of thyroid hormones may provoke serious complications such as cardiac ischaemia or arrhythmias. Providing supportive care is adequate, relatively low initial doses either IV or orally, titrated to clinical response, is prudent.

3 IV hydrocortisone 100 mg every 8 hours should be commenced, as myxoedema coma is often associated with adrenal dysfunction.

4 Hyponatraemia usually corrects with water restriction; but if severe and associated with altered conscious state, may require hypertonic (3%) saline.

5 Infection is common and should be covered with broad-spectrum antibiotic therapy.

Recovery time with treatment is highly variable, and
improvement can occur anywhere from 24 hours to many
days after commencing therapy.

Editorial Comment

Be it an elderly female with increased confusion (hypothyroid)
to a previously healthy, young patient (new-onset diabetes),
remember to think *endocrine*, as illnesses are often initially
subtle clinically but clear on simple blood tests.

Chapter 21
Acid–base and electrolyte disorders

Derek Louey

Acknowledgment

The author wishes to acknowledge the content used from the previous edition of *Emergency Medicine* which was provided by Di King.

Electrolyte emergencies

Resuscitation Evaluation—ABCD (Table 21.1)

Consider an electrolyte emergency as the cause for an acute arrhythmias, abnormal ECG, circulatory compromise, neuromuscular weakness, tetany, ventilation failure, laryngospasm, altered mental state or seizures.

Management Tip—Risk Stratification (Table 21.2)

The acuity of the disturbance and the clinical condition of the patient determines the urgency and pace of treatment. Do not make treatment decisions purely based on absolute values.

(See Table 21.1 overleaf for more details.)

CRITICAL OVERVIEW
Pathophysiology

- In health, serum electrolyte concentrations are under tight homeostatic control over a wide range of inputs or losses.
- Maintenance of electrolyte balance is achieved by altering oral intake, renal excretion or by the movement of water or electrolytes between fluid compartments.

Table 21.1 Electrolyte emergencies

Abnormality	Clinical indication	Treatment (only if clinical indication present)	Comments
Hyperkalaemia (K^+ > 6.5 mmol/L)	QRS widening; symptomatic arrhythmia (caution in digoxin toxicity)	10–20 mmol calcium chloride or calcium gluconate IV over 5 minutes (repeat until QRS narrows or patient stabilises)	Ca^{2+} temporarily stabilises membrane action potential (see text)
Hypokalaemia (K^+ < 2.6 mmol/L)	Arrhythmia	5–10 mmol potassium chloride IV bolus over 5 minutes	Continue monitoring during treatment
Hyponatraemia (Na^+ < 110 mmol/L)	Seizures or coma	1 mL/kg 3% hypertonic saline bolus over 5–10 minutes (repeat up to 2 times over 20 minutes)	Treatment may cause cerebral pontine myelinolysis and quadriplegia
Hypocalcaemia (total Ca^{2+} < 2 mmol/L)	Respiratory difficulties, hypotension, arrhythmias	5 mmol calcium chloride or 10–20 mmol calcium gluconate IV over 10 minutes	
Hypercalcaemia (total Ca^{2+} > 3.5 mmol/L)	Coma	Commence rapid rehydration with IV 0.9% saline	Hydration optimises calciuresis (see text)
Hypophosphataemia (PO_4^{3-} < 0.4 mmol/L)	Arrhythmias	IV K_2HPO_4/KH_2PO_4 5–10 mmol/L over 60 minutes	Risk of dangerous hypocalcaemia with IV PO_4^{3-}
Hyperphosphataemia (PO_4^{3-} < 2.25 mmol/L)	Arrhythmias Respiratory failure	Saline rehydration Dialyse (if severe hypocalcaemia also)	
Hypomagnesaemia (Mg^{2+} < 0.5 mmol/L)	Arrhythmias	IV magnesium sulfate 10 mmol over 5 minutes	Rapid administration may cause flushing and hypotension

Continued

353

Table 21.1   Electrolyte emergencies (cont.)

Abnormality	Clinical indication	Treatment (only if clinical indication present)	Comments
Hypermagnesaemia (Mg^{2+} > 5 mmol/L)	Arrhythmia Hypotension Respiratory failure	5–10 mmol CaCl or calcium gluconate IV over 10 min Consider dialysis	Ca^{2+} temporarily stabilises membrane action potential
The goal of emergency treatment is to resolve immediate life threats prior to definitive management and addressing causes (see body of text). In severe cases this may require ICU admission.			Ca^{2+} temporarily stabilises membrane action potential

Derangement can occur as a result of overwhelming losses or gains or disordered homeostatic mechanisms (renal disease, endocrinopathies or effects of drugs).

Obtaining samples

- Never decant excess blood between different specimen containers (preservative contamination).
- Never obtain specimens from a limb receiving IV fluids (dilution).
- Multiple needle entries, forceful aspiration or filling of containers, aerated collection and violently agitating samples increases the risk of haemolysis and spurious results.

Causes and mechanisms

There are various mechanisms affecting electrolyte balance. Disturbances may result from:

- water/electrolyte losses or gains at extra-renal sites (i.e. enteral/ gastrointestinal tract/drains/fistulas, parenteral/IV sites, skin)
- compartmental shifts:
  - intracellular fluid (ICF) ↔ extracellular fluid (ECF)
  - vascular compartment ↔ interstitial fluid; ECF ↔ bone pool
- disordered renal homeostatic mechanisms (glomerular function/renal failure, tubular dysfunction/channelopathy) or abnormal endocrine control
- drugs (via above mechanisms)

- changes in one electrolyte can result in changes of another by simple exchange between compartments (e.g. K^+/H^+); affecting renal mechanisms that regulate electrolyte balance (e.g. K^+/Mg^{2+}); or by a physicochemical effect on water disassociation (e.g. Cl^-/H^+).

Clinical effects

- Vary from mild and non-specific to severe and life-threatening (see Table 21.2).

Table 21.2   Electrolyte disorder risk stratification

Electrolyte	Mild	Moderate	Severe
Hyperkalaemia	> 4.5 mmol/L	> 5.5 mmol/L Muscle weakness ECG—peaked T wave, QT shortening	> 6.5 mmol/L Muscle paralysis Loss of P waves QRS widening Sine waves; symptomatic arrhythmia Asystole
Hypokalaemia	< 3.5 mmol/L	< 3 mmol/L U wave APCs, VPCs	< 2.5 mmol/L Muscle weakness Rhabdomyolysis Pseudo obstruction QRS widening QT prolongation Arrhythmia
Hypernatraemia	> 145 mmol/L	> 150 mmol/L Lethargy Weakness Irritability	> 155 mmol/L Seizures Coma Intracranial bleeding Osmotic Demyelination (pontine myelinolysis/ tetraplegia)
Hyponatraemia	< 135 mmol/L	< 125 mmol/L Nausea Malaise	< 115 mmol/L Coma Seizures

Continued

Table 21.2 Electrolyte disorder risk stratification (cont.)

Electrolyte	Mild	Moderate	Severe
Hypercalcaemia	> 2.5 mmol/L Constipation Nausea Fatigue Depression	> 3 mmol/L Polydipsia Polyuria Nausea Weakness QT shortening	> 3.5 mmol/l Confusion Coma

Hypocalcaemia	< 2 mmol/L	Paraesthesia
		Neuro-
		  psychiatric
		  symptoms
		QT prolongation
			< 1.8 mmol/L
			Tetany
			Torsades de
			  pointes
			Hypotension
			Seizures

Hypermagnesaemia	> 3 mmol/L	> 4 mmol/L
		Weakness
		Nausea
		Flushing
		Headache
		Prolonged PR
		Bradycardia
			> 6 mmol/L
			Drowsiness
			Areflexia
			Respiratory
			  failure
			Hypotension
			QRS/QT
			  widening
			CHB

Hypomagnaemia (see hypokalaemia and hypocalcaemia)	< 1.5 mmol/L Tremor	< 0.5 mmol/L Weakness Confusion Neuropsychiatric symptoms Paraesthesia Choreoathetosis Nystagmus Wide PR APCs, VPCs AF Flat T	Tetany Seizures Coma QRS widening Arrhythmias
Hypo-phosphataemia	< 0.8 mmol/L	< 0.3 mmol/L Confusion Paraesthesia Weakness	< 0.15 mmol/L Coma Seizures Hypotension Haemolysis Rhabdomyolysis Respiratory failure Arrhythmias

Table 21.2 **Electrolyte disorder risk stratification (cont.)**

Electrolyte	Mild	Moderate	Severe
Metabolic acidosis	$HCO_3^- < 18$ mmol/L	$HCO_3^- < 14$ mmol/L	$HCO_3^- < 10$ mmol/L Haemo-dynamic instability Coagulopathy Respiratory fatigue
Metabolic alkalosis	$HCO_3^- > 30$ mmol/L	$HCO_3^- > 32$ mmol/L	$HCO_3^- > 34$ mmol/L Hypoxia
Respiratory acidosis	$pCO_2 > 45$ mmHg	$pCO_2 > 55$ mmHg Confusion	$pCO_2 > 65$ mmHg Drowsiness
Respiratory alkalosis	$pCO_2 < 35$ mmHg	$pCO_2 < 25$ mmHg Paraesthesia	$pCO_2 < 20$ mmHg Tetany

Absolute levels, clinical manifestations and ECG changes may not correlate. Features depend on acuity, adaptation and concurrent abnormalities.

- Despite marked abnormalities, patient may be minimally symptomatic and only identified incidentally on laboratory testing.
- Electrolytes have varying roles in maintaining osmolar gradient and cell volume, governing the membrane potential of excitable tissue and regulating receptor signalling and enzyme function.
- The central nervous system (CNS), cardiovascular system (CVS), gastrointestinal motility (gastrointestinal tract) or neuromuscular system can be affected.

Clinical Interpretation Tip

If results are inconsistent with the clinical picture, repeat the test.

THE GENERAL APPROACH

(See specific disorders.)
- Determine severity and risk (see Table 21.1 and Table 21.2).
- Review volume status (shocked, dehydrated, overloaded).

Table 21.3 **Approximate correction factors for electrolyte abnormalities***

Situation	Correction
Hyperglycaemia	True [Na^+] = measured [Na^+] + 0.3 × [glucose]
Metabolic acidosis	Reduce measured [K^+] by 0.5 for every ↓ pH of 0.1
Metabolic alkalosis	Increase measured [K^+] by 0.5 for every ↓ pH of 0.1
Hypoalbuminaemia	Add 0.1 total [Ca^{2+}] for every 4 g/dL decrease in albumin

*All measurements in mmol/L. Correction factors are rough guides only.

- Review gastrointestinal (GI) intake and output (quantify oral intake including medications, tube feeds, vomiting, diarrhoea, malabsorption, stomal losses, surgical drains and fistulas).
- Review parenteral fluids (total parenteral nutrition [TPN]).
- Review skin losses (excessive sweating, extensive burns).
- Review medication history and potentially offending drugs.
- Review renal function and urine output.
- Consider renal tubular or endocrine dysfunction—perform urine electrolytes (see next section).
- Consider specific endocrine tests if cause is not obvious (see relevant chapters).
- With multiple abnormalities—evaluate each abnormality individually and attempt to find a unifying explanation (see Table 21.3).

Assessment Tip—Clinical Context is Important

The spectrum of likely causes differs between ED, hospitalised, postoperative or intensive-care patients (consult additional resources for other diagnostic considerations).

Urine electrolytes

Assessment Tip—Urinary Electrolytes

Urinary electrolytes are useful in determining if impaired renal-endocrine homeostatic mechanisms are contributing to or causing the derangement (see below).

- Urine electrolytes are ideally interpreted in the context of normal glomerular function, normovolaemia and cessation of offending drugs.
- Parallel changes (e.g. ↓ serum electrolyte, ↓ urine electrolyte) indicate a normal homeostatic response.
- Reciprocal changes (e.g. ↓ serum electrolyte, ↑ urine electrolyte) suggest primary renal or endocrine dysfunction or drug effect. For example, ↓ P_{osm} with ↑ U_{osm} indicates SIADH; ↓ P_{K+} with ↑ U_{K+} suggests mineralocorticoid excess.

Urine electrolytes and osmolarity do not have specific reference ranges but are interpreted in conjunction with concurrent serum levels.

MANAGEMENT

(For information on electrolyte emergencies see Table 21.1.)

- Often abnormalities are incidental. Address the *cause*, not just the abnormality. *More than one mechanism may be operating* (e.g. reduced oral intake + diuretics).
- Unless the abnormality is acute or life-threatening, gradual correction (over 48 hours) usually is recommended.
- In severe cases full clinical and biochemical resolution can take days.
- **Mild or chronic stable cases**: review and address causes, monitor abnormality.
- **Moderate cases**: as above, plus begin treatment and monitor response frequently as hospital inpatient.
- **Severe, life-threatening or resistant cases**: for example, neurological (seizures, coma), CVS (hypotension, arrhythmia) and respiratory muscle failure (hypoventilation, tetany). (See Table 21.1.) Get ICU opinion. Patients may need careful and vigilant management.
- Any replacement regimen for deficits needs to also account for ongoing losses.

Management Tip—Beware of Overtreatment

Resist the temptation to over-treat chronic **stable** abnormalities in an asymptomatic patient. Compare with recent results and interpret within clinical context. First optimise the management of the underlying medical problem.

Table 21.4   Classic electrolyte patterns

Situation	Pattern
'Drip arm'	$\downarrow Na^+$, $\downarrow Cl^-$, $\downarrow K^+$, $\downarrow$ urea, ($\downarrow$ Hb)
Chronic renal failure	$\uparrow K^+$, $\downarrow HCO_3^-$, $\uparrow$ urea, $\uparrow$ creatinine, $\uparrow PO_4^{3-}$ ($\downarrow$ Hb)
Diabetic ketoacidosis (DKA)	$\uparrow$ glucose, $\uparrow$ ketones, $\downarrow HCO_3^-$, $\uparrow$ anion gap
Hyperglycaemic hyperosmolar state	$\uparrow\uparrow$ glucose, $\uparrow\uparrow$ osmolality
Conn's syndrome	$\downarrow K^+$, $\uparrow HCO_3^-$ ($\uparrow Na^+$, $\downarrow Mg^{2+}$)
Diuretic use bulimia nervosa	$\downarrow K^+$, $\uparrow HCO_3^-$ ($\downarrow Na^+$, $\downarrow Mg^{2+}$)
Addison's disease Renal tubular acidosis type IV	$\uparrow K^+$, $\downarrow HCO_3^-$ ($\downarrow Na^+$)
Renal tubular acidosis types I and II	$\downarrow K^+$, $\downarrow HCO_3^-$
Pyloric stenosis Gastric outlet obstruction	$\downarrow K^+$, $\downarrow Cl^-$, $\uparrow HCO_3^-$ (this pattern is rare nowadays due to earlier sonographic confirmation of suspected cases)
Tumour lysis syndrome	$\uparrow K^+$, $\uparrow$ urate, $\uparrow PO_4^{3-}$, $\downarrow Ca^+$ ($\uparrow$ LDH, $\uparrow Mg^{2+}$ and $\uparrow$ creatinine)

Management Tip—Complex Disorders

Multiple biochemical abnormalities or those with co-existing renal failure may be complex to manage. Seek expert assistance. (See also Table 21.4.)

Monitoring Tip—Frequent Assessment During Acute Treatment

Serum electrolyte *concentrations* do not necessarily correlate with total body *stores.* Levels may rapidly change due to dynamic redistribution between compartments or unresolved pathology.

OSMOLARITY
PHYSIOLOGY

- Serum **osmolarity** is the serum concentration of substances to which a cell membrane is impermeable (normal value ~285 mOsm/L).

- It regulates movement of water between intra- and extracellular compartments and is controlled by antidiuretic hormone (ADH) and the thirst mechanism.

<u>Clinical effects</u>
- Increased osmolarity leads to cellular dehydration. Decreased osmolarity leads to oedema.
- The CNS is most sensitive to this effect.
- The degree of osmolar disturbance correlates with conscious state.

Hyper-osmolarity
STEPWISE EVALUATION
- If the patient is comatose, *get help* and provide supportive care.
- Review water intake and evidence of dehydration (elevated serum sodium and urea—see Hypernatraemia later in this chapter).
- This may result from osmotherapy (see management of intracranial hypertension in Chapter 27 Neurosurgical Emergencies).
- Evaluate for and treat concurrent illness generating excess endogenous osmoles (see hyperglycaemic states, DKA and lactic acidosis in Chapter 20 Endocrine Emergencies).
- In suspected poisoning, perform osmolal gap (see below).

THE OSMOLAL GAP
- This reveals unmeasured osmotically acting substances either endogenously generated or introduced exogenously.

Toxicology Tip—The Osmolal Gap and Toxic Alcohols

Measure P_{osm} directly in the lab by freezing-point depression.
Estimated $P_{osm} = 2 \times [Na^+] + [glucose] + [urea]$
(units in mmol/L)
The **osmolar gap** = measured osmolarity – estimated osmolarity
↑ *osmolar gap with normal anion gap may suggest early toxic alcohol ingestion.*

Hypo-osmolarity (see Hyponatraemia)
DISORDERS OF SERUM SODIUM
- Physiological significance: osmolar control of intracellular volume; the CNS is sensitive to imbalances in serum sodium.

- Physiological control: via regulating free water input and output (i.e. thirst mechanism, ADH at distal tubule and collecting duct).
- Major compartment: ECF (Na^+ is the most plentiful osmotically active cation and therefore water balance and water movement also have a major impact on serum sodium *concentration*).

Hyponatraemia

Perform risk stratification (see Table 21.2).

STEPWISE EVALUATION

- If the patient is comatose or having an acute seizure, *get help*. Provide supportive care (see Table 21.1).
- Verify that it is not a collection error (e.g. 'drip arm' sample [low K^+, Cl^-]).
- Verify that it is a 'true hyponatraemia' (low serum osmolality).
- Exclude hyper-osmolar states ('pseudohyponatraemia') (e.g. hyperglycaemia).
- Exclude iso-osmolar ('factitious hyponatraemia') (e.g. ↑↑ serum lipids and protein).
- Exclude chronic 'oedematous states': severe heart failure, liver cirrhosis, nephrotic syndrome.
- Exclude overshoot from desmopressin treatment for diabetes insipidus.
- Evaluate water intake: endurance events, psychogenic polydipsia, excessive sodium-free solutions (e.g. 5% glucose [confirm by urine sodium < 20 mmol/L]).
- Identify concurrent sodium loss with associated hypovolaemia: diuretics, polyuric states, GI losses, excessive sweating (with replacement by salt-poor fluid), cerebral salt wasting (CNS lesion).
- Check renal function.
- Perform urinary osmolality and urinary sodium once hypovolaemia is corrected. If $urine_{osm}$ > $plasma_{osm}$ and $urine_{Na}$ > 40 mmol/L and no other cause found, consider SIADH.

SIADH—A Diagnosis of Exclusion
• Low serum osmolality
• Urine osmolality > Plasma osmolality
• Urine sodium > 40 mmol/L
• Normal renal, hepatic, cardiac, pituitary, adrenal and thyroid function
• Absence of hypotension, hypovolaemia, oedema and ADH-influencing drugs or diuretics
• Hyponatraemia corrects with water restriction

SIADH—Causes
• Acute illness
• Drugs: opiates, NSAIDs, various psychotropics, carbamazepine, cyclophosphamide, chemotherapeutics
• CNS and psychiatric conditions
• Neoplasia
• Acute and chronic pulmonary disease
• HIV

MANAGEMENT

- If the patient is in seizures or coma, *get help* (see Table 21.1).
- If in shock or oliguric, repeat bolus IV 0.9% saline until circulatory parameters are restored.
- Hyper-osmolar hyponatraemia: address cause.
- Normo-osmolar hyponatraemia: repeat test with direct measurement method.
- In oedematous states: optimise medical management, consider vasopressin antagonists if persistent.
- If normotensive, non-oedematous, normal recent water intake and urine Na^+ < 20 mmol/L: consider persistent dehydration and repeat bolus IV 10 mL/kg 0.9% saline.
- Acute, mild, asymptomatic: 1 mL/kg 3% hypertonic saline over 30 minutes. Then fluid restrict (see below).
- Chronic, moderately severe, asymptomatic: 1 mL/kg 3% hypertonic saline over 2–4 hours use desmopressin (seek expert advice). Then restrict fluid (see below).
- Once circulatory parameters are normal and urine output is > 0.5 mL/kg/h, apply fluid restriction to < 800 mL/day.

- Address causes resulting in ongoing sodium loss (e.g. diuretics).
- Aim to increase Na$^+$ levels by 5–10 mmol/L/day.

Over-rapid correction may lead to central pontine myelinolysis and quadriparesis.

If [Na$^+$] rises too quickly despite careful fluid management, then obtain ICU opinion (may need desmopressin and 5% glucose infusion to re-lower).

- If refractory to treatment (e.g. Na$^+$ fails to rise > 2 mmol/day), seek expert assistance. Consider sodium tablets, frusemide, vasopressin antagonists. Other treatments include urea, demeclocycline and lithium.
- If mild hyponatraemia remains constant despite varying levels of water intake, consider 'reset osmostat'. No treatment is required.

Management Trap—Avoid Excessive 0.9% Saline in Hyponatraemia

Excessive fluid administration (including 0.9% saline) in normovolaemic patients may worsen hyponatraemia if free water excretion is already impaired (e.g. SIADH).

Hypernatraemia

Perform risk stratification (see Table 21.2).

STEPWISE EVALUATION

- If the patient has altered consciousness, *get help*. Provide supportive care for coma (see Table 21.1).
- Review water intake, especially for institutionalised patients and those with an altered mental state (common).
- Evaluate causes of water loss: GI losses, osmotic diuretics.
- Consider excessive sodium intake (e.g. salt poisoning, sodium-containing drugs).
- Consider diabetes insipidus (urine osmolality < plasma osmolality). Obtain expert advice. Confirm with water restriction test.

MANAGEMENT

- Mild, well patient, able to drink: oral water rehydration (DO NOT give sterile water intravenously: haemolysis).

- If symptomatic or unable to drink: admit for IV fluid replacement and treat other co-morbidities.
- If severe CNS symptoms/coma consider ICU.
- If in shock or oliguric: bolus IV of 0.9% saline until normal circulatory parameters.
- If volume overloaded (rare): IV frusemide 20–40 mg 2–4 hourly (seek expert advice) until normovolaemic.
- If severe salt poisoning: consider dialysis.
- Acute hypernatraemia (duration < 24 hours): give 3–6 mL/kg/h 5% glucose (if hyperglycaemic use 2.5% glucose). Aim for 2 mmol/L/h reduction and Na^+ 140 mmol/L within 24 hours. Monitor electrolytes 1–2 hourly and vary rate accordingly.
- Chronic hypernatraemia (duration > 24 hours):
  — give 30 mL/kg of 5% glucose (if hyperglycaemic use 60 mL/kg of 0.45% saline) over 24 hours to replenish water deficit
  — adjust rate to achieve a 10 mmol/L reduction over 24 hours (added K^+ will require a 25–50% increase in infusion rate due to increased osmolality of the solution)
  — additional fluid should be matched for other ongoing losses
  — repeat electrolytes 6- to 12-hourly depending on severity.
- Over-rapid correction may lead to cerebral oedema (headache, deteriorating GCS, seizures). Get help. Treat with 1 mL/kg 3% hypertonic saline over 30 minutes (as for acute severe hyponatraemia).
- In central diabetes insipidus (DI): give vasopressin or desmopressin (obtain expert advice).
- In nephrogenic DI (ADH resistance): obtain expert advice.

Disorders of serum potassium

- Physiological role of potassium: membrane potential of excitable tissue (especially cardiac muscle).
- Physiological control: renin–angiotensin–aldosterone at distal tubule.
- Major compartment: ICF (most plentiful cation). Readily exchanged with ECF or released by cellular damage.

HYPOKALAEMIA
Perform risk stratification (see Table 21.2).

Stepwise evaluation

- If the patient has acute arrhythmias, *get help* and place them in a monitored environment (see Table 21.1).
- Identify potassium losses: vomiting, laxatives, diuretics, sweating, post-obstructive diuresis.
- Consider transient compartmental shifts: hypokalaemic periodic paralysis (family history, thyrotoxicosis), metabolic alkalosis (VBG), salbutamol, adrenaline or insulin effects.
- Perform urine potassium once hypovolaemia corrected: urine K > 15 mmol/L = renal tubular defects or mineralocorticoid excess.
- Consider mineralocorticoid excess (e.g. Conn's syndrome [hypertension, elevated plasma aldosterone:renin levels]).

Management

- Life-threatening (acute arrhythmia): *get help* (see Table 21.1).
- Severe ([K^+] < 2.5 mmol/L) or nil by mouth: give 10–20 mmol potassium chloride in 500 mL of 0.9% saline per hour (a concentration > 40–60 mmol/L needs to be given by central line). Continuing below. Monitor levels every 2 hours and repeat above as necessary.
- Moderately severe: 40–60 mmol K^+ oral supplementation initially if able to tolerate.
- Special cases: intravenous K_2HPO_4/KH_2PO_4 if concurrent hypophosphataemia, oral potassium bicarbonate ($KHCO_3$) or intravenous potassium acetate if concurrent normal anion gap (hyperchloraemic) metabolic acidosis (NAGMA) (get expert assistance).
- Mild to moderate: 20–80 mmol K^+/day orally in divided dose (check formulation and quantities of elemental K^+).
  - With metabolic alkalosis (as potassium chloride).
  - With metabolic acidosis (as potassium acetate or citrate).
  - Address cause. Monitor K^+ twice weekly initially and adjust dose accordingly.
- Admit patient if they have ongoing losses.
- In chronic depletion, total deficit can be 200–400 mmol.

Management Tip—Hypokalaemia and Mg^{2+} and Ca^{2+}
Correcting hypomagnesaemia and hypocalcaemia (see below) is essential when treating hypokalaemia.

HYPERKALAEMIA
Perform risk stratification (see Table 21.2).

Stepwise evaluation
* Perform urgent ECG. If the patient has ventricular arrhythmia or bradyarrhythmia or wide QRS, *get help* and place the patient on a monitor (see Table 21.1).
* Verify that it is not a collection error (i.e. haemolysed sample—difficult venepuncture, elevated LDH).
* Identify altered potassium excretion and drug history: renal failure (check creatinine), angiotensin-converting enzyme (ACE) inhibitors, K$^+$-sparing diuretics.
* Specific scenarios: crush injury, rhabdomyolysis (check CK), severe haemolysis (check FBC and film), tumour lysis syndrome (see Table 21.4).
* Consider temporary compartmental shifts: metabolic acidosis (do VBG), beta-adrenergic blockers, digoxin toxicity.
* Consider mineralocorticoid deficiency (see Addison's disease—low aldosterone:renin levels).

Management
* Life-threatening (QRS widening, arrhythmia): *get help*, calcium IV (see Table 21.1); sodium bicarbonate (NaHCO$_3$) 1 mmol/kg over 30 minutes if concurrent NAGMA. Monitor K$^+$ 1–2 hourly.
* Moderate ([K$^+$] > 6.5 mmol/L): short-acting insulin 5–10 units + 1 mL/kg 50% glucose + 10 mg salbutamol nebulised. Rehydrate.
* Mild ([K$^+$] > 5 mmol/L): review cause +/− rehydrate. Consider frusemide 40 mg once hydrated and adequate urine output. Resonium 30 g PO/PR.
* Treat underlying cause. If severe renal failure with acidosis or fluid overload then consider dialysis (see below).

Most treatments only result in temporary trans-compartmental shifts of potassium. Kaliuresis, dialysis or Resonium treatment produces true elimination of potassium.

Clinical Chemistry Tip
Due to the complex interaction of parathyroid hormone (PTH) and calcitriol on bone, calcium, phosphate and magnesium abnormalities often co-exist.

Diagnostic Evaluation of Mild to Moderate Disorders of Calcium or Phosphate
This is beyond the scope of this text. If the screening tests do not reveal a cause for persistent abnormalities, outpatient review by a general physician or endocrinologist is recommended.

Disorders of calcium

- Physiological role of calcium: muscle contraction and blood clotting.
- Physiological control: parathyroid hormone (PTH) acting on bone pool, GI tract absorption and renal excretion.
- Major compartment: bone (some bound to serum albumin); in disease states, can be abnormally bound in the circulation, precipitate or be sequestered.

HYPOCALCAEMIA

Perform risk stratification (see Table 21.2).

Major Transfusion Warning—Hypocalcaemia and Citrate Toxicity
Massive transfusion leading to citrate toxicity and hypocalcaemia may be an alternative cause for refractory shock. Monitor *ionised* calcium and treat.

Stepwise evaluation

- If the patient has breathing difficulties, arrhythmias or hypotension, *get help* (see Table 21.1).
- Verify corrected total calcium based on serum albumin concentration (see Table 21.3) or request ionised calcium.

- Review dietary intake or major GI pathology affecting absorption.
- Specific clinical situations: post-thyroidectomy (reduced PTH), severe pancreatitis (precipitation), bisphosphonate overtreatment, tumour lysis syndrome (see Table 21.4), acute renal failure (check creatinine), hyperphosphataemia.
- Consider vitamin deficiency and hypoparathyroidism (measure vitamin D, PTH).
- Measure K^+, Mg^{2+} and PO_4^{3-} (hypomagnesaemia has similar clinical features).

Prescribing Tip

Note that 10 mL calcium chloride 10% (6.8 mmol Ca^{2+}) has approximately 3 times more calcium than 10 mL calcium gluconate 10% (2.2 mmol Ca^{2+}). Adjust dose accordingly and preferably give CaCl by central line.

Management
- Severe: give 5–10 mL 10% calcium gluconate (see Table 21.1).
- Moderate/chronic: give 60–120 mL 10% calcium gluconate in 1 L 5% glucose over 24 hours.
- Mild/chronic: treat the cause, elemental calcium 1500–2000 mg/day (600 mg calcium carbonate = 240 mg elemental calcium = 6 mmol calcium) + calcitriol 0.25 microg bd. Outpatient review.
- Treat concurrent hypomagnesaemia (see below).

HYPERCALCAEMIA
Perform risk stratification (see Table 21.2).

Stepwise evaluation
- Verify corrected total calcium based on serum albumin concentration (see Table 21.3) or request ionised calcium.
- Medication review (e.g. calcium supplements, thiazide diuretics [decreased renal excretion], antacid abuse, lithium, vitamins A and D overuse).
- Screen for unreported symptoms suggestive of malignancy, bone metastases or Paget's disease (e.g. bone pain/tenderness, elevated ALP).

- Examine for adenopathy and perform screening CXR for sarcoidosis.
- Exclude renal failure (elevated creatinine).
- Exclude hyperparathyroidism (elevated PTH).

Clinical Tip—Malignancy and Hypercalcaemia
Consider hypercalcaemia as a potential cause for altered mental state or new non-specific symptoms in a patient with known malignancy.

Management

- If the patient is comatose, *get help* (see Table 21.1).
- If the patient has fluid overload, severe renal failure or total $Ca^+ > 4.5$ mmol/L, get expert assistance and dialyse.
- If severe, correct dehydration until urine output is > 0.5 mL/kg/h. Monitor Ca^+, Mg^+, K^+.
- If no cardiac or renal failure, commence saline calciuresis:
  — IV 0.9% saline 1000 mL over 6 hours $+/-$ 20 mg frusemide over 2 hours
  — calcitonin 4 IU/kg if severe and rapid reduction required
  — pamidronate 60–90 mg over 2 hours (but seek expert advice if poor renal function).
- If sarcoidosis, vitamin D intoxication or lymphoma: prednisolone 20–40 mg/day.
- If hypercalcaemia is only mild or moderate: optimise hydration, address cause. Outpatient review.

Disorders of phosphate

- Physiological role of phosphate: intracellular energy production.
- Physiological control: calcitriol (interacts with calcium balance and PTH).
- Major compartments: ICF, bone.

HYPOPHOSPHATAEMIA

Perform risk stratification (see Table 21.2).

Stepwise evaluation

- This condition is usually due to chronic deficiency associated with reduced total body stores.
- Common scenarios: from malnourishment (e.g. unusual diet, chronic alcoholism).
- Consider antacid abuse.
- Specific scenarios: post parathyroidectomy (hungry bone syndrome), respiratory alkalosis (VBG).
- Measure PTH.

Management Tip—Iatrogenic Hypophosphataemia

Dangerous hypophosphataemia may occur during insulin treatment for DKA or re-feeding syndrome in underweight patients. Monitor and replace.

Management

- If the patient has arrhythmia, *get help* (see Table 21.1).
- Severe: intravenous K_2HPO_4/KH_2PO_4 40–80 mmol/L in 1 L 0.9% saline over 24 hours.
- Moderate: PO elemental phosphorus 10–20 mmol/L 4 times daily.
- Mild and asymptomatic: resume normal diet.

HYPERPHOSPHATAEMIA

Perform risk stratification (see Table 21.2).

Features are often related to associated hypocalcaemia (see above).

Causes

- Transcellular shifts: acute tissue breakdown (rhabdomyolysis, haemolysis, tumour lysis; see Table 21.4), phosphate enemas.
- Decreased excretion: severe renal failure, bisphosphonates, vitamin D excess.
- Homeostatic failure: reduced PTH.

Management

- If the patient has breathing difficulties, arrhythmias or hypotension, *get help* (see Table 21.1).

- Moderate/severe: commence urgent saline rehydration (but not in hypocalcaemia—consider dialysis).
- Chronic renal failure: seek advice.
- Mild: maintain hydration, address cause.

Disorders of magnesium

- Physiological significance of magnesium: membrane potential of excitable tissue (nerve, cardiac and skeletal muscle).
- Physiological control: regulated by GIT absorption and renal excretion, indirectly affect PTH and hence Ca^{2+}/ PO_4^{3-}.
- Major compartments: ECF (immediate), bone (large concentration but not rapidly mobilised).

Serum Magnesium—Indications for Ordering
• Abnormal ECG, arrhythmias, altered mental state or seizure
• Large GI losses
• Diuretic use or polyuric states
• If abnormal potassium, calcium or phosphate: magnesium therapy

HYPOMAGNESAEMIA

Perform risk stratification (see Table 21.2).
Clinical features are similar to hypocalcaemia (qv).

Causes

Causes of hypomagnesaemia are diuretics (common), chronic alcoholism, poor nutrition, GI malabsorption, pancreatitis (elevated lipase), hyperparathyroidism ($\uparrow Ca^{2+}$, elevated PTH).

Management

- If the patient has arrhythmias, *get help* (see Table 21.1).
- Moderate: intravenous magnesium sulfate ($MgSO_4$) 20–60 mmol in 1 L 0.9% saline over 24 hours.
- Mild: magnesium chloride ($MgCl_2$) 25–50 mmol daily.

HYPERMAGNESAEMIA

Perform risk stratification (see Table 21.2).

Causes

Acute kidney injury (renal function), iatrogenic (e.g. treatment of eclampsia), tumour lysis syndrome (see Table 21.4).

Management

- If there is cardiorespiratory compromise, *get help* (see Table 21.1).
- Stop Mg^{2+} infusion.
- If it is severe or the patient has renal failure, consider dialysis.
- For intravenous therapy (IVT), maintain urine output at > 0.5 mL/kg/h, short-acting insulin 5–10 units + 1 mL/kg 50% glucose. Monitor 1–2 hourly.

Clinical Chemistry Curiosity—Tumour Lysis Syndrome

This is due to massive cellular death in solid and haematological tumours resulting in multiple biochemical abnormalities (see Table 21.4) and renal failure. Optimal treatment is rehydration, recombinant urate oxidase and dialysis. With more effective chemotherapeutic agents, this condition may become more commonly seen in the ambulatory population.

Disorders of acid–base balance

Assessment Tip—Indications for a Blood Gas Analysis

Consider a blood gas analysis if the patient appears seriously unwell, has abnormal vital signs or is incidentally noted to have abnormal venous bicarbonate.

- Acid–base balance is regulated by a combination of passive buffering processes (intracellular protein buffers, carbonic anhydrase buffer system) and actively by **intact** respiratory and renal compensatory mechanisms that regulate the excretion of bicarbonate (metabolic base) and CO_2 (respiratory or volatile acid).
- Disorders of acid–base balance can be due to a variety of metabolic and respiratory disturbances or disorders affecting homeostatic control of pH.

- Changes in chloride can result in alterations in bicarbonate (metabolic base) by a direct effect on renal handling of bicarbonate and a physicochemical effect on water disassociation (for further reading beyond the scope of this book see the Stewart approach).

Clinical Interpretation Tip—pH, pCO₂ and HCO₃⁻

Evaluate pCO_2 and bicarbonate concurrently to determine the acid–base disturbance. Remember pH, which may be near-normal due to compensatory mechanisms.

Treatment should generally be primarily directed to the *cause* and not simply by directly manipulating the values.

Normal arterial blood gas values
- pH   7.35–7.45
- pCO_2 35–45 mmHg ('respiratory acid')
- PO_2 100 mmHg
- HCO_3^- 24 mmol/L ('metabolic base')

Normal venous blood gas values
- Normal values are pH 7.35, HCO_3^- 26 mmol/L, pCO_2 45 mmHg.
- Changes in venous pH, HCO_3^- and pCO_2 typically parallel arterial values in *non-shocked, non-hypermetabolic* patients.
- Normal VBG values effectively exclude an acid–base abnormality.

Patient Comfort Tip—VBGs

There is growing evidence that in single acid–base abnormalities with a stable relationship between arterial and venous values (e.g. DKA, acute respiratory failure, clinical response) therapeutic decisions can be achieved with serial VBG determinations.

Venous bicarbonate or total CO₂
- Normal values are venous bicarbonate 22–32 mmol/L and total CO_2 23–30 mmol/L.

• Some laboratories report total CO_2 in mmol/L. This largely approximates venous bicarbonate.

Cause of variances from normal
• ↓ indicates primary metabolic acidosis or primary respiratory alkalosis.
• ↑ indicates primary metabolic alkalosis or primary respiratory acidosis.
• Normal values do not *exclude* an acid–base abnormality. Perform a full blood gas analysis if in doubt.

DETERMINING THE ACID–BASE ABNORMALITY
(See the acid–base nomogram in Figure 21.1.)
1 Check **pH**: if < 7.4 then the patient is acidaemic; if > 7.4, the patient is alkalaemic.
   If acidaemic: is HCO_3^- < 24 (metabolic acidosis) or pCO_2 > 40 (respiratory acidosis), or both?
   If alkalaemic: is HCO_3^- > 24 (metabolic alkalosis) or pCO_2 < 40 (respiratory alkalosis), or both?
2 Is the **respiratory compensation** for a metabolic abnormality incomplete or complete? (See Metabolic Equations and Electrolytes in the Quick Reference section.)
   If pCO_2 is lower than expected $\Rightarrow$ concurrent respiratory alkalosis.
   If pCO_2 is higher than expected $\Rightarrow$ concurrent respiratory acidosis.
3 Is the **metabolic compensation** for a respiratory abnormality acute/incomplete or chronic/complete? (See Metabolic Equations and Electrolytes in the Quick Reference section.)
   If HCO_3^- is lower than expected $\Rightarrow$ concurrent metabolic acidosis.
   If HCO_3^- is higher than expected $\Rightarrow$ concurrent metabolic alkalosis.

Clinical Interpretation Tip—Acute on Chronic Pathology

ABG interpretation using standard formulas and acid–base nomograms may be misleading when a chronic abnormality precedes an acute disturbance. Compare with previous results to determine whether a new abnormality exists.

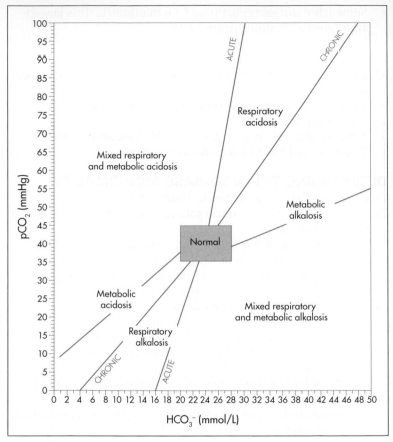

Figure 21.1 Acid–base nomogram

METABOLIC ACIDOSIS

Perform risk stratification (see Table 21.2).

This is often associated with significant pathology. Aggressively search for the cause, and treat and monitor the response (low venous HCO_3^- on serum electrolytes is a clue).

Clinical effects

- These are usually related to the cause.
- Severe metabolic acidosis can contribute to further circulatory collapse and diminished clotting function (important in shock and trauma).
- Respiratory fatigue can occur following prolonged respiratory compensation and worsening pH.

The anion gap

- A *high* anion gap (normochloraemic) metabolic acidosis (HAGMA) is due to increased endogenous or exogenous acid with conjugate base.
- A *normal anion gap* (hyperchloraemic) metabolic acidosis (NAGMA) is due to bicarbonate loss or chloride excess.

The Anion Gap—Categorising Metabolic Acidoses

anion gap = $([Na^+] + [K^+]) - ([Cl^-] + [HCO_3^-])$
The normal value for the anion gap is 10–18.

The delta gap

In a HAGMA for every 1 mmol fall in bicarbonate, the anion gap should rise 1 mmol. If it doesn't, a concurrent NAGMA may co-exist.

Delta Gap—Identifying Combined HAGMA and NAGMA

delta gap = change in anion gap – change in bicarbonate
'simplified' delta gap = Na – Cl – 36
< -6 = HAGMA + NAGMA
–6 to 6 = HAGMA
> 6 = HAGMA + metabolic alkalosis

High anion gap metabolic acidosis (HAGMA)

Stepwise assessment

- Rapidly assess the following:
  — circulatory status (HR, BP, capillary refill, urine output, lactate)
  — ketonaemia/DKA (bedside BSL and ketones, serum glucose and ketones; urinary ketones may give false negatives).

- Screen for evidence of infection and sepsis (infection symptoms, fever, ↑ WCC/CRP).
- Evaluate for cardiogenic causes of shock (injury patterns on ECG, new murmurs, poor LVF on echocardiogram).
- Ascertain history of diabetes, renal failure (creatinine), drug history and toxic ingestions.
- Other tests are:
  — electrolytes
  — serum lactate
  — serum osmolarity.

Management

1 Treat the cause.
  — Hypovolaemia: fluid challenge until vital signs and urine output restored.
  — Sepsis: fluid challenge—consider pressor support, early administration of antibiotics.
  — Cardiogenic shock: judicious fluid challenge, early pressor support, treat cause (obtain expert opinion).
  — DKA: see Chapter 20 Endocrine Emergencies.
  — Renal failure: see Box 21.1.
  — Poisoning: obtain toxicology advice.
2 Potassium deficit may be unmasked as the metabolic acidosis resolves. Monitor and anticipate need for replacement (see the section on Hyperkalaemia).
3 Repeat blood gas every few hours depending on the severity to monitor response to treatment.

Management Tip—HAGMA and Bicarbonate

Routine bicarbonate administration is generally not recommended in HAGMA. Address the *cause.*
Seek expert advice if patient critically unwell.

Box 21.1   Life-threatening complications of renal failure

- Severe hyperkalaemia (see the section on hyperkalaemia)
- Acute pulmonary oedema
- Uraemic encephalopathy

(See Box 21.2 Indications for Haemodialysis.)

Normal anion gap metabolic acidosis (NAGMA)

(This is uncommon in the ED. A detailed treatise of conditions [e.g. renal tubular acidosis] is beyond the scope of this book.)

Stepwise evaluation

- Check for bicarbonate loss from the genitourinary system or GI tract.
- Review history of diarrhoea and renal tubular acidosis.
- Look for surgical losses—fistula/stomal/drain losses.
- Review for excessive infusion of 0.9% saline ('saline induced acidosis').
- If urine osmolal gap < 150 mmol/L, consider renal causes or mineralocorticoid deficiency (see below).
- Consider Addison's disease: ↓ aldosterone:renin levels.

The urine osmolal gap

Urine osmolal gap represents hydrogen ions excreted as ammonium. In the setting of a metabolic acidosis with normal renal function, it should be > 150 mmol/L.

Urine Osmolal Gap—Renal Causes of NAGMA
urine osmolal gap = measured urine osmolality – calculated urine osmolality calculated urinary osmolality = urinary Na + urinary K + urinary urea + urinary glucose (Normal 150–400 mmol/L: < 150 mmol/L = renal causes of NAGMA)

Management

Get expert assistance. Consider the following:

- sodium bicarbonate ($NaHCO_3$) IV, sodium bicarbonate/citrate PO
- if the patient is potassium-deficient, potassium citrate/bicarbonate PO, potassium acetate IV
- total bicarbonate deficit (mmol) = (24 – existing $[HCO_3^-]$) × 2/3× bodyweight (in kg)
- replace over 4–24 hours depending on urgency.

Metabolic alkalosis

Perform risk stratification (see Table 21.2).

Stepwise evaluation

- Review diuretic use (common cause).
- Review for upper GI losses (e.g. pyloric stenosis, bulimia nervosa), less commonly lower GI loss (e.g. villous adenoma, chloride diarrhoea).
- Address perpetuating factors include dehydration and hypokalaemia.
- If the cause is uncertain, urinary chloride > 25 mmol/L suggests mineralocorticoid excess (or active diuretic effect). See Conn's syndrome ($\uparrow$ aldosterone:renin levels).
- If associated with wide anion gap, evaluate for concurrent metabolic acidosis.

Assessment Tip—Urinary Cl and Metabolic Alkalosis

With intact homeostatic mechanisms, excess bicarbonate is excreted in exchange for chloride re-absorption. A high urinary chloride > 25 mmol/L suggests abnormal renal bicarbonate re-absorption.

Management

Note: Respiratory compensation is limited. Definitely treat if pCO_2 > 50 mmHg or pH > 7.5.

- If metabolic alkalosis is associated with volume loss, it is 'saline/chloride responsive' (urine $[Cl^-]$ < 25 mmol/L). Correct dehydration with 0.9% saline or albumin (if low albumin).
- If fluid overloaded or the metabolic alkalosis is 'saline unresponsive' (urine $[Cl^-]$ > 25 mmol/L) give acetazolamide 250 mg 1–2 times/day to induce bicarbonate diuresis IV hydrochloric acid (HCl) via central venous catheter (ICU).
- Review indications of offending medications.

Management Tip—Metabolic Alkalosis and K^+

A metabolic alkalosis will not resolve unless hypokalaemia is also treated. Treat with KCl (not potassium bicarbonate or acetate).

RESPIRATORY ACIDOSIS ('HYPOVENTILATION', 'TYPE II RESPIRATORY FAILURE')

Perform risk stratification (see Table 21.2).

Clinical effects

Patients with chronic respiratory acidosis can tolerate higher levels of hypercarbia. Without increasing inspired oxygen, severe hypercarbia will cause a dangerous fall in P_AO (see alveolar gas equation in Chapter 13 Respiratory Emergencies: The Acutely Breathless Patient).

Causes

- Any cause of respiratory depression or inadequate alveolar ventilation
- Acute cardiorespiratory illness (asthma/chronic obstructive airways disease, pulmonary oedema, pneumonia)
- Central failure / CNS insults (opiates, benzodiazepines, acute space-occupying lesion)
- Trauma (head injury, flail chest, haemothorax/pneumothorax)
- Hyper-metabolic states (e.g. sepsis, thyroid storm)

Management

- Treat cause.
- Use non-invasive or mechanical ventilation (if drowsy/somnolent or severe head injury) (see the section on respiratory failure in Chapter 13).

Resuscitation Tip—Oxygen Delivery in CO_2 Retainers

Always maintain a safe oxygen saturation (SpO_2) of at least 88–92% even if CO_2 retention is of concern.

RESPIRATORY ALKALOSIS

Causes

- Physiological: late pregnancy, mountain dwellers
- Readily reversible: pain, anxiety
- Serious (within clinical context): acute cardiorespiratory illness, sepsis, pulmonary embolism, salicylate poisoning (see relevant sections)

Clinical effects
- Usually not life-threatening
- In moderate to severe cases: paraesthesia, muscle spasm and tetany (mechanism uncertain)

Management
Treat underlying cause. Rebreathing into a paper bag is not recommended due to risk of hypoxia.

LACTATE
Physiology
- The normal value of lactate is < 2 mmol/L ('significant' is > 4 mmol/L).
- Lactate is a byproduct of glycolytic activity and cleared by the liver. There are several mechanisms that result in elevation.

Diagnostic value
- Elevated serum lactate can occur with or without concurrent acidaemia.
- Elevated lactate can be a marker of systemic or regional hypoperfusion (usefulness is limited by moderate sensitivity and specificity).
- A normal lactate should not replace clinical judgment when making treatment and disposition decisions.

Stepwise clinical evaluation of elevated lactate
- If it is due to transient increase in muscle activity (e.g. exertion or seizure), no treatment is required.
- If it is chronic, and stable due to reduced metabolism (e.g. chronic liver failure), no treatment is required.
- If there is evidence of shock, commence fluid resuscitation (see Resuscitation Endpoints below).
- If there is no evidence of shock but the patient is unwell, consider type B1 lactic acidosis and treat the underlying cause (e.g. sepsis, thiamine deficiency).
- In severe type B2 lactic acidosis (drug toxicity) consider dialysis (e.g. toxic alcohols, salicylates, isoniazid, metformin).

Lactate and resuscitation endpoints

- Lactate may improve but remain persistently elevated after adequate resuscitation in shock states due to other mechanisms.
- It should not be used in isolation to diagnose or exclude ongoing hypoperfusion.

Lactate: prognosis and disposition

- A single value is not useful for disposition or prognostication and must be used in conjunction with clinical data.
- A non-resolving lactate provides some prognostic value but it is related to the inciting event and should be evaluated in combination with clinical response.

Acute kidney injury (AKI)

Acute kidney injury is defined by ANY of the following:

- rise in serum creatinine $\geq$ 26.5 micromol/L over 48 hours
- rise in serum creatinine $\geq$ $\times$ 1.5 over 7 days
- urine output $\leq$ 0.5 mL/kg/hr for 6 hours.

Subacute injury: deterioration $<$ 3 months

Chronic kidney disease: deterioration $>$ 3 months

EARLY ED ASSESSMENT AND MANAGEMENT

('Pre-renal, renal, post-renal')

1 Assess for and treat hyperkalaemia (see section on hyperkalaemia).
2 If not fluid overloaded, repeated IV fluid bolus until circulatory parameters restored and urine output $>$ 0.5 mL/kg/h.
3 If fluid overload develops, dialyse.
4 Treat sepsis or UTI: urine dipstick, urine culture, IV antibiotics.
5 Relieve obstruction and measure urine output: IDC and measure hourly urine output $+/-$ urgent renal ultrasound to exclude ureteric obstruction $+/-$ urgent nephrostomy. Beware of post-obstructive diuresis resulting in hypovolaemia, hypokalaemia.
6 Stop nephrotoxic drugs (e.g. NSAIDs, aminoglycosides, ACE inhibitors, frusemide).

PRE-RENAL (DEHYDRATION/HYPOVOLAEMIA) OR ESTABLISHED (ACUTE TUBULAR NECROSIS) RENAL FAILURE?

+ Typically in pure dehydration, plasma urea:creatinine is $> 20:1$.
+ 'Intra-renal' causes: check urine sediment for casts, protein and cells.
  (See Table 21.5.)
  Box 21.2 (also overleaf) gives indications for haemodialysis.

Table 21.5 Pre-renal versus renal failure

Cause/ mechanism	Pre-renal failure	Established renal failure (i.e. acute tubular necrosis)
Summary	Maximal water and sodium retention and maximally concentrated urine to maintain circulatory volume ($U_{Na} \downarrow$ but U_{urea}, U_{osm}, $U_{creat} \uparrow\uparrow\uparrow$)	Loss of concentrating power ($U_{Na} \uparrow$ and U_{urea}, U_{osm}, $U_{creat} \leftrightarrow$)
$P_{urea}:P_{creat}$	20:1	10–15:1
U_{Na} (mmol/L)	< 20	> 40
U_{osm} (mOsm/L)	> 500	< 350
$U_{osm}:P_{osm}$	$> 2:1$	$< 1:2$
$U_{creat}:P_{creat}$	$> 40:1$	$< 20:1$
Fe_{Na}	$< 1\%$	$> 2\%$

$$Fe_{Na} = \frac{(U_{Na} / P_{Na})}{(U_{creat} / P_{creat})}$$

$\downarrow$, decreases; $\uparrow$, increases; $\uparrow\uparrow\uparrow$, increases massively; $\leftrightarrow$, remains unchanged; P_{creat} = plasma creatinine; P_{Na} = plasma sodium; P_{osm} = plasma osmolarity; P_{urea} = plasma urea; U_{creat} = urinary creatinine; U_{Na} = urinary sodium; U_{osm} = urinary osmolarity; U_{urea} = urinary urea.

Box 21.2 Indications for haemodialysis ('too much acid, water, potassium or poison')

- Severe metabolic acidosis
- Acute pulmonary oedema—fluids challenge does not re-establish urine output
- Hyperkalaemia not responding to medical treatment (see section on hyperkalaemia)
- Acute nephrotoxic exposures (e.g. lithium, methanol, ethylene glycol)

ADVANCES IN ELECTROLYTE MANAGEMENT

Routine use of 5% + NS to reduce the incidence of hyponatraemia in sick children

CONTROVERSIES IN ELECTROLYTE MANAGEMENT

- Acute kidney injury with routine use of 0.9% saline versus balanced electrolyte solutions.
- Routine use of desmopressin in treating severe asymptomatic hyponatraemia to prevent uncontrolled rise in serum sodium.
- Treatments for refractory SIADH.
- Long-term clinical impact of untreated mild chronic hyponatraemia.
- Iatrogenic factors in the development of central pontine myelinolysis.
- Optimal fluid regimen for treatment of hypernatraemia and concurrent hyperglycaemia. The role of intravenous sterile water by central line.
- The value of the Stewart approach in assessing acid–base disturbances.
- Use of bicarbonate in severe HAGMA.
- Iatrogenic factors in the pathogenesis of cerebral oedema in DKA.
- Utility of diuretics in converting oliguric renal failure into non-oliguric renal failure.
- Indications for dialysis.

Online resources

Deranged Physiology
    www.derangedphysiology.com
LITFL
    www.litfl.com

Chapter 22
Geriatric care

Shahrzad Jahromi and David Murphy

Overview

Sensitive and effective care of the older patient is core to the mission of emergency medicine. Improved life expectancy, the growth in complexity of both acute and chronic care available for older patients, and the demographic bulge following 1945 have been key drivers in ED demand across developed countries. Older patients need unplanned care in the ED more often, stay longer and have a higher admission rate from ED to inpatient wards than younger patients.

Good care in the ED can help many older patients return home independently, and can help manage the burden of illness and frailty to carers, the community and to the health system. Providing this care is challenging in the busy, stimulating ED environment, and requires attention to comfort and dignity, early senior decision-making and close support from an aged-care multidisciplinary team.

While the broader physiological aspects of ageing are beyond the scope of this chapter, a few principles need to be considered. In a developed country, healthy ageing is marked by an extended period of preserved physiological reserve, albeit with a gradually increasing risk of cardiovascular and other pathology. Following this, however, a gradual transition to frailty occurs, the key characteristic of which is a reduced ability to recover from an insult. In frailty, the strength and elasticity of skin, muscle and bone are reduced and falls risk is increased. Cardiorespiratory reserve is reduced, especially in the context of prolonged immobility. Constipation is common, also often exacerbated by immobility, and can present in a number of ways including urinary retention and faecal overflow. Resistance to infection, especially urinary and respiratory, is reduced. Serious illness may present with subtle functional decline, falls and delirium rather than with clearly localising signs, resulting in both under- and over-diagnosis.

Editorial Comment

Get to like and be comfortable with older patients. It is a large and important part of our practice. A big tip is give them time— to answer, remember. Sit down—do not be rushed, get to know them; then quickly you will define issues: ? critically ill, ? acute deterioration, ? comorbidities, what are activities of daily living (ADL) issues, what are they worried about? It becomes rewarding for both of you— not 'another difficult geri patient'. Try it, it works!

Assessment begins with a careful history, of both presenting problem and background. While there are many reasons why an older patient may be less able to communicate, it should not be assumed that a history is not possible. Assessment of pain, using both verbal and nonverbal cues, remains possible even in advanced dementia. Collateral history at the outset from family, carers, friends, residential facility staff and the local doctor is crucial to accurate diagnosis and can save significant time and helps guide (or even avoid) investigations. If a language barrier is present, an interpreter will be of great value. Ambulance officers may well be the only source of vital information relating to living conditions and access to food. Remain alert to the possibility, however, that information from the patient, carers, facilities and even other treating staff could be inaccurate or out of date. When obtaining the history, consider the degree and time course of deviation from baseline.

Past medical history should be obtained, including history of smoking, alcohol and other drug use, visual and hearing impairment, nutritional status, dental hygiene and falls risk.

Editorial Comment

Many elderly patients are on aspirin, let alone anticoagulation. They bleed easily, especially venous bleeding—subdural haematoma may occur after minimal head trauma (due to brain atrophy and bridging veins). This is often not clinically evident within < 4 hours, or in early CT! Have a low threshold to admit and observe.

Medications are very commonly implicated in presentations to ED, whether by use or omission, so a clear pharmacological history, corroborated by carers, GP or pharmacist, should be obtained. The risk of problems rises with the number of medications prescribed and with acute illness. Avoid reliance on any single source of information: GP letters, hospital discharge letters and nursing home charts may all have errors. If you are presented with a Webster Pack, enquire regarding other medication (patches, drops, refrigerated, newly started or variable medications) that may not have been packed. Check whether medications could have been missed or extra doses taken. Maintain a low threshold for reducing, suspending or deprescribing any that could be causing harm or which are no longer likely to provide benefit. When prescribing or re-starting medications apply the principle of 'start low, go slow' (Table 22.1).

Obtaining a good social history is important for a number of reasons. It establishes the patient as a person within a family, and often as a person who has made a contribution to the community; helping you to establish rapport and prompting you to involve carers or family earlier. Find out if your patient has caring responsibilities—grandchildren, spouse, pets—as occasionally urgent support is needed. Many older patients have significant social challenges, including poverty, poor housing, isolation and lack of access to transport. Patients with a history of alcohol and/or other drug use, mental illness or other long-term chronic disease are particularly vulnerable and may face ageing-related illnesses at

Table 22.1 Examples of higher risk medications in older patients

Medication class	Adverse effect
Antihypertensives, diuretics	Dehydration, kidney injury, cardiovascular compromise
Non-steroidal anti-inflammatories	Kidney injury, gastrointestinal bleeding, fluid retention
Corticosteroids	Impaired stress response, osteoporosis
Opiates	Constipation, delirium
Psychoactive medications, sedatives, anticonvulsants	Delirium, falls
Anticoagulants	Bleeding

a younger age than usually expected. The health and other challenges faced by Indigenous Australians likewise require a range of strategies for good care. An openness to considering each person's circumstances and obtaining help, from within the ED and from the network of community and hospital services, is vital.

Ensuring consent for treatment is as important for older patients as for others. Document a reliable means of contacting the enduring guardian or appropriate surrogate decision-maker; both for general support and in case capacity is lost. Urgent care required to sustain life may need to be commenced without consent, and can be continued or ceased subsequently once more information and decision-making support is at hand.

Patients who retain capacity may refuse life-sustaining care. Where capacity is in doubt, a surrogate decision-maker is required. Some patients have an appointed *enduring guardian* to make decisions in this situation, often at the time of making a will or moving into residential care. Without this formal appointment, most states nominate a *person responsible*, in which a hierarchy is set out beginning with spouse or partner with a close continuing relationship, followed by a person who provides regular, unpaid care.

A *Resuscitation Plan*, or similar document such as a *Not for Resuscitation* (NFR) order, is likely to be the key means of conveying decisions made in this regard. Though one may exist from a previous admission, it may require renewal depending on circumstances and local rules. It should include specific consultation with the person responsible, should indicate the basis for decisions made and may contain very useful information such as treatments which may still be appropriate short of CPR, and the names of people to contact in a crisis.

An Advance Care Directive (ACD) may exist, provides information regarding a patient's wishes and values, and can help inform the preparation of the Resuscitation Plan. Though its legal status can vary depending on state and situation, in its simplest form an ACD supports the person responsible in refusing otherwise life-sustaining care.

Lastly, for patients more clearly approaching the end of life, a symptom-focused approach is clearly needed. A core domain of emergency medicine is to avoid futile or burdensome treatments, to recognise natural dying and to provide calm, empathic support to patients and families during this period.

Falls

Falls dominate traumatic presentations to ED among older people. Some falls have a single identifiable trigger—in particular consider syncope for unwitnessed falls. Most, however, are due to a combination of factors impairing postural reserve. Risk factors with limited reversibility in the ED include deficits in vision, proprioception, vestibular function, truncal strength and autonomic responsiveness. More immediately reversible factors include medications (even longstanding ones), acute illness (especially infection or hypovolaemia), the environment, footwear or pets. Non-accidental injury should also be considered, as it is frequently not disclosed. Inability to get up without assistance may be an indication of more severe injuries, and is a predictor of need for admission. The more risk factors present, the greater the likelihood of further falls.

Obtain a careful history of the circumstances of the fall and any preceding symptoms or possible environmental factors (see Table 22.2).

Intracranial injury should be considered in all patients. Age-related changes, particularly cerebral atrophy and traction on

Table 22.2 Falls assessment in the older patient

Primary survey	• Minor mechanisms may cause significant head, cervical or truncal injury.
	• C-spine protection is often difficult in the older patient due to kyphosis: avoid immobilisation where possible, provide adequate head support.
	• Cardiorespiratory compromise may be masked or exacerbated (e.g. by medications or pacemaker).
	• Pupil evaluation may be affected by surgery, drops or medications.
Cause for fall	• Check temperature, HR, postural BP, ECG.
	• Consider especially dehydration, sepsis (UTI, respiratory infection, intra-abdominal, skin), PE, CCF, arrhythmia, coronary syndrome, neurological deficit, medications, alcohol.
Secondary survey	• Skin tears: early care vital. Check head including scalp.
	• Fractures: commonly rib, spine, pelvis, radius, humerus, femur.
	• Pressure areas: consider likelihood of long-lie.

subdural bridging veins, both increase vulnerability and delay the onset of symptoms. Presentation may be subtle or gradual, typically with altered cognitive state and impaired balance. Headache is commonly absent. The original trauma may be weeks before the current presentation. Guidelines exist but have limited validation for older patients with blunt brain trauma, and in general a low threshold for brain imaging is recommended, especially in the context of anticoagulation or direct head trauma.

Fractures are the next key outcome of a fall, led by distal radius and femoral neck. Femoral neck fractures may present with classical thigh shortening and rotation, but some, in particular subcapital, are easily missed on plain X-ray and senior input should be sought. Consider pubic ramus fractures. CT is the usual second-line imaging modality if X-ray is normal. Most EDs will have a pathway for such fractures, including imaging and orthopaedic admission. Fascia iliaca compartment block, often with ultrasound guidance, is recommended and is associated with reduced need for preoperative analgesia.

Distal wrist and proximal humeral fractures are usually transmitted from an outstretched hand. While management, from ED immobilisation to orthopaedic referral, is generally similar to that for younger patients, the effect on safe mobility and ability to self-care is likely to be greater.

Vertebral fractures are also common, from stable thoracic wedge compression fractures to unstable fractures with spinal deficit. Preexisting degenerative changes both increase risk for certain injury patterns, such as odontoid C2 fractures, and make assessment of imaging difficult. Compare with old imaging if available, and have a low threshold for CT.

Next it is important to assess skin integrity. Skin tends to be thin, with reduced elasticity and with more fragile subcutaneous supports. In addition, healing may be compromised by vascular disease, diabetes, malnutrition or immune compromise. Skin tears are frequently superficial, often in areas where healing is slow, and can be extensive, but in the first hours after injury will respond very well to ED care. If left, however, skin flaps become non-viable, and prolonged open wounds may result. Obtain plastic surgery (or local appropriate service) review for deeper, contaminated or incompletely re-apposed wounds, as operative repair or skin grafting may be required (see Box 22.1).

Box 22.1   Skin tear management

Preparation: gloves and face-mask, lighting, towelling/drape.

Control bleeding, offer pain relief, assess for any deeper injury.

Topical lignocaine: drip over exposed dermal bed, identify base of flap.

Saline irrigation: be generous, use syringe and drawing up needle or soft cannula, gently wash away haematoma from bed and beneath skin flap, freeing flap from base of wound.

Gently re-appose skin flap using minimum touch, avoiding inversion.

Apply first layer: Mepitel or similar tension-relieving dressing.

Apply second layer: Mepilex Border or similar, marking recommended direction (from base towards free flap) of dressing removal.

Apply crepe, consider immobilisation in high-stretch locations.

Schedule wound review in 2–3 days.

Finally the functional impact of a fall can be significant and long lasting. Patients with significant injuries may never regain full mobility, and even those with minor injuries may require hospital admission due to difficulties in mobilisation with sling or cast, for analgesia or for loss of confidence. Crutches should be avoided in older patients.

Confusion

Confusion is often found in older patients presenting to ED, and both dementia and delirium should be systematically screened for and assessed. Tables 22.3 and 22.4 provide a structure for this.

While patterns and expected time course of dementia vary, a broad staging framework allows ED staff to identify and manage

Table 22.3   Differential diagnosis between dementia and delirium

	Dementia	Delirium
Moment of onset	Uncertain	Usually precise
Progression	Slow, chronic	Fluctuates, reversible
Vigilance	Normal	Varies between states of hyper- and hypovigilance
Orientation	Disoriented in late stages	Disoriented early

Adapted from Samaras N, Chevalley T, Samaras D, et al. Older Patients in the Emergency Department: A Review. Annals of Emergency Medicine. 2010:56(3); 261–269. https://doi.org.acs.hcn.com.au/10.1016/j.annemergmed.2010.04.015

Table 22.4   The diagnosis of delirium by the Confusion Assessment Method requires the presence of features 1 and 2 and either 3 or 4.

1	Is there evidence of an acute change in mental status from the patient's baseline?
2a	Did the patient have difficulty focusing attention, for example, being easily distractible, or having difficulty keeping track of what was being said?
2b	Did the behaviour fluctuate during the interview, that is, tend to come and go, or increase and decrease in severity?
3	Was the patient's thinking disorganised or incoherent, such as rambling or irrelevant conversation, unclear or illogical flow of ideas, or unpredictable switching from subject to subject?
4	Is there an altered level of consciousness? — Alert (normal) — Vigilant (hyperalert) — Lethargic (drowsy, easily aroused) — Stupor (difficult to arouse) — Coma (unarousable)

Reproduced from Inouye et al. Clarifying confusion: the Confusion Assessment Method: a new method for detection of delirium. Ann Intern Med. 1990.

common problems. In early dementia, various aspects of gradual functional and social decline, from isolation to medication mistakes, may lead to either a medical or a situational crisis. Anxiety or other psychiatric symptoms, particularly relatively fixed delusions, often regarding family members, are distressing and may alienate loved ones. Communication of physical symptoms is generally reliable although context can be lacking. Patients without close family or supports are particularly at risk and, even when family members are present, ED staff should be aware of the potential for abuse or neglect. Considerable community support may be available at this stage, and resources may often be coordinated from the ED, with the assistance of a dedicated aged-care emergency team if available.

As dementia progresses to the moderate stage, behavioural and psychological symptoms become more common, forgetfulness more obvious and the need for care more constant. While community services can still maintain some patients at home, an ED visit becomes more likely to lead to admission to hospital, and ultimately to a residential aged care facility (RACF). In advanced dementia, with progressive immobility, incontinence and impaired swallowing, medical crises such as sepsis and falls become more common triggers for presentation. All of these stages are very challenging for families and patients, and great care and sensitivity is required.

Delirium, a state of acute brain dysfunction marked by fluctuating impairment of cognition and attention, is easily overlooked. Although dementia is the most important underlying risk factor, delirium itself is usually due to pathology outside the nervous system. Acute infection, pain, medication changes and metabolic derangements are the commonest precipitants. Serious bacterial infection may not be accompanied by the degree of systemic response typical in younger patients. Alcohol withdrawal is another common cause, which may mimic infection and be overlooked in the ED. More than one cause is often present. It is important to note that psychiatric illness itself is generally not a cause for acute confusion.

The Confusion Assessment Method (CAM) is quick, repeatable, easy to use and validated for detection of delirium. It should be performed in all patients presenting with confusion to the ED.

Assessment and management of the confused patient in ED poses a range of challenges, not least being the tension between potentially worsening confusion in an unfamiliar hospital and discharge to a potentially unsafe, but familiar, home. Noise and light needs to be managed to allow sleep. Falls risk needs careful consideration, with measures including non-slip socks and avoidance of trip-hazards. Bed-rails should not be used for containment of agitated patients. Attention to mobility, bowels and bladder should be maintained, and prolonged immobility in bed avoided when possible. Reassurance and re-orientation, by staff, family and even by volunteer carers, is highly valuable, and pharmacological sedation reserved as a last resort. Ultimately the time spent in ED should be minimised, with transfer facilitated either to a dedicated aged care ward environment, or in the absence of acute delirium or other reason for inpatient admission, to the patient's usual environment. In some situations admission may be avoided by arrangement of early community follow-up, including geriatric or palliative care outreach to the RACF.

In delirium, extended assessment should be tailored to the likely acute cause. Full exposure and examination is needed to identify precipitants that may not otherwise be obvious, such as urinary retention, head trauma, cellulitis or surgical pathology. Urinalysis +/− microscopy/culture is an early priority, but positive findings do not negate the possibility of alternative or additional causes. Pneumonia should be considered and chest X-ray obtained. Blood cultures should be taken even in the absence of fever. Central nervous system infections, including viral encephalitis, should be considered in the setting of fever and confusion without convincing alternative focus. Electrolyte abnormalities and thyroid hyper-or hypo-function should be considered. Consider silent coronary syndrome, at minimum by obtaining an ECG, either as cause of delirium or consequence of poor perfusion. Review all medications, particularly those that may be potentially sedating or anticholinergic, as well as alcohol intake. Head CT should be considered, especially in the presence of neurological deficit or suspicion of trauma.

Treatment is addressed to the underlying cause of the delirium and management of the agitated behaviour. If there is evidence of infection, appropriate antibiotics and supportive care should be commenced. Avoid iatrogenic exacerbation where possible, such as with indwelling urinary catheters, addition of multiple medications or physical restraints. Individual nursing is probably the most effective treatment. Families can be crucial in alleviating agitation and helping to re-orient patients. Transfer to a geriatric ward specialising in delirium management should be expedited.

Antipsychotics should be avoided if possible, but small doses (risperidone 0.25–1 mg, or haloperidol 0.5–1 mg) may be needed for paranoid and persecutory delusions or aggressive behaviour. Consultation with senior ED staff or the geriatric team should always be sought if you are considering the use of parenteral sedation for a very agitated patient, as there are considerable risks from over-sedation.

Syncope

Syncope, transient loss of consciousness with spontaneous recovery, is another common presenting problem. The incidence of syncope, the risk of a serious underlying cause, and of resulting injury, all rise with age. In frail patients, a very minor illness may exceed orthostatic or cardiorespiratory reserve.

The structure for considering the causes of syncope is similar to that in younger patients, but pay special attention to the following.

* Orthostatic syncope: common, due to a combination of insufficient autonomic responsiveness, medications or hypovolaemia. Always consider bleeding and infection. Longer prodrome is typical.
* Cardiogenic: consider arrhythmia, ischaemia or pulmonary embolus. Ask about palpitations, chest pain, exertional provocation and dyspnoea. Prodrome may be brief or absent.
* Neurocardiogenic (vasovagal, or 'faint') in response to a recognisable precipitant: more common in younger patients. Best considered a diagnosis of exclusion.

Pre-syncope, or light-headedness without loss of consciousness, should be considered in a similar way. Neurological events should be considered, but are very rarely a cause for true syncope and are not generally associated with spontaneous recovery. Significant headache or abdominal pain should prompt consideration of intracranial bleeding or aortic emergency respectively.

Consider past history, any medication changes and any associated symptoms, both before and following the episode. Examination is generally similar to that for falls. All patients should have an ECG, vital signs including postural blood pressure, blood glucose and haemoglobin. A period of cardiac monitoring, at least during initial assessment, is advised. Evaluate for infection, especially UTI. Other imaging and investigations should be tailored to particular circumstances and symptoms.

Ask about social situation (including walking aids, use of alcohol, support at home) bearing in mind the ability to get help if a similar episode recurs.

There should be a low threshold for admission. Cardiology consultation for a period of monitoring is considered for older patients without a clear orthostatic relationship to symptoms. Geriatric admission is considered for a more comprehensive approach to falls risk, functional decline, impaired orthostasis and polypharmacy. Repeated syncope in ED would indicate higher risk and need for admission. Patients who are still driving should be advised to discontinue until reviewed by their GP or until specialist follow-up investigations have been arranged.

Abdominal pain

Abdominal pain is another common cause for ED presentation, and risk assessment is markedly different in older patients. Surgery and mortality rates are much higher than in younger patients. Older patients are also more likely to present with vague and poorly localised abdominal symptoms and signs.

Common diagnoses include bowel obstruction, appendicitis (with a high rate of rupture and missed diagnosis), diverticulitis and biliary pathology. Other important diagnoses to consider include malignancy, aortic aneurysm and mesenteric ischaemia.

Constipation is a diagnosis of exclusion in the ED and not generally associated with pain or tenderness; a serious cause for the patient's abdominal symptoms and signs should be actively sought. Changes in bowel habit, including 'constipation', can result from serious abdominal pathology. Diarrhoea can equally distract. While infectious gastroenteritis is common, especially in RACF, also consider faecal impaction with overflow, and, if tenderness is present, the possibility of broader abdominal pathology.

Likewise, UTI is not normally a cause for significant abdominal pain or tenderness, and can distract. Urinary retention can cause pain, however, and should be screened for on history and/or with bedside scanning. Bladderscan® or similar devices are available in most EDs. Even in classical dysuria and frequency, maintain a sufficient differential diagnosis to consider other abdominal or pelvic pathology, especially if urine microscopy is normal.

Perform a thorough history and examination, including per rectal examination, which is invaluable for diagnosing faecal impaction or bleeding. Check for scars, hernias, atrial fibrillation (risk of embolism) and masses and femoral pulses. Investigations should include full blood count, renal and liver function tests and midstream urine (MSU). Consider lactate (usually by venous blood gas) if mesenteric ischaemia is suspected, but do not rely on a normal result to exclude it. A low threshold for imaging is required in general. CT is preferred to abdominal X-ray in most situations. Check renal function before arranging a contrast scan. Bedside ultrasound enables rapid assessment for aortic size and free fluid. A good rule of thumb to remember is that all patients with a tender abdomen on palpation should have a surgical review.

Carer stress

A number of geriatric ED presentations are prompted by the inability of the family, care-workers and neighbours to maintain the patient at home or access community services. A compassionate approach is required, as caring for older family members can be very difficult. Keep in mind that subacute or acute illness may also be present, but not yet clinically apparent. Involvement of the ED social worker and referral to community geriatric/aged care assessment team (ACAT) follow-up is important.

Disposition

It is recognised that an extended stay in ED, and indeed admission to hospital, carry risks for older patients. It remains the case, however, that older patients who present with non-specific symptoms take longer to assess than is available in the usual ED timeframe. Safe discharge will usually include secondary screening for any missed acute illness, mobility assessment, an evaluation of safe transport, ensuring access to essentials in the house and careful planning of follow-up with GP, community staff, residential care staff and carers.

Many EDs have a short stay unit for use in situations where ward admission is not predicted, to facilitate observation and review by senior staff. Such a unit should have strong links with both inpatient and community services, and in many hospitals will have dedicated embedded aged-care clinicians. Some hospitals have a geriatric medical assessment unit. In many hospitals, systems have been developed to provide significant senior clinical input early in the ED and post-admission phase, including ortho-geriatric (and other surgical support) services.

As a general rule, older patients should not be discharged at night, especially alone. Individual patients may wish to go home, and a high level of caution is required to ensure capacity, that adequate care is available both getting home and once there, and that the risk of falls or deterioration is low.

For patients living at home, especially without a well-developed care network, the threshold for inpatient admission is generally low. New incontinence, confusion or loss of safe independent mobility will usually prompt admission. Single-system illness may be better under the care of a specific specialty, as in the example of syncope above. If this decline in function is due to a relatively straightforward injury or illness, then other options, from Hospital in the Home to urgent RACF respite, may be appropriate, depending on local resources.

For patients living in a RACF, the question becomes whether care required can be delivered there. This may be facilitated by a call to the GP, to staff at the facility or by referral to an outreach service or Hospital in the Home. Listen to any concerns of family members, and ensure that the plan covers reasonably anticipated problems.

Finally, providing this care to the best of your ability can be deeply satisfying. Most of us can recognise people in our life—parents, grandparents—who may need this kind of care, and most of us will one day need it ourselves. While providing it is one of the great challenges facing emergency medicine and the health system in general over coming decades, it is also an opportunity to support the health of our community.

Editorial Comment

Always 'ask': is it safe to send the patient home? Also document pre-discharge observations, test their ability to mobilise, is the patient still in pain ... be cautious and treat patients as if they were your grandparents!

Recommended readings

Samaras N, Chevalley T, Samaras D, et al. Older Patients in the Emergency Department: A Review Australian and New Zealand Society for Geriatric Medicine Position Statement No. 14 The management of older patients in the emergency department. 2008.

Australian Institute of Health and Welfare 2017. Emergency department care 2016–17: Australian hospital statistics. Health services series no. 80. Cat. no. HSE 194. Canberra: AIHW. Retrieved from: https://www.aihw.gov.au/getmedia/981140ee-3957-4d47-9032-18ca89b519b0/aihw-hse-194.pdf.aspx?inline=true

NSW Civil & Administrative Tribunal (NCAT). NCAT Guardianship Division Fact Sheet. April 2016. Retrieved from: http://www.ncat.nsw.gov.au/Documents/gd_factsheet_person_responsible.pdf

Latham LP, Ackroyd-Stolarz S. Emergency department utilization by older adults: a descriptive study. Can Geriatr J. 2014;17(4):118–125.

Published 2014 Dec 2. doi:10.5770/cgj.17.108. Retrieved from: https://www.ncbi.nlm.nih.gov/pmc/articles/PMC4244125/

NSW Ministry of Health. Assessment and Management of People with Behavioural and Psychological Symptoms of Dementia (BPSD): A Handbook for NSW Health Clinicians. May 2013. Royal Australian & New Zealand College of Psychiatrists (RANZCP). Retrieved from: https://www.ranzcp.org/Files/Publications/A-Handbook-for-NSW-Health-Clinicians-BPSD_June13_W.aspx

Chapter 23
Infectious diseases
Emma Spencer and Richard Sullivan

Acknowledgment
The authors wish to acknowledge the content used from the previous edition of *Emergency Medicine* which was provided by Dr Melinda Berry.

Antibiotic prescribing
ED doctors commence life-saving antibiotic therapies during the course of their work. Good antibiotic stewardship is as essential in the ED as it is on the wards.

- A history of allergic reaction (don't miss the presence of a medic alert bracelet), the use of antibiotics prior to presentation and the collection of appropriate and timely cultures prior to the administration of therapy are all standard-of-care considerations.
- The rise of multi-resistant organisms over the last 40 years is well known. Using inappropriate antibiotics at inappropriate doses leads to the spread of resistant organisms. Patients with infections due to resistant bacteria experience delayed recovery, treatment failure and in some cases death.
- The use of the *Australian Therapeutic Guidelines* and consultation with the infectious diseases and microbiology services in your hospital is essential.
- Antibiotics are not harmless; for example, anaphylaxis and drug interaction between antibiotics and other commonly prescribed drugs can cause death.

Antibiotic recommendations in this book are largely based on eTG Therapeutic Guidelines (can be accessed via www.ciap.health. nsw.gov.au). The doses listed in this chapter assume normal renal function and no allergies.

CNS infections
BACTERIAL MENINGITIS

Most but not all adult patients with bacterial meningitis present with two of the following:

- fever
- headache
- neck stiffness
- altered mental state.

Elderly people, immunosuppressed people, people with chronic diseases such as diabetes and people who have had antibiotics prior to their presentation may have a more insidious onset of lethargy with few other signs.

Immediate action

If an assessment of bacterial meningitis has been made (see Figure 23.1), the following empirical antibiotics should be administered within 30 minutes of this initial assessment and should NEVER be delayed for CT or lumbar puncture. Steroids should be administered immediately prior to the antibiotics or with them. Antibiotics should not be delayed if dexamethasone is not available. For adults and children > 2 months:

- ceftriaxone 4 g IV daily (or 2 g IV 12-hourly)
  PLUS
- benzylpenicillin 2.4 g 4-hourly if patient is at risk of *Listeria monocytogenes* (Box 23.1)
  PLUS
- dexamethasone IV 10 mg (child 0.15 mg/kg, up to 10 mg).
  Also:
- add vancomycin if there is otitis media or sinusitis or Gram stain shows Gram-positive diplococci (pneumococci) or Gram-positive cocci resembling staphylococci.

Cultures

As empirical antibiotics are being drawn up and administered, take samples for culture:

- two sets of blood cultures
- swabs or aspirates of skin lesions
- urine cultures

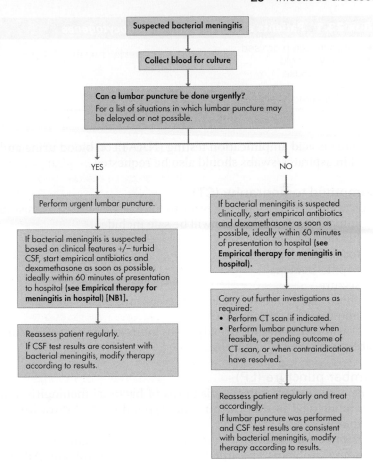

CSF = cerebrospinal fluid; CT = computed tomography
NB1: If clinical suspicion of bacterial meningitis is high, do not delay therapy while waiting for CSF test results.

Figure 23.1 Algorithm for management of suspected bacterial meningitis in adults and children

eTG complete [Internet]. Melbourne: Therapeutic Guidelines Limited; 2012 Jul.

Box 23.1 Patients at risk of *Listeria monocytogenes*
• Immunocompromised • > 50 years old • Alcohol abuse • Pregnant • Debilitated

+ nucleic acid amplification testing (NAAT) on blood urine and skin aspirates/swabs should also be requested.

Computed tomography (CT)

Indications for CT scanning prior to lumbar puncture to assist in deciding if lumbar puncture will be safe include:

+ history of CNS disease
+ focal neurological signs
+ papillo-oedema
+ seizure
+ abnormal/deteriorating level of consciousness
+ immunocompromised.

Antibiotics should already have been administered before patient proceeds to scanning.

Lumbar puncture (LP)

Early LP is essential in the diagnosis of bacterial meningitis and can be critical in determining the type, dose and duration of antibiotic.

Contraindications to LP *may* include anticoagulant therapy, bleeding problems and infection overlying the LP site. Advice should be sought *if a decision not to perform LP* is going to be made.

Note:

+ measure opening pressure
+ take off at least three bottles of CSF
+ write the clinical history clearly on the laboratory form, including HIV status, other underlying illnesses and antibiotics already given to the patient
+ ring the lab to advise that CSF is being sent to them.

HERPES MENINGOENCEPHALITIS

This is focal herpes simplex virus (HSV) infection of the cerebral cortex, especially the temporal lobe.

- Patients with herpes encephalitis are more likely to have altered mental state than those with bacterial meningitis.
- Although the distinction between meningitis and encephalitis can be blurred, encephalitis is distinguished by specific abnormalities of brain function (e.g. focal or generalised seizures, dysphasia, hemiparesis, motor or sensory deficits, altered behaviour and personality change).
- Meningitis, by comparison, is more likely to manifest as irritability and drowsiness but with intact mentation.
- **Treatment:** the disease may be hard to diagnose and patients presenting with the above should be treated as for bacterial meningitis with the addition of aciclovir 10 mg/kg IV 8-hourly to the empirical regimen until results on CSF are obtained.
- Once CSF cell count, differential, biochemistry and Gram stain are obtained, expert advice should be sought on rationalisation of the regimen.
- CT, or preferably MRI, can assist with the diagnosis acutely as inflammation of the temporal area is highly suggestive of HSV encephalitis (but may also be seen with other viruses).
- Viral DNA can be detected in CSF but it generally takes some time for the test to return, and therefore it is usually not helpful in the initial management.
- While herpes simplex is one of the most common treatable causes of encephalitis, other causes of encephalitis in Australia include autoimmune causes, varicella zoster virus, Murray Valley encephalitis, Hendra virus and enteroviruses. Empiric treatment with aciclovir should be commenced in all clinical cases while further laboratory testing is awaited. For further details see the Australian and New Zealand consensus guidelines for the investigation and management of encephalitis in adults and children (Britton et al. 2015).

Gastrointestinal infections
GASTROENTERITIS

- Typically, acute vomiting and non-bloody diarrhoea +/− abdominal cramps.
- Most commonly a self-limiting viral or non-invasive bacterial infection.
- There is no role for stool culture in uncomplicated cases.
- Fever and peritoneal signs may indicate invasive disease.
- Patients with HIV infection require particular consideration (see Chapter 24 The Immunosuppressed Patient).
- Bloody diarrhoea needs to be referred to your gastroenterology service.

Management

- Hydration (oral or IV) is the cornerstone of management.
- Adults present to the ED because they feel they are unable to tolerate liquid orally, and feel significantly better after IV fluids +/− an antiemetic.
- Empiric antibiotic treatment can be considered in patients who are immunocompromised, systemically unwell or who have severe abdominal pain, high-volume diarrhoea or blood in the stool. Any acute abdominal signs and symptoms need to be appropriately investigated.
- Use of empiric antibiotics in children with bloody diarrhoea is not recommended in specific cases as they can precipitate haemolytic uraemic syndrome. Seek expert advice.

Viral hepatitis
HEPATITIS A VIRUS (HAV)

- This acute self-limiting liver infection is transmitted by the faecal–oral route. It is endemic in developing countries and immunisation is recommended for travellers.
- The incubation period is 2–7 weeks. Clinical features include flu-like symptoms, fever, fatigue, nausea, then jaundice and dark urine. It is clinically indistinguishable from other causes of acute hepatitis.
- The diagnosis is serological.

- **Management** is supportive. Fulminant hepatitis is a rare complication of acute HAV infection but acute infection does not lead to chronic hepatitis.

HEPATITIS B VIRUS (HBV)

- This blood-borne virus is transmitted by parenteral or mucosal exposure to blood or body fluids, including sexually transmitted fluids.
- Acute infection: there can be markedly elevated prothrombin time that can indicate development of fulminant liver failure.
- Blood tests can detect HBV surface antigen, HBV core antibody and HBV surface antibody reflecting the infectivity or the immunisation status of the patient. A full panel of hepatitis serology should be ordered on anyone who is believed to have been exposed.
- Hepatitis B DNA and hepatitis B e-antigen are markers of viral replication.
- Less than 1% of patients will develop fulminant liver failure.
- The presence of HBV surface antigen beyond 6 months indicates persistent infection. Patients are at risk of progressing to cirrhosis and hepatocellular carcinoma.
- As indicated by normalisation of liver enzymes and loss of hepatitis B surface antigen, 95% of immune-competent adult patients will clear the virus over 3–4 months. The latter is replaced by hepatitis B surface antibodies. Immunity as a result of past infection is indicated by surface and core antibodies to hepatitis B. Immunity as a result of vaccination results in the development of surface antibodies only.

Immunisation has been part of the universal childhood vaccination program in Australia for more than 20 years. Adults in high-risk groups, such as healthcare workers, are also offered vaccination.

Hepatitis B immunoglobulin is also available and is used for passive immunity in non-immunised individuals following significant exposure to HBV-infected blood or bodily secretions. Vaccination is also commenced at this time. Be guided by your infectious diseases service, local post-exposure prophylaxis guidelines and *The Australian Immunisation Handbook*.

HEPATITIS C VIRUS (HCV)

This blood-borne virus is transmitted predominantly by percutaneous exposure to infected blood. It is prevalent in the injecting drug user population. Sexual contact and mother-to-infant transmission is less common than with hepatitis B infection.

- Acute infection is usually subclinical.
- Approximately 75% of those with acute HCV infection develop chronic hepatitis with the risk of cirrhosis and hepatocellular carcinoma.
- Treatment is highly successful with new direct acting antivirals. Treatment choice depends on cirrhotic status, treatment history and virus genotype. Refer to www.hepcguidelines.org.au for more information and seek expert advice.
- No vaccination is available.

HEPATITIS D VIRUS

This is found only in patients infected with hepatitis B. In developed countries, it is mostly found in the injecting drug user population. It increases the risk of fulminant hepatitis and the sequelae of chronic hepatitis.

HEPATITIS E VIRUS

Hepatitis E is an enterically transmitted self-limiting acute hepatitis similar to hepatitis A; fulminant disease is, however, more common than with hepatitis A, particularly in pregnant women. The disease is rare in developed countries.

Genitourinary infections
URINARY TRACT INFECTION (UTI)

Asymptomatic bacteriuria need not be treated, except in pregnant women. Asymptomatic bacteriuria is quite common in elderly patients.

Uncomplicated lower UTI

- Non-pregnant women
- No structural urinary tract abnormality
- No comorbidity such as diabetes
- *Escherichia coli* causes 90% of cases

Symptoms
- Burning on micturition
- Frequency
- Suprapubic discomfort
- Macroscopic haematuria

Investigations
Urinalysis and urine culture is part of the physical examination in suspected UTI.

Management (empiric for non-pregnant women)
- Trimethoprim 300 mg daily for 3 days.
- Urinary alkalinisation can give significant symptomatic relief but check drug interactions.

Pregnant women
- Treat all suspected UTIs in pregnancy. Infection in this group is associated with complications and a high risk of progression to pyelonephritis.
- Send urine for culture pre-therapy and 1 week post-therapy.
- Treatment is cefalexin 500 mg 12-hourly for 5 days (Therapeutic Goods Administration [TGA] Pregnancy Category A).
  Always consult the TGA category of risk posed by a particular antibiotic before prescribing it in pregnancy.

Men
Men with cystitis usually have an underlying urinary tract abnormality requiring investigation. Empirical treatment for cystitis is with trimethoprim 300 mg daily for 7 days.

ACUTE PYELONEPHRITIS
Symptoms of upper UTI include:
- fever, often with rigors/chills
- flank pain—bilateral or unilateral
- vomiting and dehydration are common.

Investigations
- Send urine and two sets of blood cultures to the laboratory.

- Routine imaging is not *always* necessary in uncomplicated pyelonephritis, but renal ultrasound should be performed in:
  — all men
  — pregnant women
  — diabetic patients
  — severe flank pain unresponsive to therapy
  — persistent fever
  — impaired renal function
  — severe infection.

Management
Mild infection can be treated with oral antibiotics such as amoxycillin + clavulanate 875 + 125 mg orally 12-hourly for 10–14 days, but often people present to the ED because these have failed or they are unable to keep the medication down.

- Empirical therapy for **severe infection** is:
  — gentamicin 4–5 mg/kg IV (in severe sepsis give 7 mg/kg IV) with subsequent dosing interval based on renal function + ampicillin 2 g IV 6-hourly
    OR
  — ceftriaxone 1 g IV daily if gentamicin contraindicated.
- IV fluid rehydration is essential in these cases, both for comfort of the patient and to maintain adequate circulation and protect the kidneys.
- Analgesia and antiemetics should also be administered.

Patients often feel better after a few hours and can then go home on cefalexin 500 mg 6-hourly for 10 days.

URINARY-CATHETER-RELATED INFECTION
- Asymptomatic bacteriuria and pyuria is common with long-term catheterisation.
- It should only be treated if symptomatic.
- Catheter change or removal is essential if treatment for a catheter-associated UTI is considered necessary.

ACUTE PROSTATITIS
- Tender perineum and prostate
- High fever, chills, back pain, perineal pain, dysuria, retention

- Send urine for culture
- Do not forget the possibility of a sexually transmitted infection—take a sexual history, consider testing for gonorrhoea and chlamydia and referral to a sexual health clinic

Management
- Trimethoprim 300 mg daily for 14 days in mild to moderate infection as empiric therapy (amoxycillin-clavulanate or cephalexin can also be used but adjust with microbiology results)
- Stool softeners
- For severe infection, seek Infectious Diseases advice

Sexually transmitted infection (STI)
- The presence of one STI implies potential exposure to every other STI and to pregnancy. All patients need referral to a sexual health clinic where follow-up, contact tracing, counselling and education can occur.
- Commencing treatment in the ED may have important public health benefits.
- Presenting complaints include:
  — genital lesions
  — vaginitis/vaginal/urethral discharge or dysuria
  — pelvic pain in women.

GENITAL LESIONS
Painful, vesicular lesions
- Likely to be herpes simplex infection.
- Swab the base of the ulcer and send for direct immunofluorescence/polymerase chain reaction (PCR) and culture.

Management
- Aciclovir 400 mg 8-hourly for 5 days
  OR
- valaciclovir 500 mg 12-hourly for 5 days.
- Frequent recurrences can be treated with suppressive therapy.

- Remember to provide pain relief such as topical lignocaine and oral analgesia, and beware of acute urinary retention in patients presenting with a first episode of genital herpes.

Solitary painless lesion
- Syphilitic chancre
- Diagnosis involves serology (EIA, TPPA and RPR), history, examination and PCR can also be requested
- Notifiable infection; requires referral to sexual health service

Treatment
- Benzathine penicillin 1.8 g or 2.4 million units (Bicillin L-A) or procaine penicillin 1.5 mg IM daily for 10 days (painful injection)

Wart-like lesions
- Human papilloma virus (HPV)
- Diagnosis is clinical
- Refer to sexual health clinic, gynaecologist or urologist for management

Itchy lesions
- Don't forget scabies and lice!

Management
- Topical treatments available over the counter are usually sufficient. Patient's clothing and bedding should be laundered.
- Transmission generally requires prolonged skin-to-skin contact.

VULVOVAGINITIS
- Inflamed, irritated vagina/labia with discharge.
- If discharge is from the cervix, manage as for cervicitis.
- If there is pelvic tenderness, manage as for pelvic inflammatory disease (PID; see later this chapter).
- Send swab for culture.

Trichomonas
- Not normal flora—sexually transmitted.
- Purulent malodorous discharge.
- Linked with pregnancy complications.
- **Treatment** is metronidazole 2 g PO single dose.

Candida
- Generally not sexually transmitted.
- Associated with antibiotic use, high oestrogen levels (e.g. oral contraceptive pill [OCP]) and poorly controlled diabetes.
- Clinically characterised by:
  — thick white discharge
  — pruritus
  — superficial ulceration/excoriation.
- Treatment is with topical anti-candidal creams (for 7 days in pregnancy) or a single dose of fluconazole 150 mg PO (not in pregnancy).

Bacterial vaginosis
- Polymicrobial overgrowth with anaerobes
- Generally not sexually transmitted
- Treat if symptomatic

Treatment
- Metronidazole 400 mg 8-hourly for 5 days

CERVICITIS
- Non-irritating vaginal discharge, seen to come from cervical os on speculum examination.
- Sexually transmitted infection—*Chlamydia trachomatis* and/or *Neisseria gonorrhoeae*.

Investigations
- Endocervical swab for PCR for gonorrhoea/chlamydia and culture.
- PCR for both chlamydia and gonorrhoea can also be performed.

Management
- Ceftriaxone 500 mg IM + azithromycin 1 g PO stat.

- If there is fever or pelvic pain, manage as for PID (see below).
- Refer to sexual health service for counselling, contact tracing and follow-up.

MALE URETHRITIS
- Urethral discharge or asymptomatic.
- May be detected as pyuria.
- Send first void urine for chlamydia/gonorrhoea PCR and if discharge present, swab for microscopy and culture.
- Coincident chlamydia infection in patients with gonorrhoeal urethritis leads to recommendation for treatment of both simultaneously:
  — ceftriaxone 250 mg IM + azithromycin 1 g PO stat.
- Refer to sexual health service for counselling, contact tracing and follow-up.

EPIDIDYMO-ORCHITIS
- Secondary to UTI or STI.
- If sexually transmitted, manage as for urethritis and refer to sexual health service.
- Otherwise, manage as per UTI in men.

PELVIC PAIN IN WOMEN
- Always exclude pregnancy by testing urine or blood, regardless of the history given.
- PID is common and often undiagnosed.
- **Beware a diagnosis of appendicitis or 'grumbling appendicitis' in a young woman. Urine should be sent for microculture and sensitivity and a Gonorrhoea and Chlamydia NAAT should also be requested.**

Pelvic inflammatory disease (PID)
- Thirteen per cent of women are infertile after a single episode.
- The risk of ectopic pregnancy increases 7-fold after one episode.
- It can also lead to pelvic adhesions and chronic pelvic pain.

Clinical features of PID
- Low-grade fever
- Pelvic tenderness
- Cervical discharge
- Palpable mass suggests tubo-ovarian abscess.

Most commonly PID is from a sexually acquired infection, but it can develop after termination of pregnancy or be associated with an intrauterine device (IUD) or other instrumentation of the uterus.

All PID is polymicrobial with endogenous flora.

Treatment—severe infection
- Azithromycin 500 mg IV daily
  PLUS
- ceftriaxone 2 g IV daily
  PLUS
- metronidazole 500 mg IV 12-hourly.

All women with PID should be referred to a gynaecologist for follow-up. For non-sexually acquired infection seek gynaecology and infectious diseases advice.

Needle-stick injuries and body fluids exposures
- Wash affected area/wound with water or saline.
- Irrigate affected mucous membranes/eyes (remove contacts) with water or saline.

RISK ASSESSMENT
- Determines need for testing and treatment
- Method of exposure (e.g. anal or vaginal insertive or receptive intercourse, occupational needle-stick injury, sharing of injecting equipment)
- Donor infection status or risk
- Immune status of recipient (e.g. HBV immunisation, tetanus immunisation)

BASELINE TESTING OF RECIPIENT
- Depends on risk assessment
- May include HIV antibody test, HBV and HCV serology, STI screen, pregnancy test

- Full blood count (FBC), liver function tests (LFTs), electrolytes for patients commencing post-exposure prophylaxis (PEP) for HIV
- Testing always requires appropriate counselling and follow-up

PROPHYLACTIC MEDICATION AND IMMUNISATIONS

Consider:

- HIV, HBV, HCV (see Box 23.2)
- tetanus immunisation
- prophylactic STI treatment
- pregnancy.

COUNSELLING AND FOLLOW-UP

- Occupational health service
- Sexual health service

Box 23.2　Prophylaxis for hepatitis B, hepatitis C and HIV

Hepatitis B
- Commence vaccination schedule if not immunised.
- If immune response post vaccination is unknown, test HBV surface antibody level.
- Consider giving HBV immunoglobulin to non-immune individuals within 72 hours if the source is, or strongly suspected to be, infected with HBV.
- Discuss with your infectious diseases service.

Hepatitis C
- Test with PCR at 1 month, antibody testing at 6 months.
- Refer to hepatologist or infectious diseases service for possible early therapy if PCR becomes positive and/or the patient develops acute HCV disease.

HIV
Situations where PEP may be appropriate:
- occupational exposure for healthcare workers
- sexual assault
- unprotected sex/broken condom
- contaminated injecting equipment.
  If PEP is indicated, it should commence as soon as possible; in general, PEP is not recommended after 72 hours.
  Follow protocols within your healthcare facility.
  (See also Post-exposure Prophylaxis in HIV in Chapter 24 The Immunosuppressed Patient.)

POST-SEXUAL ASSAULT PROPHYLAXIS

Refer patient to specialist sexual assault service.

Consider emergency contraception as well as STI treatment and post-exposure management as discussed earlier.

COMMUNITY NEEDLE-STICK INJURIES

The risk of HIV transmission in this situation is low. Tetanus prophylaxis is indicated.

Respiratory tract infection

See Chapter 39 Ear, Nose and Throat (ENT) Emergencies for information on upper respiratory tract infection.

LOWER RESPIRATORY TRACT INFECTION (LRTI)

(See Chapter 13 Respiratory Emergencies: The Acutely Breathless Patient.)

- Outpatient management of community-acquired pneumonia:
  - amoxycillin 1 g PO 8-hourly for 5–7 days
    OR
  - doxycycline 100 mg orally 12-hourly for 5–7 days especially if atypical organism suspected.
- Patients with moderate to severe pneumonia require inpatient management:
  - antibiotic recommendations are based on severity and local epidemiology; consult local hospital guidelines, or seek respiratory and infectious diseases advice.

Tuberculosis (TB)

- In developed countries, TB is found in migrant populations from high-prevalence countries and the itinerant population. It is also found in the Australian Indigenous population.
- Prolonged exposure to infected respiratory droplets is usually required for transmission to occur (e.g. household contacts). Patients with acid-fast bacilli seen on sputum smear are significantly more infectious than those without.
- Cellular immunity develops 3–8 weeks following exposure, causing a positive tuberculin test, and positive Interferon gamma release assay.

- TB can remain dormant for many years, 'latent TB infection' (LTBI), and may reactivate with immunodeficiency, immunosuppression and immunocompromise (including senescence of old age). In general, after exposure to TB infection, there is considered to be about a 5% lifetime risk of developing the disease. The first half of this risk (2.5%) is for progression to TB disease within 2 years of exposure. The other 2.5% risk is conferred lifelong, with an increasing risk in old age.
- Progressive primary infection can occur in the very young and immunocompromised/deficient/suppressed.
- Uncontrolled haematogenous spread causes disseminated disease.

CLINICAL FEATURES
- Anorexia, weight loss, fatigue
- Fever, night sweats
- Cough with purulent sputum +/− haemoptysis
- Pleural effusion/consolidation
- Note: Migration from a high-prevalence country and symptoms of cough lasting > 3 weeks with systemic features is highly suggestive of TB infection. Extrapulmonary TB may also occur, and should be carefully considered in patients with a chronic illness from a high-TB-prevalence country.

INVESTIGATIONS
- Sputum acid-fast staining and culture
- Specialist teams can perform PCR on relevant samples
- Chest X-ray (chest X-ray changes can be extensive despite the patient remaining comparatively well):
  — pneumonia with hilar adenopathy
  — apical changes
  — cavitating lesions
  — effusion.
- *Note:* In the immunocompromised/deficient/suppressed patient, the typical patterns of chest X-ray change are not sensitive. In end-stage HIV infection, 10% of people with pulmonary TB have a normal chest X-ray.

MANAGEMENT

TB is a notifiable disease that needs specialist management.

- Concurrent HIV infection needs to be considered.
- Public health staff perform contact tracing and prophylactic treatment of household contacts.
- Respiratory isolation (airborne precautions)/infection control should be initiated if TB is in the differential diagnosis to simplify public health measures once the diagnosis is confirmed.
- People with underlying TB can present to the ED with an intercurrent community-acquired LRTI and will need to be managed for this in addition to appropriate work-up for TB infection.
- The decision to isolate should first be addressed in the ED, and advice can be sought regarding whether this is necessary.

Severe sepsis

(See also Septic Shock in Chapter 5 Shock.)

- Sepsis is infection with a systemic inflammatory response.
- Severe sepsis is sepsis with acute organ dysfunction.
- Septic shock (high mortality, ~30%) is defined as:
  — sepsis with hypotension refractory to an initial fluid bolus OR
  — evidence of tissue hypoperfusion (lactate > 4 mmol/L).

Early aggressive resuscitation in the ED has been shown to improve outcome.

MANAGEMENT

- Prompt fluid resuscitation
  — 20–30 mL/kg fluid bolus on diagnosis.
- Take at least two sets of blood cultures simultaneously from different sites:
  — at least two sets percutaneously
  — at least one set from a vascular access device
  — culture other sites as clinically indicated.
- Administer antibiotics within 1 hour.
- Consult local protocols for guidelines on antibiotic choice.
- Insert central line and arterial line early.

Goals in the ED within 6 hours are as follows.

- Continue fluid resuscitation (crystalloid or colloid) to a central venous pressure (CVP) of 8–12 mmHg.
- Mean arterial BP > 65 mmHg using a vasopressor, such as a noradrenaline infusion once patient adequately fluid-resuscitated.
- Central venous oxygen saturation > 70% if sample from central venous catheter (CVC), or > 65% if mixed venous sample.
- Transfuse blood to haematocrit (HCT) ≥ 30% and/or dobutamine infusion (start at 2.5 microg/kg/min).
- Consult early with your infectious diseases service.
- Source control of infection; for example:
  - drainage of abscess, debridement of tissue
  - removal of foreign bodies (e.g. vascular access devices).

Meningococcal infection

- Invasive meningococcal disease is life-threatening. The course can be fulminant, with patients deteriorating within hours of the onset of symptoms.
- *Neisseria meningitidis* is a Gram-negative diplococcus with many serotypes. Vaccine is available for serotypes A, C, W, Y and also B.
- Transmission is via asymptomatic nasal carriage (~10% of the population).
- Invasive infection can manifest as meningitis sepsis. Both can be associated with a high mortality rate.

CLINICAL FINDINGS

The classic clinical findings of meningococcaemia are fever and a petechial or purpuric rash. Clinical features can be non-specific early in the course of disease, requiring a high index of suspicion and thorough clinical examination to make the diagnosis.

Early findings can also include:

- maculopapular rash that develops in the first 24 hours of illness
- myalgia which can be very painful
- cold extremities and pallor with fever.

Late signs (12–16 hours) are:
- meningism
- impaired consciousness
- shock.

Management:
- Pre-hospital antibiotics in meningococcal sepsis can be life-saving:
  — benzylpenicillin 2.4 g (child 60 mg/kg up to 2.4 g) IM or IV
    OR
  — ceftriaxone 50 mg/kg up to 2 g IM or IV.
- Draw blood cultures beforehand, but don't delay antibiotic therapy:
  — ceftriaxone 2 g IV 12-hourly.

INVESTIGATIONS
- Blood culture and *N. meningitidis* PCR
- Skin scrapings of purpuric lesions for Gram stain and culture
- CSF for culture and *N. meningitidis* PCR
- FBC, coagulation and biochemistry.

MANAGEMENT
- Antibiotic therapy as above.
- Further management as per severe sepsis.
- The local public health unit needs to be notified ASAP for all cases where invasive meningococcal disease is being considered. Discuss with your infectious diseases service.
- Droplet transmission precautions should be instituted for 24 hours after commencement of antibiotics.

CHEMOPROPHYLAXIS FOR MENINGOCOCCAL CONTACTS
This is the role of the public health department and infection control. Need for prophylaxis depends on exposure risk stratification.

Skin infections
(See also Chapter 42 Dermatological Emergencies.)

INFECTIOUS CELLULITIS

- Commonly seen in the lower limb in adults. Bilateral cellulitis is rare.
- Tinea pedis between toes is a common entry site.
- Wound-associated cellulitis is usually due to *S. aureus*, whereas 'spontaneous' cellulitis is usually group A streptococcal infection.
- Examination reveals erythema with or without lymphangitis. There may be enlarged and tender draining lymph nodes.

Management

- Management involves rest with immobilisation and elevation. Drawing a line around the border of the erythema provides some objective measure of progression or remission.
- For **mild disease**:
  — flucloxacillin/dicloxacillin 500 mg PO 6-hourly.
- **Indications for admission** to hospital include:
  — moderate to severe infection or rapidly spreading infection fever and tachycardia
  — systemically unwell patient
  — significant comorbidities such as diabetes (see below), immunosuppression, impaired lymphatic drainage of the affected area
  — cellulitis not improving with oral therapy.
- **Treatment:** flucloxacillin 2 g IV 6-hourly.
- Always consider risk factors for non-multiresistant methicillin-resistant *Staphylococcus aureus* (nmMRSA) and methicillin-resistant *Staphylococcus aureus* (MRSA) and adjust antibiotics as appropriate. Seek infectious diseases advice.

DIABETIC FOOT INFECTIONS

Diabetic foot infections are serious and can often become limb-threatening. Infection can progress rapidly. Have a low threshold for admitting these patients to hospital.

Infection can be polymicrobial and may need broader antimicrobial cover:

- amoxycillin + clavulanate 875 mg + 125 mg PO 12-hourly
  OR

- cephalexin 500 mg orally 6-hourly plus metronidazole 400 mg orally 12-hourly
  In severe infection:
- piperacillin + tazobactam 4 + 0.5 g IV 8-hourly.

BOILS AND CARBUNCLES
- Usually due to *S. aureus*.
- Incision and drainage is the main management principle.
- If there are systemic symptoms or spreading cellulitis, antibiotic therapy as for cellulitis can be used.
- Consider MRSA/nmMRSA in at-risk populations or unresolving infection.
- Follow-up of culture results is important.
- For empiric therapy give dicloxacillin/flucloxacillin 500 mg PO 6-hourly.

RAPIDLY PROGRESSING INFECTIONS (NECROTISING FASCIITIS)
Necrosis of the soft tissues can spread rapidly and be limb- and life-threatening.

It can be **polymicrobial**; for example:
- mixed aerobic and anaerobic bacteria.
  It can be a **single microbe**; for example:
- *Clostridium perfringens*
- *Streptococcus pyogenes*
- *Staphylococcus aureus*
- *Vibrio vulnificus*.

CLINICAL FEATURES
These can include:
- marked systemic toxicity out of proportion to local findings
- erythema, swelling, indiscrete margins
- severe pain
- crepitus cellulitis
- anaesthesia of overlying skin
- rapid spread (can spread widely in deep fascial planes with relative sparing of overlying skin)
- septic shock
- bullae.

MANAGEMENT

- Management requires urgent debridement of necrotic tissue and early antibiotics:
  - meropenem 1 g IV 8-hourly
    PLUS
  - vancomycin (including loading dose—consult local protocols)
    PLUS
  - clindamycin 600 mg IV 8-hourly.
- Mandatory surgical consultation and infectious diseases input at time of admission.

Wound infections

(See also Chapter 42 Dermatological Emergencies.)

- These are usually related to skin organisms and can be managed as for cellulitis (see above).
- Remove any foreign material such as sutures and clean/debride as appropriate.
- Some special circumstances are included under the following sections.

HUMAN AND OTHER ANIMAL BITE WOUND INFECTIONS

- Check tetanus immunisation status.
- Actively consider need for cleaning, debridement, irrigation, elevation and immobilisation.
- Take wound samples for microbiology.
- Routine antibiotics are recommended for:
  - wounds with delayed presentation
  - puncture wounds
  - wounds involving hands, feet or face
  - involvement of underlying structure
  - wounds in immunocompromised patients.
- If patient fits above criteria or signs of mild infection give:
  - amoxycillin + clavulanate 875 mg +125 mg PO 12-hourly for 5 days.
- If there is established moderate to severe infection, requires admission and parenteral antibiotic therapy:
  - piperacillin + tazobactam 4 + 0.5 g 8-hourly

OR

— ceftriaxone 1 g IV daily + metronidazole 400 mg PO 12-hourly.

• Therapy is modified on the basis of microbiological results and usually is 14 days total.

Water-related infections

These are complicated infections and advice should be sought from your infectious diseases service.

• Saltwater or brackish water exposure—consider *Vibrio* species infection and seek infectious diseases advice due to antibiotic susceptibility variation.
• As empiric therapy, consider addition of doxycycline 200 mg stat, then 100 mg 12-hourly to cellulitis treatment. If severe infection is present, add ceftriaxone to doxycycline.
• Freshwater or brackish water exposure can lead to infection with *Aeromonas* sp.
• Add ciprofloxacin 500 mg PO 12-hourly to cellulitis treatment.
• Coral cut infections are often caused by *Streptococcus pyogenes*, but need to consider marine organisms.
• Infection related to fish tank water can lead to *Mycobacterium marinum* infection, characterised by papular lesions.
• Requires referral for biopsy and infectious diseases expertise.

Herpes zoster (shingles)

Shingles is a reactivation of varicella (chickenpox) manifesting as a vesicular rash in a dermatomal distribution. A prodrome may precede the appearance of vesicles (e.g. pain, itch or other abnormal sensation at the site).

If more than one dermatome is involved or disease is disseminated, consider underlying immunosuppression/compromise/deficiency.

MANAGEMENT

• Antiviral therapy can reduce symptoms if commenced within 72 hours of rash onset for immunocompetent patients and

is also recommended for all immunocompromised patients irrespective of the duration of rash:
— valaciclovir 1 gram orally 8-hourly for 7 days
    OR
— aciclovir 800 mg 5 times a day for 7 days.

- Zoster of the first division of the trigeminal nerve requires special consideration as the cornea can be involved—consult an ophthalmologist.
- If disseminated disease, admit to hospital and seek infectious disease advice. IV aciclovir is required.
- Patients with shingles need pain relief to be prescribed for them.

Tetanus prophylaxis

The route of tetanus infection is commonly via contaminated puncture or laceration wounds that contain an anaerobic environment as a result of devitalised tissue. Tetanus is a preventable disease through immunisation and wound care.

The overseas traveller
TRAVELLER'S DIARRHOEA

- Commonly caused by enterotoxigenic *Escherichia coli* but Salmonella and Campylobacter are increasingly important causes.
- Norovirus is usually the cause in outbreak situations (e.g. cruise ships).
- Usually a self-limiting illness with only supportive oral rehydration necessary.
- Antibiotics can be considered in moderate to severe bacterial disease.
- Azithromycin 1 g orally as a single dose or norfloxacin 800 mg PO single dose.
- If there is fever or blood in the diarrhoea:
  — azithromycin 500 mg orally daily for 2–3 days
      OR
  — norfloxacin 400 mg PO 12-hourly for 2–3 days.
- Bloody diarrhoea should be referred to your gastroenterology service.
- Beware resistance to fluoroquinolones so seek infectious diseases advice for empiric therapy.

FEVER IN THE OVERSEAS TRAVELLER

The possible causes are numerous and may include malaria, dengue fever, typhoid, viral hepatitis, HIV (see Chapter 24 The Immunosuppressed Patient), melioidosis and other non-tropical infections such as influenza. The travel history, clinical features and epidemiological risks are particularly important. The CDC website offers global epidemiological information on important travel-related infections.

Febrile or unwell returned travellers should be referred to an infectious disease facility.

Malaria

- Fever in the overseas traveller is malaria until proven otherwise.
- Five *Plasmodium* species cause human malaria—*falciparum*, *vivax*, *ovale*, *malariae* and *knowlesi*.
- *Falciparum* causes most deaths directly related to malaria.

Presenting symptoms

- Clinical features are protean.
- Spiking fevers with temperatures up to 40°C.
- Headache, diarrhoea, abdominal pain.
- Can be non-specific 'flu-like' symptoms.
  Severe malaria is characterised by:
- altered level of consciousness and/or seizures (cerebral malaria)
- shock
- respiratory distress
- jaundice, anaemia, hypoglycaemia
- acidosis
- renal injury
- a high level of parasitaemia.

Investigations

- Rapid diagnostic tests
- Thick and thin films × three sets usually done daily for three days. *Note:* Detectable parasitaemia can lag behind symptoms:
  — thick blood film for identification of malarial parasites
  — thin blood film to determine malaria species.

Treatment

Treatment depends on the severity of disease. Intravenous artesunate is recommended for severe malaria while oral artemisinin base combination therapy used for uncomplicated or IV therapy. Primaquine may be needed to eliminate hypnozoites in some forms of malaria. G6PD needs to be excluded. Seek infectious diseases advice.

Dengue fever ('break bone fever')

Dengue can cause fever in a returned traveller and is present in Asia, Africa and the Americas. Outbreaks have previously occurred in North Queensland.

- Dengue is a mosquito-transmitted flavivirus with a short incubation period (4–7 days).
- Patients usually present with various combinations of fever, myalgia, arthralgia and rash. The rash is fine, may appear similar to sunburn and may not necessarily have been noticed by the patient. It may involve the palms and soles.
- Thrombocytopenia and leucopenia is often observed, as are elevated hepatic transaminases.
- Avoid non-steroidal anti-inflammatory medication.
- Clinically significant haemorrhagic disease and shock syndromes are seen in infants and in adults with secondary exposures. Care should be exercised in individuals who have had previous exposure to Dengue fever.
- Management is supportive and may include ICU.

Other viruses spread by mosquitoes which you may encounter include Zika and Chikungunya. Other rarer mosquito-borne infections do occur in returned travellers so seek infectious diseases advice.

Typhoid and paratyphoid fever

- Transmitted through food or water faecally contaminated with *Salmonella typhi* or paratyphi subtypes A, B and C.
- Vaccination (Table 23.1) is not completely efficacious.
- A history of vaccination does not exclude the diagnosis.

Table 23.1 Tetanus prophylaxis

Fully vaccinated (> 3 doses) in past	Time since vaccination or booster	Wound type	Give tetanus vaccination (ADT, DTP, tetanus toxoid)	Give tetanus immuno-globulin (< 24 h, 250 IU IM; > 24 h, 500 IU IM)
Yes	< 5 years	All wounds	No	No
	5–10 years	Minor clean wounds	No	No
		All other wounds	Yes	No
	> 10 years	All wounds	Yes	No
No	–	Minor clean wounds	Yes	No
		All other wounds	Yes	Yes

ADT = adult diphtheria and tetanus; DTP = diphtheria, tetanus and pertussis.
Source: Australian Immunisation Handbook.
*For immunocompromised patients, consult the handbook or seek expert advice.

- Symptoms:
  — classically, there is fever and abdominal tenderness initially with constipation
  — patient may also have confusion, rose spots (faint salmon-coloured maculopapular rash on the trunk) and hepatosplenomegaly
  — relative bradycardia is neither a sensitive nor a specific clinical finding but often looked for
  — untreated infection can lead to intestinal perforation.
- Diagnose by culturing blood and stool.
- **Treatment** is limited by widespread resistance. Laboratory testing for sensitivity is required.

Oral treatment
- Azithromycin 1 gram orally for 5 days
  or
- ciprofloxacin 12.5 mg/kg up to 500 mg orally bd for 7 days if susceptibility confirmed.

Intravenous treatment

- Ceftriaxone 2 g (child 1 month or older: 50 mg/kg), daily
- Ciprofloxacin 400 mg (child: 10 mg/kg up to 400 mg) 12-hourly until oral ciprofloxacin tolerated.

Online resources

Australian Immunisation Handbook
    https://immunisationhandbook.health.gov.au/
CIAP
    www.ciap.health.nsw.gov.au
ASHM (2016) National guidelines for post-exposure prophylaxis after non-occupational and occupational exposure to HIV). Commonwealth of Australia.
    https://www.ashm.org.au/products/product/978-1-920773-47-2
Therapeutic Guidelines Australia
    www.tg.org.au
Australasian Sexual Health Alliance. Australian STI Management Guidelines for use in Primary Care.
    www.sti.guidelines.org.au
Britton P, Eastwood K, Paterson B, et al. (2015) Consensus guidelines for the investigation and management of encephalitis in adults and children in Australia and New Zealand. Internal Medicine Journal. 45:563–575.

Chapter 24
The immunosuppressed patient

Sarah C Sasson, Judy Alford and Anthony Kelleher

Overview

Immunosuppressed patients present with emergencies related to an increased susceptibility to infection, non-infective adverse effects of immunosuppression and to their underlying condition.

- The most frequently encountered causes of immunocompromise vary according to the location and specialisation of the institution. Malignancy, human immunodeficiency virus (HIV) infection and solid-organ transplant are among the commonest conditions.
- Other causes of immunocompromise are immunosuppressive and/or cytotoxic therapy for non-malignant disease, post splenectomy, congenital immune defects and marrow failure due to drugs or infection.

Immunosuppressed patients can present with common, prolonged, recurrent or unusual infections. The signs and symptoms of infection are often diminished, and patients may present with subtle and non-specific findings and deteriorate rapidly. Fever may be the sole presenting symptom, but even that may be masked by the presence of drugs such as corticosteroids. Therefore, ***infection must be considered in the differential diagnosis of the immunocompromised patient presenting with non-specific symptoms***.

Immune system failure

The immune system consists of innate and adaptive components.

- Innate immunity stems from intact epithelial barriers, phagocytic cells (neutrophils and macrophages), natural killer cells and the complement system. Innate immunity does not require prior exposure to the infective agent for rapid activation.

- Adaptive immunity is conferred by lymphocytes and their products.
  — T-cells act against intracellular microbes and provide cell-mediated immunity.
  — Humoral immunity is conferred by B-cells and the antibodies they produce, which are active against extracellular microbes.

Failure of a component of the immune system leads to vulnerability to different infective agents.

- T-cell defects occur in acquired immune deficiency syndrome (AIDS), immunosuppressive therapy and congenital severe combined immune deficiency (SCID) and result in patients susceptible to:
  — bacterial sepsis
  — infections with intracellular bacteria (tuberculosis [TB])
  — viral infections (cytomegalovirus [CMV], Epstein–Barr virus [EBV], varicella)
  — fungal infections (candidiasis, aspergillosis), and
  — protozoal infections (cryptosporidium, toxoplasmosis).
- B-cell and humoral defects occur in haematological malignancies including myeloma, AIDS and congenital disorders such as common variable immune deficiency.
  — Patients are predisposed to infection by encapsulated bacteria (***Haemophilus influenzae type B, Streptococcus, meningococcus***), staphylococci, and enterovirus.
- Granulocyte defects including neutropenia result from chemotherapy, bone marrow aplasia or infiltration, drug reactions, myelodysplasia and rarely from congenital defects. Patients are vulnerable to infection by:
  — Gram-negative bacilli including *Pseudomonas*
  — Gram-positive cocci such as staphylococci and viridans streptococci, and
  — fungi such as candida and aspergillosis.
- Complement defects lead to susceptibility to infection with encapsulated and pyogenic bacteria, as well as predisposing to autoimmunity.
- Asplenia predisposes to severe infections due to encapsulated bacteria.

In addition to infections, fever in the immunocompromised patient may be due to malignancy, drug side effects or allograft rejection.

MANAGEMENT

Improvements in the management of the conditions associated with immunodeficiency have led to improved long-term survival and better quality of life for these patients. Nonetheless, there remains the potential for severe infections with rapid deterioration and death.

- Prompt assessment and timely, appropriate investigation is crucial; early institution of broad-spectrum antibiotics, application of treatment protocols for sepsis and the use of ventilatory support where indicated. Broad-spectrum antibiotics should be considered in less acutely unwell patients.
- Non-infective causes such as rejection must be determined, especially in transplant patients.
- Early ICU referral and a team approach involving treating haematologists, oncologists, HIV and other medical specialists and/or transplant doctors is essential in the deteriorating patient.
- The patient's wishes should be ascertained early, particularly in those with severe advanced disease or chronic progressive conditions that have been unresponsive to intervention.

Cancer patients

Cancer patients are at risk of severe infection due to immunosuppression induced by their disease and its treatment. Most at-risk are patients undergoing therapy for haematological malignancies or stem-cell transplant, who have severe and prolonged neutropenia. The risk of infection rises as the neutrophil count falls.

FEBRILE NEUTROPENIA
Clinical features

Febrile neutropenia is defined as fever with temperatures above 38.0°C in a patient with a neutrophil count $< 0.5 \times 10^9$/L or $< 1.0 \times 10^9$/L with a predicted decline to $< 0.5 \times 10^9$/L.

- Associated signs of infection may be present, such as tachypnoea, tachycardia, altered mental state, dehydration and acidosis.
- Localising signs may be absent; however, a thorough examination of the lungs, oropharynx, skin, catheters, perineum and perianal area, sinuses and urinary tract is essential and may reveal the site of infection.

Non-specific symptoms in the absence of fever may still indicate infection, especially if the patient is on high-dose corticosteroids.

Investigations

- Investigations should include:
  — urea, electrolytes and creatinine (UEC)
  — full blood count (FBC)
  — liver function tests (LFTs)
  — chest X-ray
  — urinalysis and midstream urine culture (MSU) and sensitivity if indicated
  — swabs from any skin lesions
  — sputum microculture and sensitivity (M/C/S)
- Two sets of blood cultures should be obtained, one from any indwelling catheter that may be present. Swabs should be sent from any lesions or catheter insertion sites. There should be a low threshold for the collection of specimens for culture.
- Cerebrospinal fluid (CSF) is not routinely cultured but should be if CNS infection is suspected. However, in the rapidly deteriorating patient, or in those with a coagulopathy, lumbar puncture may need to be delayed or forgone. Antibiotic administration should not be delayed by the need for lumbar puncture.
- Stool should be sent for culture if diarrhoea is present. The patient with abdominal signs will require imaging by ultrasound or computed tomography (CT); however, this should not delay surgical consultation, as signs of peritonitis are minimal in the neutropenic patient.
- CT scans of the sinuses should be obtained if there is facial pain or swelling, as severe, invasive fungal sinusitis can occur in these patients.

Management
Broad-spectrum antibiotics
Broad-spectrum antibiotics should be started immediately after cultures have been obtained. Delay in initiating appropriate antibiotic therapy is associated with increased mortality. Coverage for Gram-negatives, including *Pseudomonas*, is essential.

Recommended regimens vary between institutions. The following antibiotics are suitable:

- ceftazidime 2 g IV 8-hourly
- piperacillin 4 g + tazobactam 0.5 g IV 8-hourly
- ticarcillin 3 g + clavulanate 0.1 g IV 6-hourly
- gentamicin 4–6 mg/kg IV daily
- cefepime 2 g IV 12-hourly.

Vancomycin
Gram-positive bacteraemia due to *Staphylococcus aureus*, Strep viridans streptococci and enterococci is very common. The routine use of vancomycin is not recommended, although it should be given if the patient is in shock, is known to have methicillin-resistant *Staphylococcus aureus* (MRSA) or has a clinically infected catheter.

- The recommended dose is 30 mg/kg up to 1.5 g IV 12-hourly, with adjustment according to renal function and serum levels.
- Vancomycin is often added if fever persists beyond 48 hours.

Antifungals
Antifungals are not routinely used in the initial treatment of febrile neutropenia, unless there is evidence of fungal infection such as sinusitis. They may be introduced when fever persists beyond 96 hours, especially in patients with pulmonary infiltrates but in this case other causes of atypical pneumonias should also be considered.

A subgroup of low-risk neutropenic patients may be managed at home with oral therapy. This should only be done in consultation with the treating haematologist or oncologist.

Colony-stimulating growth factors
Recombinant colony-stimulating growth factors may be used in high-risk patients with sepsis or organ failure, after consultation with a haematologist or the patient's treating doctor.

Non-invasive ventilation (NIV)
NIV used early in the course of hypoxaemic respiratory failure may reduce the need for intubation and improve survival.

Fever in the non-neutropenic cancer patient
Cancer patients with a normal granulocyte count remain susceptible to infections when their adaptive immune response is impaired by treatment with steroids or chemotherapy, or by haematological malignancy.

- T-cell defects increase the risk of infection with intracellular pathogens including *Pneumocystis jirovecii* pneumonia (PJP), mycobacteria including non-tuberculosis mycobacteria and fungi.
- Patients with impaired humoral immunity are at risk of infection by encapsulated bacteria, often manifesting as pneumonia.

COMPLICATIONS OF TARGETED AND IMMUNOTHERAPY FOR CANCER
There has been widespread uptake of treatments targeted at specific receptors, ligands or mediators involved in tumour cell replication or killing.

- Monoclonal antibodies to tumour cell ligands enable cell killing.
- Monoclonal antibodies to tumour growth factors stop replication.
- Monoclonal antibodies to vascular growth factors stop tumour angiogenesis.
- Tyrosine kinase inhibitors interrupt mechanisms of intracellular signalling.
- Stimulation of the host immune system using chimeric antigen receptor modified T-cells and immune checkpoint inhibitors increases activity against tumour cells.

Cytokine release syndrome
This SIRS-like reaction occurs after infusions of drug targeting the immune response, leading to marked elevations in circulating inflammatory mediators, particularly IL-6. There is a spectrum of severity from fever and tachycardia, myalgias and rash,

to hypotension, bronchospasm and multiple organ dysfunction. Differentiation from anaphylaxis may be difficult, although angio-oedema is absent.

Management involves antipyretics, antihistamines, corticosteroids and fluid resuscitation.

Severe cases may need referral to intensive care for organ support. The use of antibodies directed against IL-6 carries further risks, but may be indicated in rare, life-threatening cases.

Autoimmunity

Stimulation of the host immune system can lead to immune-mediated tissue damage in various organs. A spectrum of symptoms from rashes, subclinical hepatocellular dysfunction or hypothyroidism, through to colitis, hepatitis, pneumonitis, myocarditis or pituitary axis dysfunction may occur.

The differential diagnosis includes innate autoimmune diseases, tumour related or paraneoplastic syndromes and infection.

Central nervous system toxicity

Encephalopathy, seizures, tremor, ataxia and cerebral oedema are known adverse reactions to immunotherapy with CAR T-cells and bispecific antibodies.

The differential diagnosis includes infection and metastatic disease, and antimicrobial treatment is usually required. High-dose corticosteroids are the only current treatment for neurotoxicity.

Cardiovascular toxicity

Inhibition of VEGF can cause adverse effects in the patient's vascular system:

- hypertension, ranging from mild to a severe pre-eclampsia-like syndrome
- proteinuria, altered GFR
- increased risk of thrombosis, cardiac events and cardiomyopathy.

HER2 inhibitors, a common breast cancer treatment, can cause cardiac failure.

Tyrosine kinase inhibitors can cause pulmonary hypotension, QT prolongations and systemic vascular thrombosis.

Some patients will be treated with prophylactic antiplatelet or antithrombotic drugs. The treatment of cardiovascular events should proceed as per standard guidelines. Of note, corticosteroids may worsen the risk of vascular complications.

NON-INFECTIOUS COMPLICATIONS OF CANCER AND ITS TREATMENT

Spinal cord compression

This is most common in the thoracic spine (70% of cases), although it may involve any level. It is most frequently due to metastatic breast, lung or prostate cancer, or lymphoma. An epidural abscess or discitis should be considered in patients who have had lumbar puncture or intrathecal therapy, or who are at risk of bacteraemia.

Pain usually occurs before the development of neurological symptoms. Once symptoms such as weakness, sensory loss and sphincter dysfunction begin, treatment must occur within hours to give the patient a chance of good recovery.

Investigations

- Plain films of the spine show tumour in 70–90% of cases.
- Urgent MRI will localise the lesion.

Management

1 Obtaining MRI images should not delay treatment with corticosteroids in the patient with neurological signs. An initial dose of dexamethasone 20 mg IV is followed by 4 mg IV 6-hourly.
2 Radiotherapy to the affected area is the treatment of choice, with surgery used in selected cases with spinal instability.

Hypercalcaemia

(See Chapter 21 Acid–Base and Electrolyte Disorders.)

Superior vena cava (SVC) obstruction

The SVC may be obstructed by compression, infiltration or thrombosis, and this is usually a complication of malignancy (particularly lung, breast, testicular cancer or lymphoma). Occasionally it occurs as a complication of a central venous catheter (CVC) or benign lesion (e.g. goitre, constrictive pericarditis or aortic aneurysm).

- Symptoms and signs are more prominent when the patient is supine, including periorbital and facial oedema (also trunk, arms), shortness of breath, cough, chest pain and dysphagia.
- On examination there may be neck vein distension, facial plethora, cyanosis and tachypnoea.

Investigations
- An important differential diagnosis is pericardial tamponade. A bedside ultrasound scan can rule out pericardial effusion.
- Chest X-ray usually reveals a mass in the mediastinum, which may be accompanied by pulmonary lesions or a pleural effusion.

Management
1 Treatment is directed at the tumour and involves radiotherapy or chemotherapy.
2 Elevating the head of the bed can alleviate some symptoms. Corticosteroids may be useful if the tumour is responsive.
3 SVC stenting is a further treatment option.

Tumour lysis syndrome
This occurs within days of commencing treatment for sensitive tumours, although it may occur spontaneously. Rapid cell death releases products of cell breakdown into the circulation, leading to hyperuricaemia, hyperkalaemia, hyperphosphataemia and hypocalcaemia. Renal failure and metabolic acidosis may develop. It most frequently complicates haematological malignancies and small-cell lung cancer.

The clinical manifestations include neuromuscular cramps, tetany and arrhythmias. Oliguria and acute renal failure may develop from uric acid precipitation in the renal tubules.

Management
1 Initial treatment is hydration with normal saline and treatment of hyperkalaemia.
2 Urinary alkalinisation (50–100 mg $NaHCO_3$/L fluid, urine pH > 7) is of benefit in hyperuricaemia; however, in the presence of hyperphosphataemia and hypocalcaemia, alkali therapy can exacerbate symptoms.

3 Once adequate hydration has been established, diuretics may be added to maintain a high urine output.

4 Severe cases complicated by acute renal failure may require dialysis.

HYPERVISCOSITY

Very high white blood cell (WBC) counts ($> 10 \times 10^9$/L) associated with haematological malignancies (acute leukaemias, chronic myeloid leukaemia (CML)) cause increased blood viscosity, which impairs flow in the microcirculation. The cerebral and pulmonary circulations are particularly susceptible. Hyperviscosity syndrome also occurs with high levels of paraproteinemia, especially with immunoglobulin M (IgM) paraproteins, such as in Waldenstrom's macroglobulinaemia.

- Impaired cerebral circulation causes headache, dizziness, confusion, seizures and visual disturbance. The fundi show venous engorgement and haemorrhages.
- Cardiopulmonary consequences include angina, dyspnoea, myocardial infarction and cardiac failure.
- There may be bleeding from mucosal surfaces.

Management

1 Treatment begins with hydration.
2 Patients should be referred for leukapheresis or plasmapheresis.

HIV INFECTION

Patients with HIV infection most commonly present with complications of immunosuppression and its treatment. With the improved prognosis of HIV in the era of combination antiretroviral treatment (ART), patients increasingly present with medical or surgical conditions unrelated to HIV and, while their treatment may be complicated by their HIV, their outcome and survival can be excellent.

Primary HIV infection

Within 1–6 weeks of infection (sometimes up to 12 weeks), 50–70% of patients develop a symptomatic illness. In most cases this is mild to moderate in severity and does not usually present to the ED.

- The seroconversion illness can resemble infectious mononucleosis.
- Patients develop fever, fatigue, anorexia, headache, nausea and vomiting.
- Myalgias and arthralgias, a non-exudative pharyngitis, rashes and diarrhoea are common.
- Severe cases may develop meningism or encephalitis.

Investigations

The differential diagnosis is wide, so investigations should include FBC, UEC, LFTs and monospot, along with serology for cytomegalovirus (CMV), Epstein–Barr virus (EBV), hepatitis and syphilis. In those with a recent high-risk exposure it is important to think of the diagnosis. In more severe cases, immunosuppression may be profound, and the seroconversion illness may be complicated by an opportunistic infection. Not uncommonly, other sexually transmitted infections (STIs) may occur at the same time and should be screened for.

Current HIV-1 antibody tests are usually positive by 2 weeks after the onset of symptoms (4 weeks after exposure), but earlier-generation enzyme immunoassay (EIA) tests may be negative or give indeterminate results.

Prior to antibody responses the virus can be detected by direct detection of viral p24 antigen or by nucleic acid amplification tests such as proviral DNA tests. Assays of plasma HIV-1 RNA used for monitoring HIV infection may pick up the presence of virus prior to the production of antibodies in this early stage of the infection; however, they have a substantial false positive rate in low seroprevalence settings and can give a false negative result with certain strains of the virus. Therefore, this test should not be used diagnostically.

Management

During the first 6 months of HIV infection, there is uncontrolled viral replication and destruction of CD4+ T-cells. Presentation with a severe seroconversion illness is associated with faster disease progression. There is now a strong evidence-base demonstrating that patients with HIV infection benefit from early initiation of ART (i.e. even when CD4+ T-cell counts are above 500 cells/microL) in terms of reducing related morbidity and mortality. Patients should be referred to a specialist in HIV medicine early regarding initiation of treatment, particularly those with symptomatic seroconversion.

Patients should also receive risk-reduction counselling as, with the high levels of virus circulating in these patients, they are highly infectious and likely to pass on the infection to others.

OPPORTUNISTIC INFECTIONS (OIS)

- A wide range of OIs affect HIV patients once their CD4+ T-cell counts decline. Information that helps narrow the differential diagnosis includes a recent CD4+ T count and viral load, use of antiretrovirals and prophylaxis.
- The knowledge of previous serology for infections such as CMV and toxoplasmosis is very useful, as presentations with these opportunistic infections (OIs) most often represent recrudescence of previously controlled latent infections.
- Patients presenting for the first time with late-stage disease, or those that have not sought medical care, may present with multiple opportunistic infections and/or malignancies such as lymphoma and/or CNS disease simultaneously. This should be considered in the diagnostic work-up.
- Bacterial infections are common in HIV patients, and bacterial sepsis is a more frequent cause of ICU admission than pneumonia (PJP; see below). Sources include pneumonia, catheter-related infections, orthopaedic and soft-tissue infections, urinary tract infections (UTIs) and bacteraemia of unknown aetiology.

PULMONARY INFECTIONS

The incidence of HIV-associated pneumonia changed with the use of combination ART, with bacterial pneumonia becoming increasingly common. Pneumonia in HIV patients is more often bacterial than due to an opportunistic agent and is 10 times more common in HIV patients than in non-HIV patients. The common community-acquired bacteria are the usual culprits, with most pneumonia being caused by *Streptococcus*.

Pneumocystis jirovecii (carinii) pneumonia (PJP)

Since the introduction of HAART in 1996, the incidence of PJP as an AIDS-defining illness has declined, although it remains the most frequent serious opportunistic infection. The disease occurs in patients with a CD4+ count below 200 cells/microL, particularly when antibiotic prophylaxis has not been used.

Fever, cough and shortness of breath are the usual presenting symptoms of PJP. The respiratory examination may reveal few signs other than tachypnoea and accessory muscle use. Oxygen saturations are often reduced, and severe cases may be cyanosed at presentation.

Investigations
- Chest X-ray typically reveals bilateral diffuse reticular or granular opacities. The extent of these changes may be less than expected by the degree of hypoxaemia.
- Arterial blood gas analysis assists in grading severity and planning treatment.
  — Mild to moderate cases have an arterial partial oxygen pressure (PaO_2) of > 70 mmHg on room air (A–a gradient < 35 mmHg, or O_2 saturations > 94% on room air).
  — Severe cases have a PaO_2 of < 70 mmHg on room air (A–a gradient > 35 mmHg, or O_2 saturations < 94% on room air).

Diagnosis
A provisional diagnosis is made on clinical findings and chest X-ray. Definitive diagnosis requires direct visualisation of cysts or trophic forms from respiratory specimens (induced sputum or broncho-alveolar lavage).

Management
1 Trimethoprim-sulfamethoxazole is the treatment of choice for mild to moderate PJP, in oral doses of 5 mg/kg + 25 mg/kg to 7 mg/kg + 35 mg/kg 8-hourly for 21 days.
  — If sulfamethoxazole is contraindicated, clindamycin 450 mg 8-hourly plus primaquine 15 mg daily may be used.
  — Dapsone 100 mg PO daily with trimethoprim 300 mg PO 8-hourly is a further alternative.
  — Patients who are also intolerant of trimethoprim or clindamycin can be treated with atovaquone 750 mg PO 12-hourly.

2 Severe disease is treated with intravenous trimethoprim-sulfamethoxazole 5 mg/kg + 25 mg/kg IV 6-hourly for 21 days.
  — Patients who are intolerant of or unresponsive to this may be treated with IV pentamidine 4 mg/kg up to 300 mg daily, or clindamycin 900 mg IV 8-hourly with primaquine 30 mg PO daily.
3 Pulmonary inflammation contributes to lung injury in PJP, so corticosteroids are given in severe disease. Prednisolone is given at 40 mg PO 12-hourly for 5 days, then 40 mg daily for 5 days, then 20 mg daily for 11 days.
4 Antibiotic cover for community-acquired pneumonia may be added, particularly when the patient has purulent sputum.
5 Non-invasive positive-pressure ventilation is indicated in the non-obtunded patient with hypoxaemic respiratory failure, and it may avert the need for mechanical ventilation. Unless there are clear contraindications to intubation, such as end-stage malignancy or dementia, intubation and ventilation are appropriate in the patient with severe respiratory failure, as the prognosis from a first episode of PJP is good. Recurrent episodes may be complicated by cyst formation and pneumothorax.

TUBERCULOSIS (TB)

Worldwide, this is the most important HIV-associated opportunistic pneumonia. Reactivation or primary infection can occur at high CD4+ T-cell counts (> 400 cells/microL) and the disease becomes more common with declining counts. In the severely immunocompromised, extrapulmonary sites of infection are more frequent.

Presenting symptoms are cough, haemoptysis, fever, shortness of breath, sweats and weight loss. The onset is typically insidious. The diagnosis is more likely in patients from countries where TB is endemic.

Investigations and diagnosis

Chest X-ray can show upper lobe cavitation or hilar adenopathy with diffuse infiltrates. Pleural effusions may be present. Miliary TB is uncommon in patients with poor cell-mediated immunity. Extrapulmonary manifestations or presentations are more common in patients with HIV infection.

Diagnosis remains difficult, as sputum microscopy is often negative, but PCR assays are useful, though a negative result does not exclude the diagnosis. Fine-needle aspiration of extrapulmonary sites is often diagnostic. Differentiation from atypical mycobacterial infection is essential.

Management

Treatment is specialised, involving multiple agents and complicated by interactions between antiretrovirals and antitubercular drugs. Early specialist referral is essential. If the diagnosis of open TB is considered likely, the patient must be isolated, ideally in a negative-pressure room.

CENTRAL NERVOUS SYSTEM (CNS) INFECTIONS

A number of agents infect the CNS, causing the acute or subacute onset of seizures, headache, fever, neck stiffness, confusion or focal deficits. However, symptoms may be non-specific and space-occupying lesions may be present in the absence of clinical signs. Therefore, there should be a low threshold for the performance of a CT scan and/or lumbar puncture in patients with late-stage HIV infection. With the increasing longevity of these patients and the increased risk of vascular complications, cerebrovascular accident (CVA) should be included in the differential diagnosis of CNS presentations.

Cryptococcus neoformans

This fungus causes meningitis in patients with CD4+ counts <100 cells/microL. Cryptococcal meningitis presents with the subacute onset of fever, headache, nausea and cranial nerve palsies. Cryptococcomas are rare.

Investigations

Lumbar puncture is diagnostic, with demonstration of the organism on India-ink staining or antigen testing. The CSF opening pressure is usually elevated.

Management

1 Treatment is with amphotericin B and flucytosine (seek expert consultation).

2 In cases with very high CSF pressures, urgent ophthalmology review is needed, as vision may be threatened.
3 Patients may need repeated lumbar punctures for CSF drainage.
4 Long-term prophylaxis is given with fluconazole (seek expert consultation).

Toxoplasma gondii

This protozoon is widespread in the community, but it rarely causes disease until CD4+ T-cell counts drop below 100 cells/microL. The incidence is decreased with prophylaxis with trimethoprim and sulfamethoxazole.

Presenting features are altered mental state, focal signs, headache, fever and seizures.

Investigations

The diagnosis is made by contrast CT, which shows ring-enhancing lesions, but is not diagnostic.

Toxoplasma serology is supportive, and cerebral toxoplasmosis is very unlikely in a patient with negative serology. If this is the case or if there is a poor response to therapy, consider primary CNS lymphoma.

Management

1 Treatment is with sulfadiazine 1 g PO or IV 6-hourly oral pyrimethamine 50 mg loading dose then 25 mg daily, for 6 weeks.
   — Clindamycin 600 mg PO 8-hourly is used if the patient is hypersensitive to sulphonamides.
   — If sulfadiazine is used, folinic acid 20–25 mg/day should be added to reduce marrow toxicity.
2 Anticonvulsants should be started to prevent seizures.
3 The use of steroids is not recommended, unless the lesions are associated with substantial oedema and exerting significant mass effect.

AIDS dementia

Patients with **HIV-associated dementia** exhibit a gradual decline in memory and/or psychomotor function, ataxia and personality changes. It may also present with signs of spinal cord myelopathy. The syndrome usually affects patients with CD4+ T-cell counts below 200 cells/microL but may occur earlier. Drugs, infections and metabolic derangements can exacerbate dementia in affected patients. CT scans of the brain show atrophy.

There is no specific treatment, although combination ART may improve symptoms.

Progressive multifocal leukoencephalopathy (PML)

Progressive CNS infection with JC virus (John Cunningham virus) usually occurs in patients with CD4+ T-cell counts below 100 cells/microL. PML presents with seizures, focal weakness, cranial nerve palsies, visual field deficits, cerebellar signs and confusion.

Investigations

- CT scans are relatively insensitive and, while these may reveal focal hypodensities, they are often non-contributory.
- MRI usually shows characteristic white-matter changes with cortical sparing; the absence of these changes does not exclude the diagnosis, however.
- JC virus can be identified in CSF by PCR, but this test is offered only in specialist laboratories.

Management

Combination ART may improve symptoms; however, there is no specific treatment.

GASTROINTESTINAL (GI) TRACT INFECTIONS

Candidiasis

GI tract infections frequently affect the oropharynx and/or the oesophagus, to an extent that is unusual in immunocompetent patients. Oesophageal candidiasis presents with oropharyngeal or retrosternal pain, dysphagia or odynophagia. There may be bleeding. White plaques with underlying erythema cover the affected areas.

Management

1 While simple oral candida will respond to topical treatment with amphotericin or nystatin solutions or lozenges,

oesophageal involvement requires systemic treatment with fluconazole 200–400 mg PO daily for 14–21 days or, occasionally, itraconazole 200 mg PO daily for 14 days.

2 Resistant cases may be treated with voriconazole or posaconazole.

3 Fluconazole may be used for secondary prophylaxis or maintenance therapy.

Cyclospora, Isospora, *Cryptosporidium parvum*
These may all cause chronic diarrhoea; however, frequency is less common in the era of combination ART. These infections should be considered in those presenting with chronic gastrointestinal symptoms, especially if resistant to therapy. The disease is often refractory to treatment.

Bacterial infections
Bacterial infections, especially by encapsulated organisms occur with increased frequency and severity of manifestations compared with the non-HIV-infected population. They may be more resistant to treatment than the uninfected population.

Viral hepatitis
A significant number of HIV patients, particularly those who are intravenous drug users, are also infected with hepatitis B or C. Antiretroviral drugs may worsen hepatic dysfunction and fluctuating immune function may be associated with flares of viral hepatitis. The treatment of hepatitis in the HIV patient is complex, and early specialist referral is essential. The treatment of hepatitis C has been transformed by the advent of direct-acting antivirals (DAAs). Patients with hepatitis C and HIV co-infections should be referred for DAA therapy early.

SYSTEMIC INFECTIONS
Herpes simplex
Severe mucocutaneous infections occur more frequently than disseminated infection. These may be in the form of chronic, aggressive, poorly healing perianal ulcers.

Management

Treatment is with:

- famciclovir 1500 mg PO as a single dose
- valaciclovir 2 g PO 12-hourly for 1 day
- aciclovir 400 mg PO 5 times daily for 5 days.

These drugs may be used as suppressive therapy to prevent frequent recurrences in immunosuppressed or immune-compromised patients.

Herpes zoster virus (HZV)

Recurrent HZV infections are often an early indicator of progressive CD4+ T-cell depletion. Infections usually remain dermatomal despite severe immunosuppression, though the extent of blistering may be severe and haemorrhagic. CNS infections with herpes viruses should be considered in the differential diagnosis of an encephalitic picture and treated early.

Cytomegalovirus (CMV)

Opportunistic CMV infection affects patients with CD4+ T-cell counts below 50 cells/microL.

- CMV retinitis presents with floaters, decreasing acuity and field loss. Fundoscopy reveals peripheral flame haemorrhages and exudates. However, the retinal lesions are often very peripheral and so can be missed. Dilation of the pupil and ophthalmological review are required to exclude diagnosis.
- Any part of the GI tract may be involved, with colitis, oesophagitis and gastritis being common presentations.
- CNS involvement causes encephalopathy and a polyradiculopathy.
- Interstitial pneumonitis is rare in HIV, in contrast to solid-organ transplant recipients.
- CMV adrenalitis presents with symptomatic adrenal insufficiency, hyponatraemia or hyperkalaemia.

Investigations

Detection of CMV RNA or DNA by nucleic acid testing in plasma or CSF is an aid to diagnosis. The presence of the classical inclusion bodies on biopsy of involved tissue is required for a definitive diagnosis of GI tract disease or pneumonitis.

Management

CMV infection is usually treated with valganciclovir, ganciclovir and, in problematical or resistant cases, foscarnet or cidofovir with probenecid. A specialist in HIV medicine should be consulted, along with urgent ophthalmology review in cases of suspected retinitis.

Mycobacterium avium–intracellulare complex (MAC)

This occurs in patients with CD4+ T-cell counts below 50 cells/ microL. The incidence has decreased with the use of combination ART and azithromycin prophylaxis. It presents as a systemic infection with fever, weight loss, night sweats, neutropenia, anaemia and lymphadenopathy. The diagnosis is made by performing prolonged blood culture (2–6 weeks).

Management

Treatment is with ethambutol plus either clarithromycin or azithromycin, with consideration of the addition of amikacin, streptomycin or a fluroquinolone such as levofloxacin or moxifloxacin in severely immunocompromised patients.

Malignancy in HIV/AIDS

Combination ART has changed the epidemiology of AIDS-related malignancies with the overall incidence reduced, especially primary CNS lymphoma (seen in patients with profound immunosuppression and CD4+ T-cell counts below 50 cells/microL). Most still present with advanced disease (extra-nodal, meningeal, GI tract and bone marrow disease are common) and B symptoms (fever, night sweats, weight loss). There has been improved survival with combination chemotherapy and ART.

Kaposi's sarcoma has also become much less common over the last decade. This malignancy is associated with infection with human herpes virus 8 and occurs with CD4+ T-cell counts less than 300 cells/microL.

- Skin involvement usually presents as painless, hyperpigmented purple nodules or plaques, but in pressure areas these may become painful and/or ulcerate. Especially in later disease, lesions may be more systemic, and be associated with lymphatic obstruction in the limbs and also involve the oropharynx, GI tract (causing pain, ulceration, obstruction, bleeding or perforation).

• Involvement of the lung (with pleural effusion, pulmonary infiltrates or hilar adenopathy) is a poor prognostic sign.

• Treatment consists of antiretrovirals in early stage disease, with chemotherapy in advanced disease. Systemic involvement, especially of the lung, is resistant to intervention.

Cervical cancer remains a common problem in HIV-infected women, with no impact on the disease from antiretrovirals. Treatment is as for the immunocompetent patient.

HPV may also cause premalignant and malignant changes in the anus and rectum of HIV-infected men who have sex with men (MSM).

Immune reconstitution inflammatory syndrome (IRIS)

With the widespread use of combination ART in HIV/AIDS, complications arise from the recovering immune system directing an inflammatory response against antigens associated with infectious agents.

IRIS presents as worsening signs or symptoms of infection in late-stage patients (< 100 CD4+ T-cells/microL at commencement of therapy) who have recently commenced ART. It usually manifests within 4 weeks, and may begin within days, although occasionally it develops after months of treatment. Patients with very low CD4+ T-cell counts (< 50/microL) and high pathogen loads are at highest risk.

The opportunistic infections most commonly associated with IRIS are MAC, CMV, HZV, Cryptococcus and toxoplasma. Worldwide, TB is the most common cause, with up to one-third of late-stage patients developing IRIS after starting ART. It occurs more frequently when combination ART is given in the presence of an untreated infection. For this reason ART is usually not commenced in the presence of a known opportunistic infection. Commencement of ART is usually delayed until the active infection is cleared or the patient has commenced maintenance suppressive or prophylactic therapy.

IRIS often represents a diagnostic dilemma, as the presentation is often non-specific and atypical. The differential diagnosis includes a new opportunistic infection or drug toxicity. The diagnosis is essentially one of exclusion.

PCP-associated IRIS presents with a worsening of respiratory status and occasionally unmasks clinically silent PCP. MAC- or CMV-associated IRIS presents with fevers, lymphadenopathy and systemic symptoms. CMV may present with worsening of retinitis which may result in the permanent loss of sight.

MANAGEMENT

- Prevention of IRIS by commencing ART before CD4+ T-cell counts are very low, and screening for infection with treatment before initiating ART, is preferable.
- Treatment of IRIS involves supportive care with cessation of ART in severe cases. Corticosteroids may be used to blunt the inflammatory response.

Antiretroviral drugs

The introduction of combination ART, with 3 or 4 anti-retroviral drugs, has led to improvements in morbidity and mortality in HIV/AIDS, decreased transmission and increased quality of life. Patients often have restoration of their immune function and a fall in viral load to undetectable levels.

The main classes of antiretrovirals are nucleoside reverse transcriptase inhibitors, non-nucleoside reverse transcriptase inhibitors, protease inhibitors and integrase inhibitors. entry inhibitors, chemokine (C–C motif) receptor 5 (CCR5)-blockers) have been licensed for non-first line therapy.

Specific inhibitors include:

- nucleoside reverse transcriptase inhibitors—abacavir, didanosine, emtricitabine, lamivudine, stavudine, tenofovir, zidovudine
- non-nucleoside reverse transcriptase inhibitors—efavirenz, nevirapine, etravirine, rilpivirine
- protease inhibitors—atazanavir, fosamprenavir, lopinavir, saquinavir, darunavir, tipranavir
- CCR5 inhibitors—maraviroc
- integrase inhibitors—raltegravir, dolutegravir, elvitegravir.

The protease inhibitor indinavir is now rarely used. The others are usually used in combination with low-dose ritonavir (which is a protease inhibitor) or cobicistat which act as cytochrome P450 inhibitors which increase drug levels of the protease inhibitors. It allows the doses of the protease inhibitors to be reduced.

DRUG TOXICITIES
Lactic acidosis

- Nucleoside/nucleotide reverse transcriptase inhibitors (notably didanosine and stavudine, which are now rarely used) can cause lactic acidosis via mitochondrial toxicity. Patients with a reduced creatinine clearance and lower CD4+ counts are at higher risk.
- The severity ranges from asymptomatic acidaemia to a life-threatening syndrome. Abdominal pain and distension, nausea and vomiting are common, along with myalgias, peripheral neuropathy, dyspnoea and hepatic steatosis with raised transaminases.
- Cessation of drugs may lead to resolution, or there may be progressive multisystem involvement and respiratory and circulatory failure.
- Initial lactate levels higher than 5 mmol/L may be life-threatening.

Management
1 Treatment involves cessation of ART and supportive care.
2 Riboflavin, l-carnitine and thiamine may reverse toxicity.
3 In severe cases, bicarbonate therapy and haemodialysis may be needed.

Hypersensitivity reactions
Hypersensitivity reactions are common in HIV patients. They are often minor and self-limiting and do not mandate cessation of therapy. Non-nucleoside reverse transcriptase inhibitors and antibiotics (especially trimethoprim-sulfamethoxazole) are frequent causes. The more serious Stevens–Johnson syndrome is also associated with these drugs, with widespread rash and blistering, mucosal involvement and fever.

Abacavir is associated with a life-threatening hypersensitivity syndrome, usually beginning in the first 10–14 days of treatment, with rash, fever, nausea, vomiting and abdominal pain. Patients may develop interstitial pneumonitis, hypotension and respiratory failure. The cause of this is now known to be strongly linked to the carriage of HLA-B5701. All patients being considered for abacavir therapy should be screened for the carriage of this HLA allele prior to commencement.

Nevirapine is a cause of fulminant hepatitis upon initiation of therapy, particularly in men with a CD4+ count > 400 cells/microL or women with a CD4+ T-cell count > 200 cells/microL.

Management
For severe hypersensitivity reactions, all antiretrovirals (and other potential causes such as antibiotics or anticonvulsants) should be stopped and supportive care instituted.

Other toxicities
Many other antiretrovirals (particularly protease inhibitors) can cause hepatitis.
* Atazanavir causes an isolated benign hyperbilirubinaemia.
* Pancreatitis occurs with stavudine, didanosine and lopinavir/ritonavir.
* Peripheral neuropathy, which is often painful, is associated with stavudine and didanosine.
* Myelosuppression occurs with zidovudine.
* Efavirenz has been associated with neuropsychiatric disorders.
* Tenofovir is associated with renal impairment and osteomalacia/osteopenia.

DRUG INTERACTIONS
Many drug interactions occur due to inhibition of the induction of the hepatic cytochrome P450 system especially that caused by ritonavir. Of particular note are:
* increased sedative effects from midazolam (lorazepam is unaffected)
* decreased levels of methadone, causing narcotic withdrawal
* increased levels of norpethidine, the toxic metabolite of pethidine

- a disulfiram-like reaction with metronidazole
- increased cardiovascular effects of amiodarone, diltiazem, nifedipine and sildenafil.

Systemic levels of the more potent long-acting inhaled corticosteroids can be driven high enough to induce Cushing's syndrome. Even short-acting low-dose inhaled steroids should be used with caution in patients on ritonavir-boosted protease inhibitors.

CARDIOVASCULAR COMPLICATIONS

- Long-term ART, especially with first-generation nucleoside reversion transcriptase inhibitors (NRTIs) and protease inhibitors are associated with metabolic and cardiovascular toxicities, dyslipidaemia, atherosclerosis, endothelial dysfunction and glucose intolerance with insulin resistance.
- Age-adjusted rates of coronary artery disease and myocardial infarction are elevated in HIV-positive men. The treatment of acute coronary syndromes is the same as in HIV-negative patients.

Pre-exposure prophylaxis (PrEP) in HIV

Pre-exposure prophylaxis (PrEP) involves the medium- or long-term use of antiretrovirals to prevent infection during a period of potential exposure to HIV. A combination of tenofovir and emtricitabine is the most studied regimen and is effective in preventing the establishment of viral infection in men who have sex with men, and in transgender women. It is now licenced for use as PrEP in NSW.

Due to variation in drug levels achieved in tissue cells (cervical levels are much less than rectal levels), PrEP may be less effective in female patients.

Post-exposure prophylaxis in HIV

Post-exposure prophylaxis (PEP) is the use of antiretrovirals to prevent seroconversion after potential exposure to HIV. PEP is most effective when given less than 72 hours after exposure, although there is declining efficacy after 36 hours.

- In non-occupational exposures, the HIV status of the source is often unknown. Assessment of the risk of HIV transmission requires knowledge of the risk of transmission from the method of exposure and the risk of the source being HIV-positive.

- High-risk exposures include receptive anal intercourse (1/120), sharing contaminated injecting equipment (1/50), occupational needle-stick (1/333), receptive vaginal intercourse (1/1000) and insertive anal or vaginal intercourse (1/1000).
- Although case reports of transmission exist, the risk of transmission by oral intercourse, bites, exposure to intact mucous membranes or skin and community-acquired needle-stick injury is so low it is not measurable.
- The risk of the source of exposure being HIV-positive varies between populations.
  — In MSM (men who have sex with men), the estimated HIV rates are 14% in Sydney, 9% in Melbourne, 6% in Brisbane and 5% in Perth.
  — Australian intravenous drug users (IVDUs) have lower rates of infection than overseas cohorts, with an estimated prevalence of 1%. However, IVDUs who are also MSM have a 17% rate of HIV infection.
  — The HIV rate among heterosexuals (including sex workers) is 0.1%, unless the source is from sub-Saharan Africa, where the estimated rate is 7%.

PROPHYLACTIC REGIMENS

- Choice of regimen:
  — if the risk of transmission equals or exceeds 1/1000, PEP with three drugs is indicated
  — if the risk of transmission is between 1/1000 and 1/10000, two-drug PEP is indicated
  — PEP with two drugs is considered when the risk is between 1/10000 and 1/15000; PEP is not recommended in lower-risk exposures.
- Two-drug regimens use two nucleoside reverse transcriptase inhibitors, such as emtricitabine + tenofovir.
- Three-drug regimens use either two nucleoside reverse transcriptase inhibitors and a protease inhibitor, or three nucleoside reverse transcriptase inhibitors or 2 nucleoside inhibitors and an integrase inhibitor. An example of a three-drug regimen is tenofovir + emtricitabine + efavirenz.

- Treatment duration is 28 days.
- Baseline blood testing should be performed, including FBC, LFTs and serology for HIV and hepatitis B and C. Screening for other sexually transmitted diseases may be undertaken at the first follow-up appointment, which should be within the next few days.
- Some patients require emergency contraception, immunisation for hepatitis B and tetanus immunisation.
- The need for safe behaviour to avoid further exposure and potential transmission should be emphasised.
- Repeat courses of PEP are safe and should be given as indicated.
- The use of PEP does not increase the rate of high-risk exposures.

Solid-organ transplants

The immunosuppression required for the survival of transplanted organs leaves the recipient prone to infections, which are a leading cause of mortality.

- Infections are caused by a broad spectrum of pathogens and there may be minimal signs and symptoms at presentation, followed by rapid deterioration.
- Non-infectious causes of fever (rejection, malignancy and drugs) are common in the transplant population.
- The likely cause of infection varies with the length and intensity of immunosuppression.
- The likely exposures to infection vary with the time post-transplant, with donor- or hospital-acquired infections common in the early postoperative period, and opportunistic and community-acquired infections emerging later. Patients may have had vaccinations and chemoprophylaxis.
- The unwell transplant patient may present with non-specific symptoms or fever alone.

EXAMINATION AND INVESTIGATIONS

- Examination should include a thorough search for sites of infection, including the skin, mouth and urethra. A specific diagnosis may be elusive.
- Urine, sputum and blood should be sent for culture, along with blood for serology.

- Any lesions should be swabbed.
- A chest X-ray is indicated in most cases.

MANAGEMENT

It is vital that the transplant team be involved in the patient's management as early as possible. Antibiotic therapy should be broad-spectrum; however, there are multiple potential interactions with immunosuppressive drugs. Macrolides are generally contraindicated.

INFECTIONS IN THE EARLY POST-TRANSPLANT PERIOD

Within the first month after transplant, most infections are not opportunistic. Subclinical infections suffered by the donor can be transmitted to the patient (this is uncommon and is most often a viral infection). The patient is often colonised with microbes such as MRSA, and fungi pre-operatively, and the induction of immunosuppression can precipitate clinical disease.

Injury to the transplanted organ from ischaemia and reperfusion can give rise to a site for infection, such as in the bile ducts or lung. Wounds, intravascular catheters and drains provide further sites of potential infection. The transplanted kidney is prone to pyelonephritis, the liver to abscesses, wound infections and cholangitis and the heart/lung to mediastinitis and pneumonia. These postoperative infections are mostly bacterial and may be resistant to antibiotics.

INTERMEDIATE PERIOD INFECTIONS

Unusual and opportunistic infections emerge in the 2nd to 6th months following transplantation.

- CMV can present as a systemic infection or as a pneumonitis. Nucleic acid testing (NAT) for CMV is used to detect CMV replication, allowing the diagnosis of subclinical infection and commencement of pre-emptive treatment according to standard protocols.
- Pneumonia may be caused by a wide range of pathogens. Most cases are bacterial, but fungal and viral infections also occur.
- Reactivation of latent tuberculosis can occur, often leading to disseminated disease.

- HSV is the most frequent cause of CNS disease.
- The GI tract may be infected with CMV or parasites.
- It is important to note that graft rejection also presents with fever, as do some drug reactions.

Prophylaxis has led to decreasing incidences of PJP, HSV, CMV and toxoplasmosis. The duration of prophylaxis varies between centres.

Management
- Trimethoprim-sulfamethoxazole is used to prevent PCP and common urinary, respiratory and gastrointestinal pathogens.
- Oral antiviral agents are used against CMV and HSV.

LATE INFECTIONS

After 6 months post-transplant, the risk of infection declines as immunosuppression is tapered off. Patients with rejection requiring ongoing high levels of immunosuppression will remain at risk of opportunistic infections; however, the majority of infections will be community-acquired diseases such as pneumonia. Patients are at increased risk from intracellular pathogens like mycobacteria and fungi.

Chronic viral infection may cause insidious graft injury. Recurrent disease may occur in patients who have received transplants for HCV. Renal transplants may become infected by the BK polyomavirus, causing declining graft function.

Long-term immunosuppression increases the risk of malignancy. Skin and anogenital cancers are the most common. Post-transplant lymphoproliferative disease can also develop. This has a spectrum of presentations, from an infectious mononucleosis-like illness to lymphoma.

GRAFT-SPECIFIC PROBLEMS

Acute rejection presents with systemic symptoms, including fever, along with signs of organ insufficiency. Chronic rejection develops over years, with gradual organ failure.

Heart
- The transplanted heart is denervated, the loss of vagal stimulation leading to a baseline tachycardia of 100–110 bpm.

Catecholamines and antihypertensive drugs are effective in these patients, although atropine will be ineffective.

- Myocardial ischaemia is painless, presenting as chronic cardiac failure (CCF), arrhythmias, hypotension or syncope.
- Atherosclerosis is accelerated in organs with chronic rejection.
- Routine biopsy detects most cases of rejection at an early, asymptomatic phase. More advanced rejection manifests as CCF, arrhythmias and low QRS voltages on the ECG.

Liver

- Rejection presents with fever, right upper quadrant pain and tenderness, jaundice and elevations in transaminases.
- Biliary obstruction, wound infections and cholangitis are common postoperative complications.

Kidney

- Rejection presents with fever, pelvic swelling, pain and tenderness and decreased urine output.
- Chronic rejection takes the form of nephrosclerosis, with hypertension and declining renal function.
- The kidney may be injured in trauma to the pelvis.

Lung

- Rejection presents in a similar way to infection, with fever, shortness of breath, cough and hypoxia, with infiltrates on chest X-ray.
- Chronic rejection causes bronchiolitis obliterans.

Pancreas

Drainage of exocrine secretions into the bladder predisposes to UTI, haematuria and chronic non-anion-gap acidosis (due to bicarbonate loss).

DRUG TOXICITY

Newer immunosuppression regimens using sirolimus, mycophenolate mofetil, T-cell and B-cell depletion and co-stimulatory blockade have largely replaced high-dose steroids and azathioprine.

- Corticosteroids cause decreased mobilisation and function of neutrophils, monocytes and lymphocytes.
  - There is increased susceptibility to pyogenic bacteria due to depressed leucocyte activity at sites of inflammation. These patients may have diminished clinical signs of peritonitis.
  - Patients are also at higher risk of severe infections with HSV and varicella zoster virus (VZV). The risk of infection increases with lengthy treatment and doses of > 20 mg/day (e.g. of prednisone).
  - Corticosteroids may mask fever and chronic use causes adrenal suppression. Consideration should be given to Addisonian symptoms in those on chronic corticosteroids and to increasing doses of corticosteroids in acute deterioration to ensure sufficient coverage.
- Cyclosporin suppresses cellular and humoral immunity. It has a number of adverse effects including nephrotoxicity, hypertension, hyperuricaemia and seizures, along with multiple interactions with drugs and food.
- Azathioprine is associated with neutropenia.
- Mycophenolate generally has few side effects. It may cause gastrointestinal disturbance, leukopenia and thrombocytopenia.
- Sirolimus causes an idiosyncratic non-infectious pneumonitis which resembles PCP or viral pneumonia.
- Tacrolimus may lead to nephrotoxicity, neurotoxicity, hyperglycaemia or hyperkalaemia.
- T-cell-depleting antibodies can cause fever, hypotension and pulmonary oedema, along with reactivation of viruses such as CMV and EBV.

Early discussion with the specialist caring for the patient is recommended in cases of suspected drug reactions.

Immunosuppression for non-malignant disease
PATIENTS ON LONG-TERM CORTICOSTEROIDS

Many patients with inflammatory or malignancy conditions are on long-term corticosteroids either as part of a weaning strategy or maintenance. These may include patients with malignancy (particularly with brain metastasis), chronic airways disease and immunological/rheumatological conditions such as SLE, rheumatoid arthritis.

Long term steroid use is also associated with weight gain, diabetes mellitus, hypertension, osteopenia and fractures which may be cause to present to the ED.

Additionally, patients on long-term steroids are at increased risk of infection that can be related to poor wound healing. Due to adrenal suppression corticosteroids should never be ceased abruptly and, in fact, when acutely unwell the long-term corticosteroid dependent patient may need higher 'stress doses' of exogenous steroid concurrently with other medical treatment.

Newer biological therapy

Newer immunosuppressive agents with lower toxicities have led to an expansion in the use of immunosuppression for non-malignant disease, widening the population at risk of opportunistic infection. Patients with autoimmune disease including systemic lupus erythematosus, rheumatoid arthritis, multiple sclerosis and inflammatory bowel disease may be sufficiently immunocompromised to present with similar infections to the patient with HIV, malignancy or solid-organ transplant.

Rituximab is a monoclonal antibody that depletes CD20+ B-cells. In addition to its use in haematological malignancies it is licensed for use in rheumatoid arthritis, granulomatosis with polyangiitis, idiopathic thrombocytopenia purpura, pemphigus vulgaris and myasthenia gravis. Patients are susceptible to infections related to poor humoral immunity. Rituximab can cause infusion reactions due to antibodies to monoclonal components. These may be acute or delayed. The delayed reaction is a serum sickness-like illness, with fever, arthritis and rash, which is treated with steroids.

Adalimumab, infliximab and etanercept are tumour necrosis factor (TNF) inhibitors used in rheumatoid arthritis and inflammatory bowel disease. There is increased susceptibility to tuberculosis and bacterial sepsis.

Anakinra (anti-IL-1) therapy is licensed for second-line treatment of rheumatoid arthritis and cryopyrin-associated periodic syndrome (CAPS). Ten per cent of patients can develop injection site reactions, and leukopenia and thrombocytopenia may also result.

In addition to biological agents many patients with immunological/rheumatological or inflammatory conditions are maintained on medium- to long-term immunosuppression with hydroxychloroquine, azathioprine, mycophenolate, ciclosporin, tacrolimus, methotrexate and cyclophosphamide which may be used in sequence or in combination.

Asplenia

Asplenia may result from trauma, splenectomy for idiopathic thrombocytopenic purpura (ITP), lymphoma or haematological malignancy, auto splenectomy in sickle-cell disease or functional asplenia in haematological disease, sarcoid, amyloid or autoimmune disease.

Patients without a functioning spleen are predisposed to overwhelming sepsis with streptococcus, meningococcus and haemophilus influenzae and other encapsulated bacteria. The risk is highest in the first few years after splenectomy. Early intervention in any septic presentation is essential.

Pneumococcal vaccine is routinely given; however response may be diminished in patients with severe underlying disease. Vaccinations for type B, influenza and meningococcus are also given, and patients take penicillin or macrolide prophylaxis for 2–5 years.

Summary

Primary immunodeficiency is rare and the majority of adult patients presenting to the ED will have immunodeficiency secondary to haematological malignancy, immunosuppressive therapies (for solid-organ transplant, malignant or inflammatory conditions) or chronic HIV infection. Signs and symptoms should be interpreted in the context both of the primary conditions and of the nature of the immunological deficit. Threshold for investigating for infective causes should be low especially if the cause of presentation is unclear or if symptoms are generalised. Infections may affect any organ, be acute or chronic, and pathogens may be common or opportunistic, therefore complete septic screen may only be the starting point for a broad range of investigations. These patients are medically complex, and the nature of investigations and treatment decisions should nearly always be made in consultation with the specialist care physicians.

Chapter 25
Emergency department haematology
FX Luis Winoto, Rebecca Walsh

Acknowledgment

The authors wish to acknowledge the content used from the previous edition of *Emergency Medicine* which was provided by Anthony J Dodds.

Common haematological emergencies
NEUTROPENIC SEPSIS
(See also Chapter 24 The Immunosupresed Patient.)

Severe neutropenia is defined as a neutrophil count of $< 0.5 \times 10^9/L$, but severe sepsis is unusual until the neutrophil count is $< 0.2 \times 10^9/L$.

Causes for severe neutropenia include cancer chemotherapy drugs, agranulocytosis (an idiosyncratic reaction to an otherwise non-marrow-suppressive drug) and haematological disorders causing marrow failure (acute and chronic leukaemias, myeloma, lymphoma, aplastic anaemia, etc.).

Patients presenting with a fever above 38°C require urgent investigation and therapy.

Investigations

- Investigations should be directed to possible sites of infection; however, local sites are detected in fewer than 50% of such patients.
- Suggested investigations include chest X-ray, blood cultures and urine culture.
- If there is a central line, cultures through this line are also important.

Management
- Therapy with broad-spectrum antibiotics should not be withheld while investigations are being performed but preferably after cultures taken.
- Gram-negative infections usually arising from the gut are the commonest causes but, in the presence of a central venous catheter, treatment of possible Gram-positive skin organisms should also be considered.
- Most institutions have an approved protocol to treat such patients.
  - Usually a broad-spectrum third-generation cephalosporin or piperacillin and tazobactam is combined with gentamicin until *Pseudomonas* has been excluded.
  - If the fever does not respond to this after 48 hours or a central venous catheter is present, then additional anti-staphylococcal therapy is added.

SEVERE THROMBOCYTOPENIA AND BLEEDING

Severe spontaneous bleeding with thrombocytopenia is not usually a problem until the platelet count is less than 10×10^9/L. When patients present with bleeding secondary to thrombocytopenia, an urgent assessment of the cause of the thrombocytopenia is necessary.

Differential diagnosis
1 Marrow failure (e.g. chemotherapy drugs, haematological malignancy). Such patients usually have a pancytopenia and a history of being given marrow-suppressive therapy. Urgent platelet transfusion is indicated.
2 Peripheral destruction of platelets.
   - This may be an autoimmune disorder (immune thrombocytopenia [ITP]) or less commonly an immune drug-related disorder. Heparin is a common drug cause for immune thrombocytopenia.
   - Patients presenting with ITP may have no preceding history and have isolated thrombocytopenia.
   - The disorder may be post-viral and reversible in children but commonly chronic in adults.

— If there is any doubt about the diagnosis, a marrow biopsy is indicated. This will show a normal marrow with plentiful megakaryocytes.
— **Treatment:** urgent corticosteroids (prednisolone 1 mg/kg PO daily) in conjunction with IVIg are indicated for ITP with severe thrombocytopenia, especially with bleeding. Platelet transfusion is usually not given in immune thrombocytopenia unless in the presence of bleeding and is contraindicated in heparin-induced thrombocytopenia.

3 Disseminated intravascular coagulation (DIC). DIC can occur with malignancy or severe sepsis. Treatment is aimed at the underlying cause rather than treating by platelet transfusion alone.

SICKLE-CELL DISEASE

Sickle-cell disease (SCD) is an inherited disorder due to homozygosity for abnormal haemoglobin. SCD can produce a wide spectrum of manifestations and patients may present with life-threatening complications such as vaso-occlusive crisis, stroke, aplastic crisis, acute chest syndrome and sepsis.

Acute painful crisis

This is the most common manifestation of SCD requiring hospitalisation. It is caused by vaso-occlusion of the vasculature by the abnormal sickled red cells. This can be spontaneous or precipitated by infection, stressors or dehydration.

Management

Rule out other causes of pain (e.g. avascular necrosis, cortical bone infarction or osteomyelitis; acute chest syndrome; infection).

- The mainstay of management is adequate analgesia including opiates and adjuvant non-opiate analgesia.
- A blood transfusion or exchange transfusion should not be given for uncomplicated pain crisis unless there are other indications for transfusion.

The anaemic patient

Anaemia is defined as a reduced haemoglobin (Hb) concentration in the blood. The red cell mass and the plasma volume can affect this value, so both these factors must be considered when interpreting a single value. Thus, severe dehydration can produce an elevated Hb and increased plasma volume, such as in pregnancy, can produce a falsely low Hb.

The symptoms and signs of anaemia (pallor, fainting, lethargy and anorexia) are unreliable. Anaemia may be asymptomatic and detected only on a routine blood count. The cause of anaemia can be ascertained by a logical sequence of investigations as follows. This is based on the mean corpuscular volume (MCV), which is part of an automated blood count.

MICROCYTIC (NORMAL MCV)
Common causes are as follows.
- Iron deficiency: serum ferritin low
- Thalassaemia trait: serum ferritin normal or raised

NORMOCYTIC (NORMAL MCV)
Common causes are as follows.
- Anaemia of chronic disease:
  — serum ferritin normal or raised
  — serum iron low
  — serum transferrin normal or low
  — positive inflammatory markers (erythrocyte sedimentation rate [ESR], C-reactive protein [CRP]) (e.g. chronic infection, neoplasm, renal failure)
- Bone marrow disease: (usually pancytopenia) (e.g. aplastic anaemia, marrow infiltration, marrow malignancy)
- Acute blood loss
- Haemolysis: raised reticulocyte count, positive direct antiglobulin test in immune haemolytic anaemia, low serum haptoglobin level, raised serum bilirubin and lactate dehydrogenase (LDH) levels

MACROCYTIC (RAISED MCV)
Common causes are as follows.
- Megaloblastosis: low serum B_{12} or red cell folate levels
- Secondary macrocytic anaemia (e.g. alcohol, liver disease, hypothyroidism, some marrow disorders, marked reticulocytosis)

Principles of therapy

1. Establish the cause and treat.
2. In the setting of acute haemorrhage consider activating the massive transfusion protocol.
3. In a stable patient with anaemia, red blood cell (RBC) transfusion should not be dictated by a Hb concentration alone, but should also be based on assessment of the patient's clinical status.
4. In patients with iron deficiency anaemia, iron therapy is required to replenish iron stores regardless of whether a transfusion is indicated.

Table 25.1 Commonly used blood products in emergency medicine

Product	Emergency indications
Red cell concentrate	Severe or refractory anaemia Moderate blood loss
Platelet concentrate	Thrombocytopenia with bleeding Platelet dysfunctional bleeding
Fresh frozen plasma (FFP)	Massive transfusion Severe liver disease with bleeding
Prothrombinex	Reversal of warfarin therapy
Cryoprecipitate	Massive transfusion

The patient with abnormal bleeding

Screening haemostasis tests are not warranted or cost-effective in the absence of clinical signs or history to suggest a bleeding diathesis.

The following are suggestive:

- family history of bleeding disorder
- past history of excessive bleeding with minor haemostatic insults (e.g. tooth extraction, minor surgery, minor trauma, childbirth)
- excessive local bleeding without an obvious cause
- generalised bleeding or bruising.

The usual screening tests are:

- vascular or platelet disorder—platelet count (PC), platelet function tests
- coagulation disorder—prothrombin time (PT), activated partial thromboplastin time (APTT), thrombin time (TT).

Table 25.2 Summary of the coagulation abnormalities seen in the commonly encountered acute conditions

Condition	PT	APTT	TT	PC	FDP
Severe liver disease	↑	↑	N or ↑	N or ↓	N or ↑
Heparin therapy	N	↑	↑	N	N
Coumarin (warfarin) therapy	↑	N	N	N	N
DIC	↑	↑	↑	↓	↑
Massive blood transfusion	↑	↑	N or ↑	↓	N

↑ = prolonged/increased; ↓ = decreased; APTT = activated partial thromboplastin time; DIC = disseminated intravascular coagulation; FDP = fibrin degradation products; N = normal; PC = platelet count; PT = prothrombin time; TT = thrombin time

The following is a guide to the interpretation of these tests.

PLATELET AND VASCULAR DEFECTS
Platelet count low
- Marrow failure (e.g. aplastic anaemia, malignancy) OR
- Peripheral destruction or sequestration (e.g. ITP, drug-induced immune thrombocytopenia, hypersplenism [splenomegaly], DIC)

Platelet count normal
- Primary platelet dysfunction
- Secondary platelet dysfunction (e.g. aspirin, uraemia)

COAGULATION DEFECTS
- PT prolonged, APTT prolonged, TT prolonged
  — Disseminated intravascular coagulation
  — Deficiency of fibrinogen (rarely)
  — New oral anticoagulation therapy: direct thrombin inhibitors (dabigatran etexilate)
- PT prolonged, APTT prolonged, TT normal
  — Severe liver disease
  — Lupus inhibitor
  — Congenital factor deficiencies (factor X, V, II or multiple)
  — New oral anticoagulation therapy—direct factor Xa inhibitors (rivaroxaban, apixaban)

- PT prolonged, APTT normal or slightly prolonged, TT normal
  — Oral anticoagulant (warfarin) therapy
  — Vitamin K deficiency
- PT normal, APTT prolonged, TT normal
  — Lupus inhibitor
  — Haemophilia (factor VIII or IX deficiency)
  — Other intrinsic pathway factor deficiency

Therapy

Specific therapy is usually only required if the patient is bleeding or an operative procedure is contemplated. Components available include:

- fresh frozen plasma (FFP)—DIC, massive transfusion, liver disease
- platelet concentrates—thrombocytopenia due to marrow failure
- factor concentrates—Prothrombinex (freeze-dried concentrate of human blood coagulation factors II, IX and X) for reversal of warfarin therapy or specific factor concentrates for factor deficiencies.

Anticoagulant therapy
UNFRACTIONATED HEPARIN

Heparin inhibits coagulation at a number of sites, mainly via activation of antithrombin-III. Administration is usually via constant IV infusion.

- Monitoring: the APTT is the usual method. A baseline APTT should be established, repeated 4 hours after commencing heparin, then therapeutic interval checked with laboratory. A platelet count should be done every second day.
- Reversal: for overdose or serious bleeding, stop the heparin and give protamine sulfate slowly IV (1 mg/100 units of heparin).
- Side effects: bleeding; thrombocytopenia–thrombosis (heparin-induced thrombotic thrombocytopenia syndrome [HITTS]).

LOW-MOLECULAR-WEIGHT HEPARINS

- These are often used for prophylaxis but are also commonly given for ambulatory full-dose therapy. They are usually given by subcutaneous injection.
- They have a much longer half-life than unfractionated heparin.

- They cannot be monitored by APTT testing but anti-Xa assay can be used in specific circumstances.
- They cause less bleeding and less thrombocytopenia.

VITAMIN K ANTAGONISTS (E.G. WARFARIN)

- These are oral anticoagulants that inhibit synthesis of vitamin-K-dependent clotting factors (II, VII, IX, X plus protein C and protein S).
- International normalised ratio (INR) is a standardised prothrombin ratio and is used to monitor side effects: bleeding; rash; teratogenesis.

DIRECT ORAL ANTICOAGULANTS (DOACs)

- Apixaban, rivaroxaban (factor Xa inhibitors) and dabigatran (direct thrombin inhibitor).
- Routine monitoring of levels is usually not indicated and standard laboratory coagulation tests are not reliable in predicting drug levels or bleeding risk.

Surgery in patients receiving oral anticoagulants

What to do will depend on the type of surgery and the reason for administering anticoagulants.

- For minor procedures (e.g. tooth extraction), therapy may not need to be ceased (see institutional protocols).
- For major procedures, it may be necessary to change to heparin if continuing anticoagulation is required (e.g. artificial heart valve).

Reversal vitamin K antagonists

Fresh frozen plasma or Prothrombinex will acutely reverse the effect in bleeding patients. Vitamin K will act more slowly and permanently reverse the effect, but in large doses may make it more difficult to anticoagulate the patient again.

A protocol for the management of an elevated INR is shown in Figure 25.1.

Reversal DOACs

- Apixaban, rivaroxaban
  — A specific antidote to reverse these agents in a bleeding patient is not available. In the event of haemorrhagic

Guidelines for elevated INR in adults **WITHOUT** bleeding (1)							
INR	Bleeding risk	Warfarin	Vitamin K₁	FFP	PTX-VF	Measure INR	Comments
≥ therapeutic range but < 5.0		Lower the dose or omit the next dose*					Resume therapy at a lower dose when the INR approaches therapeutic range
5.0–9.0	Low	Stop; consider reasons for elevated INR and patient-specific factors	Give 1.0–2.0 mg oral or 0.5–1.0 mg intravenous			Within 24 hours	Resume warfarin at a reduced dose when the INR is in therapeutic range
	High						
>9.0	Low	Stop	Give 2.5–5.0 mg oral or 1.0 mg intravenous			In 6–12 hours	Resume warfarin therapy at a reduced dose once INR is < 5.0
	High	Stop	Give 1.0 mg intravenous	Consider 150–300 mL	Consider 25–50 IU/kg		

Guidelines for elevated INR in adults **WITH** bleeding (1)						
INR	Bleeding risk	Warfarin	Vitamin K₁	FFP	PTX-VF	Check INR
Any clinically significant bleeding where warfarin-induced coagulopathy is considered a contributing factor		Stop	Give vitamin K₁ 5.0–10.0 mg intravenous	Give 150–300 mL If FFP is not available, give Vit K & PTX-VF Give 10–15 mL/kg	Give 25–50 IU/kg Give 25–50 IU/kg If PTX-VR is not available, give Vit K & FFP	Assess patient continuously until INR is < 5.0, and bleeding stops

Notes: *Dose reduction may not be necessary if the INR is only minimally above therapeutic range (up to 10%); INR = International Normalised Ratio; FFP = fresh frozen plasma; PTX-VF = Prothrombinex–VF

Figure 25.1 Guidelines for the management of an elevated INR in adult patients with or without bleeding
Based on Tran HA, Chunilal SD, Harper PL et al., on behalf of the Australasian Society of Thrombosis and Haemostasis. An update of consensus guidelines for warfarin reversal. Med J Aust 2013;198(4):198–199.

complications consideration may be given to the use of Prothrombinex, FEIBA or recombinant factor VIIa. Consultation with a haematologist is also advisable in this situation.
- Dabigatran
  — Idarucizumab is a non-vitamin K antagonist oral anticoagulant (NOAC) reversal agent that will only reverse the anticoagulant effects of dabigatran.

— Idarucizumab is effective for dabigatran reversal among patients who have uncontrolled bleeding or will be undergoing urgent surgery.

Blood transfusion
TRANSFUSION REACTIONS
Haemolytic
Immediate (haemolysis of donor cells usually due to ABO incompatibility). It is recognised that the majority of haemolytic reactions to red cells are due to clerical errors in transfusion practice.
- The following are manifestations of an acute haemolytic reaction: flushing, backache, chest pain, rigors, haemoglobinuria.
- Treatment:
  1. Stop the transfusion immediately.
  2. Check and monitor vital signs.
  3. Maintain intravenous (IV) access (do not flush existing line and use a new IV line if required).
  4. Check the right pack has been given to the right patient.
  5. Notify your medical officer and transfusion service provider.

Delayed (1–2 weeks after transfusion). This is due to a secondary antibody response and there is often no incompatibility at initial cross-match. The following suggest a delayed haemolytic transfusion reaction:
- fall in haemoglobin or late jaundice
- positive Coombs' test and antibody screen.

Reactions to white cell antibodies occur after previous transfusion or pregnancy ('febrile non-haemolytic reactions'). This is now very infrequent, if red cell and platelet products are leucodepleted.
- Such reactions are delayed by 0.5–3 hours after start of transfusion.
- There is a brisk rise in temperature to 38–40°C with chills and headache.
- Stop transfusion. Exclude serious adverse events. Give paracetamol orally or antihistamine IV. Recommence cautiously if reaction subsides.

Urticarial and anaphylactic reactions
- Anaphylaxis is rare—due to allergy to donor plasma.
- Occasionally occurs in IgA-deficient individuals.

- Shock—bronchospasm, laryngeal oedema, severe urticaria.
- Stop transfusion, treat with adrenaline, antihistamines and occasionally corticosteroids.
- Check haptoglobin and IgA levels.

Urticarial reaction
(Occasionally accompanied by asthma.)
- Response to antihistamines usually.
- Washed red cells may be used.

Reactions to bacterial pyrogens and bacteria
- Pyrogenic reaction:
  — extremely rare
  — clinical picture resembles leucocyte and platelet antibody reaction.
- Infected blood or platelets:
  — causes shock, fever, coma, convulsions, sudden death; beware blood removed prematurely from blood bank or heavily haemolysed supernatant or previously punctured top
  — take blood for cultures
  — treat shock and give large doses of appropriate antibiotics.

It is recognised that platelet transfusions carry an increased risk of bacterial infection because platelet donations are stored at room temperature. Central blood banks have introduced screening of platelet concentrates for infections that has reduced the risk of bacterial contamination.

Circulatory overload
- Slow or stop transfusion, treat as for cardiac or pulmonary oedema.

Transfusion-related acute lung injury (TRALI)
- TRALI is a serious pulmonary complication of transfusion. It is an immune-mediated reaction caused by donor leucocyte antibodies causing non-cardiogenic pulmonary oedema.
- Manifestation includes dyspnoea and bilateral pulmonary oedema without signs of circulatory overload within 6 hours of transfusion.
- Respiratory supportive therapy.

Air embolism

- Raised jugular venous pulse (JVP), cyanosis, hypotension, praecordial murmur.
- Treat with head down, feet up and patient on left side.
- Administer 100% oxygen.

Citrate intoxication

- Usually only in neonates, impaired liver function and massive blood transfusion.
- Muscles twitching, hypotension, ECG changes, bleeding.
- Give calcium gluconate, 10 mL of 10% by IV injection.

Massive transfusion

(See Figure 4.1 Massive transfusion guideline.)

- Hypothermia (use blood warmer)
- Deficiency of coagulation factors; check coagulation profile (use fresh frozen plasma)
- Thrombocytopenia (use platelet transfusion)
- Acidosis
- Hypocalcaemia

Infectious complications

Possible risk with nucleic acid testing (NAT):

- HIV, < 1:920 000
- Hepatitis B, < 1:100 000
- Hepatitis C, < 1:10 000
- human T-lymphotropic virus type 1 (HTLV-I), < 1:100 000
- others (e.g. syphilis, malaria, cytomegalovirus [CMV]); CMV has the highest incidence but the lowest risk to the patient unless they are immunocompromised.

Inappropriate use of blood components

There is considerable evidence of inappropriate use of blood components. Various strategies have been developed to reduce this, including guidelines, consensus conferences, monitoring, education and self-audit by clinicians. Informed consent, including the potential risks and benefits of transfusion, is a vital part of any transfusion.

Online resources

Patient Blood Management guidelines
www.blood.gov.au/patient-blood-management-pbm
Australian Red Cross Blood Service
www.transfusion.com.au
Australasian Society of Thrombosis and Haemostasis
www.asth.org.au
Consensus Guidelines for Warfarin Therapy (updated)
www.mja.com.au/journal/2013/198/4/update-consensus-guidelines-warfarin-reversal
American Society of Hematology ASH Clinical Practice Guidelines
www.hematology.org/Clinicians/Guidelines-Quality/Guidelines.aspx

Chapter 26
Gastrointestinal emergencies

Greg McDonald, Nadine Huddle and
Christopher Wong

The aim of the emergency department assessment of patients with
gastrointestinal (GI) tract emergencies is to rapidly identify and
stabilise those patients requiring urgent surgical or procedural
intervention. In pursuing this aim, the processes of assessment,
investigations appropriate to the disease and management should
be followed in an orderly and focused manner and must be performed simultaneously in the seriously ill.

Acute abdomen

An 'acute abdomen' may be defined as an acute intra-abdominal
condition causing severe pain and often requiring urgent surgery.
The causes may be:

- inflammatory (e.g. appendicitis, diverticulitis, cholecystitis,
  perforated viscus)
- mechanical (e.g. incarcerated hernia, band adhesions,
  volvulus, intussusception)
- vascular (e.g. aortic aneurysm, mesenteric infarction)
- neoplastic (e.g. carcinoma colon)
- congenital (e.g. malrotation, congenital atresia/stenosis,
  Mcckel's diverticulum)
- trauma.

ASSESSMENT
History

- Who is your patient? Age and sex are two important
  aetiological factors.
- Patients over the age of 60 years have a 60% admission rate,
  20% require surgery and 5% die within two weeks.

- Consider gynaecological disorders, especially in women of childbearing age.
- Previous medical and surgical histories and a drug history will give important clues to diagnosis and need to be considered for operative fitness
- When did the pain start? Acute onset of severe pain implies vascular events, perforated viscus or renal colic. Slower onset of pain tends to imply inflammatory causes.
- Where is the pain? Abdominal pain often localises to the site of the pathology. Has it moved? Initial visceral pain is usually diffuse and in the midline. As the disease progresses, somatic pain becomes more localised.
- What is the pain like? The colicky pain of bowel obstruction is typically episodic and gripping, with pain-free intervals. In the case of biliary and renal colic, there is constant pain which rises to a crescendo. Constant severe pain indicates advanced or serious illness.
- Which other symptoms accompany this illness? The onset of nausea and vomiting after the onset of pain suggests surgical illness. Constipation is non-specific, but absolute constipation (neither faeces nor flatus) indicates bowel obstruction. Diarrhoea, jaundice, haematuria, haematemesis or melaena suggest specific diagnoses.

Note: Only two-thirds of patients with acute surgical conditions have a classical history of illness. Children and the elderly are more likely to have atypical presentations.

Examination
General
Appearance: apprehensive and motionless with peritonitis, unsettled and agitated with colicky pain; pale and 'Hippocratic facies' consistent with advanced disease.

Check temperature, hydration, pulse and blood pressure (with postural drop).

Abdomen
- Inspection: rigid, distended or scaphoid, visible peristalsis, operative scars.
- Palpation: diffuse or local tenderness, rebound, guarding.

Note: 'Rebound' is not pathognomonic of peritonitis. It is falsely positive in up to one-quarter of patients, and subjective. Cough impulse and percussion tenderness are often more reliable.

- Percussion: local peritonism, air, fluid (shifting dullness), masses, organs.

  Note: Loss of liver dullness occurs with pneumoperitoneum.

- Auscultation: although not sensitive, you may hear peristaltic noises coinciding with colic in small-bowel obstruction; diffuse increased bowel sounds in gastroenteritis; silent abdomen or occasional tinkling sounds in late bowel obstruction or diffuse peritonitis.

Special signs

- Murphy's sign in cholecystitis; Rovsing's, psoas and obturator signs in appendicitis; Cullen's (peri-umbilical) and Grey–Turner's (flank) signs of haemorrhagic pancreatitis; costovertebral tenderness (renal punch) with pyelonephritis or perinephric abscess.
- Hernial orifices/scrotum and testes should never be forgotten.
- Rectal examination, as indicated, looking for blood (bright, melaena or occult), faecal loading, local tenderness, masses, prostatomegaly.
- Pelvic examination: incorrect and uncertain diagnoses occur much more frequently in women. A careful vaginal examination may help differentiate pelvic pathology. Ultrasonography when available is more accurate.

  Note: Cervical motion tenderness is a 'classic' sign of ectopic pregnancy and pelvic inflammatory disease, but is a subjective sign.

Other systems

Exclude non-abdominal pathology causing abdominal pain (e.g. pneumonia, pulmonary embolus and myocardial infarction).

INVESTIGATIONS
Immediate

- Urine: urine analysis, microscopy and culture, pregnancy test (if appropriate)

- Blood: haemoglobin; haematocrit (packed cell volume [PCV]); white cell count and differential; electrolytes, urea and creatinine (EUC); amylase/lipase (if appropriate); blood gases (if appropriate); group-and-hold serum/cross-match (if blood loss or operation likely)
- Stool: frank or occult blood
- Organ imaging: supine and erect abdominal X-ray; erect chest X-ray

Semi-urgent (with appropriate indications)
- Blood: liver function tests (LFTs), coagulation studies
- Stool: smear and culture for colitis, enteritis
- Organ imaging: abdominal, ultrasound CT scan, angiography
- Endoscopy: proctosigmoidoscopy, upper GIT endoscopy

Value of investigations
- **Pregnancy** should be considered in all women of childbearing years with acute abdominal pain, to exclude ectopic pregnancy in particular.
- **White cell count** and other inflammatory markers (such as C-reactive protein) are non-specific unless elevated markedly (e.g. neutrophilia above 20×10^9/L). They are often late manifestations of significant pathology.
- **Serum lipase** is the test of choice for pancreatitis. Serum amylase is frequently elevated in a variety of conditions. Lipase level of more than 2–3 times normal is more sensitive and specific for pancreatitis.
- **Abdominal X-rays** are an insensitive tool for diagnosing non-specific abdominal pain, but can be valuable in confirming specific and serious pathology. Bowel obstruction, paralytic ileus and caecal and sigmoid volvulus have typical findings. A paucity of bowel gas may be the only clue to mesenteric infarction. Remember, check for calculi and for air in the biliary tree, and to look at the psoas shadows, the size and shape of solid organs. Avoid abdominal X-rays in pregnancy.
- **Erect chest X-ray** will detect subdiaphragmatic free air, exclude pulmonary pathology and help preoperative assessment. Free air will be absent in about 20% of perforated peptic ulcers. Massive pneumoperitoneum suggests colonic

perforation. The chest X-ray is the initial investigation for Boerhaave's syndrome (oesophageal rupture).

♦ **Abdominal ultrasound** is the preferred imaging modality for women of child-bearing age and many paediatric diagnoses. It is usually indicated for right upper quadrant (RUQ) pain and cholelithiasis, obstructive uropathy, suspected abdominal aortic aneurysm and abdominal masses. It is the investigation of choice in paediatric intussusception, pyloric stenosis, appendicitis. Pelvic ultrasound is essential for the diagnosis of gynaecological and pregnancy-related diseases.

♦ **CT scanning:** spiral non-contrast CT is the initial test of choice for renal colic. Contrast CT is useful in diagnosing many acute surgical conditions (e.g. acute pancreatitis, intra-abdominal sepsis, intra-abdominal trauma). It is increasingly used to confirm the preoperative diagnosis before laparotomy.

♦ **Proctosigmoidoscopy** is a diagnostic tool in bright rectal bleeding, rectal mass and colitis, and is therapeutic in sigmoid volvulus.

Other specialised tests
♦ **Angiography** may be both diagnostic and therapeutic in intestinal haemorrhage, mesenteric ischaemia and abdominal trauma.

♦ **Endoscopy** is indicated urgently in life-threatening upper GI tract bleeding and semi-electively in stable patients with suspected peptic ulcer or other inflammatory conditions of the upper GI tract.

MANAGEMENT
Surgical emergency
Indications for urgent intervention include leaking abdominal aortic aneurysm, perforated viscus, advanced peritonitis, mesenteric infarction and strangulated bowel.

Common indications for laparotomy
'Exploratory laparotomy' is now infrequently performed. After adequate resuscitation, most patients with an acute abdomen undergo specific imaging prior to surgery. Where diagnosis is uncertain, exploratory laparoscopy may be useful.

Preoperative treatment

1 Airway/Breathing: correct hypoxaemia.
2 Circulation: intravenous access and appropriate blood tests; volume resuscitation; urinary catheter.
3 Analgesia: is a high priority in moderate to severe pain. Titrated intravenous opiates are preferred. This will not mask or delay the diagnosis, and it will help clinical assessment by reducing distress and anxiety.
4 Antibiotic prophylaxis: is required with diffuse peritonitis or if infective pathology is suspected. Ampicillin, gentamicin and metronidazole is the usual combination therapy, to cover coliforms, enterococci and anaerobes.
5 Other preparation: nasogastric tube; operative fitness (cardiorespiratory assessment); consent by surgeon.

Surgical admission

Some conditions for which admission to hospital for conservative treatment, observation and semi-elective operation is appropriate are discussed later.

Emergency department observation and disposition

Patients with mild or equivocal tenderness, minor or no laboratory abnormalities and whose condition settles can be discharged for follow-up in the community, after observation in the ED. Certain diagnoses (e.g. uncomplicated renal or biliary colic and peptic ulceration) are discharged in most cases for further investigations and referral.

Specific surgical conditions
ACUTE APPENDICITIS

This is the most common general surgical emergency. Most problems occur with extremes of age, < 5 and > 60 years, mostly due to atypical presentation and late diagnosis.

Assessment

• Classical history is vague periumbilical pain, anorexia, nausea, vomiting, pain migration to right iliac fossa, fever. However, this only occurs in about half of cases.
• Clinical features can be summarised by the Alvarado (MANTRELS) score and include:

M Migration of pain
A Anorexia
N Nausea/vomiting
T Tenderness at McBurney's point
R Rebound tenderness
E Elevated temperature
L Leucocytosis
S Shift to the left of white cell count.

- Rectal examination is no longer indicated in the diagnosis of appendicitis.
- Pelvic ultrasound is preferable to pelvic examination in excluding gynaecological pathologies.
- **Differential diagnoses:** mesenteric adenitis in children; diverticular disease/caecal carcinoma in adults; ovarian cyst, pelvic inflammatory disease, ectopic pregnancy.

Investigations

- If appendicitis is strongly suggested by clinical features, no investigations are required, other than for preoperative assessment.
- Ultrasound is preferred for evaluating right iliac fossa pain in children and fertile female patients if the diagnosis is uncertain.
- CT is more sensitive than ultrasound and may reveal alternative diagnoses; contrast is not needed with newer CT scanners.

Management

1 Surgery as soon as practical. Overnight delay in the stable patient does not significantly worsen outcome.
2 Suspected perforation/generalised peritonitis—urgent surgery.
3 Prophylactic antibiotics reduce infective complications. They should be given in the ED if peritonitis or abscess is suspected or if surgery will be delayed. Otherwise, antibiotics can be given at induction of anaesthesia.
4 Mass/phlegmon: intravenous antibiotics and fluids; nil by mouth; ultrasound/CT scan; operation at surgeon's discretion.

GALL BLADDER EMERGENCIES
Assessment
- Occur in 25% of women and 12% of men
- Past history of fat intolerance, belching and flatulence
- Right upper quadrant (RUQ) pain becoming constant and severe
- Mild fever and tachycardia; mild icterus in 10% of cases
- Tender RUQ with positive Murphy's sign (sudden increased pain on inspiration)
- Palpable gallbladder in about one-third of cases
- Complications include:
  — empyema—toxic/shocked, high spiking temperatures; palpable tender mass as disease progresses
  — local perforation—progressing fever, symptoms and signs; local mass and peritonism
  — free perforation—general peritonism
  — cholangitis—secondary to obstruction (stone disease), instrumentation procedure (endoscopic retrograde cholangiopancreatography [ERCP], cholecystectomy); ascending infection; fever/rigors (~90%); RUQ pain (~70%); jaundice (~60%)

Investigations
- Urine analysis—bilirubin; exclude renal pathology.
- White cell count—not reliable but WBC > 15 000/mL suggest more-severe disease or complication.
- LFTs—are non-specific but bilirubin > 60 mmol/L suggests common duct obstruction.
- Ultrasound demonstrates stones, debris within the gall bladder, wall thickening, masses or abscesses.
- Abdominal X-ray is not necessary but may be ordered to exclude other pathology and complications.
- Hepatobiliary iminodiacetic acid (HIDA) scan may be used if ultrasound is non-diagnostic (e.g. acalculous cholecystitis).

- Operative fitness assessment (e.g. ECG, CXR, haemoglobin [Hb], renal function).

Management
Uncomplicated biliary colic
Discharge home for outpatient investigation and referral if:
- pain resolves
- no significant local signs
- normal laboratory investigations.

Cholecystitis
1 Admit to hospital.
2 Nil by mouth and intravenous fluids.
3 Analgesia.
4 Antibiotics intravenously (ampicillin/gentamicin).
5 Endoscopic retrograde cholangiopancreatography (ERCP) is rarely indicated; but may be necessary with obstructing bile duct stone.
6 Cholecystectomy, depending on progression of conservative therapy.

Advanced/complicated disease
Examples of this are cholangitis, empyema, abscess, free perforation, septicaemia.
1 Rapid stabilisation and assessment as for 'surgical emergency'.
2 Antibiotics (ampicillin, gentamicin and metronidazole or equivalents).
3 ERCP for bile duct obstruction; urgent cholecystectomy or cholecystostomy for empyema and abscess.

DIVERTICULAR DISEASE
Fifty per cent of people over 40 years of age have diverticular disease.

Assessment
- Previous symptoms: irregular bowel habit; diffuse, non-specific lower abdominal pain
- Diverticulitis: fever; altered bowel habit; left iliac fossa (LIF) pain and tenderness with or without local peritonism; LIF or pelvic mass

- Diverticular abscess: toxic; palpable mass
- Free perforation: generalised peritonitis
- Bleeding (see Lower GI Tract Bleeding later this chapter)

Investigations

- Urine analysis and midstream urine (MSU) to exclude renal pathology
- White cell count
- Contrast CT scan is the imaging modality of choice to confirm the diagnosis and assess severity of disease
- Abdominal X-ray usually non-specific, but may reveal perforation, local or generalised ileus or large mass if CT scan is not readily available

Management

- Mild cases: stable vital signs; pain controlled, can tolerate oral fluids—may be managed as outpatients with oral antibiotics (e.g. amoxicillin + clavulanate).
- More severe cases: admit; nil by mouth; intravenous fluids; intravenous antibiotics (ampicillin/gentamicin/metronidazole).
- Complicated/severe disease (e.g. advancing peritonitis; CT findings): management as above; urgent surgical consultation.

Gastrointestinal bleeding
UPPER GI TRACT BLEEDING
Aetiology

- 50% peptic ulceration
- 5–15% erosive gastritis/oesophagitis/duodenitis
- 15% oesophageal varices
- 15% Mallory–Weiss syndrome
- 5% others (tumour, blood dyscrasias, etc.)

Note: 30% of patients with known varices will bleed from other non-variceal causes.

Assessment
History

- Amount and nature of bleeding (haematemesis/melaena)
- Symptoms of occult bleeding

- Drug history: alcohol; non-steroidal anti-inflammatory drugs (NSAIDs); steroids
- Past GI tract disease/other conditions

Examination/immediate intervention

- Airway: intubation is indicated for airway protection in massive haemorrhage.
- Breathing: correct hypoxia.
- Circulation: assess for signs of shock.
     (*Note:* Initial haemoglobin may be near-normal in spite of massive blood loss.)
- Blood: for cross-match; haemoglobin; haematocrit; electrolytes; urea/creatinine; coagulation studies; liver function.
- General: evidence of chronic liver disease and hepatic encephalopathy; abdominal examination including rectal exam with or without proctoscopy; cardiorespiratory status.

Investigations

- Nasogastric tube insertion is rarely helpful; it may be performed for:
  — stable patients as a diagnostic tool
  — profuse haematemesis to empty stomach prior to endoscopy.
- Endoscopy is the definitive investigation, and in many cases an effective immediate treatment of upper GI tract bleeding. Endoscopy within 24 hours in stable patients reduces re-bleeding rates and shortens length of stay. Information regarding the aetiology, site and prognosis of the bleeding is gained. Urgent endoscopy should be performed in cardiovascularly unstable patients and in those with profuse or persistent bleeding.

Management

1 Volume resuscitation with crystalloids and/or blood and/or clotting factors.
2 Close monitoring of vital signs, urine output and haemoglobin/haematocrit. Invasive monitoring in the ICU for patients who are cardiovascularly unstable, elderly or have cardiorespiratory disease.

3 For presumed non-variceal bleeding, commence proton-pump inhibitors (PPIs). PPIs reduce bleeding recurrence, reduce mortality and shorten length of stay for ulcer-related bleeding.

4 Urgent endoscopy on high-risk patients with shock; blood requirements > 5 units; serious underlying disease; recurrent bleeding—especially if over 60 years of age. Endoscopy within 24 hours improves outcomes for all patients.

Non-variceal bleeding

- Eighty per cent of cases will settle spontaneously; 20% will require intervention for recurrent bleeding within 48 hours.
- Poor prognostic endoscopic findings in non-variceal bleeding are: gastric ulcer, especially lesser wall; posterior site in duodenum; visible vessel; sentinel clot or black spot in ulcer base.

Definitive treatment of non-variceal bleeding:

- endoscopic haemostasis
- surgery
- angiographic haemostasis (depending on availability).

Variceal bleeding

Poor prognostic factors include large blood requirements (> 4 units), active bleeding at endoscopy and child's category C patients (advanced hepatic failure).

Further management is as follows.

1 Endoscopic banding or sclerosis is 90% effective in controlling variceal bleeding. Balloon compression prior and/or simultaneously aids sclerotherapy.

2 Vasoconstrictive drugs (e.g. octreotide, a somatostatin mimic) lowers azygous vein blood flow in patients with portal hypertension, decreasing bleeding. This is a useful adjunct when endoscopy is not readily available.

3 Sengstaken–Blakemore or Minnesota tube insertion may be used as a temporary option for failed pharmacological or endoscopic treatment. It has significant complications and is not first-line therapy.

4 Angiographic embolisation.

5 Transjugular intrahepatic portosystemic shunt (TIPS).

LOWER GI TRACT BLEEDING

Causes of profuse, bright per rectal bleeding include: diverticular disease; polyps; angiodysplasia; carcinoma/colitis/solitary ulcer; haemorrhoids; Meckel's ulcer in children.

Note: Bright or maroon rectal bleeding is usually lower GI, but can occur with profuse upper GI tract bleed.

Assessment

History, examination and immediate intervention are as for upper GI tract bleeding. Elevated urea out of proportion to the creatinine can suggest an upper GI tract site of bleeding.

Investigations

Pathology work-up similar to upper GI bleed.

Management

1 Volume resuscitation.
2 Monitor vital signs, urine output, haemoglobin/haematocrit.
3 Bleeding stops spontaneously in 75% of cases with conservative treatment.
4 Sigmoidoscopy/colonoscopy is usually done on a semi-elective basis if the patient remains haemodynamically stable.
5 If the patient remains unstable in spite of resuscitation, arrange urgent specialist referral for possible mesenteric angiogram or surgical treatment.
6 Radio-isotope scanning has a role in stable patients with uncertain sites of lower GI tract bleed.

Acute pancreatitis

The causes of acute pancreatitis are gallstones (40–50%), alcohol (25–35%), idiopathic (20%) and others which include a variety of medications (5%).

ASSESSMENT

History

- Look for potentially reversible causes.
- Acute epigastric pain through to back, associated with nausea and vomiting.

Examination/initial intervention

- Airway
- Breathing: correct hypoxaemia
- Circulation: anticipate shock; fluid resuscitate as required
- Blood: for lipase/amylase; haemoglobin/haematocrit, electrolytes; urea/creatinine; calcium; glucose; LFTs; blood gases; coagulation studies; group-and-hold
- Abdominal examination: temperature, jaundice; epigastric tenderness with or without mass; local/diffuse peritonism; Cullen's (periumbilical) and Grey–Turner's (flank) signs in haemorrhagic pancreatitis; paralytic ileus; subcutaneous fat necrosis
- Cardiorespiratory examination, especially to exclude complications (respiratory complications occur in 10–20% of cases)

Prognostic indicators

- Disease ranges from mild inflammation to severe extensive pancreatic necrosis (10–20%) and multi-organ failure, with mortality rates of > 20%.
- Assessment of severity is important for management and to predict outcomes.
- Three known severity scores are performed 48–72 hours after diagnosis. They may therefore not be useful in the ED setting, but can be used to observe progress after admission.
  a Ranson's criteria:
    o immediate—age > 55; hyperglycaemia; leucocytosis; lactase dehydrogenase (LDH); aspartate amino-transferase (AST)
    o two days—drop in haemoglobin/haematocrit; shock; hypocalcaemia; hypoxia; azotaemia (elevated urea)
    o score of 5 (at 48 hours) suggests serious illness.
  b APACHE score
  c Balthazar staging on CT scanning.

Investigations

- Amylase/lipase: levels more than three times normal confirm the diagnosis in the majority of cases. Lipase is more sensitive and specific, and is better than amylase in diagnosing chronic pancreatitis.

- Abdominal X-ray: does not need to be performed routinely, but can be used to exclude other diagnoses and complications. A 'sentinel loop' of small bowel indicates a localised ileus.
- Chest X-ray: raised left hemidiaphragm; pleural effusion; atelectasis; acute respiratory distress syndrome (ARDS).
- ECG: to exclude myocardial infarct.
- Ultrasound: should be performed to exclude gallstone pancreatitis. CT scanning with contrast may be performed within 72 hours to assess severity. It should be performed early when there is diagnostic uncertainty and in critically ill patients.

Management

1 Volume resuscitation.
2 Supplemental oxygen.
3 Monitor observations, urine output.
4 Nil by mouth; nasogastric tube for severe cases or if gastric dilation or ileus.
5 Analgesia: parenteral narcotics.
6 Insulin infusion if blood sugar level (BSL) > 15 mmol/L.
7 Observe for other complications: shock/acidosis; acute tubular necrosis; ARDS/disseminated intravascular coagulation (DIC); haemorrhagic pancreatitis; pancreatic abscess.
8 Prophylactic antibiotics: for necrotic pancreatitis or for pancreatic abscesses. Carbapenems and quinolones have best pancreatic tissue penetration.
9 Early ERCP is necessary for gall stone pancreatitis with an obstructing stone.
10 Laparotomy has up to 40% mortality. There are multiple options of invasive techniques to treat the complications of pancreatitis.

Gastro-oesophageal reflux disease (GORD)—oesophagitis

Remember: Indigestion is not a diagnosis; it is an excuse to stop thinking.

- In discussing GORD, it is crucial to consider an acute coronary syndrome. Improvement of 'indigestion' with antacids is not proof of upper GI tract pathology. 'Indigestion' is a common diagnosis in missed acute myocardial infarction (AMI). The mortality rate of missed AMI is around 30%.
- About 7% of the population reports daily heartburn. **Risk factors** for GORD include obesity, alcohol, smoking, diabetes and pregnancy. **Exacerbating factors** are chocolate/fatty and spicy foods, drugs (e.g. NSAIDs), cough medicines and bisphosphonates.
- The commonest **symptoms** of GORD are heartburn, regurgitation and dysphagia (oesophageal stricture or spasm). Atypical symptoms relate to gastric reflux, which may be 'silent' (e.g. cough/wheeze or hoarseness).
- GORD is the commonest non-cardiac cause of chest pain (~50% of cases).

ASSESSMENT
History
- Look for aetiological factors.
- Epigastric and/or chest pain, typically burning. Oesophageal spasm may occur without burning pain.
- Reflux, with or without cough/wheeze/hoarseness.
- Haematemesis/melaena.
- Cardiac risk factors and cardiac symptoms: could it be angina?
- Fatty food intolerance; belching; RUQ pain: could it be cholelithiasis?
- Weight loss; anorexia; jaundice: could it be upper GI tract malignancy?
- Malignancy/steroid use/HIV/immunosuppression: could it be infective oesophagitis?

EXAMINATION
- Airway; breathing; circulation.
- Abdominal examination: tenderness (epigastrium/RUQ); look for other causes of epigastric pain (e.g. liver, leaking abdominal aortic aneurysm). If suspicious of GI tract bleed, perform rectal exam for blood.

INVESTIGATIONS

- For uncomplicated GORD, none may be required. Do not forget an ECG. A trial of PPIs or H_2-receptor antagonists may give relief and suggest GORD, but does not rule out other diagnoses.
- Exclude other diseases: ECG/cardiac markers; CXR; LFTs; amylase/lipase; abdominal ultrasound.
- Assess complications of erosive oesophagitis (e.g. full blood count [FBC]); iron studies.

MANAGEMENT

1 Lifestyle modification: weight loss; avoid precipitating foods/ smoking; elevate head of bed about 20 cm; eat evening meal 3 hours prior to bed; smaller meals.
2 If uncomplicated GORD, commence treatment and refer to local doctor:
   a antacids after meals and at night may control symptoms
   b PPI or H_2-receptor antagonist.
3 Red flags include dysphagia/odynophagia; refractory symptoms after treatment; bleeding/anaemia; weight loss and aspiration. Consult a gastroenterologist.

Mesenteric ischaemia/infarction

Acute mesenteric ischaemia is a notoriously difficult illness to diagnose and treat. Reported mortality rates average about 70%. It is often diagnosed late because of non-specific initial symptoms and signs. By the time peritonism or advanced abdominal signs are present, extensive bowel infarction has usually occurred and the prognosis is grave. The bowel can tolerate about 4 hours of warm ischaemic time. Significant bowel necrosis occurs after 8–12 hours of ischaemia.

Mesenteric ischaemia is usually due to impaired circulation of the superior mesenteric artery (SMA): 50% is embolic, 25% thrombotic and 20% 'non-occlusive mesenteric ischaemia' (low-flow states). About 5% is due to mesenteric vein thrombosis.

ASSESSMENT

- Patients with SMA emboli will usually have a past history of atrial fibrillation or myocardial infarction.

- Patients with SMA thrombosis have evidence of other arteriovascular disease, and up to half will have experienced prior mesenteric angina.
- Low-flow mesenteric ischaemia occurs in patients with pre-existing hypotension, sepsis and vasoconstrictor infusions. The elderly and those on digoxin are particularly at risk.
- Mesenteric vein occlusion tends to occur in younger patients with hypercoagulable states and have a slower onset.
- Abdominal pain out of proportion to clinical findings is an important finding. The pain is typically acute-onset, severe, constant and generalised, sometimes colicky. It often responds poorly to analgesia. Many patients have vomiting and diarrhoea.
- Similar to other ischaemic pathologies, there are few initial physical signs. There is minimal, if any, tenderness. As the disease progresses, abdominal distension and GI tract bleeding may occur. Localised tenderness over infarcted bowel loops, diffuse peritonitis and systemic sepsis occur as the bowel becomes gangrenous and necrotic.

INVESTIGATIONS

- Most patients will have a series of screening pathology tests and abdominal and chest X-rays (see 'Acute abdomen') in the early stages in an attempt to find the diagnosis. By the time these non-specific investigations are significantly abnormal, the bowel is infarcting.
- Rising serial lactates suggest the diagnosis, but also occur late in the disease. Critically ill patients in septic shock need a work-up to assess severity and monitor resuscitation.
- The definitive investigation is an abdominal contrast CT angiogram. Whenever there is a reasonable index of suspicion of the diagnosis, this must be arranged urgently.

MANAGEMENT

1 Airway.
2 Breathing: supplemental oxygen to correct hypoxaemia.
3 Circulation: intravenous access; volume resuscitation as necessary; nil by mouth; urinary catheter.
4 Analgesia: titrated intravenous opiates.

5 Antibiotics: ampicillin/gentamicin/metronidazole, or equivalent.
6 Urgent surgical opinion/urgent radiological opinion (CT angiography can be curative, not just diagnostic).
7 Definitive treatment depends on the underlying cause and clinical situation. Many of these patients are elderly with multiple co-morbidities. Given the frequently delayed diagnosis and the background health of such patients, palliative treatment is often appropriate after discussion with the patient and family/carers.
8 Advanced peritonitis from gangrenous bowel requires urgent laparotomy if patient is not for palliative treatment.
9 Vasodilator and/or thrombolytic infusion can be administered at angiography.
10 Specific embolectomy or thromboendarterectomy by a vascular surgeon may be necessary.

Vomiting

Vomiting is a symptom, not a diagnosis. Most vomiting patients have benign, readily treated illnesses. Occasionally it is a symptom of a life-threatening problem. Management is directed at finding and treating the cause, assessing fluid deficits and controlling the symptoms.

ASSESSMENT
History

• Age: in infants and children consider pyloric stenosis, intussusception, viral gastroenteritis, reflux, sepsis and meningitis.
  Note: Children become dehydrated more quickly.
• Chest pain: acute coronary syndrome; Boerhaave's syndrome (uncommon).
• Abdomen:
  — fever; viral prodrome; contacts with gastroenteritis or suspect foods; diarrhoea—infection (e.g. gastroenteritis or food poisoning)
  — 'heartburn'; epigastric discomfort; haematemesis/melaena—peptic ulcer disease; erosive oesophagitis; oesophageal varices; Mallory–Weiss tear

- abdominal pain—colicky suggesting bowel obstruction; RUQ suggesting biliary disease; right iliac fossa suggesting appendicitis; generalised and severe suggesting peritonitis
- previous abdominal surgery and colicky pain—adhesions and bowel obstruction
- jaundice, dark urine—biliary disease; hepatitis.
- Neurology:
  - headache—migraine; meningitis or meningism; cerebrovascular event; sub-arachnoid haemorrhage
  - vertigo/'dizziness'—labyrinthitis; vertebrobasilar disease or posterior fossa lesion.
- Vision: glaucoma.
- Pregnancy: in women of childbearing age.
- Diabetic or symptoms of diabetes: ketoacidosis.
- Drugs:
  - medications—opiates; antibiotics; chemotherapy
  - marijuana abuse—cyclical vomiting syndrome (repetitive hot showers is pathognomonic).

EXAMINATION

- Airway
- Breathing: ketotic
- Circulation: vital signs; peripheral perfusion; dehydration
- Disability: mental state; Glasgow Coma Scale (GCS); pupils
- Targeted examination guided by history

INVESTIGATIONS

- Investigations depend on the clinical context and the likely aetiology. They serve two purposes: establishing the underlying cause, and assessing complications of vomiting.
- Basic tests should include FBC; EUC; LFTs; BSL; urine analysis; beta-hCG in women of childbearing age.
- Disease-specific tests depend on the suspected diagnoses.

MANAGEMENT

1 Restore fluid deficits depending on degree of dehydration and EUC results.
2 If severe dehydration/shock, resuscitate with crystalloid. Insert indwelling urinary catheter if persistent shock.

3 Otherwise, per oral/nasogastric (NG) or IV rehydration, depending on the clinical context. (Children in particular respond well to oral and NG rehydration.)

4 Anti-emetics include:

a dopamine antagonists—metoclopramide, prochlorperazine (beware acute dystonic reaction in young women and children)

b serotonin antagonists (e.g. ondansetron).

5 Disease-specific interventions as indicated.

Constipation

As in vomiting, it is important to rule out serious underlying causes of constipation. It is the commonest GI tract complaint, affecting up to 25% of people at some time. Two per cent of the population have chronic or recurrent constipation.

Causes in children are as follows.

* Functional (over 90% of cases, especially if > 1 year old)
* Change in formula or to bottle-feeding in infants
* Hirschsprung's disease
* Congenital anorectal or neurological diseases
* Cystic fibrosis
* Metabolic disorders

Causes in adults are as follows.

* Primary: functional (normal transit); slow transit; anorectal muscle incoordination
* Secondary:
  — medications (up to 40% of cases) (e.g. opioids, antidepressants, calcium-channel blockers, diuretics, iron, antihistamines, psychotropic agents)
  — irritable bowel syndrome (IBS)
  — psychological conditions (e.g. anxiety, depression)
  — anorectal structural abnormalities (e.g. anal fissure, haemorrhoids)
  — endocrine and metabolic diseases (e.g. diabetes mellitus, hypercalcaemia, hypothyroidism)
  — neurological (e.g. Parkinsonism, multiple sclerosis, spinal cord disease); autonomic neuropathy.

Note: Constipation is not a 'normal' part of ageing.

ASSESSMENT
History
- Frequency and quality of stool; effort of defecation; pain; incomplete evacuation; soiling; bleeding; nausea/vomiting; medications; urinary retention
- **'Red flags' in children:** delayed meconium; abdominal distension/vomiting; failure to thrive, recurrent pneumonia (cystic fibrosis); abnormal gait or lower limb tone; wheat intolerance (gluten enteropathy)
- **'Red flags' in adults:** age over 50 years; weight loss; rectal bleeding; family history of colon cancer

Examination
Examination is directed at finding underlying cause and confirming faecal loading.
- Airway; breathing; circulation
- Dehydration if vomiting; abdominal distension
- Abdominal examination—looking for obstruction, masses or hernia
- Anal inspection—congenital abnormality in children; anal fissure; haemorrhoids; rectal prolapse
- Rectal examination—to confirm faecal loading:
  — mandatory in an adult; may be replaced by plain abdominal X-ray in children if parents object or child distressed (level C evidence)
- Specific system examination to exclude secondary causes (e.g. neurological [altered anal tone, abnormal lower limb power/tone/reflexes])

INVESTIGATIONS
- None usually required if history of functional constipation in child.
- FBC; BSL; EUC; calcium; thyroid function; urine analysis in adults. Abdominal X-ray may be indicated to exclude obstruction and/or reveal extent of colonic loading.
- Sigmoidoscopy and/or colonoscopy (semi-elective) if 'red flags' in adult.
- Specific investigations or consultations if secondary cause suspected.

MANAGEMENT IN ADULTS

This is a possible protocol. Local preferences may apply.

1 Distal rectal vault only:
   a 1–2 Microlax enemas → wait 30–60 minutes
   b 1–2 bisacodyl enemas → wait 30–60 minutes
   c Fleet (phosphate) enema OR 20 mL lactulose in 100 mL water → retain for at least 10 minutes; may be repeated once
   d manual disimpaction (with analgesia; sedation)
   e may need admission for repeat enemas.

2 Faecal matter above rectum:
   a oral sorbitol (70%) 30 mL q2–3 hours
   PLUS
   b Fleet (phosphate) enema or lactulose enema as above → wait 4–6 hours
   c if no success (or oral sorbitol not available) → GlycoPrep-C solution 1 sachet/litre orally per hour, up to 3 litres
   OR
   Movicol 8 sachets in 1 litre over 6 hours
   OR
   oral picosulphate 1–2 sachets in a glass of water (causes greater fluid and electrolyte shifts; use cautiously in the elderly due to dehydration; renal impairment; cardiac failure).

Admission may be required for observation, repeat enemas and/or oral agents.

Patients may be discharged if they have at least one significant documented bowel action, for follow-up by their doctor in 24 hours.

The discharge plan should include dietary advice, fluid intake, exercise, toileting pattern, aperients and review of causative medications.

Editorial Comment

Constipation is *not* a diagnosis, nor is it an excuse to stop thinking. Hospital EDs often have a very helpful protocol for this very common symptom
Be aware of red flags.

Hepatic failure—portosystemic encephalopathy
FULMINANT
- Acute hepatic failure, onset within 8 weeks
- Encephalopathy, jaundice, hepatic fetor, multiple-system complications (coagulopathy, immunosuppression, renal dysfunction)

Aetiology
- Viral hepatitis
- Paracetamol overdose
- Drug reactions (e.g. isoniazid, methyldopa)

ACUTE-ON-CHRONIC
- Stigmata of chronic liver disease, jaundice, ascites, encephalopathy

Aetiology
- Alcoholic cirrhosis
- Chronic active hepatitis
- Post-necrotic
- Infiltrative
- Other

PRECIPITATING CAUSES OF ENCEPHALOPATHY
Fulminant
Encephalopathy from cerebral oedema is the hallmark of the disease. Coma has 80% mortality. It can be exacerbated by the following conditions.

ACUTE-ON-CHRONIC
- GI tract bleeding (especially upper): elevated urea/creatinine ratio is suggestive; accounts for about 25% of cases
- Reduced stool frequency
- Increased protein load
- Azotaemia/volume depletion: hepatorenal syndrome
- Hypokalaemia/alkalosis
- Hypoxaemia/hypoglycaemia

- Infection, including spontaneous bacterial peritonitis in ascites (usually coliforms or pneumococci)
- Ethanol, sedatives, opiates

ASSESSMENT
History
- Alcohol and drug history
- Rapidity of onset of symptoms
- GI tract bleeding

Examination/immediate intervention
- Airway
- Breathing: correct hypoxaemia
- Large-bore IV access
- Blood: for haemoglobin/haematocrit; coagulation studies; EUC; calcium/phosphate/magnesium; BSL; LFTs; blood gas; ammonia levels; viral serology, group-and-hold as necessary
- Dextrose: hypoglycaemia needs to be rapidly excluded and treated
- Encephalopathy: GCS; Mini-Mental State; asterixis (flap)
- Further examination: fetor; evidence of chronic liver disease/ ascites; liver/spleen/rectal examination; cause of likely decompensation, including rectal exam; complications (e.g. bleeding, cardiorespiratory, infectious disease, alcohol withdrawal)

INVESTIGATIONS
- Septic work-up, including ascitic tap if suspect bacterial peritonitis
- Blood gas
- Serum ammonia (does not correlate well with severity of illness)
- Chest X-ray
- ECG
- Head CT scan and EEG to assess encephalopathy/oedema and exclude other pathology
- Liver biopsy in some cases

Management

1 Treat precipitating causes (e.g. GI tract bleeding, constipation, volume depletion, electrolyte abnormality, infection).

2 Reduce protein absorption—oral lactulose (30–45 mL q8h); low-protein diet (20–40 g/day); oral antibiotics to treat gut flora such as neomycin or metronidazole may be used for patients intolerant of lactulose.

3 Other nutritional support (e.g. carbohydrates, zinc, magnesium).

4 Patients with potentially reversible coma will need endotracheal intubation and ICU transfer.

5 Consider reversal of portosystemic shunts in life-threatening encephalopathy not responding to treatment.

6 Liver transplant in selected patients.

Online resources

eMedicine

www.emedicine.medscape.com

Chapter 27
Neurosurgical emergencies

Rob Edwards

This chapter covers the approach to the patient who presents with headache as well as the following neurosurgical emergencies, both traumatic and non-traumatic:

- head injury
- subdural haematoma
- blunt cerebrovascular injury (BCVI)
- cervical spine injury and spinal cord injuries
- intracranial haemorrhages such as subarachnoid haemorrhage (SAH), subdural haemorrhage (SDH) and intracerebral haemorrhage (ICH)
- emergency presentations of patients with space-occupying lesions (SOLs)
- complications of ventriculoperitoneal shunts
- spinal epidural abscess.

It is helpful to consider some general concepts and principles first.

General concepts
PRIMARY VERSUS SECONDARY BRAIN INJURY

Primary brain injury is the injury that occurs at the time of the trauma. Interventions that affect primary brain injury are out of the immediate control of the emergency doctor, but are important and include public health measures aimed at prevention. Some measures that have reduced head injury include compulsory use of seat belts in cars and helmets for motorcycle riders and pedal cyclists.

Secondary brain injury occurs after the initial injury and is due to the sequelae of the original injury, such as raised intracranial pressure, hypoxia, hypercarbia or hypotension. It can be either minimised or prevented with good management.

Cerebral perfusion pressure (CPP) is the pressure that drives perfusion of the brain and is defined by the equation:

CPP = mean arterial pressure (MAP) − intracranial pressure (ICP)

Normally ICP is between 5 and 10 mmHg. Autoregulatory mechanisms will maintain constant cerebral blood flow when the cerebral perfusion varies between 50 and 150 mmHg. In some patients, such as those with severe head injury, cerebral autoregulation may be lost, thus making the brain more susceptible to hypotension. Any process that reduces MAP (e.g. hypovolaemic shock) or increases ICP (post-injury oedema, expanding intracranial haematoma or mass, and hypercarbia) will compromise cerebral perfusion, leading to secondary brain injury.

Editorial Comment

The management of concussion is complex and still evolving. There is increasing awareness of issues related to concussion, especially in sports and in research using amnesia scales. Doctors need to keep up to date on recommendations as to when people can return to sports/contact sports/work after a concussive episode.

HEADACHE

Headache is a common symptom of a neurosurgical emergency (e.g. any of the intracranial haemorrhages, space-occupying lesion). It may also be a symptom of a life-threatening non-surgical emergency (e.g. meningitis, encephalitis), or other less serious disease processes (e.g. migraine) or a non-specific manifestation of a non-neurological process (e.g. any serious infection such as pneumonia, influenza, pyelonephritis).

As headache is a frequent complaint of patients presenting to the ED, the problem is to differentiate the patients who harbour a serious cause from those who do not. Boxes 27.1 and 27.2 outline some criteria for computed tomography (CT) of the brain of both trauma and non-trauma patients.

Box 27.1   Indications for cerebral CT in mild head injury

- Glasgow Coma Scale (GCS) score < 15 at 2 hours after injury
- Abnormal alertness/behaviour or cognition despite 'normal' GCS
- Deteriorating GCS score
- Suspected open, or a depressed, skull fracture
- Age ≥ 65 years
- Vomiting (two or more episodes)
- Major mechanism of injury with significant force
- Focal neurological signs
- Persistent headache
- Anticoagulant therapy or coagulopathy
- Loss of consciousness > 5 minutes
- Persistent posttraumatic amnesia
- Consider CT if any of the following are present: large scalp haematoma or laceration, multisystem trauma, delayed presentation or re-presentation

---

Box 27.2   Indications for urgent cerebral CT in non-trauma patients with headache

- Focal neurological signs
- Altered mental status or change in behaviour
- Age > 60 years
- Nausea and vomiting
- Severe or sudden onset suggestive of subarachnoid haemorrhage (SAH)
- Absence of other demonstrable cause for headache
- History of cerebral tumour, warfarin or NOAC use or other condition (e.g. shunt, hydrocephalus, recent craniotomy)

Features which indicate that a headache is due to raised ICP are associated nausea and vomiting and headache worse on awakening in the morning and on lying down.

GLASGOW COMA SCALE (GCS)

The GCS is a widely accepted scale for assessing alteration to a patient's level of consciousness. A score is given based on three components—eye opening, verbal response and motor response (Table 27.1). In adults, the score achieved correlates well with the severity of the underlying condition. It is also useful for objectively following a patient's progress.

Table 27.1 Glasgow Coma Scale

Eye opening	Spontaneous	4
	To voice	3
	To pain	2
	None	1
Best verbal response	Alert	5
	Confused	4
	Inappropriate words only	3
	Incomprehensible sounds	2
	Nil	1
Best motor response	Obeys commands	6
	Localises pain	5
	Withdraws to pain	4
	Abnormal flexion	3
	Abnormal extension	2
	None	1

HERNIATION SYNDROMES

The cranial cavity is divided into compartments by fibrous dura mater (the falx cerebri and tentorium cerebelli). The tentorium separates the cerebrum above from the cerebellum and brainstem below. Because of the rigidity and non-expansible nature of the cranial vault, significant increases in ICP can lead to herniation syndromes where the contents of one compartment herniate across an opening in these dural structures, causing specific neurological signs. The significance of a herniation syndrome is that ICP has increased beyond the capacity of the brain to compensate, and death will ensue without urgent intervention. Raised ICP above the tentorium leads to herniation of the uncus of the temporal lobe. This manifests as dilation of the ipsilateral pupil (later bilateral), contralateral pyramidal weakness and increased tone.

Raised ICP will also lead to high blood pressure and bradycardia (Cushing response).

MANAGEMENT PRINCIPLES

The aims of treatment are to prevent secondary brain injury, treat the underlying condition, minimise symptoms and optimise neurological and functional recovery. ED management is concerned with the first three of these.

Airway, breathing and circulation (ABCs)

A patent airway is the first priority (see Chapter 2 The Airway, Ventilation and Procedural Sedation). Simple manoeuvres to maintain patency may prevent secondary brain injury from hypoxia. Airway protection is also important—patients with a GCS of 8 or less will not be able to protect their airway from *aspiration* or maintain a patent airway, and need intubation. Adequate ventilation is required to avoid *hypoxia* and *hypercarbia*. Treatment measures vary from oxygen therapy by mask to full mechanical ventilation if required. Adequate CPP relies in part on a normal blood pressure. *Hypotension* should therefore be treated with prevention of further blood loss and resuscitation with fluids and blood products.

Measures to decrease ICP

A number of interventions can reduce ICP.

- Adequate sedation and paralysis of the intubated patient with neurosurgical emergency, including at the time of rapid-sequence induction.
- Mannitol 20%, 1 g/kg (equates to 5 mL of 20% mannitol per kg) intravenous. Uses osmotic pressure to draw water out of the brain which decreases ICP. Indicated when there is severe increase in ICP (e.g. evidence of herniation syndrome, significant mass effect on CT or high ICP).
- Corticosteroids (dexamethasone) help to reduce oedema associated with space-occupying lesions. They are *not* shown to be useful in traumatic brain injury.
- Maintain normal PCO_2 (35–40 mmHg). Hyperventilation to lower than normal PCO_2 is not recommended, as this causes cerebral vasoconstriction and does not improve outcome.
- Elevate the head of the bed 30° if the spinal column has been cleared.

Surgery

The indications for surgery will be discussed specifically for each condition.

Traumatic neurosurgical emergencies
HEAD INJURY

Head injury resulting in traumatic brain injury (TBI) is the major cause of trauma-related death. Of those who survive with a residual traumatic brain injury, some are left with neurological impairment that often requires lengthy rehabilitation and may result in inability to return to work or function normally. The social and financial costs are very high. It is a relatively high-prevalence injury, and it has been estimated that in Australia there are about 150 admissions to hospital per year with TBI per 100 000 population and that peak incidence is in the age group 15–35 years.

Classification and pathophysiology

There are different ways of classifying head injury. Each is useful in that there is some relationship to treatment and prognosis. Table 27.2 outlines a classification according to the actual pathology of the injury. TBI can also be classified according to severity based on GCS (GCS 8 = severe, GCS 9–13 = moderate, and GCS 14–15 = mild or minor).

Assessment should be performed according to advanced trauma life support principles, which use a prioritised and systematised approach.

Table 27.2 Pathological lesions seen in head injury

Type of injury	Lesion
Skull fractures	Depressed (see Figure 27.1)
	Base of skull
	Linear
Cerebral contusion	
Haemorrhage	Intracerebral
	Subarachnoid
	Subdural (see Figure 27.2)
	Extradural (see Figure 27.3)
Diffuse axonal injury	
Blunt cerebrovascular injury	Rupture, dissection and occlusion of extra and intracerebral arteries

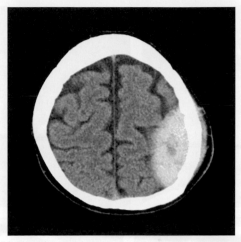

Figure 27.1 CT scan showing a left-sided extradural haematoma

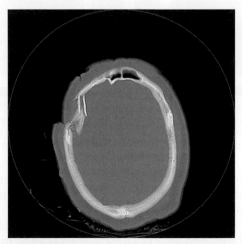

Figure 27.2 Depressed skull fracture. Bone windows of CT brain in a patient who was noted to have dysphasia after being hit on the head with a bat, due to local pressure to the speech centre of the brain.

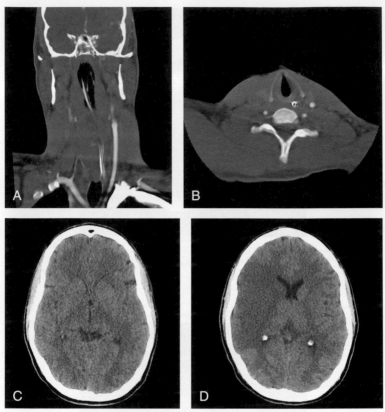

Figure 27.3 A & B. CT angiogram showing non-opacification of the right common carotid artery (CCA) and internal carotid artery (ICA) resulting from a traumatic dissection of right CCA extending up to the ICA. C & D. CT brain at time of initial imaging and after infraction of the territory of the right ICA.

Indicators of a potentially significant trauma to the head are any one of loss of consciousness, amnesia or a mechanism involving a high degree of force.

In cases where the patient may have been drinking alcohol, altered mentation and level of consciousness can be misdiagnosed as alcohol or drug intoxication. This can have lethal consequences. Where alcohol use and head injury coexist, always assume that any alteration in mental state is due to the head injury.

Clinical features

Other relevant parts of the history include the following.

- 'Lucid interval': patient regains consciousness after the primary injury then becomes unconscious later due to an expanding extradural haematoma.
- Headache, nausea and vomiting.
- Amnesia: retrograde amnesia refers to inability to remember events before the injury. Anterograde amnesia is the inability to remember information acquired since the injury. This often manifests as the patient asking the same questions over and over again. The abbreviated Westmead Post Traumatic Amnesia Scale (A-WPTAS) is an easily applied, objective tool to use on ED patients to screen for significant amnesia (www. aci.health.nsw.gov.au). The total score is a combination of the GCS and three-object recall.

On examination, local head trauma (lacerations, haematomas) may be present. The GCS should be measured (Table 27.1). Focal neurological signs such as pupillary dilation with or without hemiparesis and increased tone and reflexes indicate an uncal herniation syndrome requiring emergency management. Where there is significant increase in ICP, the Cushing reflex will lead to hypertension and bradycardia. Clues to a fractured skull base are cerebrospinal fluid (CSF) leak from the nose, bilateral periorbital bruising (raccoon eyes), CSF leak from the ear, haemotympanum and bruising behind the ear (Battle's sign).

Investigations

Urgent CT scan of the brain in severe (GCS ≤ 8) and moderate (GCS 9–13) head injuries. For mild head injury (GCS 14–15), which comprise more than 80% of head injury presentations, CT scan is more likely normal and it is accepted practice to use clinical criteria to be more selective in ordering a CT scan. See Box 27.1, above.

Blood tests such as white cell count (WCC), haemoglobin and serum chemistries are relevant though not diagnostic. Coagulation studies should be done if there is intracranial haemorrhage or if the patient is on anticoagulants. A blood group and hold should be done if the patient requires evacuation of a haematoma, as there may be significant blood loss in this procedure.

Management

A systematic trauma approach that identifies, prioritises and treats life-threatening injuries is mandatory. This will allow immediate management of life-threatening problems such as airway obstruction, lack of airway protection, hypoxia, blood loss and hypotension, thus avoiding secondary brain injury. Specific management includes the following.

Measures to reduce ICP

The specific measures (see 'Management principles' above) are appropriate for all patients with severe TBI. Mannitol 20% (1 g/kg) is usually reserved for those who have evidence of a herniation syndrome, evidence of mass effect on CT or high ICP as measured on an ICP monitor.

Surgical intervention

Surgery is required for drainage of extradural (see Figure 27.1) and subdural haematomas. If mass effect or raised ICP is present this may be required urgently. Smaller subdurals with no mass effect may be managed non-operatively. Supportive therapy is required for contusions, subarachnoid haemorrhage and diffuse axonal injury. Surgery is also required for depressed skull fracture (see Figure 27.2). In severe head injuries, insertion of an ICP monitor and monitoring of intra-arterial blood pressure to direct therapy (see above) is aimed at reducing raised ICP. To maintain adequate cerebral blood flow, a CPP of above 70 mmHg is ideal.

Analgesia

Paracetamol (IV or orally for patients who can swallow) can be used. Aspirin is absolutely contraindicated because of its antiplatelet effect. Ongoing headache unrelieved by simple analgesia is an indication for urgent CT scan in mild head injury. If stronger pain relief is required, for either headache or other injuries, titrated doses of opiate analgesia (e.g. codeine, oxycodone, fentanyl) can be given in a closely monitored situation and where CT brain is to be performed.

Other acute treatments

If seizures occur during the acute phase, phenytoin (loading dose 15–20 mg/kg IV infusion) can be given to prevent further seizures.

Alternative drugs are levetiracetam (15 mg/kg) or sodium valproate 10 mg/kg (maximum of 800 mg).

Patients with mild but significant head injury not having a CT scan should be observed until they have been normal and symptom-free for an appropriate length of time. Accepted clinical practice is at least 4 hours. Patients with an A-WPTAS score < 18 at 4 hours should be considered for admission.

When discharged, patients should be provided with written head injury advice. About one-third of patients with so-called minor head injury have disabling symptoms for several days to weeks after the head injury, including headaches, difficulty concentrating and dizziness. Patients should be warned about this.

Blunt cerebrovascular injury (BCVI)

BCVI is injury to the blood vessels (vertebral or carotid arteries) supplying the brain from blunt trauma. Improvements in vascular imaging have led to the realisation that BCVI is not rare with an estimated prevalence of 1–2% of trauma centre admissions. BCVI may lead to neurological impairment which may not be present at the time of injury and presentation but develops later (usually 10–72 hours).

The most common mechanism is high-speed deceleration from motor vehicle trauma but also direct blow to the neck, cervical spine fracture and base of skull fracture. The grade of injury varies from intimal tear to pseudoaneurysm to vessel rupture. These may lead to vessel occlusion or embolisation and subsequent ischaemic neurological events.

Patients deemed at risk for BCVI should be screened with CT cerebral angiography. Digital subtraction angiography is the gold standard but is more invasive and time consuming. Patients are deemed at high risk according to mechanism of injury, the injury itself or clinical findings (see Table 27.3).

Treatment options include medical therapy (antiplatelet agents, anticoagulation), surgical ligation or repair and angiographic interventions such as coiling and stents.

Figure 27.4 illustrates a traumatic carotid artery injury (CAI) resulting from deceleration in a head-on motor vehicle collision and the resulting infarct in the territory of the right ICA.

Table 27.3   Criteria from screening with CT angiography of neck vessels

Neurological deficit
Horner's syndrome
Base of skull fracture (especially petrous temporal bone)
Le Forte II and III fractures
Soft tissue injuries of the neck
Hanging
Cervical spine fractures
Severe traumatic brain injury (GCS ≤ 6, diffuse axonal injury)

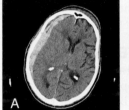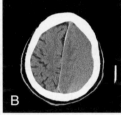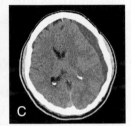

Figure 27.4 Non-contrast cerebral CT scans showing subdural haematomas of varying age. A. Acute right subdural. B. Left isodense, 10-14-day-old subdural with mass effect showing compression of the ventricle and midline shift to the right. C. Chronic left subdural.

Subdural haematoma

Subdural haematoma can present without a definite history of trauma; however, it is usually traumatic in origin. Subdural haematomas arise from injury to the bridging veins in the subdural space (between the dura mater which follows the contour of the bony skull, and the pia mater which follows the contour of the cortex of the brain). Where there is cortical atrophy this space is prominent and more at risk of subdural haematoma from an injury.

CLINICAL FEATURES

Depending on the interval between the bleed and presentation, a subdural haematoma can be acute, subacute or chronic (Figure 27.4). When large, it presents with symptoms of mass effect (see 'Space-occupying lesions', below). Other symptoms include headache, confusion and ataxia. The clinical picture can be non-specific.

INVESTIGATION

Definitive diagnosis is by cerebral CT scan. Full blood count, coagulation studies and blood group and hold should also be ordered.

TREATMENT

Appropriately manage the airway, breathing and circulation. Any coagulopathy should be reversed. Drainage is indicated if there is significant mass effect or neurological impairment.

Cervical spine and spinal cord injuries

Vertebral column injury refers to injury of any of the bones, joints and ligaments that make up the vertebral column. This may or may not be associated with spinal cord injury, which refers to injury of the spinal cord itself and is associated with neurological deficit.

The types of trauma that are high risk for spinal injury include high-speed motor vehicle crashes (particularly if there has been ejection from the vehicle), diving injuries, rugby football injuries and falls. In the elderly, falls from the standing position can easily result in cervical spine injury, especially at the C2 level. In this group, mortality is significantly higher than in younger patients.

CLINICAL FEATURES

Assessment of presence of vertebral column injury

The features of vertebral column injury are midline pain, particularly on attempted movement, and local tenderness. It may or may not be associated with a spinal cord injury (see below), which is manifest by neurological deficit. Some patients are clinically unevaluable. Patients with decreased level of consciousness or who are intubated, uncooperative or who have multiple painful and distracting injuries (e.g. severe multiple trauma) may have none of the above and require imaging with CT.

Assessment of presence of spinal cord injury

The neurological deficit can be classified according to *function* (motor, sensory or autonomic), its *distribution* (level and, in partial cord lesions, which part of the body is affected) and whether the loss of function is *complete or incomplete*.

An evaluation of motor tone, power and reflexes should be done. The initial screening sensory examination is with light touch or pin-prick. If there is other evidence of neurological deficit, test temperature and proprioception (posterior column).

When sensory loss is present, a sensory level below which sensation is lost can define the level of the injury. A working knowledge of the dermatomes of the body is required. The junction of shoulder and neck is at C4, the nipple at T4, the umbilicus at T10 and the inguinal region at L1. When the patient is log-rolled to examine the back, perianal and buttock sensory testing should be done, as well as assessment of anal tone. Sparing perianal sensation and anal tone may be evidence that the lesion is not complete and there may be some functional recovery.

Other clinical clues that suggest spinal cord injury are diaphragmatic breathing in cervical spine injury (loss of intercostal power supplied by the thoracic cord with intact diaphragm supplied by C4, C5 and C6). In males, priapism may be present, due to loss of sympathetic tone. There may also be hypotension and bradycardia due to loss of sympathetic vascular tone. Other causes of shock from trauma (haemorrhage, pericardial tamponade and tension pneumothorax) must be ruled out.

Whether or not the cord lesion is complete or partial is important for prognosis. Complete lesions have total loss of all three modalities (motor, sensory and autonomic). Partial lesions can have some residual function in any of the modalities. There are some syndromes with typical patterns of deficit indicating injury to certain parts of the cord (Table 27.4).

It should also be remembered that, in patients with a vertebral column injury, between 5% and 7% will have a second injury.

Editorial Comment

The Institute of Trauma and Injury Management (ITIM) and the Emergency Care Institute (NSW) (ECI) are advocating for the adoption of foam cervical collars in the initial management of injured adults and children requiring cervical spine immobilisation being transported by ambulance and presented to health facilities.
If cervical bony injury is identified, or if the patient cannot be cleared in ED due to competing priorities, apply a locally agreed cervical immobilisation collar such as a Philadelphia or Miami J collar, and refer to neurosurgery for advice.

Table 27.4 Partial spinal cord syndromes

Syndrome	Part of cord affected	Motor	Sensory
Brown-Séquard	Hemi-section of cord	Ipsilateral loss	Loss of ipsilateral proprioception, contralateral pain/ temperature
Anterior cord	Anterior half of cord	Bilateral motor loss	Bilateral temperature loss; intact proprioception/ vibration
Central cord		Weakness in upper limbs, sparing of lower limbs	Loss of sensation in upper limbs, lower limbs spared

Criteria for clinical clearance of cervical spine
There are two prospectively validated clinical decision rules for clearing the cervical spine clinically and without X-ray. The NEXUS (National Emergency X-radiography Utilization Study) criteria (Hoffman et al. 2000) and the Canadian C-Spine rule (Stiell et al. 2001).

NEXUS
Patients who are alert and lucid, have no midline neck tenderness, have no other significant distracting injuries (or have not received significant doses of opiates for pain) and have no neurological signs of spinal cord injury can be cleared of a cervical spine injury without X-ray. All other patients require a radiological evaluation of the cervical spine (see Imaging the Cervical Spine, below).

Canadian Cervical Spine rule
This is a more complex, three-step decision rule that is used for alert (GCS 15) and stable trauma patients where cervical spine injury is a concern. See Box 27.3.

Box 27.3   Canadian cervical spine rule

1   Are any high-risk factors present that mandate radiography?
 a   Age ≥ 65
 b   Dangerous mechanism*
 c   Paraesthesias in the extremities
 If yes, image the spine. If no, proceed to Step 2.
2   Is any one of the following low-risk factors present that allows safe assessment of the range of motion of cervical spine?
 Simple rear-end MVC or sitting position in the ED or ambulatory at any time or delayed onset of neck pain or absence of any midline cervical spine tenderness.
 If no, image the spine. If yes, proceed to Step 3.
3   Able to rotate the neck 45° left and right? If able, no radiography. If unable, image the spine.

Source: Steill et al. 2001
*Dangerous mechanisms are: fall from > 1 m or five stairs, axial load to head (e.g. diving), motor vehicle collision (MVC) > 100 km/h or with rollover or ejection, motorised recreational vehicles, bicycle collision.

Imaging the cervical spine

In patients who cannot be cleared clinically, imaging with CT scan of cervical spine is the most reliable. Plain radiology of the cervical spine has a sensitivity in the order of 50% for detecting cervical spine injuries. Anatomical detail is lacking, interpretation is difficult (especially for inexperienced doctors) and films are frequently technically inadequate.

Figure 27.5 illustrates some common cervical spine fractures and dislocations.

Magnetic resonance imaging (MRI)

CT scans are particularly useful for identifying bony and joint injury. Clinical and radiological assessment as described above will pick up the vast majority of fractures and dislocations. MRI is better for identifying ligamentous injury, however, and is useful in the further assessment of known injuries or the investigation of spinal cord injury without radiological abnormality.

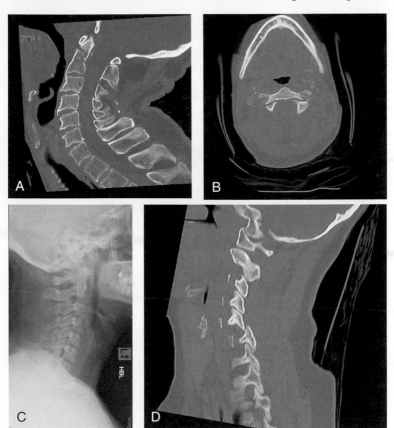

Figure 27.5 A. CT scan showing fracture of odontoid process in an elderly patient with a fall. B & C. CT showing bilateral pedicle fracture of C2 (Hangman's fracture) and plain lateral C-spine X-ray in same patient demonstrates poor sensitivity of plain cervical spine films. D. C5–C6 facet joint dislocation.

Determination of stability of vertebral column injury

The ability of the vertebral column to protect the spinal cord from abnormal movement and, therefore, injury should be evaluated. This should be done by a spinal surgeon.

The vertebral column can be considered to consist of three structural components: the anterior, middle and posterior columns.

- The anterior column consists of bone and ligaments from the anterior half of the vertebral bodies forward.
- The posterior column is made up of the neural arch (laminae and pedicles), spinous processes and posterior ligamentous complex.
- The remainder, the middle column, is from the posterior longitudinal ligament and posterior half of the vertebral body.

If at least two out of three of these columns are disrupted, the injury is considered unstable.

Treatment

In the patient with multiple injuries, vertebral column and spinal cord injuries should be managed as part of a prioritised management plan that addresses other serious injuries in context. Hypotension due to neurogenic shock should be managed with IV fluids.

Immobilisation of vertebral column

Precautions to prevent movement of the vertebral column should be instituted until it has been cleared. Elderly patients in particular are at risk of delayed respiratory complications if left lying supine for long periods immobilised in cervical collars. Cervical collars are uncomfortable and prolonged immobilisation can cause pressure areas. Every effort should be made to clear the cervical spine as soon as possible.

Patient transfers should be carried out while maintaining the position of the vertebral column. In hospital, this means use of specialised lifting techniques (e.g. log-rolling, spinal lifting technique). In each of these manoeuvres, a designated person needs to continuously maintain and monitor the position of the cervical spine.

There is no perfect splint that prevents all vertebral column movements, particularly in uncooperative patients. Cervical collars restrict but do not completely prevent cervical spine movement.

If immobilisation is required for more than a short period in the ED, a collar designed for longer term use, such as an Aspen collar, should be placed.

If intubation is required, in-line immobilisation of the cervical spine by a person designated purely for that role and intubation by an experienced operator during rapid-sequence induction has been shown to be a safe technique.

Referral and supportive care

Patients with high cervical lesions may have respiratory muscle weakness that may lead to respiratory failure. Depending on the severity, treatment for this may vary from supplemental oxygen to mechanical ventilation.

Patients with spinal cord injury should also have a gastric tube passed and an indwelling urinary catheter placed. Early transfer to a specialised spinal unit within 24 hours of injury has been shown to positively affect outcomes.

Early referral to a spinal surgeon should happen as soon as diagnosis is made. Decisions regarding the stability of a vertebral column lesion should be made by the spinal surgeon. Additionally, patients may require long-term immobilisation with skeletal traction.

Lower back pain
RED FLAGS

Does the patient have any of the following?

- History of significant trauma
- Age > 50, < 20 years
- History of cancer
- Recent bacterial infection
- IV drug use
- Immunosuppression
- Weight loss
- Severe pain when supine or at night
- Saddle (perineal) anaesthesia
- Bladder dysfunction
- Neurological dysfunction in lower limb, especially if both

If yes to any one of these, discuss with ED specialist/ neurosurgeon.

URGENT NEURO IMAGING

Required if any of the following:

- acute signs with progressive neurological deficits
- pain, signs with urinary retention, perineal numbness or bilateral signs or symptoms
- suspected neoplasm
- suspected epidural abscess.

CAUDA EQUINA SYNDROME

This is a neurosurgical emergency.

- Clinical presentation pain, bilateral weakness of legs, saddle anaesthesia (perineal numbness)
- Perianal decreased sensation, decreased anal sphincter tone
- Bowel, bladder, sexual dysfunction

Non-traumatic neurosurgical emergencies
SUBARACHNOID HAEMORRHAGE (SAH)

Early diagnosis of SAH can improve chance of survival. However, the morbidity and mortality are still significant. Up to 50% of SAH patients die and a third of survivors are left permanently disabled and dependent. While a proportion die from the initial haemorrhage, a group of patients will die from re-bleeding. The size of this latter group suffering repeat haemorrhages can be minimised if there is prompt diagnosis and treatment. Despite this, diagnosis of SAH is often missed or delayed.

In two-thirds of patients with SAH the source of bleeding is a rupture of a cerebral aneurysm. The commonest site is the anterior communicating artery.

In about 20% of patients no identifiable cause is found, and a small number have an arteriovenous malformation (AVM). A family history of aneurysmal haemorrhage increases the patient's risk of the same.

Clinical features

Sudden onset of severe headache is the hallmark of SAH. This is often associated with nausea, vomiting and symptoms and signs of meningism (photophobia, neck stiffness). Neurological deficit ranges from none to coma. Absence of meningism or neurological signs *does not* exclude the diagnosis.

The World Federation of Neurological Surgeons (WFNS) grading system for subarachnoid haemorrhage correlates with outcome and mortality (Table 27.5).

Patients may occasionally present with effects of the aneurysm before it has bled, such as warning headaches and occasionally oculomotor nerve palsy (ptosis, dilated pupil and diplopia with the eye in the down and out position).

Table 27.5 The World Federation of Neurological Surgeons (WFNS) grading system for subarachnoid haemorrhage

Grade	GCS score and motor deficit	Mortality (%)
I	GCS 15	5
II	GCS 13–14, no motor deficit	9
III	GCS 13–14, with motor deficit	20
IV	GCS 7–12	33
V	GCS 3–6	77

Investigations

Diagnosis is usually by cerebral CT scan (Figure 27.6). The ability of a cerebral CT to pick up an SAH degrades over time. If scanned within 6 hours, the sensitivity approaches 100%. Sensitivity degrades over time with only 50% sensitivity by 1 week post-bleed. If a good-quality CT done within 6 hours of the bleed is negative, it is reasonable to not perform an LP unless there is a high degree of clinical suspicion. If CT is performed

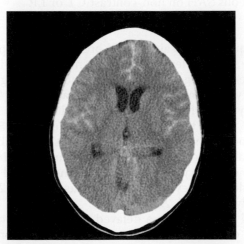

Figure 27.6 Non-contrast CT brain showing extensive subarachnoid haemorrhage

more than 6 hours post-onset and is negative, LP should be performed because of the potential lethality of a missed diagnosis of SAH.

- The LP should be examined for the presence of blood (either macroscopic or microscopic). If red blood cells are present, it is difficult to differentiate a traumatic tap from a subarachnoid haemorrhage. The CSF should be examined for breakdown products of red blood cells (oxyhaemoglobin and bilirubin) by CSF spectrophotometry.
- Oxyhaemoglobin takes 2 or more hours to develop, but bilirubin takes 12 hours to develop. A traumatic tap can give rise to oxyhaemoglobin only, but the presence of both bilirubin and oxyhaemoglobin peaks on spectrophotometry is suggestive of SAH. Because it does take 12 hours for red blood cells in CSF to break down to bilirubin, it is theoretically possible that performing an LP too soon after the occurrence of the haemorrhage may lead to false-negative LP.
- CT angiogram (Circle of Willis) is first-line imaging to determine the source of bleeding in patients with spontaneous SAH on non-contrast CT or LP.

Treatment

Ensure adequacy of the airway and breathing if the patient has a significantly reduced level of consciousness. Urgent intervention to prevent re-bleeding is by craniotomy and microsurgical clipping of the aneurysm or by angiographic endovascular occlusion of the aneurysm by a detachable coil. The re-bleeding risk is 1.5% per day and 15–20% within the first 2 weeks (Sayer et al. 2015).

Not all aneurysms are suitable for endovascular coiling. In those that are suitable for either modality of treatment, the International Subarachnoid Aneurysm Trial (ISAT) demonstrated a reduction in death or dependency with coiling versus clipping (23.5% versus 30.9%) (Molyneux et al. 2005).

Cerebral vasospasm is a delayed complication of SAH that may lead to cerebral ischaemia and worsened outcome. The risk can be minimised by using nimodipine, which should be started intravenously within 72 hours of the SAH. The patient needs to be kept adequately hydrated with IV fluids.

In the ED, effective analgesia and treatment of nausea and vomiting with antiemetic is important. Acute elevation in blood pressure should be treated to minimise risk of re-bleeding.

SPONTANEOUS INTRACEREBRAL HAEMORRHAGE

Spontaneous intracerebral haemorrhage is usually related to poorly controlled hypertension. Patients who are on anticoagulants are also at risk of intracerebral haemorrhage.

Patients usually present with sudden-onset headache and neurological impairment. Focal neurological signs are usually related to the location of the bleed. In larger bleeds, especially where there is mass effect, there is usually reduced level of consciousness or coma. Herniation syndromes may be seen, especially with posterior intracranial fossa bleeds.

Most intracerebral bleeds are treated medically with attention to the priorities of airway, breathing and circulation as well as correction of any coagulopathy (e.g. reversal of anticoagulation).

Indications for surgery include:
• posterior fossa haemorrhage with mass effect
• intraventricular blood causing acute hydrocephalus.

SPACE-OCCUPYING LESIONS

A number of non-traumatic conditions can present to the ED with the acute effects of a space-occupying lesion (SOL). These include tumours (primary and secondary tumours). Subdural haematomas may occur without a definite history of trauma. Large cerebellar infarcts can be complicated by significant swelling, rapid increase in ICP and a herniation syndrome.

Clinical features

The clinical presentation is by virtue of the enlarging size of the lesion, mass effect (local or general) or surrounding oedema (Figure 27.7). Symptoms vary greatly from just headaches, with features suggestive of raised ICP (worse on lying and in the morning, associated with nausea and vomiting), to patients with coma and herniation syndromes at the severe end of the spectrum.

The patient may present with seizures (focal or generalised). Persistent depression of GCS postictally or development of status

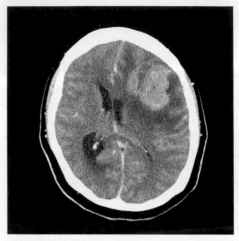

Figure 27.7 Cerebral CT scan with contrast showing left frontal enhancing space-occupying lesion with surrounding oedema resulting in marked mass effect (shift of midline to right, compression of ventricles). Patient had presented with status epilepticus and dilation of left pupil due to herniation syndrome with no previous history of seizures.

epilepticus should raise clinical suspicion and necessitate urgent cerebral CT.

Investigations
CT scan with IV contrast is first line. Box 27.2 outlines the indications for brain CT in non-trauma patients in the ED.

Management
The ED management of these conditions is guided by the same principles outlined at the beginning of this chapter. Raised ICP from tumours is often responsive to treatment with bed rest and dexamethasone. Further seizures can be prevented with levetiracetam (15 mg/kg IV infusion) or phenytoin (15 mg/kg slow IV infusion).

COMPLICATIONS OF VENTRICULAR DRAINAGE DEVICES
Patients with a ventriculoperitoneal (VP) shunt not infrequently present to the ED with shunt malfunction or complications. The

commonest of these are shunt obstruction and shunt infection. Less commonly, disconnection and migration of drainage catheter may occur. It is important to recognise these complications when they occur as, untreated, they can lead to significant morbidity or mortality.

Clinical features

The patient will usually have a clear history of having had a VP shunt inserted. Symptoms and signs are variable, but include one or more of the following: headache, decreased level of consciousness, ataxia, nausea and vomiting.

On examination the patient may have a decreased level of consciousness and, in severe cases, focal neurological signs may indicate a herniation syndrome. Papillo-oedema may be present and paralysis of upward gaze may be seen. If a shunt reservoir is palpable, inability to empty it by pressing on it would suggest a distal obstruction; if it can be compressed but is slow to refill, this suggests a proximal obstruction.

Investigation

- Plain X-rays over the course of the shunt (shunt series) will show fractured tubing, disconnections, fluid collections, migration of the shunt tubing.
- A non-contrast cerebral CT will demonstrate ventricular size (hydrocephalus, slit ventricles), other evidence of increased ICP and the position of the proximal shunt components.
- A radioisotope nuclear scan using technetium-99 can confirm obstruction and isolate its location.

Management

Supportive measures to ensure adequacy of airway, breathing and circulation. Definitive treatment for a shunt blockage is shunt revision.

EPIDURAL ABSCESS

Epidural abscess is a rare but devastating condition that is often diagnosed late, resulting in permanent neurological disability. It is estimated to account for 0.2–1.2 cases per 10 000 hospital admissions per year. Modern-day mortality is less than 10%, but persistent neurological disability is common in survivors, especially if diagnosis is delayed or the patient is elderly.

Risk factors

The pathogenesis is thought to be related to a triad of risk factors. Compromised immunity (e.g. diabetes, IV drug use, chronic medical illnesses), disruption to the spinal column (e.g. degenerative disease, surgery, epidural anaesthesia) and a source of infection (e.g. soft-tissue infections, intravenous drug use). Diabetes and IVDU are the most frequent risks. Staphylococcus is the commonest group of organism.

Clinical features

Initially fever associated with back pain, and later neurological deficit. Meningism may be present on examination. There may be tenderness over the spine. Variable degrees of motor weakness, sensory loss and loss of reflexes

Investigation

MRI is the imaging modality of choice. The white cell count is only raised in two-thirds of cases. The erythrocyte sedimentation rate (ESR) and C-reactive protein (CRP) are usually elevated, however.

Management

Urgent surgical decompression and drainage followed by a prolonged course of antibiotics.

References

Hoffman JR, Mower WR, Wolfson AB et al. Validity of a set of clinical criteria to rule out injury to the cervical spine in patients with blunt trauma. NEJM 2000;343:94–99.

Stiell IG, Wells GA, Vandemheen KL. The Canadian C-Spine rule for radiography in alert and stable trauma patients. JAMA 2001;286(15):1841–1848.

Sayer D, Bloom B, Fernando K et al. An observational study of 2248 patients presenting with headache, suggestive of subarachnoid haemorrhage who received lumbar punctures following normal computed tomography of the head. Acad Emerg Med 2015;22:1267–1273.

Molyneux AJ, Kerr RSC, Ly-Mee Yu et al. International Subarachnoid Aneurysm Trial (ISAT) of neurosurgical clipping versus endovascular coiling in 2143 patients with ruptured intracranial aneurysms: a randomised comparison on effects of survival, dependency, seizures, re-bleeding, subgroups, and aneurysm occlusion. Lancet 2005;366:809–817.

Online resources

Abbreviated Westmead Post Traumatic Amnesia Scale (A-WPTAS)
www.aci.health.nsw.gov.au

Chapter 28
Aortic and vascular emergencies
Mark Gillett

Acute aortic dissection: thoracic
OVERVIEW

Aortic dissection is the commonest aortic catastrophe, with a peak incidence between 50 and 70 years. Males are affected twice as often as females. The condition can be rapidly fatal without immediate treatment. However, diagnosis can be difficult and is often delayed.

Acute aortic dissection refers to a tear in the aortic intima that results in separation between the intima and the media. Blood flows into this space, creating a false lumen. The tear in the aortic wall may propagate proximally and/or distally, potentially involving any arterial branches from the aorta. The Stanford classification system is widely accepted, with type A (proximal) involving the ascending aorta (plus or minus the descending aorta) and type B (distal) involving the descending aorta alone. Type A generally presents at between 50 and 60 years with type B typically occurring a decade later. Mortality is higher in type A.

Complications of aortic dissection include free rupture into the chest or abdomen (usually rapidly fatal), pericardial effusion with cardiac tamponade, aortic valve regurgitation and branch occlusion causing ischaemia of bowel, kidneys, limbs or brain.

Factors associated with the condition include hypertension, stimulant abuse, inflammatory vasculitides, pregnancy and genetic conditions including Marfan's syndrome.

DIAGNOSIS

• Aortic dissection may mimic other common clinical presentations including cardiac ischaemia, stroke and acute abdominal conditions, therefore a high index of suspicion for the condition is required.

- Typically, patients present with pain in the chest, back or abdomen which is of sudden onset and tearing in quality.
- On examination, patients are typically agitated, pale and sweaty. Discernible discrepancies in limb pulses and blood pressures occurs in only approximately 30% of cases. Aortic valve regurgitation (45% of cases) is commoner in proximal dissections than in distal.
- Associated presentations may include syncope, acute coronary syndrome, cardiac tamponade, cardiac failure due to acute aortic regurgitation, stroke, limb ischaemia or mesenteric infarction.
- Chest X-ray often shows widening of the superior mediastinum and irregularity of the aortic shadow, but can be normal in up to 20% of cases.
- D-dimer levels are frequently elevated in aortic dissection; however, they are neither sensitive nor specific enough to be relied on as a stand-alone diagnostic test.
- Definitive diagnosis is by either contrast CT scanning or transoesophageal echocardiography (TOE). CT is the preferred technique in stable patients, whereas bedside TOE is ideal for critically unwell patients.

MANAGEMENT

Treatment should be instituted rapidly, as the death rate may be as high as 1% per hour for the first 24 hours. Type A dissections generally require surgery whereas type B are usually managed medically. All patients should be managed in a tertiary centre experienced in dealing with the condition. Thus, urgent transfer of the patient may be required.

- Pain is treated with IV morphine but is often very severe and difficult to control.
- Blood pressure reduction is instituted with a beta-blocker to reduce vessel-wall shear pressure. Intravenous esmolol is an ideal agent due to its rapid onset and offset of action. Alternatively, repeat boluses of IV cardioselective beta-blockers such as atenolol or metoprolol will suffice. Sodium nitroprusside can be used as an adjuvant agent to achieve further reductions in blood pressure, but should not be used without prior beta-blockade. Target parameters are pulse rate 60 bpm and systolic BP of 100–120 mmHg.

- Open surgery is indicated in type A dissections due to the high risk of life-threatening cardiac tamponade, stroke and cardiac failure related to aortic valve regurgitation. Type B dissections are generally managed medically but may be candidates for endovascular stenting in cases associated with mesenteric, renal or lower limb ischaemia.

Ruptured abdominal aortic aneurysm
OVERVIEW

Abdominal aortic aneurysm (AAA) affects approximately 2% of the population, with a peak incidence between 70 and 75 years of age and a significant male predominance. 95% of AAAs occur below the level of the renal arteries. Predisposing conditions include hypertension, smoking and connective tissue diseases such as Marfan syndrome. The most common life-threatening complications of AAA seen in the emergency department are rupture or threatened rupture.

The risk of rupture increases with aneurysmal size. The 5-year risk is 1–2% when the aneurysm is < 5 cm in diameter and rises to 20–40% when the diameter is > 5 cm.

Diagnosis

Misdiagnosis and delayed diagnosis can occur in up to 30% of cases. The differential diagnoses include renal colic, pancreatitis, diverticulitis and acute myocardial infarction.

- Ruptured AAA typically presents with severe abdominal and/ or back pain which may radiate to the groin (thus mimicking renal colic). Patients may also present with syncope.
- Examination reveals a patient who looks unwell, with tachycardia, hypotension and an acutely tender abdomen (without guarding or rigidity). A tender, pulsatile abdominal mass is felt in approximately 50% of cases only. Absent femoral pulses and an aortic bruit may sometimes be detected.
- In the stable patient, CT scanning confirms the diagnosis of AAA, including the site, the extent and the presence or absence of rupture. Its disadvantage is the requirement for the patient to move to the radiology suite.
- In the unstable patient, the diagnosis must be made on history, examination and by use of ED ultrasound.

Ultrasound is portable, safe and increasingly available in the ED. A large number of studies suggest that in the hands of emergency doctors it is both sensitive and specific in diagnosing AAA.

- While allowing easy diagnosis of AAA, however, ultrasound cannot reliably diagnose rupture as 80% of ruptures are retroperitoneal. In the 20% with free peritoneal rupture, FAST scan will be positive. Plain abdominal X-ray has a limited role, as only 60% of AAAs show significant aortic calcification and it cannot detect rupture.
- All patients suspected of AAA rupture require bloods for emergency cross-match (10 units) and estimation of haemoglobin, electrolytes, renal function, troponin and lipase. An ECG and chest X-ray should be performed if the patient is haemodynamically stable.

MANAGEMENT

- Management of **acute rupture** is rapid resuscitation while simultaneously organising immediate surgery. Patients should be monitored in an acute resuscitation area by the most senior ED staff.
- Resuscitation involves oxygen, crystalloid fluids and early blood transfusion. Type O blood may be required initially while awaiting full cross-matching. Massive transfusion protocols should be activated as large volumes of packed red blood cells, platelets and fresh frozen plasma may be required while arranging an operating theatre.
- The endpoint of fluid resuscitation is a systolic blood pressure of approximately 90 mmHg. Higher resuscitation blood pressures may increase bleeding and have been associated with worse outcomes in several studies.
- Incremental doses of IV morphine and antiemetics should be administered to control pain and vomiting.
- Ninety per cent of patients with ruptured AAAs die without surgery although the mortality with surgery is still 50%. Surgical options include open repair of the rupture with insertion of a prosthetic graft or, more recently, percutaneous endoluminal repair and stenting. The endovascular approach has been proven to have a lower short-term mortality, but

this advantage is lost over time due to increasing incidence of graft failure.

• The management of a **painful, non-ruptured AAA larger than 5 cm** is urgent surgical repair, as the risk of death from rupture outweighs that of elective repair (10%). Surgery is performed as soon as adequate CT imaging and rapid stabilisation of concurrent medical conditions have occurred.

• Suprarenal aneurysms have greater operative risk due to the need to re-implant the renal, coeliac and superior mesenteric arteries. Repair is commonly complicated by paraplegia, renal failure and mesenteric ischaemia.

Non-aortic abdominal aneurysms

Splenic artery aneurysms account for 60% of this group. They have a female predominance of 4:1 and are associated with portal hypertension and pregnancy. Rupture in pregnancy is associated with 50% maternal mortality, 95% fetal demise and delayed diagnosis. Typically splenic artery aneurysm presents with sudden onset of left upper quadrant abdominal pain associated with signs of haemodynamic shock. Treatment may be either surgery or interventional radiology.

Other sites of intra-abdominal aneurysms include hepatic, superior mesenteric and renal arteries.

Acute arterial insufficiency
OVERVIEW

Acute arterial insufficiency (AAI) is defined as sudden reduction in limb blood flow resulting in circulation inadequate to meet tissue metabolic demands. AAI is most commonly due to thrombosis associated with underlying atherosclerotic peripheral arterial disease related to premorbid smoking, hypertension, diabetes, vasculitis or hypercoagulable states. Thrombotic arterial occlusion is common in patients with previous synthetic bypass arterial grafts than occlusions involving 'native' arteries.

AAI may also be due to emboli from the heart, aorta and larger arteries. Sources of cardiac emboli include atrial fibrillation, acute myocardial infarction, prosthetic valves and infective endocarditis. Emboli tend to cause very rapid onset of symptoms and result in more catastrophic ischaemia.

Common sites of occlusion include the femoral and popliteal arteries. Less common sites are the iliac, tibial and peroneal arteries of the leg. Upper limb AAI is relatively rare and usually due to emboli or aortic dissection.

DIAGNOSIS

AAI is a time-critical condition as morbidity and mortality rise sharply with increasing delay in diagnosis and treatment. Clinical presentation is related to the site of occlusion and the relative presence of collateral circulation.

Typically, the patient presents with acute onset of severe pain (often maximal distally), paraesthesia and coldness in the limb. Loss of motor function may supervene with ongoing ischaemia. **History** should seek to ascertain the onset and duration of symptoms plus any intercurrent medical diseases.

Physical signs include loss of pulses distal to the occlusion, skin changes (including pallor, cyanosis or mottling), decreased skin temperature, loss of sensation and weakness. The presence of motor or sensory neurological signs implies prolonged ischaemia and a poorer prognosis for the limb. If AAI occurs in the presence of good collateral circulation (as occurs in chronic ischaemia), physical signs may be less florid.

Investigations may include the use of a handheld Doppler device at the bedside showing absent vascular pulses. More definitive tests include arterial duplex (B mode and Doppler) ultrasound if rapidly available. Alternatively, CT angiography is able to establish the diagnosis and facilitate angioplasty. Full blood count, biochemistry, ECG and chest X-ray should be performed to ascertain likely causes and fitness for operating theatre.

MANAGEMENT

Treatment involves IV morphine analgesia, immediate anticoagulation with IV unfractionated heparin to prevent clot progression, rapid stabilisation of any underlying medical conditions and emergency surgical revascularisation by thromboembolectomy (endovascular or open), angioplasty or arterial bypass grafting. Endovascular thrombolysis has been used in patients deemed not fit for surgery. However, the mortality is higher compared with operative treatment.

Irreversible ischaemic changes occur within 4–6 hours and revascularisation is less effective after 8–12 hours.

Atheroembolism

Atheroembolism is a subset of AAI in which fibrin/platelet deposits embolise from proximal atherosclerotic lesions to distal-end arteries. It is associated with invasive arterial procedures such as cardiac catheterisation.

Patients develop signs of arterial insufficiency involving the extremities. Affected areas are painful, tender and may be either dusky or necrotic.

Treatment is unsatisfactory as anticoagulation, emergency surgery and thrombolysis all fail to reduce morbidity. Low-dose aspirin therapy should be started and vascular surgery review organised.

Chronic arterial insufficiency

The most common presentation is intermittent claudication associated with reduced pulses and trophic skin changes. Critical chronic arterial insufficiency is associated with ischaemic pain at rest and ankle systolic BP of less than 50 mmHg. Calculating an ankle/brachial index (ankle systolic BP divided by arm systolic BP) helps predict severity. A ratio of < 0.9 is abnormal and < 0.4 is indicative of severe disease.

The investigation of choice is arterial duplex ultrasound.

Chronic management revolves around cessation of smoking, regular exercise, aspirin, control of associated medical problems such as cardiac failure and a trial of alpha-blocking drugs.

Editorial Comment
Never ignore marked or unrelieved pain as a possible indicator of a vascular complication—ischaemia, aneurysm, dissection, compartment syndrome—or the need for urgent referral.

Further reading

Emergency Clinics of North America, Nov 2017;3(4).

Chapter 29
Orthopaedic emergencies
John Raftos

Acknowledgment
The author wishes to acknowledge the content used from the previous edition of *Emergency Medicine* which was provided by Peter Locke.

Editorial Comment
Ensure the patient understands the need for follow-up, confirmation of a diagnosis/formal X-ray report and the need for review if healing/pain/function is not to plan. Ignore this, and you could be sued. These patients commonly present to the ED. Respect pain and swelling—suspect fracture. Remember: 1. you are not a radiologist; and 2. not all fractures are visible even on good films.

General principles
RESUSCITATION AND DETECTION OF OTHER INJURIES

Orthopaedic injuries often occur in multiple-injury patients. Resuscitation and identification and management of life-threatening injuries during the primary survey usually takes precedence over the identification and management of orthopaedic injuries which should be identified and managed during the secondary survey once the patient has been stabilised. Exceptions include:

- major pelvic fractures—may cause life-threatening haemorrhage which must be controlled in the primary survey
- femoral shaft fractures—may involve 1–2 L of blood loss and should be reduced and splinted during the primary survey.

ANALGESIA

Most fractures and dislocations cause severe pain that requires urgent analgesia on presentation to the ED. Appropriate initial analgesia may include:

- inhaled nitrous oxide or methoxyflurane or intranasal fentanyl
- intravenous morphine (0.1 mg/kg for children, 2.5 to 5 mg aliquots for adults)
- oxycodone 5–10 mg orally
- immobilisation with a plaster slab, traction splint, Zimmer splint, sling, etc.
- regional anaesthesia (fascia iliaca block [FIB], femoral nerve block for femoral neck, shaft fracture).

DETECTION OF ASSOCIATED INJURIES

A thorough anatomical knowledge is necessary to suspect and detect injuries to tendons, nerves, blood vessels and other viscera that are commonly associated with bony injuries.

EARLY REDUCTION OF FRACTURES

Some displaced fractures and dislocations should be reduced urgently to prevent serious permanent sequelae. These injuries (and their sequelae) include:

- traumatic hip dislocation (sciatic nerve injury, avascular necrosis, heterotopic calcification)
- true knee joint dislocation (popliteal artery injury with lower limb ischaemia, common peroneal nerve injury)
- supracondylar fractures of the elbow (median nerve, radial artery injury)
- elbow dislocation (ulnar nerve injury, heterotopic calcification)
- displaced pelvic fractures (ongoing haemorrhage)
- ankle fracture/dislocation (ischaemic necrosis of compressed skin, usually over one of the malleoli)
- shoulder dislocation (traction injury of the brachial plexus, axillary artery injury, recurrent dislocation).

EARLY REDUCTION OF DISLOCATIONS

Joint dislocation causes injury to the structures supporting the joint. Prolonged dislocation increases the likelihood of recurrent dislocation. Early reduction reduces the risk of recurrent dislocation and is effective analgesia. Most patients require little or no analgesia once the dislocation has been reduced and their time in the ED is minimised with early reduction.

PROCEDURAL SEDATION FOR ED REDUCTION OF DISLOCATIONS AND FRACTURES
(See also Chapter 2 The Airway, Ventilation and Procedural Sedation.)

Performed by appropriately qualified ED specialists and registrars, procedural sedation is a safe technique for the reduction of most dislocations and the urgent reduction of some fractures in the ED. **Ketamine** or the combination of **inhaled nitrous oxide and intranasal fentanyl** are the preferred agents for use in children. The combination of **propofol and fentanyl** is ideal in adults because its short duration of action minimises the duration of altered consciousness and allows early discharge. **Morphine** and **midazolam** is an adequate alternative in adults but has a longer duration of action.

Safe procedural sedation requires appropriate staffing with an airway-skilled doctor, other than the doctor who will perform the procedure, to perform the sedation and monitor the patient. Continuous ECG, oxygen saturation and expired CO_2 monitoring should be in place and advanced airway and resuscitation equipment should be at hand.

APPROPRIATE CONSULTATION AND REFERRAL
Each hospital has its own arrangements for referral of patients who need specialist orthopaedic assessment. If the patient needs orthopaedic assessment in the ED, then the orthopaedic registrar should be contacted. If outpatient orthopaedic referral is necessary, then this is provided either at a hospital fracture clinic or in the rooms of the orthopaedic surgeon on call if there is no fracture clinic.

INJURIES OF THE HAND AND WRIST
(See also Chapter 37 Hand Injuries and Care.)

The management of hand injuries is the domain of specialist hand surgeons. Fractures of any of the bones of the hand or carpus should generally be reviewed by a hand surgeon as should any laceration of the hand or wrist with the potential for nerve or tendon injury, nail bed injuries, crush injuries, burns, hand infections and high-pressure injection injuries. Arrangements for consultation with and referral to a hand surgery unit will vary from hospital to hospital and should be clearly laid out in the ED.

Upper limb injuries
CLAVICLE FRACTURE
Assessment
- This is most commonly caused by falls onto the outstretched hand, less commonly by direct-force injury.
- Patients usually present with pain, tenderness and deformity and are reluctant to move the affected arm.
- Fractures of the medial and middle thirds usually heal without sequelae. Fractures of the outer third may be complicated by delayed or mal-union.
- Plain X-rays usually adequately demonstrate clavicle fractures.

Management
- Orthopaedic registrar assessment in the ED is necessary for:
  — angulated or displaced fractures
  — fractures of the outer third which may need open reduction and internal fixation.
- Management of undisplaced fractures of the medial and middle thirds is:
  — a triangular sling or proprietary shoulder immobiliser
  — simple analgesia, and
  — referral to the fracture clinic or orthopaedic surgeon's rooms.

ACROMIOCLAVICULAR (AC) SUBLUXATION/ DISLOCATION
Assessment
- This is most commonly caused by a fall onto the tip of the shoulder or an impact on the tip of the shoulder during contact sport.
- Subluxation of the AC joint is associated with rupture of the acromioclavicular ligament and generally requires symptomatic treatment only.

- Dislocation of the AC joint is associated with rupture of the acromioclavicular ligament and the stronger coracoclavicular ligament and may require open reduction and internal fixation, especially in sportspeople.
- Plain X-rays of the shoulder will show widening (subluxation) or displacement (dislocation) of the AC joint. Comparative X-rays of the normal side and weight-bearing views may help with diagnosis.

Management
- Symptomatic management (triangular sling/proprietary shoulder immobiliser, ice, simple oral analgesia) is appropriate for subluxation.
- Patients with dislocation should be referred to the fracture clinic or orthopaedic surgeon for consideration of open reduction and internal fixation.

STERNOCLAVICULAR SUBLUXATION/DISLOCATION
Assessment
- Caused by:
  — a direct blow to the sternum or medial clavicle or
  — transmitted force from a blow to the posterolateral shoulder causing anterior dislocation of the clavicle or to the anterolateral shoulder causing posterior dislocation.
- Anterior dislocation of the medial clavicle causes pain and localised deformity.
- Posterior dislocation of the medial clavicle has the potential to injure or compress the trachea and the major vessels and nerves that underlie the sternoclavicular joint, causing dyspnoea, chest pain, altered sensation in the arm or vascular abnormality in the arm.
- Plain X-rays are not sensitive for sternoclavicular dislocation. CT scan should be performed for diagnosis and to detect any injury or compression of intrathoracic structures.

Management
- All patients with sternoclavicular dislocation should be seen by the orthopaedic registrar in the ED.

- Subluxations and some anterior dislocations may be treated symptomatically.
- Posterior dislocations and most anterior dislocations will require reduction under general anaesthesia.

ANTERIOR DISLOCATION OF THE GLENOHUMERAL (SHOULDER) JOINT
Assessment

- The mechanism of injury is a forced abduction and external rotation of the arm at the shoulder or a fall onto the hand forcing the humeral head anteriorly. It occurs most frequently at sport or in the surf in young people and in falls in older people.
- Every dislocation damages the rotator cuff and/or bony structures of the shoulder and so recurrent dislocation is common. The incidence of recurrent dislocation after an initial dislocation is about 50% and increases after each subsequent dislocation which tends to occur with decreasing force. The likelihood of recurrent dislocation is reduced by prompt reduction.
- The patient complains of pain in the shoulder and the arm is held immobile. Inspection usually reveals prominence of the tip of the shoulder and loss of the deltoid contour with an apparent hollow subacromially. Diagnosis may be difficult in obese individuals.
- Examine the patient for common complication of shoulder dislocation:
  — circumflex axillary nerve injury with loss of sensation over the deltoid and loss of deltoid function (usually masked by pain pre-reduction)—test for sensation in the 'nurse's cape' distribution over the deltoid
  — fracture of the humeral head or neck—inspect the humeral head and neck and the greater tuberosity carefully on X-ray
  — posterior cord brachial plexus injury with weakness of wrist extension through the radial nerve—test the function of the wrist and the hand, especially wrist extension
  — axillary artery injury—palpate the radial pulse.

• Plain X-rays will identify the great majority of shoulder dislocations. The humeral head usually lies in the subcoracoid position. Look for avulsion fracture of the greater tuberosity and fracture of the humeral neck. Patients with greater tuberosity avulsion should have standard reduction by ED staff. Patients with humeral neck fracture need orthopaedic consultation.

• CT scan may be necessary for the patient with a painful immobile shoulder and inconclusive X-rays.

Management

• Some emergency doctors may opt to reduce recurrent shoulder dislocations without preliminary X-rays but this should not be regarded as standard practice.

• Standard management for shoulder dislocation is prompt reduction in the ED. Reduction may be performed with or without procedural sedation. When procedural sedation is used, the preferred agent in children is ketamine and in adults propofol and fentanyl.

• Reduction techniques that do not involve traction are preferred because they are said to reduce the likelihood of recurrent dislocation. Techniques include:

— the Spaso (after Spaso Miljesic) technique—with the patient supine the arm is lifted vertically with gentle traction and an assistant thumbs the humeral head while gentle external rotation is applied

— the Stimpson technique—the patient lies prone on a bed with traction applied with weights to the extended arm

— the Kocher manoeuvre—counter-traction is provided by an assistant with a towel in the axilla, the operator applies axial traction using the flexed forearm as a fulcrum, followed by external rotation to 90°, and then adduction of the upper arm across the chest wall and internal rotation

— the Milch technique—with the patient supine on a bed, the arm is fully abducted and gentle external rotation is applied while an assistant thumbs the humeral head

— the Hippocratic method—with the patient supine on a bed place the stockinged foot in the axilla for counter-traction, hold the arm at the wrist in both hands, and apply traction to the straight arm.

- Reduction is usually heralded by a palpable 'clunk'.
- Once reduction has been achieved:
  — perform post-reduction X-rays to assess position and the possibility of bony injury
  — re-examine for neurovascular injury
  — immobilise the arm in a triangular sling/shoulder immobiliser
  — advise the patient to avoid abduction for at least one week
  — referral to the GP for follow-up is usually adequate if there is no evidence of associated fracture or neurovascular injury
  — discuss referral to a specialist shoulder surgeon with patients with recurrent dislocation.
- Successful reduction is generally a function of good technique and adequate sedation. The use of excessive force may result in humeral neck fracture, especially in older patients. If reduction is difficult, review the adequacy of sedation and/or seek orthopaedic assistance. Never apply excessive force.

POSTERIOR DISLOCATION OF THE GLENOHUMERAL (SHOULDER) JOINT
Assessment

- Posterior shoulder dislocation is uncommon (about 1% of all shoulder dislocations) and the diagnosis is often missed because the humeral head appears to be located on anteroposterior X-ray.
- The mechanism of injury is a forceful impact to the anterior aspect of the shoulder or tetanic muscle contraction during seizure or electric shock.
- The shoulder is painful and the patient is reluctant to move the arm which is held adducted and internally rotated.
- The shoulder joint may appear located on the anteroposterior X-ray but careful inspection will show the 'light bulb sign' (the usually asymmetrical appearance of the humeral head becomes symmetrical because of internal rotation) or the humeral head overlapping the glenoid. The lateral X-ray will show the head of the humerus posterior to the glenoid.
- CT scan should be performed when the anatomy is not clearly seen on plain X-ray.

Management

Reduction under procedural sedation in the ED is usually successful—axial traction is applied while the arm is abducted to 90° and then externally rotated.

HUMERAL HEAD AND NECK FRACTURES

Assessment

- The majority of fractures of the upper humerus occur in falls onto the outstretched hand in older patients.
- Fractures most commonly involve the surgical neck of the humerus but may also involve the anatomical neck, the greater and lesser tuberosities, and the articular surface, all either alone or in combination.
- The history is usually of a fall onto the outstretched hand causing pain, swelling and later bruising about the shoulder. Bruising and/or reluctance to move the shoulder may be the only clinical features in older patients with dementia.
- X-rays of the shoulder are usually diagnostic. Look for associated shoulder joint dislocation, angulation, displacement, involvement of the articular surface and displacement of the greater tuberosity.

Management

- Most patients with upper humerus fractures should be reviewed by the orthopaedic registrar in the ED to determine appropriate treatment.
  - Surgical treatment with replacement hemiarthroplasty should be considered for adults with significant intraarticular involvement.
  - Surgical treatment with closed reduction or open reduction and internal fixation should be considered for younger patients with significant displacement or angulation and for displaced avulsion fractures of the greater tuberosity.
  - Epiphyseal fractures in younger patients often require closed reduction under general anaesthesia.
  - Uncomplicated fractures of the neck of humerus are treated conservatively in a triangular sling/shoulder immobiliser or in a collar and cuff if there is impaction requiring gravitational reduction.

- Older patients may be significantly disabled by immobilisation of one arm—social work involvement is necessary to make appropriate care arrangements while the disability persists. Overnight/medical assessment unit admission allows analgesia to be optimised and social arrangements to be made.

HUMERAL SHAFT FRACTURES
Assessment
- Humeral shaft fractures are caused by direct-force injuries, torsion or falls onto the outstretched hand.
- The patient presents with upper arm pain and is reluctant to move the arm which is generally supported by the other hand.
- X-rays of the upper arm are usually diagnostic. Look for displacement, angulation and the presence of a 'butterfly' fragment.
- The radial nerve may be contused in the radial groove in fractures of the middle third of the humerus—always test extension of the wrist and fingers. The injury is usually a neuropraxia which will recover over 6 weeks to 6 months. Vascular injury is uncommon.

Management
- The orthopaedic registrar should review all humeral shaft fractures in the ED.
- Management includes the following.
  - Standard management of humeral shaft fractures is immobilisation in a 'hanging slab'—apply ample padding, especially around the elbow, using an appropriate-width plaster slab. Start in the axilla and continue the slab under the flexed elbow, over the outer surface of the upper arm and well onto the shoulder. Wrap with a gauze bandage and support in a sling or collar and cuff.
  - Some humeral shaft fractures will require open reduction and internal nail fixation. These may include those with a butterfly fragment and those associated with multiple injuries.
  - Supply appropriate analgesia and arrange review at the fracture clinic or orthopaedic surgeon's rooms.

SUPRACONDYLAR FRACTURES OF THE HUMERUS

Assessment

- Supracondylar fracture is most common in children, with peak incidence at age 8 years, and is usually caused by a fall onto the outstretched hand.
- The patient presents with a painful, swollen elbow and is reluctant to use the arm which is usually supported by the other hand.
- Assessment should include a full neurovascular examination of the hand looking for complications of the fracture.
  - Brachial artery injury: the brachial artery may be compressed or, in severe cases, there may be intimal damage or rupture. Check the radial pulse and capillary refill in the fingers.
  - Median nerve injury: check sensation in the radial palmar 3½ fingers and motor function in the abductor pollicis.
  - Increased tissue pressure/compartment syndrome: haemorrhage and oedema around the fracture site may cause vascular compromise that is detected by regular vascular checks of the hand and forearm.
  - Volkmann's ischaemic contracture: is a disabling ischaemic injury of the muscles and nerves of the forearm caused by arterial injury or compartment syndrome following supracondylar fracture.
- X-rays will demonstrate a supracondylar fracture line. Look for displacement, angulation, comminution.

Management

- Urgent orthopaedic review is needed if there is evidence of vascular compromise.
- All supracondylar fractures should be reviewed by the orthopaedic registrar in the ED. Those with significant displacement or angulation will need closed reduction under general anaesthesia. Those with vascular compromise will need urgent reduction and Vascular Surgical assessment.
- Comminuted fractures in adults may require open reduction and internal fixation.
- Undisplaced fractures without significant swelling can be managed, after orthopaedic registrar review, with a collar

and cuff, oral analgesia and referral to the fracture clinic or orthopaedic surgeon's rooms.

ELBOW DISLOCATION
Assessment

♦ Elbow dislocation occurs in both children and adults, usually as the result of a fall onto the outstretched hand. The radius usually dislocates posteriorly in response to forced hyperextension.

• The patient presents with a painful, swollen elbow and is reluctant to use the arm which is usually supported by the other hand.

• Assessment should include a full neurovascular examination of the hand looking for complications of the fracture.

— Ulnar nerve injury: check sensation in the ulnar palmar 2½ fingers and motor function in adduction and abduction of the fingers.

— Brachial artery injury: the brachial artery may be compressed or, in severe cases, there may be intimal damage or rupture. Check the radial pulse and capillary refill in the fingers.

— Median nerve injury: check sensation in the radial palmar 3½ fingers and motor function in the abductor pollicis.

— Increased tissue pressure/compartment syndrome: haemorrhage and oedema around the fracture site may cause vascular compromise that is detected by regular vascular checks of the hand and forearm.

• X-rays usually demonstrate the dislocation clearly. Intra-articular bone fragments are common and their origin is often unclear. Look for these carefully—they may inhibit reduction.

Management

• Elbow dislocations are generally reduced in the ED under procedural sedation. Most will reduce with axial traction on the forearm which is held in 30° flexion while the assistant thumbs the olecranon process. If this is not successful, then, with traction still applied, extend the elbow to unlock the coronoid process. An intraarticular bony fragment may prevent reduction—these patients will need open reduction.

- Test range of elbow movement post-reduction—a full, smooth range suggests successful reduction, resistance to movement suggests intraarticular bone fragment or soft tissue entrapment.
- Post-reduction X-rays are performed to show alignment and the position of any intraarticular fragment.
- Repeat the neurovascular examination post-reduction to ensure that none of the nerves has been entrapped in the reduction.
- Support the reduced elbow in a long arm plaster back slab and refer to the fracture clinic/orthopaedic surgeon's rooms for review.

OLECRANON FRACTURES
Assessment

- These fractures are caused either by a fall onto the elbow or forcible contraction of the triceps.
- There is usually pain and swelling over the olecranon.
- X-rays clearly demonstrate the fracture in most cases. Look for displacement and the position of the fracture relative to the joint.

Management

- All olecranon fractures require orthopaedic registrar review in the ED.
- Management usually depends on the integrity of the extensor mechanism. If the mechanism is intact and the fracture undisplaced, treatment consists of immobilisation in a long arm slab supported in a sling/shoulder support and review at the fracture clinic or orthopaedic surgeon's rooms. If the extensor mechanism is disrupted, then open reduction and internal fixation is usually necessary.

PULLED ELBOW
Assessment

- Occurs in children aged 1–6 years when the radial head slips out from under the annular ligament as a result of axial traction when there is a sudden tug on the arm by either child or parent while the parent is holding the child's hand.

- The parent indicates that the child is not using the affected arm which is usually held limply by the side or semi-flexed. There is often, but not always, tenderness over the radial head.
- X-rays are not necessary when the history is clear.

Management
- Reduction is achieved without anaesthetic—the operator, having gained the child's and parent's confidence, holds the elbow in one hand with the thumb over the radial head while the other hand fully supinates and then flexes the forearm. Reduction is usually palpable.
- The child does not usually begin to use the arm again immediately. Review about 15 minutes post-reduction usually shows that full movement has returned. No follow-up is necessary.

RADIAL HEAD AND NECK FRACTURE
Assessment
- These structures may be injured by direct force but the most common mechanism of injury is a fall onto the outstretched hand.
- The patient presents with pain in the elbow and pain on movement. Supination and pronation are usually limited by pain. Firm palpation over the radial head reveals tenderness.
- Most of these fractures are undisplaced and do not require manipulation.
- The outstanding feature on X-ray is a positive 'fat pad sign', indicating the presence of an elbow joint effusion:
  — visible posterior elbow joint fat pad
  — anterior bowing of the usually straight anterior fat pad
  — a blood/fat level in the anterior fat pad.
- On X-rays, look for angulation in the normally smooth arc of the radial neck and intraarticular fracture of the radial head.

Management
- Undisplaced fractures of the radial head or neck are treated with triangular sling or shoulder immobiliser and referral to the fracture clinic or orthopaedic surgeons' rooms.

- Angulated fractures of the radial neck and displaced intraarticular fractures of the radial head should be reviewed by the orthopaedic registrar in the ED and considered for open reduction and internal fixation.

RADIUS AND ULNA SHAFT FRACTURE
Assessment

- Isolated fracture of the shaft of one of the forearm bones is usually caused by direct-force injury. Fractures of both bones are much more common and are caused by transmitted forces from falls onto the outstretched hand. The position of the hand and arm at the time of the fall will determine the pattern of the fractures.
- The patient presents with pain, swelling, deformity and limitation of movement of the forearm.
- X-rays will demonstrate the pattern of the fracture. Both bones are usually broken or there is a pattern of fracture of one bone with dislocation of the other (Monteggia, Galeazzi fracture/dislocations) so views that include the whole of the forearm including the elbow and wrist joints are essential. Look for angulation, displacement and comminution.

Management

- All fractures of the shaft of the radius and/or ulna should be reviewed by the orthopaedic registrar in the ED.
- Management depends on patient's age, the site of the fracture and the degree of angulation and displacement.
- A significant proportion of radial/ulnar shaft fractures will require either closed reduction under general anaesthesia or open reduction and internal fixation.

DISTAL RADIUS AND ULNA FRACTURE
Colles' fracture
Assessment

- Colles' fracture, first described by Abraham Colles in 1814, is defined as a fracture of the distal radius within 2.5 cm of the wrist joint with dorsal and radial angulation and dorsal displacement.

- It is caused by falls onto the outstretched hand and is commonest in older women.
- The patient presents with pain, swelling, and deformity ('dinner fork' deformity) of the wrist after a fall. There is tenderness over the distal radius.
- X-rays show a transverse fracture of the distal radius. Look for angulation, displacement, comminution, intraarticular involvement.

Management

- Management depends on the nature of the fracture.
    — Fractures with minimal displacement and angulation are adequately treated by immobilisation with a short arm slab with the wrist in the neutral position.
    — Fractures that demonstrate features of instability (comminution, radial shortening, intraarticular involvement) may require open or closed reduction and internal fixation because they are at increased risk of mal-union.
    — Displaced and angulated Colles' fractures that are not unstable are managed with closed reduction and plaster immobilisation.
- Colles' fracture reduction is performed in the ED at some institutions. Procedural sedation and regional nerve block are the preferred anaesthetic options in the ED. Some institutions still use intravenous regional anaesthesia (Bier's block) which should be performed only by senior medical staff with a thorough understanding of its complications.
- Complications of Colles' fracture include:
    — mal- or non-union, especially with unstable fractures
    — median nerve compression
    — Sudeck's atrophy
    — rupture of the extensor pollicis longus tendon
    — residual wrist stiffness and pain.

Editorial Comment

In any wrist injury (especially after a fall), look for/exclude dislocated lunate (pressure damage to median nerve) which needs urgent reduction and is often missed early.

SMITH'S FRACTURE
Assessment

- Defined as a full-thickness fracture of the distal radius 1–2.5 cm from the wrist with volar displacement and angulation. Also known as a reversed Colles' fracture.
- It is caused by falls onto the outstretched hand with forced supination and by injuries that cause forced hyperflexion at the wrist (fall onto the back of the hand, handlebar injuries).
- The patient presents with pain, swelling and deformity (often described as 'garden spade' deformity) of the wrist after a fall. There is tenderness over the distal radius.
- X-rays show a transverse fracture of the distal radius. Look for angulation, displacement, comminution, intraarticular involvement.

Management
All Smith's fractures should be reviewed by the orthopaedic registrar in the ED and most will require closed reduction.

Barton's fracture/dislocation
Assessment

- Barton's fracture/dislocation is an intraarticular fracture of the distal radius in which impingement of the carpus causes displacement of either the volar (more common) or dorsal rim of the radius.
- X-ray shows an intraarticular fracture of the distal radius with either volar or dorsal displacement and angulation of the intraarticular rim of the radius, the carpus having been effectively driven into the distal radius.

Management
Closed reduction may be attempted but the carpus tends to hold the fragments apart and so many of these fractures will require open reduction and internal fixation.

Scaphoid fracture
Assessment

- The scaphoid is the most frequently fractured carpal bone.

- Scaphoid fractures are usually the result of a fall onto the outstretched hand.
- About 70% of fractures involve the middle third ('waist') of the scaphoid, 10–20% involve the distal pole and 5–10% involve the proximal pole.
- The patient presents with pain and perhaps swelling of the wrist after a fall. Presentation may be delayed days or weeks after an apparent 'sprain' does not resolve. Examination reveals tenderness in the anatomical 'snuff box' and pain on axial compression of the thumb.
- X-rays (with scaphoid views) usually reveal a transverse fracture of the scaphoid but may be normal. If clinical suspicion is high and the X-rays are negative there are several options.
  — Apply a scaphoid plaster and re-X-ray after 10 to 14 days.
  — Perform a CT (or MRI) scan of the wrist.
  — Perform a radionuclide bone scan of the wrist.
- The chosen option will depend on patient preference and availability of imaging.

Management

- All scaphoid fractures should be reviewed by the orthopaedic or hand surgery registrar in the ED to determine the need for internal fixation.
- Management is either immobilisation in a scaphoid plaster slab or open reduction and internal fixation. Fractures displaced by more than 1 mm are usually internally fixed. Some surgeons routinely internally fix proximal pole fractures because of their increased incidence of non-union and avascular necrosis.
- The main complications are as follows.
  — Avascular necrosis: occurs in 15% to 30% of scaphoid fractures, most commonly in proximal pole fractures—the more proximal the fracture, the more likely is avascular necrosis.
  — Delayed and non-union: most common in proximal pole fractures.
  — Osteoarthritis: results from avascular necrosis, mal-union and non-union and leaves the patient disabled with a painful, stiff wrist.

- Delayed diagnosis and immobilisation of scaphoid fracture significantly increases the likelihood of avascular necrosis and non-union—obtain further imaging (CT, MRI, bone scan) for patients with snuff box tenderness but normal initial X-ray.

Gamekeeper's/skier's thumb
Assessment
- This injury involves rupture of the ulnar collateral ligament of the thumb metacarpophalangeal (MCP) joint because of forced abduction and hyperextension of the thumb in motorcyclists, skiers and footballers.
- The patient presents with pain and swelling at the MCP joint and examination reveals laxity of the joint in abduction.

Management
Management is immobilisation in a thumb spica and referral to the fracture/hand clinic or orthopaedic/hand surgeon's rooms for consideration for surgical repair.

Fifth metacarpal fracture
Assessment
- The 'boxer's fracture' is a fracture of the neck of the fifth metacarpal from punching a person or a wall or occasionally from a fall directly onto the fifth metacarpal knuckle.
- X-rays reveal a fracture of the neck of the metacarpal, usually with volar angulation.
- Test for rotational deformity by asking the patient to flex the fingers—if there is significant ulnar or radial deviation of the flexed little finger, then reduction is necessary.

Management
- Reduction is best performed with a proximal digital block.
- Immobilisation is best maintained with a gutter slab that holds the wrist slightly extended, the MCP joint in 70–90° flexion and the interphalangeal joints in extension (the 'position of safe immobilisation', POSI).
- Punch injuries may also cause dislocation of the head of the fifth metacarpal which often requires reduction under general anaesthesia and internal fixation.

Metacarpal and phalangeal fractures

Assessment

- These fractures are usually caused by direct-force trauma.
- Examine for rotational deformity and associated injuries:
  — open fracture
  — tendon injury
  — digital nerve injury
  — nail bed injury.
- X-rays of the hand adequately demonstrate most metacarpal and phalangeal fractures. Look for angulation, displacement and tendon avulsion fractures.

Management

- Isolated, uncomplicated metacarpal fractures with minimal angulation and displacement can be safely treated with immobilisation in a volar slab in the position of safe immobilisation:
  — wrist slightly extended
  — the MCP joint in 70–90° flexion and
  — the interphalangeal joints in extension.
- Refer patient to the fracture/hand clinic or orthopaedic/hand surgeon's rooms.
- Isolated, uncomplicated phalangeal fractures with minimal angulation and displacement can be safely treated with immobilisation by 'buddy strapping' and referred to the fracture/hand clinic or orthopaedic/hand surgeon's rooms.
- Painful subungual haematoma should be treated by trephining the nail by gently pressing the tip of a red-hot paperclip onto the middle of the nail over the haematoma.
- Angulated or displaced fractures, those with rotational deformity, open fractures and those complicated by tendon, nerve or nail bed injury need review in the ED by the orthopaedic or hand surgery registrar.

Dislocations of the interphalangeal and metacarpophalangeal joints

Assessment

- Dislocations of the finger joints are usually caused by forced hyperextension and the dislocation is usually dorsal.

- Always X-ray deformed fingers before attempting reduction because displaced fractures give a similar external appearance to dislocations.

Management

- Most finger dislocations are easily reduced. Digital nerve block may be used but many dislocations can be reduced without anaesthesia. The technique involves applying axial traction to the distal part while pressing with the thumb of the other hand over the base of the dislocated bone.
- Failed reduction may occur when the head of the proximal bone is 'button-holed' through the volar plate necessitating open reduction.
- Always obtain a post-reduction X-ray to exclude avulsion fractures.
- Examine active movements of the finger post-reduction to detect rupture of the middle slip of the extensor tendon in distal interphalangeal dislocations.
- Buddy strap the reduced finger and encourage active movement.

MALLET FINGER

Assessment

- Mallet finger is caused by avulsion of the insertion of the extensor tendon mechanism from the dorsal base of the distal phalanx. It usually occurs in ball sports when the ball strikes the tip of the finger, forcing it into hyperflexion.
- The patient presents with pain and swelling at the distal interphalangeal joint and examination reveals weak or absent active extension.
- X-ray reveals a dorsal avulsion fragment. Look for the degree of separation and amount of joint surface involvement.

Management

- Definitive management depends on the degree of separation and joint surface involvement. The majority of patients are adequately treated with a mallet finger splint (splinting the joint in mild hyperextension) for 6 to 10 weeks.

- Apply a mallet finger splint and refer the patient for early review in the Hand/orthopaedic Clinic or the Hand/orthopaedic Surgeon's rooms.

BOUTONNIÈRE DEFORMITY
Assessment

- Boutonnière ('buttonhole') deformity results from avulsion of the central slip of the extensor tendon from the base of the middle phalanx. The lateral bands then migrate towards the volar surface causing flexion at the proximal interphalangeal joint and extension at the distal interphalangeal joint.
  The central slip disruption may be caused by laceration, dislocation of the interphalangeal joint or forced flexion of the extended finger.
- Most patients present with a tender, swollen proximal interphalangeal joint.
- X-rays may show an avulsion fragment adjacent to the dorsal base of the middle phalanx.

Management
All patients with boutonnière deformity should be referred urgently to the hand surgery/orthopaedic registrar for prompt surgical treatment.

DIGITAL NERVE INJURIES
Assessment

- All patients with any injury, especially lacerations, of the hand and fingers should be carefully examined for nerve injury before any anaesthetic agent is given.
- Sensory loss from digital nerve injury usually affects a quadrant of the finger.

Management

- Hand surgeons will usually attempt surgical repair of any digital nerve injury proximal to the distal interphalangeal joint. Any patient with digital sensory loss following a hand or finger injury should be referred to the hand surgery registrar for consideration of operative repair.

- Patients with lacerations should be treated with tetanus immunoprophylaxis and intravenous antibiotics pending hand surgery review.

TENDON INJURIES IN THE HAND

Assessment

- The majority of tendon injuries in the hand are associated with skin lacerations.
- Tendon injury must be suspected with any hand or finger laceration and its presence must be confirmed/excluded by the following.
  - Testing tendon function/finger movement.
  - Careful inspection of the wound for signs of tendon injury—remember that many tendon injuries are not visible in the wound because the injury has occurred with the finger in a different posture.
  - If the laceration is in a position where tendon injury may have occurred and the laceration appears to extend past the deep fascia, then tendon injury should be suspected.
  - Be wary of partial tendon laceration which will go on to rupture.

Management

Urgently refer all patients with actual or possible tendon laceration to the hand/orthopaedic registrar for formal exploration with a bloodless field and operating microscope in the operating theatre.

Pelvic fractures

Pelvic fractures occur in three broad settings:

1. As a result of simple falls from standing in older patients—these are usually undisplaced fractures of the pubic rami or acetabulum and usually do not require active treatment.
2. Avulsion fractures in adolescents and young adults.
3. As a result of major forces (falls from a height, vehicle accidents) in young and old patients—displaced pelvic fractures often cause life-threatening haemorrhage requiring urgent resuscitation and active definitive treatment.

PELVIC FRACTURES IN THE ELDERLY
Assessment

- These fractures occur as a result of falls from standing and include fractures of the pubic rami and undisplaced fractures of the acetabulum.
- The patient presents with hip pain, often localised to the groin in pubic ramus fractures, and is unwilling to bear weight.
- X-rays will often demonstrate undisplaced fractures of the pubic rami or acetabulum.
- CT imaging or radionuclide bone scan will detect occult fractures in patients who are unwilling to mobilise but have apparently normal X-rays. Always CT scan the hips and pelvis of older patients who have fallen, have apparently normal X-rays and are still unable to bear weight.

Management

Management includes:
- adequate analgesia
- orthopaedic registrar assessment
- admission to hospital under the orthogeriatric or geriatric team
- initial bed rest
- prophylaxis against thromboembolic disease
- early mobilisation
- social work involvement to facilitate return to home
- falls assessment.

PELVIC AVULSION FRACTURES

- Anterior superior iliac spine avulsion:
  - occurs in athletes and young people as a result of forceful contraction of the sartorius
  - is treated by rest from exercise for 2–6 weeks.
- Ischial tuberosity avulsion:
  - occurs in athletes as a result of forceful contraction of the hamstrings
  - may require lengthy rehabilitation and surgical treatment.

- Anterior inferior iliac spine avulsion:
  - occurs in athletes as a result of forceful contraction of the rectus femoris
  - is treated by rest from exercise for 2–6 weeks.
- Posterior iliac spine avulsion:
  - occurs in weightlifters
  - may require lengthy rehabilitation.

MAJOR PELVIC FRACTURES
Assessment
- These injuries occur as the result of major trauma:
  - falls from heights
  - motorcycle and motor vehicle crashes
  - crush injuries
  - industrial accidents.
- They may be complicated by:
  - life-threatening haemorrhage from arteries and venous plexuses within the pelvis and sacrum
  - bladder injuries
  - urethral injuries
  - gynaecological injuries
  - rectal injuries
  - neurological injury to the sacral nerves.
- A plain X-ray of the pelvis is a standard element of the primary survey for trauma management and will show most haemodynamically significant pelvic fractures. Look for continuity of the three circles (pelvic inlet, two obturator foramens), sacral fracture, sacroiliac dislocation. Major pelvic fractures usually involve double breaks in the pelvic ring—if one is identified, look for the second.
- CT scan gives accurate visualisation of pelvic and sacral fractures but should not be performed if the patient is haemodynamically unstable.

Management
- Management of major pelvic fracture in the primary survey includes:
  - ABC—identification and management of other life-threatening injuries

- — resuscitation—crystalloid or blood
- — analgesia with intravenous morphine
- — pelvic haemorrhage control:
  - ○ reduction and immobilisation in the ED—sheet tied around the pelvis, proprietary pelvic immobiliser
  - ○ urgent transfer to the angiography suite for radiological identification and embolisation of bleeding points
  - ○ transfer to the operating theatre for pelvic packing if embolisation is unsuccessful
  - ○ transfer to the operating theatre once stable for closed reduction and application of external fixator immobilisation.

Lower limb injuries
FEMORAL NECK FRACTURES
Assessment

- These fractures are common in the elderly, most commonly caused by a simple fall from standing. They can occur with minimal or no apparent trauma in osteoporotic patients and as pathological fractures, especially with metastatic breast carcinoma.
- Most femoral neck fractures are clinically obvious. The patient is unable to stand or mobilise after a fall and there is characteristic shortening and external rotation of the affected limb. Be wary of the impacted fracture in which the limb may appear normal and the patient may be able to bear weight, albeit with pain and a limp.
- X-rays will usually identify the femoral neck fracture. Look for position of the fracture, alignment, displacement, features of pathological fracture.
- When X-rays do not show an obvious fracture but there is pain or inability to mobilise, perform a CT scan or radionuclide bone scan to identify an occult fracture.

Management

- Regional analgesia—FIB or femoral nerve block.
- Patients with femoral neck fractures tend to be elderly with significant co-morbidities. Many hospitals have joint

orthopaedics/geriatrics (orthogeriatric) admission policies that provide thorough peri-operative medical assessment and management. Ensure that all co-morbidities are identified, assessed and optimised pre-operatively by appropriate investigation and consultation.

• The management of femoral neck fracture is operative. Best mortality and morbidity outcomes are achieved with operation within 24 hours of injury.

Hip joint dislocation

Hip dislocation occurs in two circumstances: traumatic and prosthetic.

Traumatic hip dislocation

Assessment

• This is a medical emergency because of the risk of injury to the femoral head and sciatic nerve and requires urgent reduction.

• Usually caused by a high-velocity impact on the flexed, abducted knee as in motorcycle crashes and impact from the dashboard in high-speed motor vehicle crashes (MVCs) or in falls from significant heights.

• Often associated with other injuries in the pelvis and knee with intra-abdominal and thoracic injuries.

• Of all traumatic hip dislocations, 80–90% are posterior, 10% are anterior and the remainder are central.

• Major complications are:
— avascular necrosis of the head of the femur
— sciatic nerve injury
— myositis ossificans.
The likelihood of all of these complications is reduced by early reduction.

• The patient presents from a high-velocity impact with a shortened, internally rotated and adducted leg.

• Urgent assessment should include:
— primary survey (ABCDE, resuscitation)
— look for injuries in other organ systems
— examination of the knees and femoral shafts for associated injuries

  — assessment of sciatic nerve function—test dorsiflexion
    and plantarflexion at the ankle and sensation over the
    lateral border of the foot.
  — palpate the arterial pulses of the leg and foot.
- X-rays usually demonstrate the dislocation adequately—
  always obtain X-rays of the pelvis, femur and knee joint. Look
  for associated pelvic, femoral, patellar or tibial fractures.

Management

Reduction may be performed in the ED under procedural sedation
if the patient is otherwise stable. In unstable patients, the dislocation is reduced in the operating theatre after life-threatening
injuries have been controlled.

Prosthetic hip dislocation

Assessment

Does not cause sciatic nerve or femoral head injury but should still
be reduced promptly to relieve pain.

Management

- Usually reduced in the ED with procedural sedation. With the
  patient supine in bed, an assistant provides counter-traction
  to the pelvis while the operator stands on the bed and flexes
  the hip and knee to 90° and then applies vertical traction.
  X-ray to confirm successful relocation and re-check sciatic
  nerve and vascular function.
- Perioperative dislocations, that is dislocations in the first
  6 weeks following hip replacement surgery, should be
  reduced by the orthopaedic surgeons in the operating theatre.

FEMORAL SHAFT FRACTURES

Assessment

- The mechanism of injury usually involves significant force as
  in MVCs, falls or sporting accidents, and occurs most often
  in young adults. The fracture may be transverse, oblique or
  spiral.
- Clinically the thigh is swollen and tender and the leg may be
  angulated and/or shortened.

- X-rays of the whole of the femur and the hip and knee joints are needed.
- Complications include:
  — blood loss of up to 2000 mL
  — fat embolism
  — vascular and nerve injury (uncommon).

Management
- Urgent management should include:
  — primary survey (ABCDE, resuscitation)
  — look for injuries in other organ systems
  — aggressive fluid resuscitation
  — urgent blood cross-match
  — consider CT angiogram for arterial injury
  — consider femoral nerve block for analgesia
  — early reduction and immobilisation in a traction splint reduces pain and haemorrhage.
- Most femoral shaft fractures in adults are treated with open reduction and internal fixation. Children are usually treated in gallows traction.

DISTAL FEMORAL FRACTURES
Assessment
- Includes supracondylar and condylar fractures. Occur with major trauma in MVCs and falls and with minimal trauma in older and/or osteoporotic patients.
- Examination shows that the knee is swollen (with lipo-haemarthrosis in condylar fractures) and deformed with decreased range of movement.
- X-rays usually define these fractures well. Look for displacement, angulation and effusion and a blood/fat level in the knee joint.
- Consider CT angiogram for arterial injury.

Management
Give adequate intravenous analgesia and immobilise in a long leg plaster slab while awaiting urgent orthopaedic registrar review.

RUPTURE OF THE QUADRICEPS TENDON
Assessment

- Usually occurs in men from early middle age onwards when an axial force is applied to the leg with the knee fixed in flexion.
- The patient presents with pain around the knee after a fall and is unable to mobilise.
- Careful examination reveals a visible and palpable gap in the suprapatellar tendon immediately above the upper pole patella.
- X-rays often show avulsion flakes from the superior border of the patella.
- Ultrasound confirms the diagnosis.

Management

Management is surgical repair of the tendon. Immobilise the knee in a Zimmer splint or long leg plaster slab and ask the orthopaedic registrar to see the patient in the ED.

PATELLAR FRACTURES
Assessment

- Caused by direct-force injury to the patella in falls from standing and from the dashboard in MVCs or from sudden forceful contraction of the quadriceps.
- The patient presents with a painful knee after the accident. Knee joint effusion is often, but not always, present.
- X-rays should include anteroposterior, lateral and 'skyline' views. Undisplaced linear fractures may be difficult to see on plain X-ray—obtain a CT scan of the knee when there is significant pain but no evident fracture on plain X-rays. Look for a knee joint effusion with blood/fat level which is diagnostic evidence of a fracture.
- The orthopaedic registrar should review the patient in the ED.

Management

Management depends on patient age and the integrity of the quadriceps mechanism.

- If the mechanism is intact, management is usually with immobilisation in a Zimmer splint or long leg plaster.

- Open reduction and internal fixation is standard management if the mechanism is disrupted.

PATELLAR DISLOCATION
Assessment

- Patella dislocation most commonly occurs in adolescent females but is also common in young males, especially during sport. Dislocation is usually lateral and is caused by either a force applied to the medial patella or forceful contraction of the vastus lateralis with the knee flexed. Congenital predisposition is present in more than 50% of cases, with excessive external rotation at the hip joint being the most common precipitant. Recurrent dislocation is common.
- The diagnosis is usually apparent with obvious lateral dislocation of the patella.
- Pre-reduction X-ray is not necessary when the diagnosis is clear.

Management

- Reduction is often achieved without anaesthesia with the operator gently extending the knee fully while pressing on the lateral patella with the thumb. If the patient is reluctant to allow this, then procedural sedation should be used.
- Post-reduction knee X-rays (anteroposterior, lateral, skyline) are performed to detect associated avulsion fractures.
- The leg should be immobilised with the knee straight in a Zimmer splint for 3 weeks to allow the medial ligaments to heal. The patient is referred to the fracture clinic/orthopaedic surgeon's rooms and to a physiotherapist for strengthening of the vastus medialis.

TRUE DISLOCATION OF THE KNEE
Assessment

- True dislocation of the knee is a medical emergency because it is commonly associated with popliteal artery injury and the risk of amputation.
- The mechanism of injury often involves significant force as in high-speed MVCs, pedestrian/car accidents and falls but rotation on a planted foot at sport can cause dislocation, especially in heavy individuals.

- Associated injuries:
  — up to 30% of knee dislocations are open
  — popliteal artery injury occurs in up to 79% of knee dislocations
  — common peroneal nerve injury with foot drop occurs in up to 40%
  — compartment syndrome occurs because of swelling around the knee joint and upper leg and its presence increases the risk of nerve and muscle ischaemia and amputation.
- The risk of amputation because of arterial injury increases if reduction is delayed.
- Three of the four major ligaments of the knee must be ruptured for the knee to dislocate.
- Examine for:
  — distal pulses, capillary refill, colour, temperature
  — common peroneal nerve injury—dorsiflexion of the foot and toes, sensation between the first and second toes dorsally
  — increased compartment pressure.
- Urgent X-rays confirm the diagnosis of knee dislocation.

Management
- Management should include:
  — primary survey (ABCDE, resuscitation)
  — look for injuries in other organ systems
  — urgent orthopaedic registrar review in the ED
  — prompt reduction in the ED using procedural sedation
  — post-reduction immobilisation in a long leg plaster slab
  — urgent CT angiography and vascular surgery consultation in all cases.
- If reduction is delayed for more than 8 hours, the likelihood of distal amputation is about 80%.

TIBIAL PLATEAU FRACTURE
Assessment
- Classically described as 'bumper bar fractures', these injuries are common in pedestrians struck by cars but also occur in falls from standing in the elderly and occasionally at sport. The causative force is usually applied to the knee

laterally, driving the lateral femoral condyle into the lateral tibial plateau and opening the knee medially. The lateral tibial plateau is more frequently injured than the medial. Lateral tibial plateau fracture may be associated with medial collateral ligament (MCL) and anterior and posterior cruciate ligament (ACL, PCL) tears as the knee opens up from a laterally applied force.

- The patient complains of knee pain, usually has a knee joint effusion and is unable to bear weight.
- Tibial plateau fracture is easily missed on plain X-ray. Look for a knee joint effusion with a blood/fat level.
- CT scan of the knee should be performed on any patient with knee pain and inability to mobilise and will detect tibial plateau fractures that are poorly delineated on plain X-rays.
- Examine for popliteal artery and common peroneal nerve injury.

Management
- Management depends on patient age and degree of displacement.
- Immobilise the knee in a Zimmer splint or long leg plaster slab and obtain orthopaedic registrar review in the ED.

ACUTE KNEE PAIN

The cruciate ligaments (anterior and posterior, ACL and PCL), collateral ligaments (medial and lateral, MCL and LCL), and the medial and lateral menisci are frequently injured at sport and in accidents in which linear and/or torsional forces are applied to the knee. Injuries to the ACL, PCL and the menisci, along with fractures of the distal femur, proximal tibia and patella, will usually cause acute knee effusion (lipo-haemarthrosis). Acute inflammatory and infective monoarthropathies (gout, pseudogout, septic arthritis are the most common) often also present with acute painful knee joint effusion.

TRAUMATIC KNEE PAIN
Assessment
- All patients with acute knee injuries should have plain X-rays of the knee (anteroposterior, lateral and skyline) to demonstrate fractures:
  — tibial plateau fracture, femoral condyle fracture, patella fracture

- — avulsion fractures:
  - ○ of the tibial spine in cruciate ligament injury
  - ○ avulsion flakes from the upper pole patella in quadriceps ligament rupture
  - ○ avulsion flakes from the femoral condyles in MCL and LCL injuries
  - ○ vertical avulsion flake from the proximal lateral tibia (Segond fracture, indicative of ACL tear).
- • A careful history of the mechanism of the knee injury points to the probable derangement.
  - — A linear force applied to the lateral knee will open the joint medially and compress the bones laterally, resulting in, with increasing amount of force:
    - ○ MCL tear—the most common knee ligament injury. Occurs most frequently in football tackles, skiing. There will be tenderness over the MCL above and/ or below the medial joint line. Test for laxity to valgus strain—grade 3 injuries involve complete rupture, cause medial joint laxity and may require surgical repair. Grade 1 and 2 injuries are partial tears, there is no laxity and they usually heal without surgery.
    - ○ MCL tear plus medial meniscus tear—also occurs most commonly at football and skiing. As well as features of an MCL tear, there will be a knee joint effusion and tenderness over the medial meniscus at the medial joint line. Usually requires arthroscopic repair of the medial meniscus.
    - ○ MCL tear plus medial meniscus tear plus ACL tear— also occurs most commonly at football and skiing. As well as the features of MCL and medial meniscus injury, there will be laxity to anterior stress. Usually requires arthroscopic ACL reconstruction.
    - ○ Lateral tibial plateau fracture plus MCL tear.
  - — PCL tear is usually caused by hyperextension of the knee, most commonly at football or skiing. There will be a knee joint effusion and laxity to posterior strain.
  - — Rotational forces, as in changing direction on a planted foot, cause meniscal tears and cruciate ligament injuries.

- Examination of acute knee injury is often difficult because of pain and swelling but should always include the following.
  - Inspect for the presence and size of effusion. Compare with the other, normal knee; remember to milk the prepatellar bursa and test for patellar tap. Effusion suggests internal derangement and is unusual in isolated collateral ligament injuries.
  - Palpate for tenderness. Tenderness over the MCL and LCL above and below the joint line suggests collateral ligament injury. Tenderness in the joint line suggests internal derangement.
  - Test range of movement. A 'locked' knee is usually caused by acute or exacerbation of chronic meniscal tear.
  - Test for collateral ligament integrity. Laxity to valgus strain suggests MCL tear, laxity to varus strain suggests LCL tear.
  - Test for cruciate ligament integrity.
    - Anterior drawer sign: supine on bed, hip at 45°, knee at 90°, sit on patient's foot and pull tibia forwards—laxity suggests ACL tear.
    - Lachman test: supine on bed, knee flexed to 20–30°, tibia lifted upwards—laxity suggests ACL tear.
    - Posterior drawer sign: supine on bed, knee at 90°, sit on patient's foot and push tibia backwards—laxity suggests PCL tear.
  - Test for meniscal injury.
    - Apley grind test: prone on bed, knee at 90°, apply axial force through leg and rotate.
    - McMurray's test: patient supine on bed, knee at 90°, thumb over joint line, rotate lower leg—pain and palpable click indicates meniscal injury.

Management

Initial management of knee ligament and meniscal injuries includes:
- analgesia
- consider aspirating a tense haemarthrosis for pain relief

- immobilise in a Zimmer splint
- refer to fracture clinic or orthopaedic surgeon's rooms for further assessment and management.
- consider ordering outpatient MRI scan.

NON-TRAUMATIC KNEE PAIN

- All patients with knee pain, effusion and no history of injury should have plain X-rays of the knee along with screening blood tests (blood count, ESR, CRP, urate).
- Aspiration of knee effusion fluid for cell count, microscopy, culture and crystals should always be performed to exclude a diagnosis of septic arthritis.
- Septic arthritis requires admission to hospital for urgent surgical lavage and intravenous antibiotics.
- Acute gouty arthritis should be treated with oral prednisone 1 mg/kg up to 50 mg daily for 3–4 days +/– a non-steroidal anti-inflammatory agent.

TIBIA AND FIBULA SHAFT FRACTURES

Assessment

- Often seen in the younger age group during active adolescence and adulthood.
- Swelling and deformity are usually obvious.
- Open fractures are common.
- Usually require reduction under anaesthesia with external and/or internal immobilisation.

Management

- Management includes:
  - analgesia, usually with intravenous morphine
  - orthopaedic registrar review in the ED
  - test for distal neurovascular compromise
  - reduction of deformity should be performed urgently in the ED with procedural sedation if there is evidence of distal vascular compromise
  - urgent attention to open injuries with lavage and antibiotics
  - immobilisation in a long leg plaster slab.

Editorial Comment

BEWARE COMPARTMENT SYNDROME with tibial shaft fractures. The anterior compartment of the lower leg is the most common site of compartment syndrome which may occur with any tibial shaft fracture. The outstanding symptom is pain out of proportion to that expected with the fracture, often accompanied by altered sensation in the foot or toes. Most tibial fractures immobilised in plaster will not require opiate analgesia. Urgent orthopaedic assessment with a view to early fasciotomy is necessary.

ISOLATED FIBULAR SHAFT FRACTURES
Assessment

+ These fractures are usually the result of direct-force trauma but may be associated with diastasis of the tibiofibular ligament, especially if the fibular fracture is at the neck of the fibula.
+ X-rays of the tibia and fibula should always include the knee and ankle joints. Look carefully for evidence of tibiofibular diastasis if an apparently isolated fibular fracture is present.

Management

Isolated fibular fractures may be treated with either a firm bandage or a short leg plaster slab and referral to the fracture clinic or orthopaedic surgeon's rooms.

ANKLE LIGAMENT INJURIES
Assessment

+ Common cause of presentation to EDs.
+ Usually caused by trips applying torsional force at the ankle joint. Inversion injury is the most common.
+ The lateral ligament of the ankle comprises:
  — anterior talofibular ligament
  — posterior talofibular ligament
  — calcaneofibular ligament.
+ The medial (deltoid) ligament of the ankle consists of superficial and deep components.

- Seventy-five per cent of ankle injuries are ligament injuries without fracture and 90% of these involve the lateral ligaments; 90% of lateral ligament injuries involve its anterior talofibular portion.
- The great majority of ankle ligament injuries are partial (grade 1 and 2) tears which will heal to full strength with conservative treatment. Full (grade 3) tears of more than two ligaments often result in persistent ankle instability and so will often require surgical reconstruction. Assessment of instability is difficult at the acute presentation because of pain and swelling.
- The patient presents with a painful, often swollen ankle.
- The decision to image the ankle depends on the independently validated Ottawa ankle rules: if there is pain in the malleoli and any one of:
  — inability to bear weight both immediately and for four steps in the ED
  — bone tenderness over the distal 6 cm of the fibula or the tip of the lateral malleolus
  — bone tenderness over the distal 6 cm of the tibia or the tip of the medial malleolus
  then plain anteroposterior and lateral X-rays of the ankle should be performed.

Management

For a patient with no evidence of fracture on ankle X-rays, management should include the following.
- Adequate analgesia.
- Explanation that pain, bruising and swelling in ankle ligament injuries usually persists for 3–6 weeks and that sporting activity should be deferred for 4–12 weeks. Ankle strapping should be used for sport up to 6 months after injury.
- Apply a firm (tubigrip) bandage.
- Ice for 48 hours and elevate while sitting until swelling subsides.
- Most patients will need crutches for the first few days.
- Active weight bearing can be resumed when pain permits, usually in 3–5 days.
- Arrange physiotherapy referral.

- Arrange review by the general practitioner for assessment of instability after one week. If the GP finds instability, then an MRI scan is performed to determine the extent of ligament injury.

ANKLE DISLOCATION
Assessment

- This is a common injury and is usually associated with ankle fractures.
- The patient presents with pain, swelling and obvious deformity at the ankle joint.
- Distal neurovascular function is usually preserved but the skin is stretched tight over one of the malleoli and this may lead to ischaemic necrosis of the skin if reduction is delayed.

Management
Management should include the following.
- X-rays should be performed before reduction to differentiate between ankle joint and subtalar dislocations.
- Urgent reduction under procedural sedation in the ED. Most dislocations reduce easily with manual traction on the foot.
- Immobilisation in a short leg plaster slab.
- Post-reduction X-rays to reveal the associated fractures.
- Urgent orthopaedic registrar review in the ED.
- Associated fractures will usually require open reduction and internal fixation.

ANKLE FRACTURES
Assessment

- Ankle fractures are common and usually result from trips and over-balancing.
- Management depends on the integrity of the ankle mortice.
- Pott's classification:
  — uni-malleolar, lateral or medial
  — bi-malleolar, lateral and medial
  — tri-malleolar, lateral, medial and posterior.
- The mortice is unstable if there is evidence of:
  — talar tilt or shift

— displacement of any of the malleoli
— bi-malleolar fracture
— tri-malleolar fracture
— uni-malleolar fracture with ligament injury at the opposite malleolus.

Management

• Stable fractures in anatomical position are usually treated conservatively in a short leg plaster slab with referral to the fracture clinic or orthopaedic surgeon's rooms.
• Unstable fractures are usually treated with open reduction and internal fixation.
• The orthopaedic registrar should review all ankle fractures in the ED.

ACHILLES TENDON RUPTURE

Assessment

• Achilles tendon rupture is usually a sporting injury and occurs in adults from the 20s with forceful contraction of the posterior compartment muscles, often when pushing off at tennis and squash and in sprinters.
• The patient reports a sudden severe pain at the base of the leg. There is often an audible snap and the patient describes feeling as though they have been hit in the calf and is unable to walk or stand on the toes.
• The Thompson test is usually diagnostic. The patient either lies prone or kneels on a chair facing away. The operator squeezes mid-calf—the foot plantarflexes with an intact Achilles tendon, but does not move when the tendon is ruptured.
• Ultrasound confirms the diagnosis, demonstrates partial rupture and differentiates between Achilles tendon rupture and calf muscle tears.

Management

• Consult the orthopaedic registrar.
• Non-operative management is increasingly common.

TALUS FRACTURES

Assessment

- Flake avulsion fractures are common with ligamentous injury of the ankle and foot and are usually treated as ligamentous injuries.
- Fractures of the neck and body of the talus require substantial force (falls from a height, compression of the foot against the firewall in high-speed MVCs) and may lead to ischaemic necrosis of the talus.
- Most talus fractures will be visible on plain X-rays of the foot and ankle. CT scanning is indicated for patients with foot pain and swelling with apparently normal X-rays.

Management

Patients with talar fractures should be reviewed by the orthopaedic registrar in the ED. Displaced fractures will require open reduction and internal fixation.

CALCANEUS FRACTURES

Assessment

- Calcaneus fractures are common, are usually the result of a fall from height and are bilateral in up to 20% of cases.
- May be a part of the complex of injuries caused by dissipation of energy from a fall onto the feet:
  — calcaneus fracture
  — ankle fractures
  — tibial plateau fracture
  — proximal femoral fracture
  — thoracolumbar vertebral fracture (with 10–20% of calcaneus fractures)
  — atlas and base-of-skull fractures.

- Assess all of these areas for pain and tenderness and image any areas of concern.
- Plain X-rays will demonstrate most calcaneus fractures.
- Once a calcaneus fracture has been identified, obtain a CT scan of the calcaneus to demonstrate articular involvement, comminution, subluxation.

Management
- Calcaneus fractures should be reviewed by the orthopaedic registrar in the ED.
- Displaced and intraarticular fractures will need open reduction and internal fixation.
- Patients with bilateral fractures will need hospitalisation because they are unable to mobilise.

MAJOR FRACTURE/DISLOCATIONS IN THE FOOT
Subtalar dislocation
Assessment
- Subtalar dislocation occurs with major forces as in falls from a height or compression of the foot against the firewall in high-speed MVAs.
- May lead to avascular necrosis of the talus.
- Usually identified on plain X-rays.
- Requires CT imaging to identify associated fractures and articular involvement.

Management
- Urgent reduction is necessary if there are features of distal vascular compromise.
- Initial reduction may be performed under procedural sedation in the ED or under general anaesthesia in the operating theatre.

Chopart fracture/dislocation
Assessment
- The Chopart fracture/dislocation is essentially a dislocation of the midfoot on the hindfoot. It is an uncommon injury, caused by major forces as in falls from a height or compression of the foot against the firewall in high-speed MVCs.

- There is fracture and dislocation about the talonavicular and calcaneocuboid joints.
- Plain X-rays may appear normal.
- CT imaging should be performed if there is pain and swelling of the foot with apparently normal X-rays. It will clearly identify the complex of injuries.

Management
- Urgent reduction is necessary if there are features of distal vascular compromise.
- The orthopaedic registrar should review all midfoot and hindfoot fractures in the ED.
- Management is by open reduction and internal fixation.

Lisfranc fracture/dislocation
Assessment
- The Lisfranc fracture/dislocation is essentially a dislocation of the forefoot on the midfoot. It is caused by major forces, as in a heavy weight falling on the foot.
- The key to the injury is the articulation of the base of the second metatarsal with the midfoot, anchoring the forefoot and preventing lateral movement. Lisfranc fracture/dislocation occurs when lateral and rotation forces cause fracture of the base of the second metatarsal and disrupt Lisfranc's ligament, allowing lateral dislocation of the forefoot.
- X-rays of the foot may appear normal. Look carefully for fracture of the base of the second metatarsal and lateral displacement of the metatarsals.
- CT imaging should be performed if there is pain and swelling of the foot with apparently normal X-rays.

Management
- Urgent reduction is necessary if there are features of distal vascular compromise.
- The orthopaedic registrar should review all midfoot and hindfoot injuries in the ED.
- Management is usually by open reduction and internal fixation.

OTHER METATARSAL INJURIES
Fifth metatarsal fractures
Assessment

- Fractures of the base of the fifth metatarsal are common. The two types of this fracture should be differentiated because their management differs. Both are caused by inversion injuries of the foot.
- The 'Jones' fracture is a transverse fracture of the base of the fifth metatarsal and usually requires immobilisation in a boot or short leg plaster because of a tendency to non-union.
- The 'Pseudo-Jones' fracture is an oblique fracture of the base of the fifth metatarsal caused by avulsion of the insertion of peroneus brevis. It usually heals well and is usually treated symptomatically in a firm bandage.

Management
Initial management includes:
- a firm bandage or a short leg plaster slab
- crutches
- referral to the fracture clinic or orthopaedic surgeon's rooms.

Stress fractures
- The second and third metatarsals are prone to stress fracture because they have little mobility in the forefoot.
- The patient will complain of persistent forefoot pain without history of injury.
- There is often a history of recent increase in walking or running.
- X-rays are often normal.
- MRI scan and/or radionuclide bone scan will demonstrate these fractures.
- Advise rest and refer to the fracture clinic or orthopaedic surgeon's rooms.

PHALANGEAL FRACTURES IN THE FOOT
Assessment
Toe fractures are common and are caused by direct injury. The big toe and the little toe are the most exposed and the most frequently injured.

Management

- Fractures are usually minimally displaced and are best treated by buddy strapping.
- Painful subungual haematoma should be treated by trephining the nail by gently pressing the tip of a red-hot paperclip onto the middle of the nail.
- Open fractures of the toes require assessment in the ED by the orthopaedic registrar for lavage under general anaesthesia and intravenous antibiotics.

INTERPHALANGEAL AND METATARSOPHALANGEAL JOINT DISLOCATIONS
Assessment

- These are caused by direct injury and are usually easily reduced.
- X-ray all deformed toes before attempting reduction because of the possibility of fracture.

Management

- Most toe dislocations are easily reduced. Digital nerve block may be used but many dislocations can be reduced without anaesthesia, depending on patient preference. The technique of reduction involves applying axial traction to the distal part while pressing with the thumb of the other hand over the base of the dislocated bone.
- The relocated toe should be buddy-strapped and the patient mobilises normally.
- Open dislocations, fracture/dislocations, and failed reductions should be reviewed by the orthopaedic registrar in the ED.

Chapter 30
Urological emergencies
Daniel Gaetani and Edmond Park

Acknowledgment

The authors wish to acknowledge the content used from the previous edition of *Emergency Medicine* which was provided by Phillip C Brenner.

Balanitis
KEY PRESENTATION/CLINICAL FEATURES

- Infection of foreskin: bacterial or fungal
- Associated with poor hygiene, diabetes, oedematous conditions (e.g. congestive heart failure, nephrotic syndrome)
- Gradual-onset pain, tenderness or pruritus of glans/foreskin, associated with erythema and purulent exudate[1]

MANAGEMENT

- Soap washes; soaking in antiseptic solution or antibiotic ointment (e.g. neomycin); topical clotrimazole 1% and consider hydrocortisone 1%.[2]
- PO antibiotics are sometimes needed, and if whole of shaft involved then IV antibiotics.

COMPLICATIONS

- Phimosis secondary to adhesions
- Paraphimosis secondary to oedema[1]

Common post-procedural problems
EXTRACORPOREAL SHOCKWAVE LITHOTRIPSY (ESWL)
Key presentation/clinical features
Complications that commonly present to the ED include incomplete stone fragmentation resulting in urinary tract obstruction

leading to pain and haematuria, and parenchymal injury resulting in subcapsular haematoma or haemorrhage again resulting in pain.[3]

Investigations

- Urinalysis (UA) and midstream urine (MSU)
- Electrolytes, urea, creatinine (EUC), full blood count (FBC)
- X-ray of kidneys–ureters–bladder (KUB) relevant to establish size of stone fragment passing down ureter or presence of Steinstrasse (a series of stone fragments in a line)
- Measure diameter of largest fragment in millimetres

Management

- Analgesia: intravenous (IV) opioids; indomethacin 100 mg 12-hourly per rectum (PR).
- Fever with temperatures $> 38°C$ is an absolute indication for admission and indicates an infected, obstructed system requiring likely decompression by a double-J stent or nephrostomy.
- Anuria or raised creatinine due to bilateral disease or solitary kidney is similarly an emergency requiring admission.
- If patient is pain-free, discharge with indomethacin suppositories 100 mg 12-hourly PR (if no history of ulcer or other contraindication to NSAIDs) and oral opioids such as oxycodone 5 mg 6-hourly PO or codeine phosphate 30 mg/paracetamol 500 mg combination tablets.

TRANS-RECTAL ULTRASOUND PROSTATE BIOPSY (TRUS BIOPSY)

Key presentation/clinical features

This is performed in the office under ultrasound control or as a day-only procedure. The needle is passed trans-rectally and hence is prone to bacterial seeding and sepsis, which may be life-threatening.

Complications

- Sepsis: patients with any fever (temperature $> 37.5°C$) must be admitted for intravenous ampicillin and gentamicin (or ciprofloxacin if allergic to penicillin). Take blood and urine cultures and initiate resuscitation, and refer to ICU if there are signs of hypotension or anuria.

- Haematuria: only requires treatment if it precipitates retention or is massive. Use a 22 Fr three-way irrigation catheter.
- Retention: usually due to preexisting prostatism. Pass a small (14 Fr or 12 Fr) Foley catheter. If this is not possible, use a small suprapubic stab catheter (12 Fr).
- Rectal bleeding can also occur within the first 72 hours, and only requires intervention if massive brisk bleeding is encountered.[4]

PLACEMENT OF INDWELLING URETERIC STENTS
Key presentation/clinical features
Indwelling ureteric stents are placed by cystoscopic guidance to re-establish and maintain ureteric patency following ureteric obstruction secondary to tumour, fibrosis or nephrolithiasis.[5]

Complications
- Haematuria: microscopic haematuria commonly occurs secondary to irritation of bladder mucosa. Macroscopic haematuria can occur, and does not require intervention unless massive or precipitates retention.[6]
- Urinary tract infection (UTI): as a foreign body, indwelling ureteric stents colonise bacteria within two weeks of placement. Diabetes and chronic renal impairment increases the risk of UTI. A short course of antibiotics can reduce stent colonisation, however early stent removal is the most important factor in reducing risk of UTI.[7]
- Stent migration: Occurs in 4% of patients most commonly due to inadequate stent length. Flank pain or UTI occur. Abdominal X-ray shows an inadequate proximal or distal ureteric coil. Urological consultation required.[6]

Epididymo-orchitis
KEY PRESENTATION/CLINICAL FEATURES
- Commonest cause of scrotal pain.
- Commonest in 19- to 35-year-olds:
  - < 35 years: usually gonorrhoea or chlamydia; in men who have sex with other men, may be *Haemophilus*, coliforms
  - > 35 years: obstructive cause (urethral or prostate); infected urine extension via vas deferens to epididymis; coliforms from urinary tract infections (UTIs)

— but do not use age as only discriminator; > 35 years can be sexually transmitted infection (STI).

- Other causes are *Pseudomonas aeruginosa*, *Mycobacterium tuberculosis*, viral mumps, cryptococcal causes, amiodarone.
- There can be sudden pain, swelling to the epididymis/testis of < 6 weeks' duration; associated urethritis.
- Tender epididymis and/or testis.

DIFFERENTIAL DIAGNOSIS
- Testicular torsion
- Undisclosed trauma
- Fournier's gangrene
- Strangulated inguinal hernia

INVESTIGATIONS
Bedside
Urinalysis.

Pathology
- MSU
- Urine chlamydia and gonorrhoea PCR
- Urethral swab: white cell count (WCC) > 5/mm³ indicates urethritis.

Imaging
- Colour Doppler ultrasound: reveals epididymal involvement, characteristic features; to assess flow into testicle.

MANAGEMENT
Supportive
- Bed rest
- Scrotal support

Specific
- Antibiotics IV (see local therapeutic antibiotic guidelines)
  — For suspected STI:
    ○ ceftriaxone 500 mg IV or with 2 mL of 1% lignocaine IM injection for 3 days
      PLUS

- ◦ azithromycin 1 g PO as single dose
  PLUS
- ◦ a further single dose of azithromycin 1 g PO in 1 week
  OR
- ◦ doxycycline 100 mg 12-hourly for 14 days
— For suspected non-STI:
- ◦ trimethoprim 300 mg daily for 14 days
  OR
- ◦ cephalexin 500 mg 12-hourly for 14 days
  OR
- ◦ amoxycillin + clavulanate 500 mg + 125 mg 12-hourly
  for 14 days
— If unwell (whether STI or non-STI suspected):
- ◦ gentamicin 4–6 mg/kg as single dose, then determine a
  maximum of 1–2 further doses based on renal function
  (see Antibiotic Guidelines 2017 for further details;
  www.ciap.health.nsw.gov.au/home.html)
  PLUS
- ◦ ampicillin or amoxycillin 2 g 6-hourly
  OR
- ◦ if patient is penicillin-hypersensitive, gentamicin alone
  is usually adequate
- ◦ if gentamicin is contraindicated, ceftriaxone as single
  agent 1 g once daily or cefotaxime 1 g 8-hourly
- • Discuss with urology if follow-up is needed, otherwise
  discharge with GP follow-up

COMPLICATIONS
- • Abscess formation
- • Testicular infarction
- • Chronic pain and infertility

Fournier's gangrene
KEY PRESENTATION/CLINICAL FEATURES
- • Necrotising fasciitis of scrotum, penis or vulva, usually from
  peri-anal infection or UTI extending from peri-urethral glands.
- • Mixed aerobic/anaerobic microorganisms (anaerobic
  Streptococcus, Gram-negative rods, anaerobes, *Bacteroides
  fragilis*, *Escherichia coli*).

- Can progress very rapidly and dramatically, with a mortality of 22–40%.[8]

HISTORY

- Risk: much more common in men; diabetes; obesity; immunocompromised individuals; alcohol abuse; chronic steroid use
- Severe pain sometimes out of proportion to clinical findings

EXAMINATION

- Patient is febrile, unwell, confused, signs of septic shock; can begin from anterior abdominal wall
- Haemorrhagic, discoloured, necrotic, indurated, bulla formation in scrotal or perineal region
- Crepitus

INVESTIGATIONS

Bedside

Venous blood gas to assess lactate in septic patient (lactate > 4 mmol/L is associated with higher mortality).

Pathology

- FBC, EUC, glucose
- Blood cultures
- Wound swab if relevant.

Imaging

- Should not delay urgent surgery if diagnosis is very likely.
- CT can reveal air in fascial planes or deep-tissue involvement.

Management

- The first priority is urgent surgical/urological referral, as debridement is the specific management.
- Sepsis resuscitation:
  — early antibiotics within 1 hour of presentation: meropenem 1 g 8-hourly IV + clindamycin 600 mg 8-hourly IV + vancomycin 30 mg/kg loading dose

followed by 1.5 g 12-hourly (dose adjust in renal impairment) IV (see Antibiotic Guidelines 2017, www. ciap.health.nsw.gov.au/home.html).
— IV volume resuscitation with normal saline—can start with 10–20 mL/kg, then reassess.
— as a guideline, aim of sepsis management is mean arterial pressure (MAP) > 65 mmHg, urinary output > 0.5 mL/kg/h, no confusion, lactate clearance.
— intubation for obtunded patient or inadequately ventilating patient
— inotropes (noradrenaline, starting at 0.05 microg/kg/min) after adequate volume challenge (at least 2000 mL) and ensure ongoing volume resuscitation occurs concurrently.
- Supportive care:
— narcotic analgesia required
— glucose control if hyperglycaemic in a diabetic patient (use half the recommended insulin dose in patients not usually on insulin (e.g. < 0.5 U to 0.5 U/kg/h).
- Hyperbaric oxygen therapy could be considered by the surgeons, if available, *after* surgical debridement.
- Intravenous immunoglobulin controversial.[8]

COMPLICATIONS
Septic shock; multi-organ dysfunction.

Hydrocele
KEY PRESENTATION/CLINICAL FEATURES
- Fluid collection between the visceral and peritoneal layers of tunica vaginalis of the scrotum or along the spermatic cord.
- Causes are:
— idiopathic—commonest
— reactive collection secondary to infection; trauma; neoplasia (any inflammatory condition of the scrotum or its contents).
- Fluid trans-illuminates with torch and is usually painless.
- May be asymptomatic or have symptoms related to secondary cause.

INVESTIGATIONS
Depend on whether secondary cause is thought likely.

Imaging
Depends on suspected cause: scrotal ultrasound to confirm diagnosis or look for secondary causes.

MANAGEMENT
+ Depends on cause.
+ Indications to consider intervention for hydroceles include:
  — inability to distinguish from indirect inguinal hernia
  — failure of resolution after reasonable period of observation
  — unable to assess testis reliably
  — hydroceles secondary to disease (infection, tumour)
  — patient preference.

Paraphimosis
KEY PRESENTATION/CLINICAL FEATURES
+ Inability to retract the pulled-back foreskin over the head of the penis in uncircumcised males, producing oedema and venous obstruction.
+ May occur in elderly uncircumcised males who have the foreskin pulled back for catheterisation and it is then not retracted afterwards.
+ Cannot occur in circumcised males.

INVESTIGATIONS
None are usually required.

MANAGEMENT
+ Consider the need for procedural sedation before attempting retraction (dorsal penile nerve block using lignocaine *without adrenaline* is an alternative; inject around base of penis).
+ Apply ice packs for > 5 minutes or alternatively grasp the distal penis with a gloved hand, and squeeze circumferentially for several minutes until swelling has improved. Then use lignocaine gel lubricant and gentle *continuous* traction

(over minutes if needed), holding the shaft of the penis and slowly retracting the foreskin.

- If unsuccessful, involve urology for surgical correction.

COMPLICATIONS
- Venous obstruction leading to compromised arterial flow, infarction and necrosis.
- Urethral obstruction secondary to swelling.

Phimosis
KEY PRESENTATION/CLINICAL FEATURES
- Inability to pull the foreskin back from the head of penis; can produce secondary ballooning of foreskin, urine retention, balanitis
- Congenital or acquired (from recurrent balanitis and adhesions)

MANAGEMENT
- Congenital phimosis usually resolves with age.
- Urological consultation should be sought to discuss management options for acquired cases: non-operative (e.g. topical corticosteroids and stretching exercises) versus operative (e.g. circumcision for acquired cases).

Priapism
- Low flow/veno-occlusive (commonest): painful, reduced venous outflow can lead to ischaemia, thrombosis from venous stasis; late erectile dysfunction occurs.
- High flow/arterial (rare): arterial laceration (can be trauma from direct injection), leading to uncontrolled inflow of arterial blood; long-term erectile dysfunction is unlikely.

KEY PRESENTATION/CLINICAL FEATURES
Causes
- Toxicological:
  — cavernosus injection (prostaglandin E_1 or papaverine)
  — psychotropics—phenothiazines (e.g. chlorpromazine), butyrophenones (e.g. haloperidol); selective serotonin reuptake inhibitors (SSRIs)

— rarely, sildenafil (Viagra), tadalafil (Cialis), vardenafil (Levitra); cocaine; anticoagulants; tetrahydrocannabinol (THC)
- Haematological: sickle-cell anaemia (in children too), leukaemia, myeloma, polycythaemia
- Spinal trauma
- Idiopathic
- Trauma causing arterial laceration (high-flow)

HISTORY
- Low-flow priapism is painful.
- High-flow priapism is painless, with associated trauma.

EXAMINATION
- Look for trauma.
- Urine retention.
- Ask about penile implants.
- Low-flow form will usually have a soft glans; high-flow form will have an engorged glans.

INVESTIGATIONS
Bedside
Consider intracavernous blood gas if unsure if low- or high-flow form (low-flow pH < 7.25)—involve urologist first.

Pathology
Consider investigating possible underlying causes such as haematological malignancy or sickle-cell anaemia.

Imaging
Duplex ultrasound for high-flow; look for arterial laceration, then angiography can be used to embolise.

MANAGEMENT
Urgent involvement of urology.

Pharmacological
(Urologist should perform or supervise.)

Intracavernosal injection of phenylephrine 1 mL of 500 microg/mL every 5 minutes until resolution

Needle aspiration
(Urologist should perform or supervise.)
- Aseptic technique
- Consider procedural sedation
- Local anaesthesia technique:
  — direct infiltration
  — penile nerve block (inject around base of penis; never use adrenaline-containing solutions).
- Insert 23-gauge butterfly needle laterally at 2 or 10 o'clock and at a 45° angle to the skin (not perpendicular to the skin, to avoid damage to the urethra and dorsal neurovascular bundle). Aspirate slowly (often ~30 mL aspirated); only one side needs to be aspirated, as shunts connect both sides.
- If retumescent, consider intracavernosal injection of phenylephrine 1 mL of 500 microg/mL every 5 minutes until resolution or up to 1 hour, after discussion with a urologist. This procedure must be performed in an environment with continuous cardiac and blood pressure monitoring, and should be avoided in patients at risk of complications if absorbed systemically.

COMPLICATIONS
- Penile ischaemia/necrosis
- Long-term erectile dysfunction

Prostate disease
PROSTATITIS
Clinical features
- Causes: *E. coli* is commonest; consider sexually transmitted infections (e.g. chlamydia trachomatis) in younger males
- Increased urine frequency; urine retention; perineal or low back pain
- Fever; very tender, enlarged prostate

Investigations
- Urinalysis

- MSU (pyuria, bacteriuria, PCR for chlamydia)
- FBC, EUC; blood cultures if septic and unwell
- CT of pelvis with IV contrast can have characteristic findings.

Management
- Antibiotics as for UTI (see section on management of UTIs later in this chapter)
- Analgesia

Complications
- Bacteraemia, epididymitis, chronic bacterial prostatitis, prostatic abscess and metastatic infection (seeding to vertebral discs or sacroiliac joints)

BENIGN PROSTATE HYPERTROPHY
Clinical features
- Prostatism: difficulty initiating urine stream, poor urine stream, inadequate emptying, post-void dribbling, nocturia.
- Very enlarged bladders can develop when there is a chronic degree of urine retention with bladder-wall stretching.
- Usually presents to the ED with urine retention or UTI.

Investigations
- Urinalysis +/−MSU
- EUC, consider prostate-specific antigen (PSA; can be elevated in prostatitis), digital examination

Management
- (For acute retention, see the section on urine retention later in this chapter.)
- Urologist follow-up is required.
- Medical treatment includes alpha-1 adrenergic antagonists and 5 alpha reductase inhibitors, which have proven to be effective in meta-analyses.[9]

Complications
- Chronic urine retention causing hypertrophied enlarged bladder and renal impairment.

- If patient presents post-trans-urethral resection of prostate (post-TURP), issues include:
  — bleeding
  — infection
  — post-TURP syndrome: hyponatraemia with confusion
  — impotence
  — retrograde ejaculation.

PROSTATE CANCER

- Adenocarcinoma in > 95% of cases; peripheral gland involvement in 70%.
- Metastases: osteoblastic (not lytic) to the lumbosacral area, pelvis, spinal cord, ribs, thoracic spine, brain.
- Consider cord compression in these patients if they present with gait instability, urine retention, constipation or lower-limb weakness.

Renal/ureteric calculus
KEY PRESENTATION/CLINICAL FEATURES

- Typically occurs between 20 and 50 years of age, though can also occur in children; it is commoner in men (~3:1).
- Risk factors are dehydration, family history, inflammatory bowel disease, diseases associated with hypercalcaemia or hyperuricaemia, myeloproliferative disorders.

HISTORY

- Sudden, severe flank pain radiating to the groin or testis with nausea, vomiting.
- Patient is restless, unable to keep still and prefers to stand.
- Lower ureteric stones can present with ill-defined lower pain and an extreme desire to pass urine when the bladder is empty; that is, may present with retention but without urine in bladder.

EXAMINATION

- Pallor, fever if infection present.
- Patient can be tachycardic, hypertensive from pain.
- There is usually a lack of abdominal tenderness; if found to be peritonitic on examination, look for differential diagnoses.

DIFFERENTIAL DIAGNOSIS

- Ruptured abdominal aortic aneurysm (AAA): around 40% can present with haematuria; suspect if it is a first presentation of flank pain in an older patient (> 60 years).
- AAA below the age of 50 is very uncommon.
- Pyelonephritis, testicular torsion, ovarian torsion.
- Gastrointestinal causes: diverticulitis, retrocaecal appendix, pancreatitis, bowel obstruction.
- Herpes zoster in L1 nerve root.
- Musculoskeletal cause: radicular back pain from disc prolapse.
- Opioid-seeking patient.

INVESTIGATIONS

Bedside

- Urinalysis: 90% of cases have micro- or macroscopic haematuria—meaning that 10% have *negative* urinalysis results.
- In AAA, ultrasound study by accredited staff.

Pathology

- MSU
- FBC
- EUC, liver function tests (LFTs), lipase, beta-hCG
- Consider calcium and uric acid levels if there is recurrent calculus.

Imaging

- Stones are 90% radio-opaque (uric acid stones are radiolucent).
- CT of kidneys–ureters–bladder (KUB): sensitivity 97%, specificity 96%; reveals other diagnoses (e.g. AAA, appendicitis, diverticulitis), size and position of calculus, complications of calculus, and identifies presence of dual collecting system.
- Plain KUB: sensitivity about 58–62%. The ureter runs across the tips of the transverse processes of L2–L5, the upper and lower sacroiliac joint and next to the ischial spine; the ureteric orifice is medial, near the coccyx.
- Intravenous pyelogram (IVP): sensitivity approximately 96%; can reveal size and assess for renal function; use if CT KUB is not available.

- Renal ultrasound: sensitivity approximately 70%, but operator-dependent; stone size cannot be estimated.
- MRI: no radiation, therefore possible use in pregnant patients. (Note that the effects of magnetic exposure on the fetus in the first trimester are not known; a risk/benefit discussion with the radiologist and the patient is advised.) There may be a lack of availability; MRI can miss small stones and is an expensive technique.

MANAGEMENT
Supportive
- Analgesia with combination opioids and NSAIDs:
  — opioids—faster-acting initial analgesia (e.g. morphine 2.5–5 mg); titrate to response; do not use pethidine
  — indomethacin 100 mg 12-hourly PR (check for contraindications).
- Intravenous fluids if the patient is dehydrated or septic; note that there is no credible supporting evidence for the use of greater-than-maintenance IV fluids to assist stone passage.
- A Cochrane Systematic Review in 2014 showed medical expulsion therapy (alpha$_1$-blockers; e.g. tamsulosin) increases stone passage and decreases time to expulsion, in patients with distal stones which are < 10 mm in diameter.[10]

Editorial Comment
Recently, the use of alpha blockers has become more controversial.

Specific
- Stone size and likelihood of being passed within 1 month:
  — < 5 mm will pass itself in 90% of cases
  — 4–6 mm, > 50% will pass
  — > 7 mm, 5% will pass.
- Stone location:
  — proximal ureter, 25% will pass
  — mid-ureter, 45% will pass
  — distal ureter, 70% will pass.

- Interventions include:
  - percutaneous radiological nephrostomy: drains obstructed kidney
  - ureteroscopic removal/stent
  - open surgery for large stones
  - extracorporeal shockwave lithotripsy (ESWL).
- Renal calculi:
  - if < 2 cm can be treated with ESWL; larger renal calculi are best managed with percutaneous nephrolithotomy.
- Ureteric calculi:
  - if in upper half of ureter, can be pushed back into kidney for ESWL
  - if in lower half of ureter, can be removed with ureteroscope.
- Advise admission if:
  - patient is septic (or has fever with temperatures > 37.5°C)
  - there is impaired renal function (creatinine > 0.2 mmol/L)
  - there is persisting pain
  - stone is > 5 mm
  - patient has a single kidney
  - there is extravasation of contrast from renal pelvis on imaging (rare); this indicates ruptured renal pelvis from high-grade obstruction; can mimic an 'acute abdomen' from other causes.
- Advise discharge if:
  - patient is pain-free and stone is < 5 mm
  - none of the above criteria for admission are present
  - can get patient to strain urine with fine sieve to see if stone is passed.
- Arrange follow-up with urologist—liaise locally regarding type of repeat imaging: either plain KUB or repeat CT KUB to ensure passage of stone.

COMPLICATIONS
- Obstructed kidney (can be painless): this is an emergency requiring urgent intervention
- Ruptured renal pelvis from obstruction mimics 'true acute abdomen'

- Urosepsis
- Renal impairment
- Bleeding

Testicular torsion

KEY PRESENTATION/CLINICAL FEATURES

- Peak incidence is in newborns and in puberty or a young teenager; 75% occur under the age of 20 years and it is rare after age 30—but can occur at any age, as the anatomical abnormality (enlarged tunica vaginalis preventing testicular anchoring—'bell-clapper deformity') that predisposes is present from birth.
- Presents with lymphatic and venous obstruction followed by arterial occlusion.
- Complete torsion is a 360° turn or greater; the more turns, the shorter the time to ischaemia.

HISTORY

- Sudden severe lower abdominal or scrotal pain in a previously well patient; often nausea, vomiting present.
- Some patients report previous short-lived (< 2 hours) episodes of the same type of pain.
- Can present without sudden onset of pain.

EXAMINATION

- Fever can occur uncommonly.
- Always assess testes in paediatric patients with abdominal pain or a distressed, crying infant.
- Look for a high-riding, abnormally lying, swollen, exquisitely tender testis (only with 360° torsion) with scrotal swelling.
- The presence of cremasteric reflex and symptom relief with scrotal elevation, are *unreliable signs* in excluding torsion.
- There may be minimal findings if torsion is $< 360°$.

DIFFERENTIAL DIAGNOSIS

- Epididymo-orchitis
- Torsion of testicular appendage

- Strangulated hernia
- Haematocele/hydrocele
- Henoch–Schönlein purpura (vasculitis)
- Idiopathic scrotal oedema

INVESTIGATIONS
Surgical exploration when torsion is the most likely diagnosis.

Bedside
Urinalysis.

Imaging
Colour Doppler ultrasound.
- Compare blood flow with that on 'normal' side; if reduced, suspect torsion. An untwisted testis can have hyperaemia.
- Sensitivity is quoted to be as low as 82% up to 88.9% sensitive and 98.8% specific; the technique is operator-dependent. Note that *normal flow does not exclude torsion and should only be considered in equivocal cases, after consultation with urology.*

MANAGEMENT
- Surgical exploration: if testis is viable, then orchidopexy should be performed; the other testicle should be fixed as well.
- If urological services are unavailable within a reasonable timeframe (< 6 hours), then perform manual untwisting (turn right testicle clockwise, left testicle anticlockwise) under procedural sedation. If successful, patient will have reduced or no pain. All patients still need urological assessment at the time of presentation.

COMPLICATIONS
The salvage rate depends on the number of turns and the time to surgery.
- Salvage rate is 100% if surgery is < 4 hours from onset; 80–90% if within 6 hours; 20–50% at 10–24 hours.
- Despite salvage, long-term damage such as reduced volume, sperm and motility can occur.

TORSION OF TESTICULAR APPENDAGE

- Peak incidence 10–13 years of age; a common cause of scrotal pain at age 3–13 years (tort more often than testes in this age group).
- An embryological peduncle < 5 mm with no function can twist.
- The 'blue dot sign' is a tender blue spot on scrotum viewed with trans-illumination, and considered pathognomonic.

Urinary tract infections (UTIs)

Include: asymptomatic bacteriuria, urethritis, cystitis, pyelonephritis.

CAUSES

- More than 90% of cases are caused by Enterobacteriaceae (e.g. *E. coli*) and *Enterococcus faecalis* (previously classified as *Streptococcus faecalis*).
- *Staphylococcus saprophyticus* (skin-commensal) is a cause of simple cystitis in young sexually active females.
- Consider non *E. coli* infection post-instrumentation or after prolonged recent hospital admission.

Risk factors

- Frequent sexual intercourse
- Previous UTI
- Pregnancy
- Foreign body in urinary tract (e.g. calculus, catheter)
- Diabetes mellitus
- Anatomical/functional urinary abnormality
- Immunosuppressive state (e.g. HIV, transplantation, chemotherapy, corticosteroid use)

KEY PRESENTATION/CLINICAL FEATURES

Urethritis

History
Dysuria.

Examination
Urethral discharge.

Cystitis
History
- Dysuria, increased urine frequency
- Suprapubic pain

Examination
- Patient should look well.
- There may be suprapubic tenderness.
- Obviously blood-stained urine can be present.

Pyelonephritis
History
- Dysuria, increased urine frequency; sometimes lack of urinary symptoms
- Flank or lower back pain
- Nausea/vomiting

Examination
- Fever; assess whether patient looks well or unwell.
- Assess for features of systemic inflammatory response; temperature $< 36°C$ or $> 38°C$ respiratory rate > 20/min; heart rate > 90 bpm or $pCO_2 < 30$ mmHg; WCC < 4 or $> 12 \times 10^9$/L.
- Hypotension or relative hypotension in elderly patient (e.g. BP < 110 mmHg in 80-year-old).
- Symptomatic light-headedness on standing indicates a need for ongoing admission.
- Flank tenderness or abdominal tenderness.

DIFFERENTIAL DIAGNOSIS
Pyuria
Previous recent antibiotics; renal calculi; non-specific urethritis in males; renal tract neoplasm; catheter; prostatitis; renal tuberculosis (TB).

Urethritis
Urethral trauma.

Cystitis
Vulvovaginitis.

Pyelonephritis

- Renal: calculus
- Gastrointestinal tract: appendicitis, diverticulitis, acute abdomen of any cause
- Gynaecological: ectopic, ovarian cyst rupture, endometriosis
- Vascular: AAA rupture
- Musculoskeletal: radicular pain

INVESTIGATIONS

Regarding nitrites on urinalysis:

- only coliform bacteria reduce urinary nitrate to nitrite (*Enterococcus* spp. and *S. saprophyticus* do not)
- overall there can be a high false-negative rate (i.e. patient has UTI but no nitrites on urinalysis).

Urethritis

Bedside

Urinalysis.

Pathology

- Swab for STI culture
- MSU and chlamydia/gonorrhoea PCR

Cystitis

Bedside

- Urinalysis:
  - leucocyte esterase test for WCC: reported 48–86% sensitive, 17–93% specific
  - positive predictive value in symptomatic patients is 50%; negative predictive value is 92% (is a reasonable screening test if negative; however, in elderly individuals do not rely on it if UTI is considered a possible diagnosis).
  - if nitrites are positive, sensitivity for urinalysis increases.

Pathology

MSU:

- Significant bacteriuria is $> 10^5$ bacteria/mL (colony-forming units/mL); this indicates infection rather than contamination.

- Asymptomatic bacteriuria is the above amount grown, but no symptoms in patient.
- Symptomatic patient with bacterial count $> 10^5$ has a very high probability of infection.
- Asymptomatic patient with bacterial count $> 10^5$ and pregnant should be treated.
- Asymptomatic geriatric patient with significant bacteriuria is common in functionally impaired elderly people and should not be treated.
- Bacteriuria and pyuria in catheterised patients is common and is usually asymptomatic; however, symptomatic patients (e.g. haematuria, fever, rigors, flank or pelvic pain) require treatment. Ideally the catheter should be removed permanently (to improve antibiotic effectiveness, as superinfection with resistant organisms can occur when left in situ) or be replaced if it has been in situ > 2 weeks. Following insertion of the new catheter, urine should be collected for culture and sensitivity. Empiric antibiotics should be commenced while awaiting sensitivities, and duration of treatment is 7 days (14 days if delayed response) (see the Cystitis section later in this chapter for options). In the case where the catheter cannot be replaced, urine should be collected from the side port of the drainage system to reduce contamination, and empiric antibiotics started.

Editorial Comment

Unnecessary urinary catheterisations and hospital-acquired urinary infections must be very much avoided.

Pyelonephritis
Bedside
Urinalysis.

Pathology
- MSU
- FBC, EUC, beta-hCG in women $+/-$ LFTs; $+/-$ lipase
- Blood cultures

Imaging

- Consider if calculus or obstruction is suspected.
- In ongoing fevers despite appropriate antibiotics.
- Renal ultrasound can be performed as an outpatient in stable patients with a very likely diagnosis; assesses for abscess, hydronephrosis, anatomical abnormalities.
- CT KUB if calculus is suspected.

MANAGEMENT

Urethritis

Fully treat if STI is suspected.

Cystitis

- Antibiotics
  - send urine for culture, but no need for any pathology or imaging in these patients
  - no need for consideration of IV antibiotics.
- Non-pregnant females:
  - trimethoprim 300 mg daily for 3 days
    OR
  - cephalexin 500 mg 12-hourly for 5 days
    OR
  - nitrofurantoin 100 mg 12-hourly for 5 days
    OR
  - amoxycillin + clavulanate 500 mg + 125 mg 12-hourly for 5 days.
- Pregnant females (doses as above):
  - cephalexin (class A)
    OR
  - nitrofurantoin (class A)
    OR
  - amoxycillin + clavulanate (class B1).
- Males:
  - trimethoprim 300 mg daily for 14 days
    OR
  - cephalexin 500 mg 12-hourly for 14 days
    OR
  - amoxycillin + clavulanate 500 mg + 125 mg 12-hourly for 14 days.

Pyelonephritis

Supportive care

♦ If patient is unwell or has features of sepsis, commence sepsis package:
  — early empiric antibiotics within 1 hour, after collection of blood cultures
  — if severe sepsis, use 10–20 mL/kg normal saline (consider maximum 2000–3000 mL)
  — consider inotropes (noradrenaline 0.05 microg/kg/min) for hypotension refractory to IV fluid resuscitation (aim for MAP > 65 mmHg, lactate clearance, urine output > 0.5 mL/kg/h), and ensure ongoing volume resuscitation occurs concurrently (Surviving Sepsis Guidelines, 2016).

♦ Analgesia (paracetamol, NSAIDs, PRN opioids IV/PO).

Specific antibiotics

♦ If pyelonephritis mild with low-grade fever and no vomiting:
  — amoxycillin + clavulanate 875 mg + 125 mg 12-hourly for 10 days
    OR
  — cephalexin 500 mg 6-hourly for 10 days
    OR
  — trimethoprim 300 mg nocte for 10 days.

♦ If resistant to above or *Pseudomonas aeruginosa* is the cause:
  — norfloxacin 400 mg 12-hourly for 10 days
    OR
  — ciprofloxacin 500 mg 12-hourly for 10 days.

♦ If severe, use:
  — gentamicin 4–6 mg/kg for 1 dose, then determine dosing interval for maximum 1 or 2 doses based on renal function (see Antibiotic Guidelines 2017; www.ciap. health.nsw.gov.au/home.html for details of gentamicin doses)
    PLUS
  — amoxycillin or ampicillin 2 g 6-hourly IV.

♦ If patient is hypersensitive to penicillin, gentamicin alone is usually sufficient.

♦ If gentamicin is contraindicated, use as a *single* drug:
  — ceftriaxone 1 g daily IV

OR
— cefotaxime 1 g 8-hourly IV.
- The above regimens do not adequately cover for *P. aeruginosa* or enterococci.
- Change to PO administration when able; total duration of treatment should be 10–14 days, then send urine for culture 48 hours after finishing antibiotics.

Complications
- Septic shock
- Renal abscess
- Bacteraemia and seeding of other organs
- Secondary stone formation from certain bacteria: *Proteus* or *Klebsiella* (struvite/staghorn calculus)

Urine retention
KEY PRESENTATION/CLINICAL FEATURES
Causes
- Obstruction: prostatomegaly; rectal constipation; blood clot; urethral stricture; post-TURP bladder neck stenosis; recent instrumentation.
- Neurogenic: spinal injury; cauda equina syndrome (*painless* retention).
- Toxicological (in younger patients): any drug with anti-cholinergic effects (e.g. antipsychotics, tricyclic antidepressants, first generation anti-histamines); alpha-adrenergics.
- Infection: UTI.
- Painful genital condition: herpes; trauma.

HISTORY
- Look for underlying cause.
- Sudden onset, preceding urinary symptoms or worsening prostatism.

EXAMINATION
- Degree of bladder distension (can be quantified with bedside bladder scan pre and post voiding).
- Rectal examination to assess constipation, prostate size, perianal sensation, tone.

- Always perform, and document, a detailed neurological assessment to consider a neurological cause, including saddle sensation, anal tone, lower limb power and reflexes.

DIFFERENTIAL DIAGNOSIS

- Pelvic haematoma will present as a suprapubic mass and retention, but the bladder is empty and no urine will be obtained from suprapubic puncture.
- Any cause of lower abdominal peritonitis will give the impression of retention, but bladder is empty from anuria. Irrigate 50 mL in and out of an indwelling urinary catheter (IDC) to confirm correct IDC position and emptiness of bladder.
- Lower abdominal mass, such as diverticular phlegmon, ruptured AAA or pelvic malignancy.

INVESTIGATIONS

Bedside

- Urinalysis for UTI.
- Bladder scanner if in doubt: normal bladder capacity is approx. 400 mL maximum; patients with a chronic degree of retention from prostate disease can have larger capacities, > 1 L.

Pathology

EUC, FBC, coagulation profile if patient is on anticoagulants.

Imaging

Urgently indicated if a neurogenic cause is being considered (MRI of spine).

MANAGEMENT

- Catheterisation options
  - IDC: try 16F then the less-flexible 18F. Consider using a coude-tip catheter in patients who are predicted to be difficult to catheterise (or use this as first choice if available). Keep a firm hold on the shaft of the penis with slight traction upwards, perpendicular to the supine patient. Always note residual volume; rapid

decompression of volume of > 1000 mL can cause bladder-wall bleeding. Also monitor for post obstructive diuresis with decompression of large bladder volumes.
— Suprapubic catheter (SPC). liaise with urology before attempting insertion; should be done under ultrasound guidance; involve senior staff.
— Only urology specialists should ever attempt introducer-based catheterisation.
• Patients can usually be considered for discharge with a leg bag and education with referral to a urologist/urology trial of void clinic.
— Regarding trial of void (TOV)
  ○ measure pre- and post-void residual volumes, which should be < 150 mL.
• Clot-based retention
— Patients report frank haematuria and passage of clots, usually in the context of prostate/bladder cancer or recent urological procedure.
— Always assess if patient is on anticoagulation and assess the risk/benefit of reversing it if needed; consult appropriately.
— Consult with urology.
— Catheterisation should occur with a 3-way catheter (larger-diameter, stiffer catheters with a 60 mL balloon) placed using the same technique as for a normal IDC—avoid overly aggressive attempts. Following insertion, manually irrigate bladder with 60 mL syringe and normal saline, until urine becomes clearer, in order to dissolve clots, then connect to continuous irrigation to help wash out clots. Consult urology or urology ward about protocol for bladder irrigation.
• Investigate/manage any underlying condition.

COMPLICATIONS
• Transient loss of bladder tone occurs after significant retention; this can take 1–3 days to normalise, therefore the catheter should be left in for at least that long before TOV if patient has acute retention; in patients who have acute on chronic retention, the IDC should be left in situ until urology follow-up.
• Renal impairment.

- UTI.
- Post-obstructive polyuria:
  — occurs in patients who present with acute on chronic retention
  — requires admission under urology
  — give IV fluids as per urology, but as a guide the IV fluid rate needs to match the prior hour's urine output plus maintenance if nil by mouth (NBM)
  — EUC needs to be closely monitored.

Urological trauma
KIDNEY
Key presentation/clinical features

- The kidney is the commonest genitourinary organ injured (80% blunt and < 15% penetrating).
- Markers for significant injury include:
  — hypotension (systolic blood pressure < 90 mmHg)
  — flank bruising, pain or tenderness
  — posterior rib or spine fractures
  — macroscopic haematuria.

Differential diagnosis
For haematuria in trauma: lower urinary tract trauma (ureter, bladder, urethra).

Investigations
Bedside
Urinalysis
- If microscopic haematuria:
  — perform urgent imaging if there is:
    ◦ hypotension at any time from trauma
    ◦ suggestive injury (fall from > 3 m, flank bruising, direct blow, injury from deceleration > 60 km/h)
    ◦ suggestive associated injury (fractured lumbar vertebrae; fractured lower ribs)
  — in blunt trauma with low suspicion of urological trauma, there is no need for imaging but urinalysis should be repeated in 1–2 weeks to check for resolution; if there is ongoing haematuria, then consider CT KUB with IV contrast

to assess for non-traumatic, preexisting renal disease
— in penetrating trauma, always perform imaging.
• If macroscopic haematuria:
  — always investigate
  — can be from any part of urinary tract.

Pathology
• FBC, EUC, coagulation studies, venous blood gas analysis (VBG)
• Blood group and hold

Imaging
• IV-contrast-enhanced CT KUB: assess the contralateral functioning kidney; delayed or absent function in affected kidney; contrast extravasation.
• IVP if CT is not available: assess contralateral kidney function and possible ureteric involvement.
• MRI: use if available in those with contrast allergy; results are as good as CT.
• A negative ultrasound does not exclude renal injury.

Management
Supportive care
• Trauma assessment to look for other injury
• Trauma resuscitation if required
• Analgesia
• Tetanus if a penetrating injury

Specific care
• Conservative
  — for stable patients with functioning kidney and minor extravasation.
• Surgical exploration acutely if:
  — unstable patient due to haemorrhage
  — major extravasation due to shattered or bisected kidney
  — renal peduncle disruption
  — continued subacute haemorrhage or ongoing transfusion requirements
  — urinoma with sepsis.

Complications
- Haemorrhagic shock
- Renal impairment
- Kidney loss

URETER
- Rare; in children trauma to the ureter can occur from deceleration injury
- Usually penetrating and associated with more severe injuries
- Diagnosed on IV-contrast-enhanced CT KUB
- Usually diagnosed at laparotomy for other injuries

BLADDER
Key presentation/clinical features
- The majority of bladder injuries are associated with pelvic fracture; about 10% of pelvic fractures occur with bladder injury.
- Occasionally a stab wound or seat belt injury will rupture a full bladder.
- Most injuries are to the dome; blunt injuries can result in large lacerations.
- Suspect based on mechanism and associated injuries (e.g. displaced pelvic fractures).
- The patient may have difficulty voiding.
- Suprapubic bruising, tenderness, peritonism.
- Haematuria.

Differential diagnosis
Frank haematuria from kidney or ureter or urethra.

Investigations
Bedside
Urinalysis: macroscopic haematuria in the majority of cases.

Pathology
- EUC, FBC, coagulation studies, VBG
- Blood group and hold

Imaging

- Retrograde cystogram: 350 mL of water-soluble contrast introduced into the bladder, then look for extravasation (indicates rupture), both during administration and after drainage.
- CT cystography: assess surrounding structures.
- Perform IV-contrast-enhanced CT KUB to assess the upper urinary tract.

Management

- Manage all aspects of the trauma patient—prioritise injuries and need for intervention.
- If no blood at meatus: gently pass a 16F or 18F catheter (IDC is preferred over SPC).
- If blood at meatus, a urethrogram must be performed first before catheterisation.
- Minor extraperitoneal rupture may be managed with catheter drainage alone.
- Bladder body injury can be managed with prolonged use of an IDC.
- Major extraperitoneal rupture, all intraperitoneal rupture and dome injuries must be explored and repaired.

URETHRAL TRAUMA
Key presentation

- Consider blunt (fall astride) injury or penetrating injury.
- Is more common than bladder trauma.
- The risk in males with anterior pelvic fractures including pubic symphysis diastasis increases with the number of pubic rami fractured and the degree of displacement (especially displaced superior pubic ramus fracture), and also if there is sacroiliac involvement with the pubic ramus fracture.
- In females, usually occurs only with major pubic symphysis diastasis; often with associated vaginal bleeding.
- No displaced pelvic ring fracture makes urethral injury very unlikely in the absence of direct trauma.

Clinical features

- Urine retention; frank haematuria; blood at urethral meatus; scrotal/penile 'butterfly bruising'; palpable penile fracture; high-riding prostate on rectal examination.
- Some patients have no initial physical signs, then blood at meatus.

Investigations

Retrograde urethrogram to assess for complete tear.

Management

- If there is high clinical suspicion, displaced anterior pelvic fractures on X-ray or frank haematuria—consult urology urgently, and do not pass an IDC.
- For minor/incomplete injury: IDC is carefully placed under radiological control.
- For major injury: SPC and urethroplasty/re-anastomosis to repair.
- Penetrating urethral trauma is very unlikely if all the following are present: no meatal blood; normal urination or easy catheter insertion; normal urinalysis.

Complications

- Urine retention
- Strictures
- Haemorrhage

SCROTUM/TESTIS

Key presentation/clinical features

- In paediatric patients, consider non-accidental injury.
- Intratesticular bleeding can lead to intra-capsular pressure rise and subsequent necrosis.

History

- Mechanism
- Pain

Examination

- Exclude other, more significant associated trauma

- Scrotal bruising and swelling
- Assess for testicle size, tenderness, lie
- Consider penile, bladder or pelvis trauma depending on mechanism

Injury patterns
- Scrotal wall haematoma
- Tunica vaginalis haematoma (haematocele)
- Intratesticular haematoma (or subcapsular)
- Testicular rupture

Investigations
Bedside
Urinalysis.

Imaging
Colour Doppler ultrasound: assess degree of injury. This technique can underestimate; a normal ultrasound does not rule out the need for exploration.

Management
- Supportive (ice bags, analgesia).
- Surgical exploration indications:
  — if uncertain about the degree of trauma after clinical and ultrasound examination
  — for testicular injury/rupture/haematoma
  — if tunica albuginea disrupted
  — for large haematocele
  — for penetrating trauma.

Complications
Risk of orchidectomy with conservative management for significant injury.

PENIS
Key presentation/clinical features
- Amputation often self-inflicted or patient was psychotic at the time.

- Fractured penis is traumatic rupture of the corpus cavernosum: the patient hears a loud 'snap' like the breaking of a glass rod, associated with direct injury to the erect penis; it collapses immediately and develops a large swelling on the affected side. Rarely the urethra ruptures as well.

Investigations

Bedside

ECG and venous blood gas if toxicological features are associated.

Pathology

- FBC, blood group and hold if there is significant blood loss
- Psychiatric- or toxicology-based pathology if indicated

Imaging

Discuss with urologist.

Management

- Stop ongoing bleeding if present.
- Look for other injury/concomitant overdose if patient has an abnormal mental state.
- Wrap severed penis if recovered in sterile saline-soaked gauze, place in sterile bag and then put on ice.
- Urgent urology referral +/− psychiatric referral is required.
- Suspected fractured penis should be referred urgently to urology for urgent repair.

Complications

- After reattachment: stricture, urethral fistula, skin loss, impotence.
- After fractured penis: if no repair, 50% have impotence and traumatic curvature of the penis.

Varicocele
KEY PRESENTATION/CLINICAL FEATURES

- Dilation of the pampiniform plexus of the spermatic cord veins; commoner on left than on right; occurs predominantly in post pubertal males.

- If isolated right-sided varicocele or painful varicocele, look for inferior vena cava obstruction.
- Can be asymptomatic or patients can experience a dull ache, particularly on standing, that is relieved with recumbency.
- There is an association with men who are infertile, and can lead to testicular atrophy.

DIFFERENTIAL DIAGNOSIS
Other scrotal conditions such as epididymitis.

INVESTIGATIONS
Imaging
Ultrasound to assist diagnosis.

MANAGEMENT
- Goals of treatment include analgesia (NSAIDs and scrotal support in older males) and referral to urologist to discuss improving testicular function and fertility (particularly in younger males).
- Surgical versus conservative management is determined on an individual basis.

References
1. Edwards SK, Bunker CB, Ziller F, et al. (2013) European guideline for the management of balanoposthitis. *International Journal of Sexually Transmitted Diseases and AIDS* 25:615.
2. Pulido-Perez A, Suarez-Fernandez R (2017). Circinate Balanitis. *New England Journal of Medicine* 376:157.
3. Pengfei S, Yutao L, Jie Y, et al. (2011) The results of ureteral stenting after ureteroscopic lithotripsy for ureteral calculi: a systematic review and meta-analysis. *Journal of Urology* 186:1904.
4. Loeb S, Vellekoop A, Ahmed HU, et al. (2013) Systematic review of complications of prostate biopsy. *European Journal of Urology* 64:876.

5. Betschart P, Zumstein V, Piller A, et al. (2017) Prevention and treatment of symptoms associated with indwelling ureteral stents: A systematic review. *International Journal of Urology* 24:250.

6. Nevo A, Mano R, Baniel J, et al. (2017) Ureteric stent dwelling time: a risk factor for post-ureteroscopy sepsis. *British Journal of Urology* 28:1385

7. Ringel A, Richter S, Shalev M, et al. (2000) Late complications of ureteral stents. *European Journal of Urology* 38:41.

8. Stevens DL, Bisno AL, Chambers HF, et al. (2014) Practice guidelines for the diagnosis and management of skin and soft tissue infections: 2014 update by the Infectious Diseases Society of America. *Clinical Infectious Diseases* 59:147.

9. Dahm P, Brasure M, MacDonald R, et al. (2017) Comparative Effectiveness of Newer Medications for Lower Urinary Tract Symptoms Attributed to Benign Prostatic Hyperplasia: A Systematic Review and Meta-analysis. *European Journal of Urology* 71:570.

10. Campschroer T, Zhu Y, Duijvesz D, et al. (2014) Alpha-blockers as medical expulsive therapy for ureteral stones. *Cochrane Database Systematic Reviews* CD008509.

Recommended readings

Flores S, Herring A. Dorsile Penile Block: Clinical Key Ultrasound-guided dorsal penile nerve block for ED paraphimosis reduction. American Journal of Emergency Medicine. 1 June 2015.

Roberts JR, Price C, Mazzeo T. Penile block: Clinical Key Intracavernous Epinephrine: A Minimally Invasive Treatment for Priapism in the Emergency Department. Journal of Emergency Medicine. 1 April 2009.

Chapter 31
Wounds

Ania Smialkowski

Wound assessment
WOUND HISTORY
- Circumstances surrounding injury
- General medical history including medications:
  - immunosuppression (immunomodulating medications, steroids, systemic diseases such as cancer, HIV etc.)
  - anticoagulation
  - smoking/tobacco use
  - malnutrition
  - diabetes, renal disease, cardiac disease, peripheral vascular disease
- History of wound-healing problems
- Chronicity
- Previous diagnostic tests or investigations
- Previous treatments

WOUND EVALUATION AND EXAMINATION
- Location
- Size
- Extent of defect
  - Is there any tissue loss?
  - Depth of wound (fat/tendon/muscle/bone visible?)
- Surrounding tissue
  - Cellulitis, inflammation, induration
  - Colour, pigmentation
  - Oedema
- Condition of wound bed
  - Odour
  - Granulation tissue
  - Slough, fibrin, pus, exudate

— Necrotic tissue or skin edges, eschar
— Foreign bodies, maggots
— Tunnelling, sinuses

Wound debridement

• Debridement involves the removal of obviously contaminated, foreign, devitalised or dead material from a wound bed.
• This can involve simple irrigation for lightly contaminated wounds.
• For heavily contaminated or devitalised wounds this requires some form of anaesthesia and extensive removal of tissue.
  — For smaller wounds can use local anaesthetic +/– procedural sedation in ED.
  — Dilution is the solution to pollution: irrigate with litres of saline.
  — May require mechanical debridement with scissors or a blade. Surgical scrubbing brush is also a good instrument.
• For heavily contaminated wounds, they still require debridement in ED, followed by appropriate dressings and referral to appropriate surgical team for definitive debridement and management.

Basic dressings

Wounds can be:

• dry and therefore need moisture
• moist—ideal condition for healing and re-epithelialisation
• wet and therefore need drying out.

DRESSINGS FOR DRY WOUNDS THAT NEED MOISTURE

• Hydrogel
  — Hydrophilic gel: good for keeping wound moist but also absorbs moderate amount of exudate to promote autolytic debridement
  — Examples are IntraSite Gel, Solugel, Woundaid Gel
  — Good for ulcers, infected wounds, granulating wounds or cavities

- Hydrocolloid
  — Impermeable to gases/liquids, keeps moisture in wound
  — Examples are Comfeel, DuoDERM
  — Leave on wound for 3–7 days
  — Good for incision lines, superficial burns, nearly epithelialised wounds

DRESSING FOR EXUDATIVE WOUNDS THAT NEED DRYING OUT

- Foam
  — Non-adherent foam most used for highly exudating wounds (wicks moisture)
  — Examples are Biotain, Mepilex, AMD foam
  — Good for pressure ulcers, any other ulcers
- Packing gauze
  — Usually soaked in betadine or saline
  — Change daily or more frequently (e.g. BD or TDS) for highly exudative wounds
- Hydrofibre dressing
  — Examples are Aquacel or Aquacel Ag
  — Absorbs fluid from wound bed and creates a soft gel to maintain moisture

Basics of wound closure
SUTURE MATERIAL
See Table 31.1.

SUTURE SIZE
Sutures are assigned a number or size according to their tensile strength. The more zeros a suture has, the less strength it has (e.g. a 2-0 suture has more strength than a 5-0 suture). General guidelines for size of suture to use are as follows.

- Face: 5-0 or 6-0. All non-absorbable sutures should be removed around 5 days.
- Scalp: 3-0, 4-0 or 5-0, or skin staples. Remove after 10–14 days.
- Torso (chest, abdomen and back): 3-0 or 4-0.
- Limbs: 3-0 or 4-0. Non-absorbable sutures should be removed after 7–14 days depending on area. Leave longer over mobile areas such as joints.

Table 31.1 Types of suture materials

Absorbable	Non-Absorbable
Monocryl, PDS, Maxon: monofilament suture used for deep layer sutures under the skin; not usually removed	Prolene, Novafil: monofilament suture, has memory (difficult to get knots squared); used to approximate skin edges
Vicryl, Polysorb: braided suture used for deep layers under the skin and tying off vessels	Nylon, Ethilon: monofilament suture; used to approximate skin edges
Fast Gut: very fast-absorbing gut suture, used for approximation of skin edges, commonly used in children and facial wounds	Silk—braided suture: generally used as a temporary suture (e.g. to secure a drain or a tension suture)
Vicryl Rapide: fast-absorbing braided suture used for approximation of skin edges; commonly used for facial wounds, children (any wound), elderly (any wound)	

SUTURE TECHNIQUE

- The object of wound closure is to obtain tension-free approximation of the skin edges.
- Sutures should be balanced and placed evenly with equal bites taken on either side of the wound edge.
- You can use interrupted sutures or running sutures if appropriate for the wound.
  - Most common is to use interrupted simple sutures.
  - Can also use mattress sutures (vertical or horizontal) to ensure good wound edge eversion.
  - Continuous running suture runs the entire length of the wound.
  - If wound is gaping, buried interrupted deep sutures with a non-absorbable suture (Monocryl, PDS, Vicryl) can be used to minimise skin tension.
- Ensure sutures are not too tight as they can cause wound-edge necrosis as the skin edges swell post-procedure.
- Appropriate dressings. Consider immobilisation or compression where appropriate for limbs and over joints.

— For example, large wounds or skin tears over the knee should be protected with immobilisation in something like a Zimmer splint until sutures are removed.

Lacerations, abrasions and bites
LACERATIONS

- Examination.
  - Any signs of neurovascular involvement should be discussed with appropriate surgical team.
  - Document neurovascular findings prior to infiltration with local anaesthetic.
- Washout and debridement under local anaesthetic and analgesia.
- Assess wound depth.
  - Generally not many important structures above fascia.
  - Identify any structures or foreign material visible in base of wound.
  - If in doubt, call senior for help, take a photo (with patient consent) and call appropriate surgical team for advice.
- X-ray if foreign body seen or suspected.
- Closure without tension with appropriate sutures.
  - Avoid non-absorbable sutures in children.
- Supportive dressings.
  - Non-adhesive dressings on wounds.
  - Can use steri-strips across wound for extra support if some tension on closure, or wound across highly mobile area.
  - May need compression with crepe bandage for limbs or bleeding potential (anticoagulation) to minimise haematoma.

ABRASIONS

- Usually contaminated (dirt, gravel)
- Must clean and remove all debris (otherwise heal with tattooing)
- May need analgesia +/– local anaesthetic for adequate cleaning and debridement
- Dress with non-stick dressings until re-epithelialises (usually 14–21 days)

— Jelonet or Bactigras (need to change < 48 hourly)
— Mepilex silicone dressing (change 1–2 times weekly)
— Silver such as Acticoat or Mepilex Ag (change 2–3 times weekly)

BITES

- Even small, superficial wounds can cause significant infection
- Humans > cats > dogs in order of severity of infection
- Cats: sharp teeth and nails that puncture
  — Often seeds deep infection, particularly around joints
- Thorough debridement and irrigation early are critical to prevention of infection
- Loose closure with monofilament non-absorbable suture
  — If small wound that is not bleeding, can leave open and allow to heal by secondary intention (ugly scar can always be excised)
- ADT
- Empirical antibiotics
  — IV Tazocin or Augmentin for established infection (any sign of pus)
- Refer to appropriate surgical team for definitive management if deep or extensive
- Usually require regular wound monitoring even after closure (regular dressings with community nurse or GP or appropriate wound clinic)

Skin tears
ASSESSMENT

- Partial thickness
  — Epidermal depth only
- Full thickness
  — Epidermis and dermis involved with exposure of underlying subcutaneous tissue
- Location
- Size
- Surrounding skin
- Haematoma/bleeding

MANAGEMENT

- ADT.
- Basic wound first aid: clean wound with sterile saline.
  — May need to infiltrate with local anaesthetic as this can be painful, especially in large areas.
  — Use local anaesthetic with adrenaline in all areas except the fingers and toes.
- Unfold skin flaps and roll out edges to approximate wound edges as best possible.
- If referring for further management by surgical team, dress with:
  — double-layer Jelonet or Bactigras
  — absorbent dressing such as Combine or Zetuvit
  — wrap limbs from distal to proximal with Webril or Velband and crepe bandage with light compression.
- Elevate limbs.
- If skin tear is small and partial thickness, can be managed in ED using same principles:
  — basic wound first aid with local anaesthetic/adrenaline and/or analgesia
  — unroll edges and skin flaps to approximate wound edges
  — use skin adhesive (glue) to secure skin edges that are able to be approximated
  — dress with Mepitel or Jelonet or Bactigras as primary dressing
  — secondary dressings include absorbent pad (combine or similar), wrapping limbs with compression bandages (Velband/Webril and crepe from distal to proximal)
  — use Tubigrip compression for lower limbs (from toes to knees to prevent lower limb oedema)
  — discharge home with GP follow-up:
    ○ antibiotics for 5 days
    ○ dressings stay intact for 5 days before review (unless soiled/wet), essential to keep clean and dry
    ○ keep limbs elevated as much as possible.
- If large skin tears, refer to appropriate surgical team.

Pressure ulcers

- Susceptible areas include all bony prominences, but especially ischial tuberosity, sacrum, greater trochanter, heel.

- Those at risk include elderly, those in long-term care facilities, paraplegics, quadriplegics, neurologically impaired.
- Many aetiological factors, almost always a combination of inadequate pressure care and intrinsic/patient factors.
- Classification:
  Stage 1: Non-blanchable erythema on skin
  Stage 2: Partial-thickness skin loss (usually presents as blister, abrasion, shallow ulcer)
  Stage 3: Full-thickness skin loss down to but not through fascia
  Stage 4: Full-thickness skin loss involving underlying muscle, fascia, bone, tendon, joint capsule, ligaments etc.
  Unstageable: Full-thickness skin loss, depth unknown
- Management principles:
  — patient evaluation
    ◦ history and examination
    ◦ pressure care assessment
    ◦ bloods including screening for anaemia, diabetes, malnutrition, immunocompromise
    ◦ imaging looking for osteomyelitis if suspected.
  — Referral to appropriate medical team for medical optimisation.
  — Referral to surgical team where appropriate.
  — Local infection control and dressings.
    ◦ Clean and debride wound.
    ◦ Dressings can include packing gauze for deep cavities or hydrogel or other absorbent dressings (depending on amount of exudate and size of wound).
- Referral to wound CNC for dressing advice is usually appropriate.

Chapter 32
Pain management in the emergency department

Jennifer Stevens and Tiffany Fulde

'... we reckon the fastest track to becoming a university
professor through publication would be to show
how bad we are at prescribing for pain.'
EmergencyPedia. We Suck—6 Tips for Controlling Pain
in the Emergency Department. Posted on 14 May 2015
by Andrew Coggins.

Overview
KEY OBJECT-IVES IN PAIN MANAGEMENT
IN THE EMERGENCY DEPARTMENT

(Adapted from Australasian College for Emergency Medicine
2015.[1])

The ED team:

- has standardised processes to document the severity of pain
  and the ongoing management of pain
- ensures that patients are well informed about their pain
  management options and are involved in the decision-making
  process concerning pain management
- communicates with a patient's chronic pain or addiction
  management health provider when appropriate
- advocates for quality pain management for patients in the ED
  and on discharge from ED
- ensures that pain assessment and management take into
  account issues such as culture, gender, age, substance
  use, chronic conditions, cognitive, behavioural and/or
  sensory impairment, in order to ensure optimal care in all
  circumstances.

KEY CLINICAL INDICATORS RELATED TO BEST-QUALITY PAIN MANAGEMENT IN ED

(Adapted from National Institute of Clinical Studies 2011.[2])

* **Assessment and documentation of pain:** see assessment section.
* **Timeliness to intervention:** ED length of stay is reduced when time to initial analgesia is reduced. It is not dependent on reduction in pain scores.[3]
* Where oral analgesia is appropriate, do not withhold it just because the patient will be nil by mouth for procedural sedation or surgery.
* Giving analgesia early for abdominal pain does not interfere with diagnosis or clinical judgment.[4]
* **Reassessment of pain** to determine the effect of treatment and assess for adverse effects: regularly reassess **AND DOCUMENT** the patient's pain every 5–15 minutes if severe, or every 30–60 minutes if less severe.

PAIN HISTORY AND ASSESSMENT

'Pain is an unpleasant sensory and emotional experience associated with actual or potential tissue damage or described in terms of such damage.'[5]

Acute pain is a normal sensation that alerts us to possible injury and resolves as the injury resolves.

* Somatic: well localised sharp or aching, often with local tenderness. Origin in free endings (nociceptors) of mainly Aδ fibres in skin and deep tissues (muscle, bone, fascia, peritoneum).
* Visceral: less well localised, dull, crampy or colicky, and tenderness may be localised or more diffuse. Origin in free endings of mainly C fibres of viscera (e.g. intestines, heart).

For example, appendicitis may present initially as visceral pain (poorly localised and dull) but progress to somatic pain (localised to the right lower quadrant [RLQ] and sharp) as inflammation spreads to the fascia.

Chronic non-cancer pain may occur after an initial injury or illness but does not resolve as the injury or illness resolves. Sometimes there is no prior injury or illness. Three months is often used as the time when pain is called chronic but the lack of an ongoing source of nociception is at least as important a part of the definition as duration.

Neuropathic pain requires a clinical scenario that includes a potential for nerve injury, pain that is burning or shooting, paroxysmal or spontaneous, sometimes with altered sensation. Neuropathic pain may be acute or chronic.

Key Questions for a Pain History
Presenting complaint
• Location of pain
• Time of onset
• Nature of onset (acute versus gradual, traumatic versus atraumatic)
• Character
• Severity
• Associated factors (including any neurological symptoms or 'red flags')
• Exacerbating and relieving factors
• Chronicity
• Previous treatments (including if non-effective)
• Previous investigations
• Functional losses
Full medical and surgical history
Medication history—including allergies and over-the-counter remedies

Pain scales are unidimensional (used primarily for acute pain and also for cancer pain) and multidimensional (used primarily for chronic pain).

- Unidimensional:
  — Numeric Rating Scale (NRS). A scale of 0–10 where 0 represents 'no pain' and 10 represents 'worst pain imaginable'. It correlates well with the Visual Analogue Scale (VAS) which is used primarily for research.
    ∘ Mild pain, 1–3: noticeable but has little effect on day-to-day functioning.
    ∘ Moderate pain, 4–6: interferes with some areas of functioning.
    ∘ Severe pain, 7–10: significant interference; pain has become a central concern.

- Unidimensional scales for the nonverbal patient:
  — Pain Assessment in Advanced Dementia Scale (PAINAD).
    It measures on a scale of 0–2 across five behavioural
    domains to give a score form 0–10 making it easy to
    understand for those used to the NRS (Figure 32.1).
  — Faces Pain Scale. Used for children from age 4 years
    (Figure 32.2).

		Pain Assessment in Advanced Dementia (PAINAD) Scale		
Items*	**0**	**1**	**2**	**Score**
Breathing independent of vocalisation	Normal	Occasional laboured breathing Short period of hyperventilation.	Noisy laboured breathing. Long period of hyperventilation. Cheyne-Stokes respirations.	
Negative vocalisation	None	Occasional moan or groan Low-level speech with a negative or disapproving quality.	Repeated troubled calling out. Loud moaning or groaning. Crying.	
Facial expression	Smiling or inexpressive	Sad. Frightened. Frown.	Facial grimacing.	
Body language	Relaxed	Tense. Distressed pacing. Fidgeting.	Rigid. Fists clenched. Knees pulled up. Pulling or pushing away. Striking out.	
Consolability	No need to console	Distracted or reassured by voice or touch.	Unable to console, distract or reassure.	
			Total**	

*Five-item observational tool (see the description of each item below).

**Total scores range from 0 to 10 (based on a scale of 0 to 2 for five items), with a higher score indicating more severe pain (0 = "no pain" to 10 = "severe pain").

Figure 32.1 PAINAD scale
Warden V, Hurley A, Volicer L. Development and psychometric evaluation of the Pain Assessment in Advanced Dementia (PAINAD) scale. J Am Med Dir Assoc 2003;4(1):9–15.

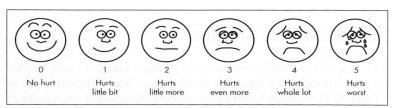

0	1	2	3	4	5
No hurt	Hurts little bit	Hurts little more	Hurts even more	Hurts whole lot	Hurts worst

Figure 32.2 Faces Pain Scale
Hockenberry MJ et al. Wong's essentials of pediatric nursing, ed 9, St Louis, 2013, Mosby.

- Multidimensional:
  - Brief Pain Inventory (BPI). It assesses pain intensity, response to medications, and interference with mood, work, sleep, social and other functions. It provides much more information about context and is used primarily for chronic pain.

Analgesia

Most analgesic drugs have significant side effects. Doing no harm and responding to a patient's pain are both important goals.

MULTIMODAL ANALGESIA VERSUS INAPPROPRIATE POLYPHARMACY

Multimodal analgesia aims to layer interventions and drugs to give synergistic analgesic action while minimising side effects. Inappropriate polypharmacy combines medications with synergistic side effects without proven increases in efficacy (e.g. combining opioids and benzodiazepines for pain).

Multimodal analgesia includes non-drug techniques such as:

- ice and elevation
- immobilisation
- reassurance
- heat packs
- oral glucose for infants
- placebo or contextual response (for example, paracetamol 1 g orally as an initial dose may not reach therapeutic levels for analgesia in some patients; however, enquiring about pain and responding rapidly with administration of a low-side effect drug like paracetamol may provide a placebo response that may legitimately be utilised for mild to moderate level pain).

NON-OPIOID MEDICATIONS

Paracetamol

This is a useful medication in mild to moderate pain and as part of a multimodal package for severe pain. At therapeutic doses (Table 32.1), toxicity is very rare. Rectal administration results in variable blood levels. Intravenous administration results in higher and more predictable blood levels in patients who are unable to

Table 32.1   Paracetamol administration

Route	Oral, intravenous, rectal (variable absorption)
Adult, and children over 12 years dose	1 g qid
Paediatric dose	10–15 mg/kg q4h; max 100 mg/kg/day or 4 g per day whichever is less
Elderly dosing	Consider 1 g tds over 80 years

have oral formulations or have severe pain. Intravenous administration is as effective as opioids for pain from renal colic.

Anti-inflammatories

These are highly effective for somatic and visceral inflammatory pain. They are significantly opioid sparing and in fact have equivalent efficacy to opioids, including for simple fractures in both adults and children.[6,7] A single standard dose of anti-inflammatories is equivalent to approximately 10 mg subcutaneous morphine.

Anti-inflammatories have a low incidence of side effects with short-term use in selected patients.

DO NOT use in patients who are likely to be defending their renal blood flow/glomerular filtration rate (a process that involves prostaglandins); for example:

- cardiac failure, even if well compensated
- renal impairment or longstanding diabetes
- hypovolaemia
- advanced age.

DO NOT use anti-inflammatories where there is a major bleeding risk; for example:

- major trauma
- head or spinal cord injury.

Other contraindications are relative and depend on the context. Coxibs (e.g. celecoxib and intravenous parecoxib) do not affect platelet function and are associated with a lower rate of gastrointestinal side effects than the non-specific anti-inflammatories, especially if co-administered with proton pump inhibitors.

Thromboembolic side effect rates vary with patient comorbidities and with the individual drug (e.g. diclofenac > ibuprofen, naproxen and celecoxib), and are dose dependant.

Aspirin-sensitive asthma is a contraindication for NSAID use but coxibs may still be used.

An increased rate of miscarriage and malformation is associated with NSAID use in early pregnancy. NSAID use after 30 weeks' gestation is associated with an increased risk of premature closure of the fetal ductus arteriosus and oligohydramnios. Fetal and neonatal adverse effects on the brain, kidney, lung, skeleton, gastrointestinal tract and cardiovascular system have also been reported after prenatal exposure to NSAIDs.

This list of possible complications is not exhaustive. This group of drugs remain highly useful in the ED when used wisely (see Table 32.2).

Paracetamol combined with an NSAID is more effective than either medication alone.

Ketamine

Ketamine (see Table 32.3) has a history of use for procedural sedation in EDs. It reduces dose and cardiorespiratory complication rates of propofol sedation when added in a 1:1 dose ratio and has a lower rate of cardiorespiratory side effects than when opioids are

Table 32.2 NSAID dosing

Oral ibuprofen in adults	200–400 mg tds
Oral ibuprofen in children	4–10 mg/kg/dose tds; max 400 mg/dose
Oral celecoxib in adults	100 mg bd or 200 mg daily
Intravenous parecoxib in adults	40 mg IV as a single dose

Table 32.3 Ketamine dosing

IV ketamine for adult and paediatric analgesia	0.1 mg/kg q 5 minutely up to a maximum of 0.3 mg/kg
IM ketamine for paediatric analgesia	0.5 mg/kg
Doses are different for procedural sedation	Requires specific training and monitoring

the adjunct with propofol. There is an increased rate of non-life-threatening side effects, primarily hallucinations and dizziness.

There is increasing interest in sub-dissociative doses as primary or rescue analgesia. Analgesic efficacy for severe pain is similar to systemic opioids and cardiorespiratory side effects of opioids are reduced when ketamine is used as an adjunct for analgesia. Ketamine is also opioid sparing in severe pain. However, hallucinations, dizziness and drowsiness occur at rates up to 50% and although not dangerous the psychiatric side effects can be extremely distressing for some patients. Postoperative literature would suggest that ketamine for analgesia is most likely to be useful when pain is severe, for patients who are opioid tolerant or dependent and when cardiorespiratory depression is a risk.

Methoxyflurane

Methoxyflurane (see Table 32.4) is a volatile anaesthetic that was removed from use as a general anaesthetic agent because of dose-dependent renal toxicity. It is now available in many countries as a self-administered handheld inhaler for analgesia and procedural sedation. Safety for single use is well established in adults and children but with use restricted in those with established significant renal impairment. Staff safety with multiple exposures has also now been established. Onset time is 5 minutes with a peak at 15 minutes. Headache and dizziness are the most common side effects. Cognitive recovery occurs within 30 minutes. It has efficacy with minimal side effects for pre-hospital and in-hospital analgesia, for dressings and other minor procedures. Efficacy requires good patient education and cooperation, thereby limiting use in younger paediatric patients in particular.

LOCAL ANAESTHETIC TECHNIQUES

Local anaesthetic techniques have an important role in trained hands within the ED for local infiltration and regional blockade.

Table 32.4   Methoxyflurane dosing

Methoxyflurane self-administration age > 5 years	3–6 mL dose, maximum 15 mL/ week; do not use on consecutive days

The use of a fascia iliaca block in elderly patients with a fractured neck of femur improves analgesia, is opioid sparing and reduces the burden of delirium in these high-risk patients. The use of dental blocks will be explained in the section on dental pain.

Systems to ensure competency and safe administration of regional techniques are very important. Regional blockade requires cardiorespiratory monitoring, intravenous access and safety equipment and drugs for use in overdose or intravascular injection. Do not use adrenaline-containing solutions where end arteries are involved (i.e. fingers, toes, nose, ears, penis).

Aspirin and NSAIDs are not contraindications to peripheral regional nerve blockade but if other anticoagulants (e.g. warfarin or the NOACs) have been ingested recently enough to be therapeutic then a decision should be made by a senior and experienced clinician about the risk–benefit ratio for the individual patient's circumstances.

BENZODIAZEPINES

Benzodiazepines are life-saving drugs when used for withdrawal syndromes and have a short-term role in selected and closely monitored cases of anxiety, but their use for pain and 'muscle relaxation' is not supported by evidence. Opioids and benzodiazepines are synergistic with respect to respiratory depression. Patients with psychiatric comorbidities have the highest rates of death with this combination. Use of benzodiazepines for pain should be actively avoided.

ANTINEUROPATHIC AGENTS

Antineuropathic agents include the gabapentinoids (pregabalin and gabapentin) and tricyclic antidepressants.

MIGRAINE DRUGS

See special situations.

Opioids

Route of administration should be oral in preference to systemic. Fasting patients (nil by mouth) may be administered oral analgesia unless they have (or are suspected of having):
- bowel obstruction
- perforated viscus

- compromised swallow
- compromised airway.

Patients in severe pain may require systemic bolus administration initially.

Intravenous bolus dosing has traditionally been with morphine at doses of 0.05 mg/kg, with a maximum of around 0.2 mg/kg.

Use of fentanyl at 1 microg/kg, then 0.3 microg/kg every 5 minutes is growing as it has a shorter onset and duration of action, has a lower risk of accumulation than morphine in patients with renal impairment and may cause less nausea and vomiting. Bolus doses should be significantly reduced in the elderly for both morphine and fentanyl.

Dose for adults is most closely predicted by age. For postoperative patients aged 20 and over using intravenous patient-controlled analgesia (PCA) use is best predicted by the following formula:[8]

average first **24 h** morphine requirement (mg) = 100 − age

This implies that a 60 year old will require half the dose of a 20 year old to achieve similar analgesia with moderate to severe pain. This should be seen only as an indicator of the large difference in dosing requirements at different ages only, and adjustments should be made for opioid tolerance, comorbidities such as renal and hepatic impairment, weight and current illness severity.

The very elderly should be started with very low doses.

Slow-release opioid use increases side effects, including respiratory depression and death, when used for opioid-naïve patients for acute pain. Use should be actively discouraged within EDs unless the patient will be admitted to a monitored environment in select situations and even then, only using those agents with a lower effect on respiratory function, like tramadol or low-dose tapentadol. Fentanyl patches in particular have been associated with deaths when used for non-cancer pain. Opioid-naïve patients with non-cancer pain should not be discharged from the ED on slow-release opioids.

Prophylactic antiemetics are likely to be unnecessary unless the patient has a history of nausea and vomiting associated with opioids or travel sickness.

Laxatives should always be prescribed concurrently with opioids unless there is a contraindication (e.g. bowel obstruction). Stimulant laxatives such as senna are particularly useful for opioid-induced constipation, but stool softeners should be added in most cases. Large doses of senna or bisacodyl in breastfeeding women can cause diarrhoea in their breastfed infant.

Discharge prescribing principles. Surgery, and to a lesser extent ED visits, are now recognised as gateway events to unplanned long-term opioid use. Although most opioids are prescribed by general practitioners, most are started in hospitals.

Transition to unplanned long-term opioid use or abuse is reduced by:

- use of non-opioid alternatives
- dispensing a minimum number of opioid tablets with GP follow-up if it is thought additional supply may be required.

Opioid stewardship in EDs require an acknowledgment that for some patients a first prescription of an opioid for an acute episode can be a trigger event for long-term use and dependence. Patients with psychiatric comorbidities are at particularly high risk.

Side effects of short-term use:

- respiratory depression and exacerbation of sleep apnoea
- falls and increased fracture rate; this may be up to four times the non-opioid rate
- constipation
- nausea and vomiting
- itch
- urinary retention.

Side effects of longer term use—rates increase with regular daily use, increasing daily dose, length of use and polypharmacy:

- depression, and treatment resistance in established depression
- dry mouth and tooth decay
- increased cardiovascular mortality with increased rates of AMI and CCF
- hypothalamic–pituitary axis suppression with decreased testosterone
- sexual dysfunction
- opioid-induced hyperalgesia
- dependence, abuse and withdrawal.

Individual opioids differ substantially.

• Genetic variability in metabolism affects all opioids but has been particularly implicated in deaths with codeine use. Approximately 10% of the population in the United Kingdom and 30% of the Hong Kong Chinese population are poor metabolisers and therefore experience poor analgesia with codeine (CYP2D6 polymorphism).

• The opioid receptors are the primary targets for morphine, fentanyl, hydromorphone, methadone and oxycodone. These drugs therefore exhibit respiratory depression that is strongly dose-dependent. They also cause significant dose-dependent gastrointestinal side effects. Extreme caution should be used when using these drugs with other sedative drugs.

• Tramadol is not structurally an opioid, but it does bind weakly to opioid receptors. It also inhibits reuptake of serotonin and noradrenaline. At usual doses it causes less respiratory depression and constipation than the above listed opioids, but similar level of nausea and vomiting. Caution should be used in combination with other drugs that increase serotonin levels. CYP2D6 polymorphism also results in slow metabolism and reduced analgesia.

• Tapentadol is an opioid and also a noradrenaline reuptake inhibitor. Analgesic efficacy is similar to oxycodone but with lower rates of respiratory depression (this may not hold for doses above 100 mg and for elderly patients), nausea, vomiting and constipation.

Dependency. All opioids can result in dependence. Tramadol is often cited as being the least likely; however, they have all been associated with abuse, dependence and death, as have other analgesics such as ketamine and even anti-inflammatories.

Dose conversion. The Faculty of Pain Medicine has created an excellent free conversion app accessed via the following link:[9] http://fpm.anzca.edu.au/documents/opioid-dose-equivalence.pdf

Unintentional bias in prescribing. Significant variance in prescribing for pain exists. In EDs in the United States (US), opioid prescription has been found to be comparable for patients of varying ethnic backgrounds where there is a clear and verifiable diagnosis, but to be significantly higher for white patients where the diagnosis is unclear. This is thought to be one reason for the significantly higher use of opioids and associated higher death rate from opioid use and abuse in the white community in the US.

Figures from New Zealand show opioid dispensing for European patients to be double that for Māori and Pacific Islander patients, and five times that for Asian patients.

Elderly patients with fractured neck of femur receive less analgesia if they have dementia despite evidence that pain levels are similar to cognitively intact patients.

These examples of disparities in treatment of pain should act as alerts to other unmeasured disparities that are likely to exist. It is essential to be aware of how bias may influence prescribing (unintentional or not), and ensure analgesia is appropriate.

Clinical Pearls

Major trauma
- Dose reduction is necessary in volume-depleted patients.
- Ketamine is often a good choice (greater cardiac stability).
- Remember nonpharmacological techniques including splinting fractures.

Non-specific back pain

- Exclude red flags first:
    - history of significant trauma
    - age > 50 years, < 20 years
    - history of cancer
    - recent bacterial infection
    - IV drug abuse
    - immune suppression (IMMB, transplant, corticosteroids)
    - weight loss
    - severe pain when supine and/or at night
    - saddle anaesthesia
    - bladder dysfunction
    - neurological deficit in lower limb.
- Patients with non-specific back pain in the ED require education and encouragement to remain active.
- In randomised controlled trials, exercise alone has been shown to prevent back pain.

— Patients with persistent back pain benefit most from active involvement in treatment (e.g. exercise) as opposed to passive treatment (e.g. acupuncture, massage).
— Exercise programs should be individually tailored and include strengthening and stretching components.
♦ Patients with moderate to severe chronic back, hip and knee pain had better pain and functional outcomes and fewer side effects with non-opioid analgesia than with opioid analgesia in a recent 12-month follow-up randomised control trial.[10]
♦ Regular paracetamol.
♦ NSAIDs.
♦ Minimise opioid use and provide only a small supply for discharge, if any. Use early GP follow-up rather than providing larger amounts for discharge.

Dental pain

♦ Non-opioid (paracetamol, ibuprofen) analgesics provide equivalent analgesia to opioid analgesics.
♦ By the time of presentation to ED many patients will have tried most readily available analgesics, including combinations with codeine.
♦ Repeat dosing to achieve therapeutic levels, or for synergistic effect, may still offer some benefit.
♦ Local anaesthesia (nerve blocks) are a useful tool in experienced hands.
— Longer-acting agents (e.g. bupivacaine + adrenaline) are recommended over shorter agents (lignocaine).
— Local anaesthetic is less effective in infected tissues due to lower pH, and these patients should be discussed with a specialist prior to infiltration.
— Inferior alveolar block for ipsilateral mandibular teeth to midline.
— Mental nerve block for ipsilateral mandibular teeth from 2nd premolar to midline.
— Buccal infiltration for maxillary teeth in area that local anaesthetic is deposited.
♦ See block techniques at http://onlinelibrary.wiley.com/doi/10.1111/1742-6723.12266/full

Renal colic

- Renal colic is prostaglandin mediated; therefore, NSAIDs are the first-line analgesics. Evidence shows NSAIDs are more effective, with fewer side effects than opioids in patients with renal colic.[11]
- Regular paracetamol should also be given, with IV paracetamol having a similar efficacy to opioids for this indication and being of particular use in the vomiting patient. When compared to each other, the route of paracetamol administration is not related to efficacy.
- Opioids may be used as a second-line treatment to provide immediate relief pending the onset of NSAID-analgesia.
- IV fluids may worsen pain due to renal capsular distension.
- There is no evidence that anti-spasmodics (e.g. Buscopan) are effective.
- Patients may require admission to achieve adequate analgesia.

Migraine pain

- If a patient with recurrent migraines presents to an ED exclude red flags first (see Table 32.5). It usually indicates a particularly severe episode with failure of usual therapy.
- Nonpharmacological measures against migraine:
  — cold packs over the forehead or occiput
  — hot packs over the neck and shoulders
  — neck stretches and massage
  — rest in a quiet, dark room.
- Pharmacological treatments are usually more effective when administered early and a large single dose tends to work better than repetitive small doses.
- The main drug groups for acute treatment for migraine are non-opioid simple analgesics and triptans. (See Table 32.5.).
  — Try a non-opioid analgesic first
    ° aspirin 900–100 mg PO/ibuprofen 400–600 mg PO OR
    ° naproxen 500–750 mg PO/paracetamol 1 g PO
  — Triptans (serotonin 1B/1D agonists) are effective for acute migraine and act at the pathophysiological mechanism of action for headache (thus are migraine 'specific').

- ○ Choice of agent should be individualised, including factors such as route of administration. No efficacy-evidence strongly supports one agent over another.
- ○ Beware serotonin toxicity in patients taking other scrotonergic medication, including SSRI and SNRIs (although not an absolute contraindication).

- Overuse of analgesics can lead to medication overuse headache.
- Avoid opioids.
- IV or IM antiemetics have been shown to be as effective as triptans in treating acute migraine.
  - Dopamine receptor antagonists metoclopramide (IV) (NNT [number needed to treat] = 4), chlorpromazine (IV/IM) [NNT = 2] and prochlorperazine (IV/IM) are effective single agents.
    - ○ *Note:* Monitor for prolonged QT interval.
  - PO antiemetics are not useful as monotherapy, but PO metoclopramide may be a useful adjunct to reduce migraine-induced gastric stasis and improve PO absorption of other analgesics.
- There is limited evidence relating to ondansetron and granisetron in this setting, although both drug side effects include headache.
- Ergotamine and dihydroergotamine (serotonin 1B/1D receptor agonists) have also been used, sometimes in combination with caffeine.
  - Parenteral dihydroergotamine may be combined with metoclopramide for severe migraine, but should not be used as a sole agent.
  - There are considerable associated side effects (worsening nausea and vomiting, vascular occlusion, rebound headaches) and contraindication in vascular disease (cardiac, cerebrovascular and peripheral disease).
  - Ergotamine has been found to be indicated for relatively few patients.
- IV or IM dexamethasone may be a useful adjunct to reduce risk of early headache recurrence.

Table 32.5   Migraine—exclude headache red flags first

Headache red flags:
* sudden onset
* > 50 years of age
* increased frequency or severity of headache
* new onset of headache with an underlying medical condition
* headache with concomitant systematic illness, focal
* neurological signs or symptoms (papillo-oedema)
* headache subsequent to head trauma.

Cancer pain

Pain is one of the top two reasons for cancer patients to present to ED. Cancer pain may be due to the disease or its treatment (e.g. radiotherapy, surgical, side effects from chemotherapy) and may have elements of neuropathic and nociceptive pain (including inflammation, ischaemia and compression). Prevalence of pain increases with advanced stages of cancer, but severe pain can occur in any stage of the disease.

The most important aspects to include in a multidimensional assessment of cancer pain are intensity, temporal pattern and treatment-related factors (exacerbation/pain relief).

TEMPORAL PATTERN

* Continuous
* Intermittent pain
  — Incident (associated with known precipitant)
  — Non-incident (breakthrough, spontaneous)
* End-of-dose failure (occurs just prior to scheduled opioid dose)

A neurological examination including for signs of spinal cord compression and muscle wasting is an important part of the physical examination. Increased or altered pain patterns should cause high suspicion of disease progression, recurrence or complications from treatment.

Opioid analgesia using the WHO analgesic ladder (Figure 32.3) is effective in 80–90% cancer patients. Opioids should be given orally, with morphine, oxycodone and hydromorphone first-line agents. Continuous pain should use regular around-the-clock dose

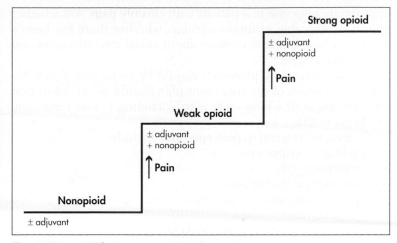

Figure 32.3. WHO Analgesic ladder for cancer pain
*Parala-Metz A, Davis M (2013) Cancer Pain. http://www.clevelandclinicmeded.com/
medicalpubs/diseasemanagement/hematology-oncology/cancer-pain/*

regimens (immediate release [IR] or sustained release [SR]) with
IR opioids charted as a rescue dose for intermittent pain (dose
10–20% of total daily opioid dose). In end-of-dose failure, the regular dose should be titrated rather than reducing the dose interval.

Cancer pain and analgesia may be associated with significant
side effects. Opioid rotation results in resolution of side effects
and improved pain control in > 50% of patients.[15] Other options
include adding adjuvant analgesia or other drugs for symptom-
control, slow dose titration and changing route of administration.
Where possible this should be done in consultation with the patient's usual treating team.

CHRONIC PAIN PATIENT AND CHRONIC OPIOID USE
Patients with chronic pain or those who use long-term opioids,
including as part of an opioid substitution program, should have a
full assessment. In the assessment of an exacerbation of a chronic
pain complaint, the repeated use of the NRS may be unhelpful.
Eliciting a pain score of 9/10 in acute pain would usually result
in early administration of medications and this may not be the

appropriate response in a patient with chronic pain. Ask whether pain is manageable or unmanageable, whether there has been a change in function, and enquire about social circumstances and psychological state.

The usual treating physician should be contacted if possible and confirmation of the treatment plan should occur. Education and discussion of a long-term plan, including opioid reduction, can begin in ED.

Criteria for referral to pain specialist include:

- debilitating symptoms
- escalating needs
- poor response to therapy
- high-dose opioid use (especially > 100 mg morphine equivalent/day)
- major physical or psychological disability.

Consider a multidisciplinary ED management plan for patients with repeated presentations. Many EDs will have systems in place to alert ED staff to a complex medical history in these cases.

Stay alert for red and yellow flags.

Patients taking regular opioids (chronic pain and opioid-replacement regimens) presenting to ED with acute pain should have their regular dose opioids continued as a baseline, especially if going for a painful procedure, with additional analgesia titrated. Contact appropriate specialists for advice including anaesthetics, pain specialist and drug and alcohol as appropriate.

There is little or no evidence of a benefit with opioids in chronic non-cancer pain and a large amount of high-quality evidence of harm so commencing opioids for chronic non-cancer pain is inappropriate in an ED setting.

Patients on an opioid substitution program should have their usual dose and the time last taken confirmed by the prescriber as soon as possible. Prevention of withdrawal should be a high priority. Analgesia will usually require continuation of usual opioid plus non-opioid analgesics and often extra opioid.

There is high-quality evidence for use of opioids in an opioid substitution program in the circumstances of drug abuse to reduce patient and community harms.

References

1. Australasian College for Emergency Medicine (2015) Quality standards for emergency departments and other hospital-based emergency care services.
2. National Institute of Clinical Studies (2011) Emergency care acute pain management manual. National Health and Medical Research Council, Canberra. https://www.nhmrc.gov.au/guidelines-publications/cp135
3. Sokoloff C, Daoust R, Paquet J, et al. Is adequate pain relief and time to analgesia associated with emergency department length of stay? A retrospective study BMJ Open 2014;4:e004288. doi: 10.1136/bmjopen-2013-004288.
4. Manterola C, Vial M, Moraga J et al. (2011) Analgesia in patients with acute abdominal pain. Cochrane Database Syst Rev(1): CD005660
5. International Association for the Study of Pain (2018) IASP Taxonomy.
6. Parish E. Ibuprofen as effective as morphine for fracture pain in children, study shows. BMJ 2014;349:g6581
7. Chang AK, Bijur PE, Esses D, et al. Effect of a Single Dose of Oral Opioid and Nonopioid Analgesics on Acute Extremity Pain in the Emergency Department. JAMA 2017;318(17):1661–7.
8. Macintyre PE, Jarvis DA. Age is the best predictor of postoperative morphine requirements. Pain 1996 Feb;64(2):357–64.
9. ANZCA Faculty of Pain Medicine. Opioid Dose Equivalence. http://fpm.anzca.edu.au/documents/opioid-dose-equivalence.pdf
10. Krebs E, Gravely A, Nugent S. Effect of opioid vs non-opioid medications on pain-related function in patients with chronic back pain or hip or knee osteoarthritis pain. JAMA 2018;319(9):872–882.
11. Pathan S, Mitra B, Straney L, et al. Delivering safe and effective analgesia for management of renal colic in the emergency department: a double-blind, multigroup, randomised controlled trial. Lancet 2016 May 14;387(10032):1999–2007.

Recommended readings

National Institute of Clinical Studies. 2011, Emergency care acute pain management manual. National Health and Medical Research Council, Canberra.

Agency for Clinical Innovation (2018) Chronic Pain in the ED. Online. Available: https://www.aci.health.nsw.gov.au/__data/assets/pdf_file/0008/394046/ED-Flow-Chart-Chronic-Pain_1.pdf

Randall C, Clinch D. Evaluation of acute headaches in adults, American Family Physician. 15 Feb 2001.

Chapter 33
Paediatric emergencies

Melinda Berry and Arjun Rao

Recognition of the sick child

Identifying the sick child can be difficult even for experienced staff. The younger the child, the more difficult it can be, particularly when trying to exclude focal and serious bacterial infections. The following guidelines provide a useful approach to detecting serious illness in the child less than 36 months of age. Single signs are not as useful as considering the full complement of symptoms and signs and may be misleading; combinations of serious symptoms are very concerning. Similarly, repeated assessment of children over time during a period of observation is more useful than a single evaluation. No child should be sent home from the ED without having had a thorough assessment, consideration of appropriate investigations and an appropriate period of observation.

In paediatrics, it is always safest to start with the assumption that the parents are always right. It is crucial for a successful consultation to listen to the parents and get a clear understanding of their concerns. It can be especially useful to understand what specifically led them to present at the particular time that they did. Appropriate involvement of children in conversation and history taking often yields useful information. The social and family situation has a large impact on the environment the child will be discharged into and must be considered in any disposition decisions.

Features that will help you recognise and safely manage the sick child include:

1 A good history:
— important and usually doesn't take long to elicit
— may reveal important signs even though child now appears normal
  ° e.g. cyanosis after coughing episode, apnoea or seizure

- ask about antibiotic use as this may mask significant infection
- elicit specifically what the parents/carers are worried about.

2 Initial impression:
- appearance/activity
- work of breathing
- perfusion
- the 3 'Os': Observation, Objective signs, Opportunistic approach.

3 Observation over time:
- children's clinical state can change rapidly
- a period of observation can make it much clearer whether a child is getting better or getting worse
- pressure of ED overcrowding and lack of beds should not influence clinical decisions about needing to admit children or keep for a period of observation.

4 Close follow-up:
- ensure that parents/carers feel comfortable about going home
- give clear parameters for what to expect and when to return
- consider how easy it will be for them to return if needed.

The sick baby

Infants under 3 months are a group that pose particular challenges in assessment and management. New parents may not know what is normal for their baby, especially when it comes to changes in feeding and sleeping routines. It can be difficult to rely on clinical assessment alone. Infants in this age group are more susceptible to serious bacterial infections. Congenital disorders may also present in this age group, including congenital cardiac disease.

AIRWAY

Babies may present with noisy breathing and stridor. Stridor present from birth may indicate laryngomalacia or tracheomalacia. These are often benign and resolve with growth but severe cases where there is concern of obstructed breathing may warrant admission for observation and saturation monitoring. Referral to a paediatrician or ear, nose, throat (ENT) surgeon may be warranted and direct visualisation of the airway with nasendoscopy or laryngeal bronchoscopy (LBO) is useful in some babies.

BREATHING

Respiratory viral illnesses such as respiratory syncytial virus (RSV) bronchiolitis can be more severe in babies and can cause apnoea. If they present early in the illness remember they may get worse before getting better and have a low threshold for admission. Similarly pertussis in the age group is a particular concern because of the propensity to cause apnoea. Consider admission and observation for any baby under 6 months who presents with suspected pertussis. All parents and close relatives should receive pertussis vaccination prior to the delivery of the infant.

CIRCULATION

Cyanotic congenital heart disease is usually picked up at birth but acyanotic congenital heart disease may present with cardiac failure in babies. It can be confused with primary respiratory illness if the potential for a cardiac diagnosis is not considered. Difficulty feeding with sweating and pallor may indicate a cardiac cause of respiratory distress. Listen for a murmur, palpate for a displaced apex beat and look for peri-orbital and sacral oedema. Palpate for a liver and finally feel for femoral pulses. Babies with a duct-dependent coarctation can present in the first few weeks of life with shock as the duct closes. Supraventricular tachycardia can also present in this age group and can be difficult to differentiate from sinus tachycardia. A 12-lead ECG should be done. Some useful features are abnormal P-waves, 'machine gun regularity' of complexes, short PR interval or delta wave (the last two indicate pre-excitation). In babies with suspected sepsis, blood pressure is maintained and persistent tachycardia is particularly concerning as a sign of shock and should never be ignored.

NEUROLOGICAL DEFICIT

'Irritability' in babies comes with many connotations of severe illness and should be characterised more completely to help aid refining the diagnosis. Babies who present unsettled and irritable may require admission for observation. Consider urinary tract infection—send a urine for culture. In the more unwell cases think of meningitis and sepsis. Measuring and plotting a head circumference can be useful. These babies should always be discussed with a senior before discharge. See The Unsettled Crying Baby later in this chapter for other potential differentials to consider.

INFECTION

Young babies are immunologically immature and more susceptible to serious bacterial infection. Have a low threshold for investigation (full septic work-up including lumbar puncture) and management. If a baby is very sick, prioritise administration of empiric antibiotics over waiting to collect specimens of urine and CSF for culture. See The Child with Fever section later in this chapter for a suggested approach to fever in this age group.

The child with stridor

Stridor is a high-pitched sound produced during inspiration because of upper airway obstruction. Children are more susceptible to stridor than adults because their airway is smaller. Children may have chronic stridor due to laryngomalacia or other congenital airway abnormality. The most common cause of acute stridor is croup. Other considerations and management are listed below. The overriding principle for the management of children with airway obstruction is minimal handling. Children with severe airway obstruction may 'tripod' and it is important to leave them in this position and not lie them flat.

CROUP

* Laryngotracheitis due to viral infection
* Causes a distinctive seal-like barking cough
* Usually 6 months to 4 years of age

GRADES
+ Mild: barking cough with stridor only when crying
+ Moderate: stridor at rest
+ Severe: stridor with recession

MANAGEMENT
+ Keep child calm, upright in carer's lap
+ Nebulised adrenaline for stridor at rest with respiratory distress (moderate to severe)
  — 1:1000 adrenaline nebulised 0.5 mL/kg up to 5 mL
+ Steroids
  — All children presenting to ED with croup should receive steroids
  — Dexamethasone 0.15 mg/kg or prednisone 1 mg/kg single dose
  — If oral steroids not tolerated give budesonide 2 mg nebulised

DIFFERENTIAL DIAGNOSES TO ALWAYS CONSIDER
+ Bacterial tracheitis
  — Febrile
  — May look toxic
  — May present early in illness
  — Child becomes more unwell over hours, which emphasises the benefit of observation in uncertain cases
+ Epiglottitis
  — Soft low stridor
  — Usually febrile
  — Drooling
+ Retropharyngeal abscess
  — Usually febrile
  — No barking cough
  — May be unable to extend neck—won't look at the ceiling
+ Anaphylaxis
  — Usually associated rash/urticaria
  — No infective symptoms
  — May have known allergies

- Foreign body aspiration
  - Ask specifically in history about this possibility (sudden coughing or choking episode, missing objects)
  - Sudden onset stridor with no infective symptoms
  - Brief period of cyanosis at onset

The child with respiratory distress

Respiratory distress in children can be seen as tachypnoea, sub-costal recession, tracheal tug, nasal flaring and grunting. Much of the respiratory exam can be completed by observation alone. The most common cause of respiratory distress in infants is viral bronchiolitis. The most common cause of respiratory distress in young children is viral-induced wheeze and asthma.

BRONCHIOLITIS

- Usually affects infants < 12 months
- Usually begins with viral upper respiratory tract infection
- By day 2–3 has evolved into a lower respiratory tract infection
- Inflammation in the small infant's airways causes air trapping
- Infant has respiratory distress with widespread crackles and wheeze
- CXR and blood tests are not routinely required
- Routine virological testing (e.g. nasopharyngeal aspirate [NPA]) has no role in management of individual patients

Risk factors for more serious illness
- Gestational age < 36–37 weeks
- Chronological age < 10–12 weeks
- Chronic lung disease
- Congenital heart disease
- Chronic neurological condition
- Failure to thrive
- Exposure to cigarette smoke

Indications for admission
- Presence of risk factors for more serious illness
- Apnoea episodes

- Oxygen requirement (SaO_2 persistently $< 92\%$)
- Feeding reduced such that NG feeding or IV fluids are required
- Moderate to severe work of breathing
- Poor social supports or geographic isolation
- Early phase of illness

Treatment is supportive
- Oxygen for sats persistently $< 92\%$
- Hydration: 2/3 maintenance IV or NG
- Humidified high-flow nasal cannula
  - For moderate to severe respiratory distress and hypoxia
  - Suction and NG insertion at commencement of therapy
  - Start at 2 L/kg up to a maximum of 5 L
  - Titrate FiO_2 for sats $\geq 92\%$
  - Effect should be seen within 1–2 hours, otherwise escalate therapy (CPAP, paediatric intensive care unit [PICU] consult, transfer)

Differential diagnoses to always consider
- Pneumonia (if significant fever, more unwell looking, grunting)
- Heart failure (hepatomegaly, abnormal heart sounds)
- Foreign body aspiration (sudden onset with coughing)
- Pertussis (contacts, unvaccinated, paroxysmal cough)

VIRAL-INDUCED WHEEZE AND ASTHMA
Toddlers and children of preschool age frequently develop wheeze that is precipitated by a viral upper respiratory tract infection (URTI). Some of these children will have a history of atopy and some will go on to be diagnosed with asthma once they reach school age. The benefit of steroids for wheeze in toddlers is unclear and evidence continues to emerge to inform guidelines. The authors' approach is to withhold steroids for simple viral-induced wheeze in well toddlers not requiring admission and without an atopic or family history. Otherwise the management is much the same as for asthma.

Airway inflammation and bronchospasm
- Present with cough, wheeze or difficulty breathing
- Most children (75%) have infrequent intermittent asthma
  — Isolated episodes lasting 3–7 days
  — At least 6 weeks symptom-free in between episodes
  — Triggered by viral URTI
- Some children (20%) have frequent intermittent asthma
  — Episodes more frequently than 6 weeks
  — Symptom-free between episodes
  — May benefit from preventive therapy especially seasonally
- Some children (5%) have persistent asthma
  — Symptoms on most days
  — Require preventive inhaler and close follow-up

Differential diagnoses to consider
- Inhaled foreign body
- Pneumonia
- Heart failure

High-risk patients
- Chronic lung disease or history of prematurity
- Congenital heart disease
- Previous PICU admissions
- Frequent presentations or representations
- Brittle asthma
- Already on maximal therapy

Mild asthma
- Minimal work of breathing at rest
- Able to talk or cry normally
- Oxygen sats > 94% in room air
- Management
  — Prednisone 1–2 mg/kg
  — Salbutamol 6 puffs (< 6 years) or 12 puffs (> 6 years)
- Usually able to be managed at home

Moderate asthma

- Mild to moderate work of breathing (suprasternal, intercostal, subcostal recessions, nasal flaring, use of accessory muscles)
- Talking in phrases
- Sats 90–94% in room air
- Management
  — Prednisone 1–2 mg/kg
  — Salbutamol 6 puffs ($<$ 6 years) or 12 puffs ($>$ 6 years) 20 minutely $\times$ 3
- Observe for 3 hours post salbutamol
- May be able to be discharged home if improved

Severe asthma

- Moderate to severe work of breathing
- Talking in words at best
- Sats $<$ 90%
- Peri-arrest if bradycardic or drowsy
- Summon senior help/retrieval service/PICU
- Management
  — Oxygen for sats $>$ 94%
  — Continuous nebulised salbutamol until improved
  — IV steroids: hydrocortisone 4 mg/kg or methylprednisolone 1 mg/kg
  — Consider high-flow oxygen
  — IV $MgSO_4$ 0.2 mmol/kg/dose (max 8 mmol) over 30 minutes
  — If not improving, load with aminophylline 5 mg/kg over 30 minutes

PNEUMONIA

Fever and cough with tachypnoea, tachycardia and grunting are common clinical features of pneumonia. The classic (but not universal) history involves a relatively sudden deterioration after a period of being well with a viral URTI. Some children, particularly with lower lobe pneumonia, may present misleadingly with abdominal pain. There may be increased work of breathing. Examination involves inspection, palpation and percussion in addition to auscultation. Auscultatory signs may be subtle, and focal crackles are not sensitive or specific for pneumonia.

Pneumonia can induce poor feeding and subsequent dehydration. Children may have diarrhoea. Pneumonia can cause significant sepsis.

Admission to hospital may be required for the following reasons:

- hypoxia with oxygen saturations consistently < 92%
- dehydration
- moderate increase in work of breathing
- signs of systemic sepsis—drowsy, mottled, tachycardic
- high-risk patients (e.g. congenital heart disease, chronic lung disease)
- failure of outpatient therapy.

Antibiotic therapy

Phenoxymethyl penicillin bd or amoxycillin 25 mg/kg 8-hourly for 5 days

- If IV therapy is required:
  — benzylpenicillin 60 mg/kg 6-hourly
- For severe disease:
  — cefotaxime 50 mg/kg 8-hourly or ceftriaxone 50 mg/kg daily PLUS
  — flucloxacillin 50 mg/kg 6-hourly.
- If atypical pneumonia suspected:
  — azithromycin 10 mg/kg (up to 500 mg) PO or IV.

The child with fever (Figure 33.1)

Fever is one of the most common causes of presentation to an ED. Most fevers are due to viral infections, but care must be taken to exclude a bacterial infection. Diagnosis can often be difficult, particularly in the younger child. The febrile child without a clear focus presents a real challenge. In children who are fully immunised the risk of serious bacterial infection is low, although pneumococcal and meningococcal infection are incompletely covered and should always be considered in any child who is unwell. How aggressively to investigate and administer empiric antibiotics is based on risk stratification that takes into account age, signs of

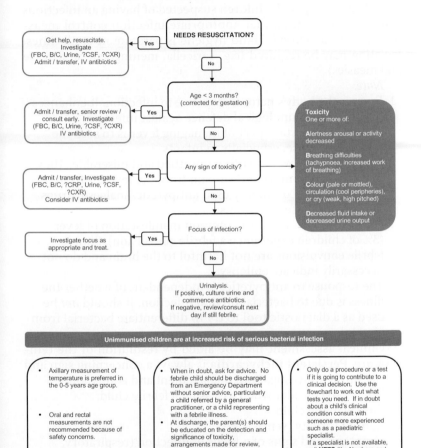

 Infants and Children: Acute Management of Fever, second edition
PD2010_063
Issue date: October 2010 **Review Date:** October 2015

Figure 33.1 Assessment and initial management of children < 5 years old presenting with fever (> 38°C axillary)

toxicity and any focus of infection. When in doubt, err on the side of caution. A number of institutions have implemented paediatric sepsis pathways, though the challenge is finding a tool with a high positive and negative predictive value when the disease has a low prevalence.

When dealing with children suspected of having an infectious disease, it is essential that appropriate infection control measures are implemented. Hand hygiene is paramount at all times. Isolation may be required (e.g. varicella, meningococcal disease and measles).

Note:

1 Fever is the body's natural response to infection. It enhances the child's immunological defence against infection.

2 The most important part of managing fever is to seek the underlying cause, especially in infants.

3 Children with fever are often unsettled and miserable. They may have discomfort and/or pain from the fever or from the cause of fever. Commonly used antipyretic/analgesic drugs may relieve these symptoms.

4 Febrile convulsions are a common manifestation of fever (3% of children experience a febrile convulsion). Simple febrile convulsions are not harmful to the brain and do not necessarily indicate epilepsy.

5 The response to antipyretics is independent of whether the illness is due to bacterial or viral infection. It should *not* be used as a diagnostic tool to try to differentiate bacterial from viral infection.

Clinical assessment may be aided by resolution of the temperature. **Persistent tachycardia** is always a concerning sign and should prompt investigation, management and admission.

Factors to consider when assessing a febrile child:

- the age of the child
- signs of toxicity (sepsis)
- symptoms and signs of a focus of infection (respiratory, meningitis, urinary tract, ears/throat).

Neonates and young infants may not have the characteristic signs of serious infection (the temperature can be high or low) and localising features may be absent. They can deteriorate rapidly. They may be infected with organisms from the birth canal, especially Group B Streptococcal organisms; a history of maternal Group B Streptococcal colonisation and the subsequent administration of antibiotics during labour should be sought.

Febrile children under 1 month of age will need a full septic work-up including lumbar puncture and treatment with empiric intravenous antibiotics. A more risk-stratified approach may be applied to the 1–3 month age group.

Older infants/toddlers localise infection better than neonates, but may still be pre-verbal. They are frequently exposed to infectious diseases in group childcare and get viral infections. The incidence of previously 'typical' bacterial infections (pneumococcus, meningococcus and *Haemophilus influenzae*) has been significantly lessened by immunisation.

IS THE CHILD TOXIC?

Toxicity is a term used to describe the clinical picture produced by the body's response to exotoxins and endotoxins (the lipopolysaccharide cell wall of Gram-negative organisms). It is often difficult to detect. The best approach to evaluating a child for toxicity is to use the 'ABCD' approach:

A is for arousal, alertness and activity.

B is for breathing difficulties.

C is for poor colour (pale/mottled) and poor circulation (cold peripheries, persistent tachycardia).

D is for decreased fluid intake (less than half normal) and decreased urine output (fewer than four wet nappies a day).

Abnormality of any of these signs places the child at higher risk of serious bacterial illness. The presence of more than one sign increases the risk. In communicating a concern about toxicity it is useful to add objective findings such as heart rate and respiratory rate to your ABCD assessment.

INVESTIGATIONS

The decision whether or not to perform investigations is not always simple but is generally dependent on the child's age and the clinical presentation. The 'full septic work-up' includes a full blood count, blood culture, chest X-ray, urine microscopy and culture and lumbar puncture. All children who are toxic with a potential for underlying serious bacterial infection should have a 'full septic work-up' as should very young children, especially those less than 1 month of age. Successful vaccination has led to a marked reduction in cases of bacterial meningitis and lumbar puncture in children is being done less often. It should always be considered in children where there is the possibility of meningitis or where the child is on antibiotics and may have partially treated meningitis. In all cases ensure appropriate observation, review and, if in doubt, seek further consultation. The dilemma of when and where to treat and which antibiotic to use depends on the individual and the local environment. It is better to err on the side of over-investigating and treating particularly when infants are involved.

Children with a definite focus of infection should have specific management of that focus unless they are very young or toxic. Very young and toxic children require empiric antibiotics and a full septic work-up in that order. Remember, in some conditions such as meningococcaemia, delay in the administration of antibiotics may result in a poor clinical outcome.

The most common cause of serious bacterial illness in infants is urinary tract infection and if the child is toxic, consider the possibility of underlying pyelonephritis. An ultrasound examination of the kidneys may be very useful in making the diagnosis and directing treatment.

TREATMENT

Figure 33.1 outlines one possible approach to management of the febrile child. As shown in the figure any child who is toxic requires urgent resuscitation. In particular, they are at risk of septic shock and require urgent attention to prevent circulatory collapse. This involves rapid intravenous or intraosseous access, the delivery of boluses of normal saline or another isotonic crystalloid solution such as Hartmann's solution and perhaps inotropic support. Recent evidence has suggested that a more cautious approach to fluid resuscitation in septic children may be warranted but conclusive recommendations around this are still pending. In such cases, urgent consultation with paediatric specialists and intensivists should be obtained. The child should ultimately be transferred to an appropriate facility to deal with the situation.

Antibiotic choice depends on your patient population and local resistance rates. The antibiotics listed in Table 33.1 are suggested only as a starting point; we strongly recommend you discuss this with a senior colleague, a paediatrician or your infectious disease consultant.

WHAT ELSE COULD IT BE?

Always think of underlying metabolic, cardiac and endocrine problems. A simple viral illness may provoke an acute metabolic decompensation in these patients.

Table 33.1 Empiric antibiotic guidelines

Condition	Age	Antibiotic
Suspected bacterial sepsis (not critically ill)	< 3 months	IV ampicillin 50 mg/kg 6-hourly + IV gentamicin (see local dosing guidelines)
	> 3 months	IV cefotaxime 50 mg/kg up to 2 g, 6-hourly OR IV ceftriaxone 50 mg/kg up to 2 g, 6-hourly
Severe sepsis (sepsis + organ dysfunction)	All ages	IV cefotaxime 50 mg/kg up to 2 g, 6-hourly OR IV ceftriaxone 50 mg/kg up to 2 g, 6-hourly PLUS IV vancomycin (see local dosing guidelines) PLUS IV gentamicin (see local dosing guidelines)
Meningitis (suspected or proven)	< 3 months	IV ampicillin 50 mg/kg (6-hourly age adjust) PLUS IV cefotaxime 50 mg/kg, 6-hourly
	> 3 months	IV cefotaxime 50 mg/kg up to 2 g, 6-hourly OR IV ceftriaxone 50 mg/kg up to 2 g, 6-hourly

Sydney Children's Hospital Network fact sheets, schn.health.nsw.gov.au

PROLONGED FEVER OF UNKNOWN ORIGIN

Most children in whom fever has been prolonged for 7 days or more will be found to have infectious diseases. The most common infection to consider is Epstein–Barr virus infection; however, other viruses may be found as the cause for fever. Autoimmune disorders, Kawasaki disease and malignancy should be considered. In these cases early consultation and hospital admission should be considered.

FOLLOW-UP

All children who are discharged home from the ED with fever should be followed up the next day in an acute review clinic, the ED or by the family doctor. This is to detect progression of infection, response to treatment and results of investigations.

Parents should be provided with a fact sheet and encouraged to look for signs of toxicity every 4–6 hours, and to seek clinical review if the child becomes toxic or unwell. Clear communication from a doctor with empathy for the parents may enhance safety and improve the functioning of stressed families.

COMMON INFECTIONS

Consider the following.

- Preschool children normally experience 6–8 URTIs per annum.
- Antibiotics neither cure viral URTIs nor prevent complications.
- Exclude common and dangerous causes:
  — otitis media
  — tonsillitis
  — bronchiolitis
  — pneumonia
  — meningitis
  — urinary tract infection.
- Decongestants and antihistamines are of dubious value.
- Take an immunisation history.
- Paediatric symptoms are often non-specific—fever, diarrhoea, off feeds etc.

The common exanthemata (measles, rubella/German measles, varicella, scarlet fever, erythema infectiosum and roseola infantum) are not always easy to diagnose, and may have significant morbidity and mortality. You should be familiar with the classic presentations. If in doubt, consult.

The use of paracetamol in febrile illnesses is controversial (fever has an active role in the anti-infection cascade). Vigorous control of fever will not necessarily prevent febrile convulsions. Fever control may be of assistance in a child who is in obvious discomfort in whom the fever exceeds 38.5°C (> 38.0°C axillary). Remember there is a real risk of hepatotoxicity with paracetamol overdose so limit the daily dosage to 60 mg/kg (maximum 3 g/day) and do not use for more than 72 hours. If fever is persistent, the child should be reassessed.

Aspirin for the management of fever is contraindicated in childhood.

The child with abdominal pain

Abdominal pain may be difficult to assess in a young child. Examination requires a general, gentle approach and warm hands to gain the child's trust. Often, asking the child to take deep breaths, move or even palpate their own abdomen will provide invaluable clues. Consider analgesia to aid examination.

INTUSSUSCEPTION

Intussusception classically presents in the 6 months to 3-year-old age group. It frequently follows a minor viral illness, where a lymphoid follicle in the terminal ileum gets carried into the colon, dragging mesentery with it. This is what forms the 'sausage-shaped' mass in the right upper quadrant. The affected bowel becomes oedematous, obstructed and, over the following hours, can become ischaemic and perforate.

The clinical features of early intussusception can be very similar to other more benign illnesses such as gastroenteritis or constipation, leading to missed or delayed diagnosis which can be life-threatening. Intussusception should always be considered as a differential diagnosis in young children who have abdominal symptoms, unexplained distress or lethargy.

Typical presentation features are intermittent abdominal pain causing screaming, pallor and vomiting, usually without diarrhoea. Increasing lethargy develops between exacerbations of pain. The abdomen can be tender and the sausage-shaped mass may be palpable in the right upper quadrant. Blood in the stools and shock are traditionally considered late presentations, but may occur surprisingly early. X-ray is not routinely done but may reveal an area of paucity of gas or obstruction. Abdominal ultrasound is diagnostic.

Treatment involves air enema reduction under surgical supervision and radiological visualisation. Cases that present late or may have perforation require reduction (and repair) in theatre.

APPENDICITIS

Appendicitis can occur at any age but is rare under 5 years. Up to 50% of younger children will not present with the classic signs and symptoms of anorexia, fever, poor appetite and right iliac fossa pain and tenderness. They often have a short history (< 24 hours). Children under 3 years often present with perforation. Retrocaecal and pelvic appendicitis can also be difficult to diagnose. Diarrhoea can be seen with a pelvic appendicitis and can distract clinicians away from the diagnosis. Having said that, careful clinical history and thorough clinical examination employing observation, documentation of objective signs and an opportunistic approach are the cornerstone to diagnosis. Remember to elicit the obturator (pelvic appendicitis) and psoas (retrocaecal appendicitis) signs. Observing the child's ability to walk, hop or jump on the spot can be useful. Blood work including WCC and CRP are of limited diagnostic value, especially with a short history but can help in uncertain cases. Abdominal ultrasound can be useful and may show an inflamed, enlarged (> 6 mm), non-compressible appendix or free fluid. Definitive treatment is surgical excision, though a more conservative approach using intravenous antibiotics is currently being investigated.

INGUINAL HERNIAS

Inguinal hernias are common in the first year of life and need early correction as they are liable to become incarcerated. Surgical referral should be made at the time of diagnosis. Gentle reduction using analgesia is often possible in the ED. If the hernia is irreducible, urgent surgical review is indicated.

HIRSCHSPRUNG DISEASE

Hirschsprung disease is absence of intramural ganglion cells, usually in the rectosigmoid region. It is four times more common in males. It presents early in life with increasing constipation and abdominal distension from the newborn period to early childhood. Absent passage of meconium in the first 24 hours after birth can suggest the diagnosis. Rectal examination often reveals explosive release of stool under pressure. Abdominal X-ray shows faecal loading. The complications are enterocolitis and perforation. Definitive diagnosis involves a bowel biopsy and treatment is surgical resection of the aganglionic segment.

TESTICULAR TORSION

Abdominal pain should always prompt examination of the genital area.

Testicular torsion is a surgical emergency as the compromised blood flow can result in ischaemia and loss of the testicle. Classical features are:

1 sudden onset of unilateral scrotal pain
2 nausea and vomiting
3 elevated and horizontal lie of the affected testis
4 absent cremasteric reflex on the affected side.

The diagnosis can be difficult to make due to complicating factors such as the presence of a secondary hydrocele, prior episodes of torting and detorting, or torsion that has occurred following trauma. Torsion of a testicular or epididymal appendage can be difficult to distinguish from torsion of the testis. Scrotal ultrasound is unhelpful and may only delay surgical exploration. Urgent surgical assessment is indicated.

The child with vomiting
PYLORIC STENOSIS

Pyloric stenosis occurs from 1 week to 3 months of age, with males four times more commonly affected than females. They present with increasing vomiting, dehydration and hypokalaemia, with a hypochloraemic metabolic alkalosis. A pyloric mass can often be felt, particularly at the end of a test feed; ultrasound or barium meal can confirm this. The child needs IV fluids and operative treatment after the electrolyte imbalance has been corrected.

INTESTINAL MALROTATION

Bile-stained vomit is always concerning for intestinal malrotation leading to midgut volvulus. It most commonly presents in the neonate. There may be no other signs in the early stage but urgent surgical consultation is indicated as the twisted intestine may become gangrenous within 6 hours.

GASTROENTERITIS

Gastroenteritis is a common childhood complaint, the commonest complication of which is dehydration. Most cases will be viral. Bloody diarrhoea often suggests a bacterial cause.

Organisms to consider include:

- viruses—rotavirus, enteroviruses, enteric adenovirus, Norwalk (norovirus)
- bacteria—*Salmonella*, *Shigella*, *Campylobacter*, *Yersinia*, *E. coli*
- protozoa—*Giardia*, amoebae.

Clinical manifestations include vomiting, diarrhoea, fever and abdominal pain. The diarrhoea with rotavirus and adenoviruses often lasts for 5–12 days, and that of bacterial diarrhoea (especially *Campylobacter*) is often bloodstained. *Giardia* infection commonly causes an epidemic and is complicated by asymptomatic carriers. Beware of attributing vomiting without diarrhoea to gastroenteritis.

ASSESSMENT

Assessment should include: 1. confirmation of the diagnosis and exclusion of differential diagnoses; and 2. determination of the degree of dehydration. Evidence of sepsis is important, especially in the young infant. Of children under 3 months of age with *Salmonella*, 5–10% are bacteraemic. *Salmonella* can also cause focal infections in children with sickle cell anaemia. Abdominal X-ray commonly shows multiple fluid levels representing ileus: it is rarely helpful unless obstruction is suspected. Stool culture is advisable when bacterial or parasitic infections are suspected.

Signs of dehydration

Signs of dehydration can become more evident with the extent of fluid imbalance, but are altered in hypernatraemia. Percentages of fluid loss give a guide to the rate at which fluids need to be given, but frequent reassessment of the child's fluid state is vital.

- Mild dehydration:
  — 3% dehydration manifests with reduced urine output and thirst but no clinical signs.
- Moderate dehydration
  — 5% presents with sunken eyes, dry mucous membranes and reduced skin turgor
  — 7% manifests with a more severe presentation of the above signs and irritability, lethargy and tachycardia.
- Severe dehydration:
  — 10% presents with marked lethargy, irritability and even coma, plus cardiovascular compromise with tachycardia, hypotension, coldness and sweating.

These signs are difficult to appreciate at times and even experienced clinicians are only able to determine mild/moderate/severe dehydration rather than percentages. Serial weights performed on the same set of scales without the contribution of clothing/nappies are accurate but rarely available.

What else could it be?

- Surgical conditions
  — Intussusception
  — Appendicitis
- Infections
  — Urinary tract infection
  — Sepsis, otitis media
  — Haemolytic uraemic syndrome:
    ° an uncommon condition is the presenting usually 5–10 days after gastroenteritis, caused by enteropathic *E. coli*
    ° can also occur after URTI
    ° manifest by microangiopathic haemolysis, low platelets, raised urea, poor urine output, hypertension and renal failure
- Diabetic ketoacidosis
- Metabolic disorders
- Head injury (raised intracranial pressure)

TREATMENT

Rehydration via the oral route is the best route to provide fluids for children. Try oral rehydration solution in small frequent sips at a rate of 1 mL/kg every 10 minutes. Dispensing by oral syringe is often effective where a child does not wish to drink. Oral rehydration ice preparations are available and may be more readily accepted by children.

Ondansetron has been demonstrated to decrease the chance of vomiting with rehydration in gastroenteritis. A single dose may be given as a therapeutic trial. Other antiemetics which may cause dystonic reaction are generally avoided, especially in small children.

If this fails, commence nasogastric tube rehydration with an oral rehydration solution. If this is not tolerated, commence IV rehydration, remembering to check the glucose and sodium levels. Daily volumes to replace the fluid deficit and volumes for maintenance requirements should be calculated separately, added together then divided by 24 to get the hourly rate (see section on fluid therapy).

Frequent reassessment to monitor progress is important.

Antibiotics (third-generation cephalosporins) are recommended for *Salmonella* in the young septic infant, those with a prolonged severe course of illness or with documented typhoid infection (***Salmonella typhi***). Otherwise they do not convey any benefit as they do not shorten the course or reduce the infectivity of the patient with *Salmonella*. *Campylobacter* infection should be treated with azithromycin or ciprofloxacin only if the symptoms are prolonged. *Giardia* infection causing symptoms should be treated with metronidazole.

WHEN NOT TO TREAT AT HOME

- Dehydration
- Diagnosis in doubt
- Family not coping
- Persistent vomiting
- No consultation available
- Deterioration
- Anticipated deterioration
  Think again if:
- vomiting bile or blood

- severe abdominal pain
- toxic, high fever
- abdominal signs: distension; tenderness, guarding; mass, visceromegaly
- neonates
- failure to thrive.

FLUID THERAPY

Children can rapidly become dehydrated because of their small size and large, insensible fluid loss (they have a high surface-area-to-volume ratio). The aim of fluid therapy is to continue maintenance fluid intake and replace fluid in the dehydrated child. Common causes of fluid loss are gastroenteritis, fever, blood loss and poor oral intake in respiratory distress.

Maintenance fluids

- Maintenance fluids can be estimated using:
  — 100 mL/kg for the first 10 kg
  — 50 mL/kg for the next 10 kg
  — 20 mL/kg for every subsequent kg.
- Maintenance fluids should be 0.9% saline + 5% dextrose or similar isotonic fluid.
- Potassium 20 mmol per 500 mL can be added for ongoing maintenance fluids as long as the potassium is in the normal range, renal function is normal and the child is passing urine.

Rehydration

Acute resuscitation of the child with cardiovascular compromise (i.e. shock) should include a bolus of 20 mL/kg of crystalloid fluid such as 0.9% sodium chloride or Hartmann's solution. Recent evidence has suggested a more cautious approach to fluid resuscitation in septic or severely dehydrated children may be warranted but conclusive recommendations around this are still pending. Hypotonic solutions such as half normal (0.45%) and quarter normal (0.225%) saline should *not* be used for resuscitation and never be given as a bolus.

Once shock has been addressed, rehydration can commence in a slower, controlled fashion. Most centres have moved away from low-sodium-containing fluids for rehydration and use 0.9% sodium chloride + glucose 5% or similar isotonic preparation.

Volume required to replace the fluid deficit can be estimated using:

$$\% \text{ dehydration} \times \text{weight} \times 10 = \text{total deficit in mL}$$
(replace over 24–48 hours, don't replace > 5% over a 24-hour period)

Remember:
- serum electrolytes, urea, creatinine should be checked if rehydrating intravenously
- reassess the child clinically and monitor the urine output to see if the fluid therapy is appropriate.

The child with diabetic ketoacidosis (DKA)

DKA may be the presentation for first diagnosis of type 1 diabetes. In patients with known type 1 diabetes, DKA is the result of increased insulin requirement or failure of insulin delivery.

PRESENTATION
- Polyuria
- Polydipsia
- Nausea/vomiting
- Abdominal pain
- Fatigue
- Weight loss
- Hyperventilation (Kussmaul breathing)
- Altered mental state, confusion
- Dehydration and shock

COMMON MISDIAGNOSES
Beware of the following common misdiagnoses:
- hyperventilation misdiagnosed as a chest infection
- polyuria misdiagnosed as urinary tract infection
- nausea and vomiting misdiagnosed as gastroenteritis.

DIAGNOSIS
- Diagnosis of DKA:
  — blood glucose > 11 mmol/L and
  — venous pH < 7.3 or bicarbonate < 15 mmol and

— ketonaemia or ketonuria.
- Other tests include UEC, CMP (calcium, magnesium, phosphate), BSL, VBG, osmolality.
- First diagnosis type 1 diabetes will need further tests (coeliac screen, antibodies, thyroid testing).
- Other tests may be needed according to intercurrent illness or precipitant.
- Don't forget to correct the serum sodium for the hyperglycaemia.

corrected Na = measured Na + (BSL − 5.5) / 3

MANAGEMENT

This is a guide and not a substitute for local hospital guidelines.

1. Fluid resuscitation

Children with DKA are usually dehydrated. It is often difficult to estimate the percentage of dehydration due to fluid shifts and osmotic diuresis. The dehydration has usually occurred over days and involves compensatory fluid and electrolyte shifts and losses. It can be deleterious to try to correct this too quickly. In general it is safe to aim to correct a 3–5% deficit over 48 hours using 0.9% sodium chloride or Plasma-Lyte 148.

Fluid boluses should be reserved for children with reduced perfusion and shock. Tachycardia is often due to acidosis rather than shock, so look for prolonged capillary refill time and/or a thready pulse.

Use 0.9% sodium chloride 10 mL/kg and reassess the need for another. It is rare to need more than two boluses, so consult widely before administering a third.

Do not give potassium in the fluid bolus.

2. Potassium management

Children with DKA usually have a total body depletion of potassium, even though the serum potassium may be normal or elevated. This is due to extracellular shift of potassium in the acidotic, insulin-depleted state. Administration of insulin can cause rapid shift of potassium into cells with a precipitous fall in serum potassium that can be life-threatening.

K needs to be checked at least hourly in the initial stages.

If there is renal impairment, consult early with endocrinology before administering potassium.

K < 3.5 mmol/L

Start maintenance fluids + KCl 40 mmol/L

Wait until K is up to normal range before starting insulin infusion.

K 3.5–5.0 mmol/L

Start maintenance fluids + KCl 40 mmol/L

Insulin infusion commences after an hour of IV fluids.

K > 5.0 mmol/L

Commence insulin infusion.

Commence maintenance fluids without potassium until K < 5.0 mmol/L.

If K > 7.0 mmol/L with ECG changes—give 10% calcium gluconate 0.5 mL/kg over 3–5 minutes.

3. Insulin

Insulin needs to be given as an intravenous infusion of Actrapid insulin.

There is no reason to start with an insulin bolus; in fact, it is worth waiting until after an hour of IV fluid resuscitation before commencing the insulin infusion. Some endocrinologists may elect to start with subcutaneous insulin in mild cases or where acidosis is not present.

Infusion rate can commence at 0.05–0.1 units/kg/h.

Blood sugar level needs to be checked hourly.

Add glucose 5% to maintenance fluids once BSL < 15 mmol/L.

Higher glucose concentrations may be required to maintain BSL 5–10 mmol/L; continued glucose and insulin administration is still required to clear the ketones.

Hypoglycaemia (< 4.0 mmol/L) should be treated by stopping the insulin infusion for 30 minutes, giving a 2 mL/kg IV bolus glucose 10% then restarting the insulin infusion at half the previous rate.

4. Precipitant

In an established stable type 1 diabetic, there must be a reason that they have developed DKA. They either have an increased insulin requirement or insulin deficit. Increased insulin requirement can be from intercurrent illness. The most common reason, however, is a failure of insulin delivery through non-compliance or insulin pump failure. These need to be addressed.

5. Complications
Cerebral oedema
Raised intracranial pressure from cerebral oedema is a sudden and unpredictable complication of DKA. It usually occurs in the first 24 hours of treatment. The onset of headache in DKA patients may herald the onset.

Increased risk is associated with:
- severe dehydration
- severe acidosis with low potassium
- hypernatraemia
- deteriorating conscious state
- severe hyperosmolality on presentation (> 320 mosm/L).

Management
- Elevate the head of bed to 30°.
- Reduce IV fluid rate by at least one-third.
- Administer mannitol 1 g/kg IV over 10 minutes.
- An alternative to mannitol is 3% saline 5 mL/kg over 10 minutes.
- Intubation and hyperventilation may be required.
- Involve PICU as early as possible.

The child with seizure

Seizures are common in children. Most seizures are associated with a fever in young children, or mild head injury. Most seizures are brief and self-terminating. If the seizure continues beyond 5 minutes, it may not stop spontaneously. If the child arrives in the ED with ongoing seizure, it can be assumed to be a prolonged seizure, and efforts to terminate the seizure should be undertaken without delay. Phenytoin has been the mainstay of second-line treatment for status epilepticus in children and at time of publishing remains so; however, large multicentre randomised trials from Australia/New Zealand, the United Kingdom and the United States are currently being analysed comparing the effectiveness of alternative agents such as levetiracetam.

MANAGEMENT OF ONGOING SEIZURE

- Maintain the airway.
- Apply high-flow oxygen via face mask with reservoir.
- Check BSL: if BSL < 3.0 mmol/L, give 2 mL/kg IV glucose 10%.
- Midazolam 0.15 mg/kg IV
  OR
- Midazolam 0.3 mg/kg intranasal/buccal if no IV access.
- If still fitting after 5 minutes post midazolam give second dose.
- If still fitting after 5 minutes post second dose midazolam:
  — obtain intraosseous access if still unable to get IV access and give:
    ○ IV phenytoin 20 mg/kg (max 1.5 g) over 20 minutes
      OR
    ○ *levetiracetam 20–40 mg/kg (evidence pending).*
- If seizure is ongoing despite these measures, involvement of ICU/anaesthetics/paediatrics/emergency senior staff is required.

The most common cause of fits in children is febrile seizures which are benign. Febrile seizures have the following characteristics:

- age 6 months to 5 years
- fever > 38°C
- absence of CNS infection or inflammation
- absence of metabolic abnormality that might produce seizure
- no history of afebrile seizures.

Simple febrile convulsion:

- generalised (not focal)
- short duration, less than 10 minutes (most < 5 minutes)
- single, isolated seizure in a 24-hour period, usually 1 per illness.

Complex febrile convulsion:

- may have focal onset
- may last > 10 minutes
- may occur more than once in a 24-hour period.

Differential diagnoses to always consider:

- meningitis
- encephalitis
- head injury
- toxic ingestion

- electrolyte disturbance
- metabolic disorder
- afebrile seizure.

The child with a rash

Parents commonly present to emergency with concern about a rash. It is not expected that you will be able to 'spot diagnose' every rash that presents to the ED but it is useful to be familiar with some of the common viral exanthemata of childhood. An approach employed by the authors is as follows.

1 Apart from the rash, what else are the carers worried about? For example, a febrile, lethargic and listless child who is clinically tachycardic and dehydrated is very different from a well, alert, interactive, child whose only concern is the rash.

2 Is this a 'killer rash'? Actively exclude the following concerning diagnoses.

   a Meningococcal sepsis: child is usually unwell, rash may start as blanching maculopapular, but rapidly progresses to petechiae and purpura. The child will be febrile, unwell and tachycardic. If there is concern about this diagnosis, have a low threshold to investigation (meningococcal PCR) and treat (ceftriaxone IV).

   b Kawasaki disease: this is an autoimmune disease that can lead to coronary artery aneurysms. Key diagnostic features are fever for five days, erythematous rash, lymphadenopathy, oral mucosal changes and conjunctivitis with peri-limbic sparing. Peeling of the skin of the fingers may occur later. Thrombocytosis may be seen on bloods. Treatment is with admission for intravenous immunoglobulin (IVIg) and high-dose aspirin under a paediatrician.

   c Stevens-Johnson syndrome/toxic epidermal necrolysis: a spectrum of disease triggered by medication or infections that causes a severe rash with mucosal ulceration. It is thought to be an immune reaction and is a medical emergency. Therapy is largely supportive with differing practice in regard to immune-modulating therapy such as steroids and IVIg.

   d Staphylococcal scalded skin syndrome: caused by *S. aureus* exotoxins that cause epidermal detachment leading to painful erythroderma and fluid-filled blisters with desquamation. Treatment involves antibiotics and supportive care.

3 Is this a classic viral exanthem of childhood? These include the following.

a Measles: cephalocaudal spread of erythematous macular rash with cough, conjunctivitis and coryza. The child may be unimmunised and have a known contact.

b Rubella: similar to measles with cephalocaudal spread of rash, not as unwell looking as children with measles.

c Scarlet fever: caused by group A streptococcus, features include sandpaper rash, circumoral pallor and strawberry tongue. The most common site of infection is the throat but remember to check for other sources including perianal streptococcal infection.

d Parvovirus B19 (slapped cheek syndrome or 'fifth disease'): classic erythematous rash on cheek (stage 1), followed by spread to trunk and proximal extremities (stage 2), then central clearing of the macular lesions leading to a lacy reticular rash (stage 3); low-grade fever and URTI in prodromal phase but afebrile with rash. Isolation from school is unnecessary.

e Human herpes virus 6/roseola: high fevers with no source found which usually resolves by 72 hours (but may last up to 6 days). Rash appears after defervescence and lasts 1–3 days.

f Chickenpox/varicella: coryzal prodrome followed by typical vesicular rash. Immunised children may have a more attenuated illness with low-grade temperature and occasional vesicles.

g Hand-foot-and-mouth disease; coxsackie and other enteroviruses: febrile prodrome followed by maculopapular and blistering rash around mouth, in nappy distribution and on palms and soles. Accompanied by pharyngitis and oral ulcers, usually at the back of the throat.

h Herpes gingivostomatitis: high fevers, vesicular stomatitis with gingivitis and oral ulcers with drooling. Consider treatment with antiviral medication (valaciclovir 20 mg/kg/dose tds for 7 days) if detected within 72 hours.

4 Is this a vasculitic rash? Cutaneous vasculitis can have many different causes and presentations. Only a minority of cases are associated with a systemic vasculitis. Henoch-Schönlein purpura is an example of a vasculitic rash associated with systemic illness. These children have 'palpable purpura' usually on dependent areas and lower extremities. It may be associated with nephritis and abdominal pain.

5 Is this an inflammatory rash such as dermatitis or eczema?

6 Is this a birthmark or vascular malformation?

Common causes of neonatal rash (https://www.aafp.org/afp/2008/0101/p47.html) are:

1 Erythema toxicum neonatorum: most common pustular rash in newborns, appears during second or third day with small papules surrounded by erythema; fades over a week but may recur.

2 Cutis marmorata: mottling of the skin in response to cold in an otherwise well newborn.

3 Harlequin colour change: dependent erythema with contralateral blanching that lasts for 30 seconds to 2 minutes.

4 Transient neonatal pustular melanosis: similar to erythema toxicum but with no surrounding erythema, vesicopustular, may have pigmented macules, affects all parts of the body including palms and soles.

5 Acne neonatorum: comedones on the forehead, nose and cheek; usually resolves spontaneously without scarring within months.

6 Milia: small white papules on the face but may occur in other areas; usually resolves spontaneously in the first few months.

7 Miliaria: also appears in the first month but more vesicular (small, 1–2 mm), and vesicles rupture with desquamation; resolves in hours to days.

8 'Cradle cap': sebhorrhoeic dermatitis involving the scalp but may also involve face and neck, and can be similar to atopic dermatitis; usually self-limiting but treatment options involve emollients and tar-containing shampoos.

The limping child

The most common reason for a child to limp is as a result of injury. Usually the history and physical examination +/− imaging make diagnosis straightforward. Sometimes trauma can be occult or concealed. Seemingly minor trauma can cause an injury such as a toddler's fracture. The child may have fallen because they have a limp for a non-traumatic reason.

Most children that present to the ED with a non traumatic limp have a benign cause and the most common of these is transient synovitis of the hip.

TRANSIENT SYNOVITIS 'IRRITABLE HIP'

- Usually affects children in the 3–10 age group.
- Around half will have had an URTI in the last 1–2 weeks.
- The child looks well and is afebrile or has a low-grade temperature.
- Partial weight-bearing is usually possible.
- There is obvious discomfort with internal and external rotation of the hip.
- Alternative diagnoses should always be considered.
- Most of these children do not require investigation if they present in the first 24–48 hours and can be safely managed with ibuprofen, rest and GP follow-up.

  Diagnoses to always consider are as follows.

1 Trauma
   — History of trauma may be unclear, misleading or coincidental.
   — Toddler's fractures can occur after seemingly minor trauma.
   — Non-accidental injury may have occurred.
   — Plain X-ray is useful to detect most fractures.

2 Septic arthritis
   — Factors that increase the likelihood of septic arthritis, as opposed to transient synovitis, are:
     ◦ temperature $> 38.5°C$
     ◦ refusal to weight-bear at all
     ◦ elevated CRP, ESR > 40 mm/h and/or WCC $> 12 \times 10^9$/L.

3 Osteomyelitis
   — Subtle signs can make diagnosis difficult.
   — Constitutional symptoms may be present.

— Localised bone tenderness and/or warmth over infection.
— Raised inflammatory markers sensitive but not specific.
4 Malignancy
— Haematological malignancies can cause bone and joint pain.
— There may be other signs or symptoms of pallor or bruising.
— FBC usually helps to make this diagnosis.
5 Inguinoscrotal cause (appendicitis, testicular torsion)
— Usually detected by a complete physical examination.
6 Legg-Calvé-Perthes disease (avascular necrosis of the femoral head)
— Affects predominantly boys and in the 4–8 years age group.
— Usually mild, dull, chronic pain.
— Restricted range of hip movement due to synovial hypertrophy.
— X-ray is usually diagnostic but may be normal early in the disease.
— Some children will require a bone scan or MRI.
7 Slipped upper femoral epiphysis (SUFE)
— Occurs in the adolescence 9–16 years age range.
— Associated with obesity.
— May have a history of trauma.
— Plain X-ray usually diagnostic.

The baby with jaundice

Mild jaundice is common in neonates as they have a high red cell turnover and reduced hepatic clearance of bilirubin. 'Physiological' unconjugated bilirubin levels usually reach a peak at day 3 and resolve over 1–2 weeks. This is usually benign but high levels can cross the blood–brain barrier and cause bilirubin-induced neurological dysfunction (BIND).

Jaundice in the first 24 hours of life:
• not physiological and requires urgent medical review
• suggests haemolysis from ABO/Rh incompatibility.

Jaundice that is noticed on day 2–4 is usually physiological and benign as long as:
• jaundice is mild and confined to head, neck and upper trunk

- not low birth weight or premature
- baby is well
- baby is passing normal coloured urine and stool
- there are no other abnormalities.

If these criteria are not met, measure serum bilirubin (SBR) (un/conjugated).

Measured SBR should be plotted on the appropriate graph for gestational age to determine thresholds for phototherapy and exchange transfusion. If the child is dehydrated from poor feeding or unwell from sepsis, these issues also need to be addressed.

Prolonged jaundice (jaundice > 14 days):

- should be investigated
- measure conjugated and unconjugated
- conjugated bilirubin > 20 micromol/L or > 20% of total SBR is abnormal and should be investigated urgently.

Physiological jaundice (slow maturation of glucuronyl transferase among other factors) and 'breast milk' jaundice (competitive use of glucuronyl transferase) should be considered diagnoses of exclusion; they are not diagnoses of convenience. Continue to monitor the child and/or arrange for follow-up until either a cause is found or the jaundice disappears.

The unsettled crying baby
FEEDING

Feeding problems can be the result of any illness from a cold to congestive cardiac failure. They can also be due to difficulties with attachment, maternal milk supply and oral anatomy.

History and examination are paramount to: 1. elucidate a cause (infection, surgical condition, etc.); or 2. assess effect (weight loss, dehydration etc.).

It is important to be familiar with basic feeding practices and to be able to support a breastfeeding mother through a crisis when her child is unwell. Milk allergies and intolerances are not common. Resist changing milk formulas for the lack of better inspiration. Rather than give inappropriate advice, refer the infant and mother to their local doctor, paediatrician, community health centre or, in some instances, an appropriate mothercraft centre.

THE INCONSOLABLE INFANT

These families often present at night. Listen to the parents. Don't be dismissive—they are at the end of their tether, sometimes dangerously so for the child. Occasionally, a potentially serious cause may be found. Remember that if the child is not sleeping, the parents are usually not sleeping either.

Consider physical causes of pain and discomfort, especially treatable conditions such as:

• intussusception/malrotation volvulus
• otitis media
• dental problems (rarely 'teething')
• hair tourniquets (check toes and fingers)
• peptic ulceration (oesophagitis secondary to clinical reflux)
• missed fractures (intentional or accidental)
• stones—renal/gall bladder
• infection (paradoxically, sepsis often leads to quietening)
• ischaemic heart disease (anomalous coronary arteries—rare).

There is a group of children (infants) for whom no physical cause can be elucidated. Their parents require immense support.

Consider admission if:

• there is a physical condition to treat
• children are at risk from tired, frustrated carers.

Always acknowledge carers' concerns and frustrations. This often resolves 50% of problems. Ensure adequate, appropriate, definitive and close follow-up if you intend sending the child home.

Trauma in children
MAJOR TRAUMA

The priorities for assessing and managing paediatric trauma patients are the same as for adult trauma patients. A systematic ABC approach is required.

Drug doses and equipment sizes need to be adjusted for the size of the child.

The child's airway is smaller so can obstruct more easily. Children have a higher rate of oxygen consumption and less oxygen reserve, so children can desaturate faster than adults.

Children have a soft, pliable chest wall. This means that blunt chest trauma in children is more likely to result in lung contusion than rib fracture. This is important to keep in mind, as the absence of rib fractures does not exclude significant lung injury. Likewise, if rib fractures are present, then there was a large force involved in the trauma.

Children will vigorously defend their circulation by increasing their heart rate and vasoconstricting peripherally. This occurs long before the child becomes hypotensive. A child may have lost a lot of blood and still have a 'normal' blood pressure, albeit with a narrow pulse pressure, but they will have poor capillary refill and be tachycardic. Hypotension is a late sign.

Abdominal viscera have less protection in children compared with adults because the child's rib cage does not extend as distally and the abdominal wall is thinner.

Mild head injuries are common. Children are more likely to vomit or even have a brief seizure at the time of a mild head injury, even when the head injury is relatively benign. These are features of concussion, and these children should at least have a period of observation with clear verbal and written discharge advice.

Persistent vomiting, prolonged or delayed seizure, headache, abnormal behaviour, signs of skull fracture or neurological deficit are all features that suggest a CT head is indicated and senior staff should be involved. Skull X-ray and head ultrasound are unhelpful, as though they may show a skull fracture, they do not determine the need for neurological intervention.

Head injury decision rules such as CHALICE (see Medcalc. com) or those contained in the NSW Paediatric Head Injury Clinical Practice Guidelines can help with risk stratification and decisions around observation and imaging (Table 33.2).

With a greater surface area relative to their mass, children can lose heat easily. It is much easier to keep a child warm than to have to actively warm them, so measures need to be taken early to prevent heat loss.

Imaging the paediatric trauma patient involves a higher risk-to-benefit ratio than in adults because there are greater long-term consequences from any radiation exposure. This needs to be weighed sensibly against the need to detect important injuries.

Table 33.2 Injury risk stratification

	Low risk (all features)	Intermediate risk (any feature / not low or high risk)	High risk (any feature)
History			
Witnessed loss of consciousness	Nil	< 5 minutes	> 5 minutes
Anterograde or retrograde amnesia	Nil	Possible	> 5 minutes
Behaviour	Normal	Mild agitation or altered behaviour	Abnormal or drowsiness
Vomiting without other cause	Nil or 1	2 or persistent nausea	3 or more
Seizure in non-epileptic patient	Nil	Impact only	Yes
Non-accidental injury (NAI) suspected	Normal	No	Yes
Headache	Nil	Persistent	Persistent
Co-morbidities	Nil	Present	Present
Age	> 1 year	< 1 year	Any
Mechanism			
MVC (pedestrian, occupation or cyclist)	Low speed	< 60 km/h	> 60 km/h
Fall	< 1 m	1–3 m	> 3 m
Force	Low impact	Moderate impact or unclear mechanism	High-speed projectile or object
Examination			
Glasgow Coma Scale (GCS)	15	14–15 (fluctuating)	< 14 or < 15 if under 1 year old
Focal neuro abnormality	Nil	Nil	Present

Continued

Table 33.2   Injury risk stratification (cont.)

	Low risk (all features)	Intermediate risk (any feature / not low or high risk)	High risk (any feature)
Injury			*High-risk feature (e.g. scalp haematoma in < 1 year of age [see below])

* *High-risk injury:* a) penetrating injury, or suspected depressed skull fracture or base of skull fracture; b) scalp bruise, swelling or laceration > 5 cm, or tense fontanel in infants < 1 year of age.

Placement			
Observation area	Anywhere in ED	Acute area in ED	Acute (obs area) or resus bay

Observations			
• Respiratory rate / sats • Pulse/BP • Temp • GCS, pupillary response & size, limb strength • Pain assessment • Sedation score	Hourly observations until discharge	Half-hourly obs for 4–6 hours until GCS 15 sustained for 2 hours then hourly obs till discharge **Revert to half-hourly obs/ continuous monitoring if signs of deterioration occur.**	• Continuous cardio-resp and sats monitoring • BP and GCS every 15–30 minutes

Taken from the NSW Paediatric Head Injury CPG based on CHALICE.

ORTHOPAEDIC TRAUMA

The patterns of fractures in children relate to the developing bone structure and vulnerable growth plates. As ligaments tend to be the stronger component in the paediatric skeleton, fractures occur more readily than 'sprains'.

Paediatric bone can bow, buckle or greenstick fracture as well as fracture completely. These types of fractures can be subtle on X-ray and need to be deliberately sought.

Paediatric bone is growing, and cartilaginous areas are becoming ossified. Paediatric X-rays show growth plates and ossification centres. These change with the age of the child. Growth plates can be mistaken for fractures, or the fracture may involve the growth plate. An ossification centre that has shifted may be an indication of a fracture. If unfamiliar with what is a normal X-ray in a child at a given age, use references and consult senior colleagues.

Fractures that involve the growth plate are best described using the Salter-Harris classification:

Salter-Harris 1	S	Separated/slipped growth plate fracture
Salter-Harris 2	A	Above towards metaphysis
Salter-Harris 3	L	Lower involving articular surface
Salter-Harris 4	T	Through growth plate to articular surface
Salter-Harris 5	ER	Rammed/compression of growth plate

Radial head subluxation, or 'pulled elbow', is a common injury in the 1–4 years age group. It can occur from a common simple event such as a toddler falling over while an adult is holding their hand. Alternatively, there may be no history of a 'pull', just sudden distress in the child and not using one arm. Often, the radial head can be easily relocated at triage. Pronation and supination with the elbow flexed to 90° ('supination/flexion manoeuvre') results in a click that can be felt over the radial head. Another option is to cup the elbow with the thumb placed over the radial head, and to fully pronate ('hyper-pronation manoeuvre').

Forearm fractures are common in children. If it is a simple buckle fracture, it can be safely managed with a forearm splint and follow-up with the GP.

Supracondylar fractures are a common injury in children when they fall onto an outstretched hand. An elbow effusion may be palpable and seen on X-ray as an enlarged anterior or a posterior fat pad. A posterior fat pad is always abnormal. If undisplaced, the fracture may not be seen. The presence of an elbow effusion is a sign of a fracture, and management is immobilisation with follow-up in a fracture clinic. Displaced supracondylar fractures should be discussed with an ED senior or orthopaedic service.

The toddler fracture is a non-displaced tibial shaft fracture that results from a rotational force in the fall-prone toddler. It presents as non-weight bearing in that leg and tenderness may be elicited in the tibia. The X-ray may look normal. If the diagnosis is unclear, other differentials need to be considered as for a child with a limp. Management is backslab immobilisation with fracture clinic follow-up with repeat X-ray in 10 days.

Non-accidental injury

Whenever a child presents to the ED, consideration must be given to the social circumstances in which they live. Every child should be living in an environment where they thrive because they are safe, well cared for, nurtured and loved. ED presentation may be an opportunity to recognise a family under stress and provide much needed support, or link the family in with community support services.

Non-accidental injury of children occurs in families from all cultural and economic groups. Sometimes it is obvious that non-accidental injury has occurred. Unfortunately, non-accidental injury of children can also be insidious. The following are some features in history and examination that increase the likelihood that non-accidental injury may be occurring.

FEATURES IN HISTORY

- Inadequately explained delay in seeking medical attention
- Injuries not consistent with mechanism described or developmental stage of child
- The explanation for the injury varies significantly
- Multiple presentations to different healthcare services seeking medical attention

EXAMINATION

- Multiple injuries at different stages of healing
- Bruising in mouth, ears, inner aspects of upper arm, buttocks
- Fractures that don't fit the mechanism, metaphyseal corner fractures, rib fractures, multiple fractures at different stages of healing
- Head injuries: skull fractures, bilateral eye injuries, retinal haemorrhages, frenulum tears
- Burns on the buttocks and perineum (from dunking in boiling water) or discrete burns in other areas consistent with cigarette burns

- There is vaginal or anal bleeding or injury in the absence of an adequate explanation

MANAGEMENT

- Diagnose and treat the injuries.
- Actively seek evidence of other potentially associated injuries.
- Document extensively and precisely.
- Admit the child to hospital for protection and ongoing management.
- Consider the need for protection of siblings or others that may be at risk.
- Consult the local child protection unit.
- Avoid having the child interviewed on multiple occasions.
- Notify the statutory authority in those places that have mandatory notification laws.

Pain management in children

Reducing psychological distress in children is an important component of pain management. Distraction therapy can be very powerful at mitigating pain. It can be useful when used alone or alongside pharmacotherapy. Simple measures such as keeping the parents close and the use of bubbles, music and videos should be considered. Pharmacotherapy may still be required and should not be withheld from children in pain.

In babies under 3 months of age oral sucrose is proven to help with painful procedures (25%, 0.05 mL to 0.5 mL per dose; can be repeated up to maximum of 5 mL in 24 hours).

Paracetamol 15 mg/kg works well in most children for fever and mild pain. It works synergistically with opiates, so can also be part of more severe pain management. Ibuprofen 10 mg/kg is an alternative.

Oxycodone 0.1 mg/kg is the recommended oral opiate and should be administered in combination with paracetamol. Codeine is no longer recommended in children under 12 years of age due to the huge variability and unpredictability in metabolism to morphine.

Intranasal fentanyl 1–2 micrograms/kg is a great way to give quick onset, strong analgesia without needing to use a needle. Morphine 0.1 mg/kg IV can be titrated to the child's comfort once IV access is established.

Vaccination schedule

NSW Immunisation Schedule
from 1 July 2018

AGE	DISEASE	VACCINE
CHILDHOOD VACCINES		
Birth	Hepatitis B	H-B-VAX II **OR** ENGERIX B
6 weeks	Diphtheria, tetanus, pertussis, *Haemophilus influenzae* type b, hepatitis B, polio	INFANRIX HEXA
	Pneumococcal	PREVENAR 13
	Rotavirus	ROTARIX
4 months	Diphtheria, tetanus, pertussis, *Haemophilus influenzae* type b, hepatitis B, polio	INFANRIX HEXA
	Pneumococcal	PREVENAR 13
	Rotavirus	ROTARIX
6 months‡	Diphtheria, tetanus, pertussis, *Haemophilus influenzae* type b, hepatitis B, polio	INFANRIX HEXA
12 months	Meningococcal ACWY	NIMENRIX
	Pneumococcal	PREVENAR 13
	Measles, mumps, rubella	MMR II **OR** PRIORIX
18 months	Diphtheria, tetanus, pertussis	INFANRIX **OR** TRIPACEL
	Measles, mumps, rubella, varicella	PRIORIX TETRA **OR** PROQUAD
	Haemophilus influenzae type b	ACT-HIB
4 years	Diphtheria, tetanus, pertussis, polio	INFANRIX-IPV **OR** QUADRACEL
ADOLESCENT VACCINES - SCHOOL VACCINATION PROGRAM		
Year 7	Diphtheria, tetanus, pertussis	BOOSTRIX
	Human papillomavirus (2 doses)	GARDASIL 9
Years 10 - 11 (In 2018)	Meningococcal ACWY	MENACTRA
ADULT VACCINES		
Pregnant women	Influenza (Annually-any trimester)	INFLUENZA
	Pertussis (Third trimester, ideally 28-32 weeks)	BOOSTRIX **OR** ADACEL
65 years and over	Influenza (Annually)	FLUAD **OR** FLUZONE HIGH DOSE
	Pneumococcal (One dose)*	PNEUMOVAX 23
70 years (Catch-up for 71-79 years until 31 October 2021)	Zoster	ZOSTAVAX
AT RISK GROUPS		
6 months and over with medical risk conditions†	Influenza (annual)	INFLUENZA
All children 6 months to < 5 years (In 2018)		
Aboriginal people 15 years and over		
Aboriginal people 15-49 years with medical risk factors	Pneumococcal*	PNEUMOVAX 23
Aboriginal people 50 years and over		
65 years and over		

† Refer to the current online edition of The Australian Immunisation Handbook for all medical risk factors and conditions
* Refer to the current edition of The Australian Immunisation Handbook for timing of doses
‡ at risk children require an additional dose of pneumococcal (Prevenar 13)

June 2018 © NSW Health. SHPN (HPNSW) 180491

Online resources

Australian Medicines Handbook Children's Dosing Companion July 2018
https://childrens.amh.net.au.acs.hcn.com.au

Advanced Paediatric Life Support algorithms
https://apls.org.au/page/algorithms

Royal Children's Hospital Melbourne Clinical Practice Guidelines
https://www.rch.org.au/clinicalguide

Sydney Children's Hospitals Network Clinical Policies
http://www.schn.health.nsw.gov.au/our-policies/index/clinical

NSW Health Clinical Excellence Commission Sepsis Tools
http://www.cec.health.nsw.gov.au/patient-safety-programs/
adult-patient-safety/sepsis-kills/sepsis-tools

Newborn Skin: Part 1. Common rashes
https://www.aafp.org/afp/2008/0101/p47.html

Australian Asthma Handbook
http://www.asthmahandbook.org.au/

Australian Immunisation Handbook
https://immunisationhandbook.health.gov.au

Chapter 34
Gynaecological emergencies
Nikki Woods

Acknowledgment
The author wishes to acknowledge the content used from the previous edition of *Emergency Medicine* which was provided by Sally McCarthy.

General principles
- History includes last normal menstrual period (LMP), past pregnancy history, sexual activity, contraception, pregnancy signs and symptoms, preventive health strategies (Pap smear, breast examination) as well as characteristics of presenting symptoms (commonly pain, abnormal vaginal bleeding +/− pregnancy, vaginal discharge, fever).
- Investigations often will involve quantitative serum beta-human chorionic gonadotrophin (beta-hCG; see Table 34.1) and pelvic ultrasound.
- Management includes excluding pregnancy for every female of reproductive age, and early attention to vital signs, anticipating that certain conditions are associated with immediately life-threatening presentations.
- Sensitivity and attention to patient comfort mandates conducting gynaecological history and pelvic examinations in a private area (when the patient's condition is stable), using a chaperone, and offering analgesia early.

Common presentations
PAIN
Ruptured ectopic pregnancy
- **Incidence** of ectopic pregnancy is increasing worldwide, mainly due to the increased incidence of pelvic inflammatory disease (PID) caused by *Chlamydia trachomatis* and assisted

Table 34.1   **Interpretation of quantitative serum beta-hCG results**

Reference intervals

	Serum beta-hCG (U/L)	
Females	< 2.0	Pre-menopausal
	< 10	Post-menopausal
Males	< 2.0	

Pregnancy test

	Serum beta-hCG (U/L)	Interpretation
	< 2	Negative (if taken after first missed period)
	2–25	Borderline result (suggest repeat in 48 hours)
	> 25	Consistent with pregnancy

Pregnancy staging

Weeks since LMP	Approximate hCG range (U/L)	Comment
3–4	0–130	Week prior to first missed period
4–5	75–2 600	Week after first missed period
5–6	850–20 800	
6–7	4 000–200 000	
7–12	11 500–289 000	
12–16	18 300–137 000	
16–29	1 400–53 000	Second trimester
29–41	940–60 000	Third trimester

LMP = last normal menstrual period

reproductive techniques. Ectopic pregnancy occurs in 2% of reported pregnancies.

- **Risk factors** include past history of tubal damage or tubal surgery, previous ectopic pregnancy, PID, assisted reproductive techniques, increasing maternal age, smoking, progesterone-only contraception, intrauterine contraceptive device (IUD), endometriosis.
- **History** includes abdominal pain (90%), missed period (80%), vaginal bleeding (79%), which is rarely heavy,

shoulder tip pain (which indicates rupture) and syncope. Patients commonly present between the fifth and eighth week following the LMP. Note that 10% present with no pain and no bleeding, and 10% present with pain but no bleeding. Presenting signs of *ruptured ectopic pregnancy* include abdominal tenderness, adnexal tenderness and, less frequently, syncope and hypovolaemic shock.

Investigations
Diagnosis is made by a positive beta-hCG (see Table 34.1) and an ultrasound negative for intrauterine pregnancy (in the presence of a serum beta-hCG of > 1500 IU.) Be aware that heterotopic pregnancy—an ectopic pregnancy together with an intrauterine pregnancy—occurs in approximately 1 in 3800 pregnancies, and up to 1 in 100 in those who have undergone assisted reproduction.

Other investigations include a full blood count (FBC) and cross-match in any haemodynamically unstable patient. Blood group and Rh factor should be determined on all patients.

Management
* **Haemodynamically unstable patients:** oxygen, large-bore cannula, IV fluid resuscitation (preferably packed cells), cross-match blood, urgent obstetrics and gynaecological (O&G) consult for operative management.
* **Haemodynamically stable patients:** insert IVC, perform group-and-hold (G&H), O&G consult. Management may be expectant, medical or surgical, depending on initial serum titre of beta-hCG and trend in titres, tubal size and local practice.

Acute salpingitis (PID)
(See also the section Pelvic Inflammatory Disease in Chapter 23 Infectious Diseases.)
* Encompasses endometritis, salpingitis, tubo-ovarian abscess and/or pelvic peritonitis.
* Risk factors include history of previous episode, multiple sexual partners, instrumentation, adolescence and the presence of an IUCD.
* Often sexually acquired. Infection is usually due to *Chlamydia trachomatis* or *Neisseria gonorrhoea*.

- May result from mechanical interruption of the normal cervical barrier (e.g. post-termination, postpartum, postoperative infection), or in association with IUDs.
- Presenting symptoms can be vague. May include pelvic or lower abdominal pain, purulent or mucopurulent vaginal discharge, low-grade fever, generalised malaise, dyspareunia and abnormal vaginal bleeding. There is no correlation between extent of disease and symptom severity.
- On examination there may be abdominal tenderness and adnexal and cervical motion tenderness (95% sensitivity).

Investigations

Diagnosis is made by a combination of clinical findings and some or all of the following: positive microbiology from endocervical swabs or positive urine PCR (for *N. gonococcus* and *Chlamydia*), leucocytosis, ultrasound documenting inflammatory adnexal mass or retained products.

Management of acute salpingitis

1 **Severe infection or systemically unwell** or requires removal of retained products or IUD: admit for IV antibiotics.
   — Sexually acquired: doxycycline 100 mg PO 12-hourly, metronidazole 500 mg IV 12-hourly plus ceftriaxone 1 g IV 8-hourly while awaiting culture results.
   — Non-sexually acquired: ampicillin 2 g IV 6-hourly, metronidazole 500 mg IV 12-hourly plus gentamicin 4–6 mg/kg IV once daily.
2 **Milder infections** may be discharged on oral therapy.
   — Sexually acquired: azithromycin 1 g PO stat dose, doxycycline 100 mg 12-hourly PO for 14 days plus metronidazole 400 mg PO 12-hourly for 14 days.
   — Non-sexually acquired: amoxycillin + clavulanate 875 mg + 125 mg PO 12-hourly, plus doxycycline 100 mg PO 12-hourly, both for 14 days.
3 Must treat sexual partner(s).
4 *Chlamydia* and *Gonorrhoea* are notifiable diseases.
5 If associated with IUD or retained products, removal is necessary.

Long-term sequelae may include tubo-ovarian abscess, chronic pelvic pain, dyspareunia, infertility and increased risk of ectopic pregnancy.

Adnexal cyst or mass complications
Ruptured ovarian cyst
- Ovarian cysts are asymptomatic until complications occur.
- Physiological cysts such as corpus luteum cysts (in pregnant or non-pregnant women) and follicular cysts rupture at different points in the menstrual cycle, giving a clue to aetiology:
  - Rupture of a follicular cyst with the extrusion of an ovum occurs mid-cycle, and gives rise to the unilateral pain of mittelschmerz. Discomfort may last 2–3 days, and may be associated with mild general malaise and/or vaginal spotting.
  - Corpus luteal cyst rupture in the non-pregnant woman occurs just prior to menses and is usually associated with some intraperitoneal bleeding, which may be significant. Ectopic pregnancy must be excluded.
  - In pregnancy, the corpus luteum may persist until 10 weeks, so that spontaneous rupture typically occurs during the first trimester.
- Presenting symptoms and signs are unilateral pain and adnexal tenderness; fever and leucocytosis are uncommon (approximately 20%). Diffuse peritoneal irritation occurs with spillage of fluid into peritoneal cavity.

Investigations
- Ectopic pregnancy must be excluded: serum beta-hCG and pelvic ultrasound.

Management
- Resuscitation with IV fluid resuscitation if haemodynamically unstable
- Exclude pregnancy
- Analgesia: NSAIDs if not pregnant
- Laparoscopy may be indicated if the cyst is > 5 cm in size, or there is severe pain or a large amount of free fluid.

Torsion of ovarian or tubal mass

- More common in women < 30 years of age. Usually, but not always, associated with a diseased ovary or fallopian tube. Torsion occurs when these structures twist on their supportive appendages, causing compromise to their vascular supply.
- Clinical presentation may be non-specific. Features include sudden onset of sharp, unilateral pain which is intermittent and which becomes increasingly severe. There may have been previous similar episodes. There may be associated nausea, vomiting, low-grade fever and leucocytosis and, infrequently, amenorrhoea or abnormal vaginal bleeding.
- Examination findings vary from unilateral lower abdominal tenderness to peritonitis.

Investigations
- Ultrasound reveals reduced perfusion of the torted mass.

Management
- Analgesia, resuscitation as appropriate and laparoscopy or laparotomy.
- Complications include ovarian necrosis and shock.

Editorial Comment

Torsion of ovary is the equivalent to a torsion of testicle but often not thought of; for example, appendicitis, subsequent misdiagnosis and treatment delay.

Other gynaecological causes of lower abdominal or pelvic pain

- **Endometriosis:** initially the pain is cyclic and associated with menses. Later it can become continuous as adhesions develop. Dyspareunia and infertility are also common. Diagnosis is made at laparoscopy.
- **Uterine perforation:** typically after intrauterine instrumentation, may present acutely due to intraperitoneal irritation secondary to intraperitoneal blood or as delayed diffuse pain with diffuse peritonitis.

- **Severe dysmenorrhoea:** manage with anti-prostaglandins (e.g. NSAIDs) and paracetamol.
- **Denial of pregnancy and unanticipated labour:** estimated at 1 in 2000–5000 births, the diagnosis is made when the woman presents in labour, putting both mother and fetus at risk.
- **Vulvovaginitis:** common causes are infection, irritation, allergy, systemic disease. Treatment depends on the likely cause.

BLEEDING

In early pregnancy
Ectopic pregnancy
See Ruptured Ectopic Pregnancy section earlier this chapter.

Spontaneous abortion or miscarriage
- Approximately 25% of all pregnancies are associated with bleeding in the first trimester; 50% of these will be due to a failed pregnancy.
- Presenting symptoms include intermittent vaginal spotting progressing to heavy bleeding with passage of clots and gestational tissue; midline, cramping abdominal discomfort occurring after bleeding has commenced. On examination there may be midline, suprapubic tenderness on deep palpation, uterine enlargement consistent with pregnancy or the abdominal examination may be unremarkable.
- Shock or bradycardia can occur due to products sitting in the cervical os. These will require urgent gentle removal after direct visualisation on speculum examination. Vaginal speculum examination is necessary to assess the cervical os (i.e. open or closed?).
- Several stages of spontaneous miscarriage are recognised:
  — threatened miscarriage—cervical os closed; no products passed
  — incomplete miscarriage—cervical os open; bleeding $+/-$ products passed
  — complete miscarriage—cervical os open or closed; products of conception expelled
  — inevitable miscarriage—cervical os open; no products passed
  — missed miscarriage—cervical os closed; no products passed.

Investigations
- Confirmation of pregnancy with serum beta-hCG level
- Assessment of state of cervical os
- Ultrasound examination to confirm diagnosis and exclude ectopic pregnancy (if not already known to have intrauterine pregnancy)
- Assessment of Rh factor status

Management
- Assessment of vital signs, and monitoring of blood loss
- Analgesia
- May require dilation and curettage (D&C) after consultation with O&G
- Administration of Rh (anti-D) immunoglobulin if Rh-negative
- Miscarriages are frequently associated with grieving, and referral for counselling should be offered to the patient

In later pregnancy (antepartum haemorrhage, > 20 weeks' gestation)
Placental abruption and placenta praevia
- **Placental abruption.** Separation of normally located placenta from the uterine wall is usually associated with characteristically dark vaginal bleeding, uterine pain and tenderness. Complications include fetal distress or death (15%), disseminated intravascular coagulation (DIC), maternal haemorrhage.
- **Placenta praevia.** Implantation of the placenta over, or near, the cervical os in the second or third trimesters. Bleeding in this situation is usually associated with painless fresh vaginal bleeding, which may become severe with cervical probing. The uterus is typically non-tender. There may be a history of several small 'warning' bleeds.

Assessment
- Vaginal or speculum examination is contraindicated until the placenta position is identified.
- FBC, coagulation screen, Rh factor and cross-match.
- Urgent ultrasound to assess placental position, fetal gestation, presentation and liquor volume. However, 50% of placental

abruptions are not seen on ultrasound. The diagnosis is often clinical.

Management of antepartum haemorrhage
* Maternal and fetal monitoring
* Resuscitation with IV fluids $+/-$ blood
* Urgent obstetric consultation; massive antepartum haemorrhage requires urgent delivery, usually by caesarean section
* Analgesia if required
* Anti-D if indicated.

Bleeding in the non-pregnant woman
* History should include questions to elucidate the cause and severity of the bleeding. There may be history of PID, vaginal trauma, abnormal Cervical Screening Test, previous cervical surgery, recent instrumentation or childbirth.
* The timing of bleeding is important (postcoital, intermenstrual), as are associated symptoms (e.g. pelvic pain, fever, dyspareunia, dysmenorrhoea).
* Symptoms and signs of systemic disease should be sought (e.g. bleeding diathesis, symptoms of hypothyroidism).
* Assessment of blood loss may be difficult, but menorrhagia is indicated by anaemia, use of 2 pads concurrently or tampon plus pad, pads/tampons changed every 1–2 hours when flow is heaviest, episodic flooding with staining of clothes or sheets, frequent clots, duration > 7 days.
* Differential diagnosis is shown in Box 34.1.

Investigations
* Exclude pregnancy
* Exclude pelvic infection: first pass urine PCR $+/-$ swabs
* FBC and coagulation studies
* Consider TFTs
* Consider pelvic ultrasound

Management
* Resuscitation if necessary
* Supportive treatment

Box 34.1   Differential diagnosis of abnormal bleeding in the non-pregnant patient

- Ovulatory bleeding
- Anovulatory bleeding or dysfunctional uterine bleeding (DUB)
- Uterine and ovarian pathology:
  — fibroids
  — pelvic inflammatory disease
  — endometriosis
  — polycystic ovary syndrome
  — endometrial polyps
  — endometrial carcinoma
- Genital trauma or foreign body
- Iatrogenic cause:
  — IUD
  — Drugs (e.g. anticoagulants, chemotherapy)

- Specific treatment depending on identified cause $+/-$ O&G consultation or follow-up

---

Editorial Comment

Abnormal vaginal bleeding is a common ED presentation. In the non-pregnant female get a gynaecological opinion—even by phone is suitable, especially as hormonal regimens or other agents such as tranexamic acid may be indicated.

Other complications of later pregnancy (> 20 weeks' gestation)
PREECLAMPSIA AND ECLAMPSIA

- **Preeclampsia** is a multisystem disorder, unique to pregnancy, which is usually associated with hypertension and significant proteinuria. It rarely presents before 20 weeks' gestation and is more common in nulliparous women.
  — Hypertension in pregnancy is a systolic BP $\geq$ 140 mmHg and/or diastolic BP $\geq$ 90 mmHg.
  — Features of severe preeclampsia are BP > 160/110 mmHg, proteinuria > 300 mg/day, hyperuricaemia, serum creatinine > 0.09 mmol/L.

— Other features include liver pain, elevated transaminases or bilirubin, persistent headaches, visual disturbances, hyperreflexia or clonus, thrombocytopenia.
- **Eclampsia** is the onset of seizures in pregnancy or the postnatal period, usually preceded by preeclampsia.
  — Preeclampsia and eclampsia may occur up to 4 weeks postpartum.

Investigations
- FBC, blood film (haemolysis), coagulation studies, EUC, LFTs, uric acid, group-and-hold
- Urinalysis for proteinuria $+/-$ 24-hour urine collection
- CT of the brain may be indicated only to rule out a differential diagnosis or complication

Management
Severe preeclampsia and eclampsia are medical and obstetric emergencies.
1 Seizure prophylaxis or treatment.
  — Magnesium sulfate loading dose = 4 g IV over 15 minutes.
  — Followed by an infusion of magnesium sulfate 1 g/h IV.
  — Monitor serum magnesium levels 6-hourly and assess for clonus and deep tendon reflexes 1- to 2-hourly.
2 Blood pressure control.
  — Intravenous labetalol 20 mg is the antihypertensive of choice. This dose can be repeated every 5–10 minutes. If unavailable, intravenous hydralazine can be used, 5–10 mg IV over 5–10 minutes. The aim is for a diastolic BP of 90–100 mmHg.
3 Urgent obstetric consultation.
4 Fetal monitoring: ideally continuous cardiotocography (CTG) monitoring.
5 General resuscitative measures: maintenance of airway, oxygen therapy, IV access, nurse patient on left side, IDC and fluid balance monitoring.
6 Delivery is indicated in severe preeclampsia or in a fetus > 37 weeks' gestation.

TRAUMA IN LATE PREGNANCY

The risk to the pregnancy in 'minor' trauma is significant, with preterm labour occurring in 8%, abruption in 1% and fetal death in 1% of occurrences. In severe trauma, the fetal death rate rises to 20% or greater.

It is important to remember that there are two patients; however, the survival of the fetus is dependent on optimal management of the mother. Maintaining maternal oxygenation and tissue perfusion is the primary goal.

Assessment and management

- Maternal primary survey and resuscitation (ABCs with cervical spine precautions).
- Left lateral tilt if > 20 weeks' gestation (while maintaining cervical spine stability) to displace uterus and prevent vena caval compression.
- Perform secondary survey, including assessment of the uterus +/− vaginal exam. If mother unstable, resuscitate and treat cause.
- Monitor mother and fetus (cardiotocography [CTG] ideally).
- Continue CTG monitoring for at least 4–6 hours. Consider ultrasound.
- Check Rh factor status.

All patients with minor trauma should be admitted to hospital for at least 24 hours.

CARDIOPULMONARY RESUSCITATION IN LATE PREGNANCY

In cardiac arrest, all the principles of basic life support (BLS) and advanced life support (ALS) apply; see Chapter 1 Cardiopulmonary Resuscitation. Specific considerations include:

- Call for help immediately—obstetrician, neonatologist, anaesthetist.
- Tilt the pelvis to the left (shoulders flat to enable cardiac compressions and a wedge under woman's right hip).
- Secure the airway early.
- Perform chest compressions slightly above the centre of the sternum.

- Consider **early** (within minutes of cardiac arrest) to proceed to a resuscitative hysterotomy if gestation is estimated to be > 24 weeks.

Prescribing in pregnancy

- All drugs should be avoided if possible during the first trimester.
- Drugs should be prescribed in pregnancy only if the expected benefit to the mother is thought to be greater than the risk to the fetus.
- Drugs that have been extensively used in pregnancy and appear to be usually safe (category A) should be prescribed in preference to new or untried drugs; and the smallest effective dose should be used.
- For information regarding specific drugs, MIMS should be consulted.

Anti-D prophylaxis

$Rh_o(D)$ immunoglobulin (anti-D) is administered for prophylaxis against haemolytic disease of the newborn. All Rh(D)-negative women should be offered anti-D in the following clinical situations.

- **First trimester (dose 250 IU IMI):** chorionic villous sampling, miscarriage, termination of pregnancy and ectopic pregnancy.
  There is insufficient evidence to suggest that threatened miscarriage before 12/40 necessitates anti-D.
- **Second and third trimester (basic dose 625 IU IMI):** obstetric haemorrhage, amniocentesis, cordocentesis, abdominal trauma or any other suspected intrauterine bleeding or sensitising event.

Postcoital contraception: morning-after pill

- Give levonorgestrel 1.5 mg orally as a stat dose.
- If administered within 72 hours of unprotected intercourse, pregnancy rate is approximately 1.1%.

Advice given with emergency contraception should include risk of failure, risk of sexually transmitted infections (STIs) and appropriate follow-up and counselling regarding ongoing contraception.

Online resources

Australian Resuscitation Council (ARC) guidelines
www.resus.org.au

eTG Therapeutic Guidelines
www.ciap.health.nsw.gov.au

MIMS Online
www.ciap.health.nsw.gov.au

Royal Women's Hospital, Melbourne
www.thewomens.org.au

Guidelines for the use of Rh(D) Immunoglobulin (Anti-D) in Obstetrics in Australia
www.ranzcog.edu.au

Chapter 35
Sexual assault and domestic violence

Nikki Woods and Sophie Blake

(Adult) sexual assault
Nikki Woods

Sexual assault is a crime which occurs against men and women of all ages and all cultural backgrounds. It has long-lasting impact which must be addressed as quickly as possible to alleviate trauma and prevent or reduce long-term psychological difficulties. Victims may seek care immediately or after a delay.

A person who has experienced sexual assault needs timely, competent and compassionate medical care and the option of referral to a forensic medical service.

It is important to remember that a victim of sexual assault has been forced, coerced or manipulated into sexual acts. All procedures must recognise this fact and ensure that the patient feels in control of what is happening to them.

The needs of the patient vary greatly. The aim of the clinician is to respond to these needs in a way that can facilitate recovery from this traumatic experience. The patient may want the following.

- **Medical attention and/or information:** (e.g. treatment of physical/genital injury or pain, emergency contraception, STI prophylaxis, hepatitis B vaccination, HIV PEP, mental health assessment). If a medical examination is appropriate, the medical officer will clearly explain the nature of the examination to the patient, including the right to have a support person present.
- **Forensic examination:** it is important to stress that the patient can elect to have a forensic examination and then decide *later* whether and when this information is given to the police. Sexual assault forensic examiners may be either medical

officers or nurses who have undertaken specialist training and usually work at a dedicated sexual assault service facility.

- **Information, advice or counselling only:** in the acute setting and referral for ongoing follow-up.

Treatment after sexual assault should be provided as a matter of urgency due to the time constraints of the collection of forensic evidence and clinical management (e.g. the provision of post-coital contraception).

People who have been sexually assaulted often want reassurance that they are physically unharmed and this is just as important as the collection of forensic evidence.

KEY POINTS

- Your response matters. Offer crisis counselling and support (including practical information and assistance) to assist the patient to deal with the crisis. The period of crisis immediately following the assault offers a good opportunity to engage the client in counselling in an attempt to prevent future long-term problems.
- Privacy and confidentiality are important and should be respected.
- Ask and ring for advice (see resources at the end of this chapter, especially with children < 16 years).
- The police should be contacted only if the patient wishes to report the assault and make a statement. The exception to this is if the assault is a domestic violence assault and fits the criteria for mandatory reporting. Health workers working within NSW Health must report to NSW Police regardless of the victim's views where the victim is a patient and:
  - there are serious injuries such as broken bones, stab and gunshot wounds
  - there are guns and weapons (the perpetrator has access to, is/was carrying a gun and is threatening to cause physical injury to any person; or the perpetrator is using or carrying a weapon [including guns, knives or any other weapon])
  - there are reasonable fears for public safety
  - in the hospital (i.e. an offence has occurred on NSW Health premises where workers are threatened because of their professional role).

- Medical assessment includes examination and treatment of any injuries, consideration of emergency contraception, tetanus prophylaxis, STI prophylaxis, HIV PEP, hep B PEP.
- Use the sexual assault investigation kit (SAIK) as provided.
- Referral for a forensic examination should be offered if they wish and if the assault has occurred within the previous 7 days. Time is of the essence with regards to evidence collection. If there is going to be a delay in transferring the patient to a sexual assault service, advise the patient how to preserve any evidence (e.g. advise not to shower, eat/drink, brush teeth, urinate) depending on the nature of the assault if at all possible. Keep clothing worn immediately after or during the assault unwashed and place in brown paper bags.
- Meticulous documentation is important with diagrams if relevant.
- Follow-up regarding injuries, pregnancy, sexually transmissible diseases and other general medical matters should be arranged for patients (as relevant to the history of the assault), and should be conducted in a private and sensitive manner.

USEFUL CONTACTS AND RESOURCES FOR PATIENTS

- NSW Rape Crisis hotline (1800 424 017); www.nswrapecrisis.com.au
- Victims Access Line (1800 633 063) provides information, referral and support to victims of crime.

USEFUL CONTACTS AND RESOURCES FOR DOCTORS

- Sexual Assault Services (NSW Health): https://www.victimsservices.justice.nsw.gov.au/sexualassault/Pages/sexual_assault_contactus.aspx#SexualAssaultServices(NSW Health)
- Education Centre Against Violence (ECAV): (02) 9840 3737, www.ecav.health.nsw.gov.au (for publications and details about training).

Domestic violence
Sophie Blake

OVERVIEW

Within their life span, 1 in 3 Australian women will have experienced physical and/or sexual violence perpetrated by someone known to them. Domestic and family violence (DFV) is a universally gendered social issue which typically uses behaviours of power and control which can significantly impact a woman's physical health and social and emotional wellbeing. It is an unbiased social epidemic that affects all women irrespective of their age, class, culture, socioeconomic status or religion.

In Australia, Indigenous females are estimated 35 times more likely to be hospitalised due to DFV-related assaults than other Australian females.

Though it is acknowledged that DFV also impacts a proportion of males and can be experienced by persons who identify as part of the lesbian, gay, bisexual, transgender, intersex or queer (LGBTIQ+) community, this chapter will be applying interventions with a women- and child-centred trauma-informed focus. However, the principles for child protection, risk assessment and safety planning can be applied universally to DFV affecting patients of all sexes and sexual orientation in the acute health setting.

Emergency departments are critical points of contact for individuals to be afforded an opportunity to access intervention and support around domestic and family violence. This chapter will aim to provide a practical approach to identifying and responding to DFV as a health professional in the ED irrespective of urban or rural context. It will cover guidelines and tools for best practice principles to respond effectively to DFV including:

• How do I identify domestic and family violence?
• How do I speak to a patient who is a victim of DFV?
• Risk assessment and safety planning
• Clinical documentation
• Child protection and mandatory reporting
• Quick point survival guide
• Online resources
• References

HOW DO I IDENTIFY DOMESTIC AND FAMILY VIOLENCE?

No two domestic violence presentations are ever the same and they rarely present as a singular issue. They are notoriously complex and often rely on the practitioners' ability to pick up on subtle or more obvious indicators as they present themselves. On some occasions you will encounter situations in which patients disclose when triaged that a domestic assault has occurred and is the direct mechanism for presentation or cause for obvious physical injury. However, other presentations are less obvious and may appear 'vague' or unclear. The patient might be completely unassuming until the *right questions are asked at the right time.*

We cannot see domestic violence and it is often hidden; it is important to never assume anything of a person's situation.

In the absence of mandatory screening for domestic and family violence across all hospital EDs, it is not always possible to identify domestic assaults. We therefore need to educate our multidisciplinary teams to raise awareness in being able to identify potential indicators in our patient's behaviour and respond accordingly.

As a general rule of thumb, trust your instincts:

If it doesn't sound right, doesn't look right, doesn't feel right—then it probably isn't.

There are many indicators of injuries in a presentation that may be flags for physical assault as a result of DFV. Below is a list of indicators from the Domestic Violence Resource Centre Victoria that may be used as a *guide only*; it is not exhaustive nor absolute.

The woman may have:

- bruising on the chest and abdomen
- multiple injuries
- minor laceration
- injuries during pregnancy
- ruptured eardrums
- delayed seeking medical attention
- patterns of repeated injury.

Other behaviours that might indicate the woman is experiencing physical, emotional or psychological abuse may include:

- appearing nervous, ashamed or evasive
- describing her partner as controlling or prone to anger

- seeming uncomfortable or anxious in the presence of her partner
- being accompanied by her partner, who does most of the talking
- giving an unconvincing explanation of the injuries
- having recently been separated or divorced
- appearing tearful and having difficulty engaging in questions specific to the injury.

Utilising the skills in your allied health team is an important part of responding effectively to DFV. Your social workers are your greatest resource in 'frontline' responses to domestic and family violence and trauma-informed care.

Talk to your nursing staff. In particular your educators, clinical nurse specialist (CNS), clinical initiatives nurse (CIN) and triage nurses hold a wealth of experience and knowledge and can assist in creating safe spaces and interventions with patients while in the ED. The physiotherapist can also provide pathways for conversations and intervention, in that they treat many patients with soft tissue and orthopaedic injuries that may be related to domestic assaults. Interventions are most effective when they have a collaborative approach.

DFV presentations often have coexisting issues such as mental health, homelessness and drug and alcohol concerns. Be mindful that before you explore the DFV, where applicable you must first:

- refer to, and consult with, the appropriate specialty teams; in particular mental health and drug and alcohol
- allow *time* for the patient to have appropriate mental health or other drug and alcohol clearances.

HOW DO I SPEAK TO A VICTIM OF DOMESTIC AND FAMILY VIOLENCE?

Knowing how to start a conversation with your patient around confirmed or suspected assault or DFV can certainly be daunting. However, when we break it down, there are key principles of verbal and nonverbal communication, coupled with common sense, that can help you build rapport with your patient.

Start with the basics

- Where is the perpetrator? If they are with the patient, you will need to consider her safety and yours: never ask a patient about domestic or family violence in the presence of the suspected perpetrator. Sometimes we need to be creative to manoeuvre an opportunity for vital time alone with the patient.

For example:

— 'I'll ask you to step out for 10 minutes while I complete my examination.'
— 'The nurse needs to take her to another room for a blood test; we'll come and get you when she's done.'
— 'I'll ask you to sit out in the waiting room while she goes for an X-ray.'

- Privacy: although best practice is to speak in a private space, this is not always possible in the chaos of an ED where more often than not the space is divided by nothing more than a curtain. Sometimes this needs a pragmatic approach.
- Maintain good eye contact, sit down and show the woman that you are genuinely interested in what she has to say.
- Be even and measured in your tone of voice. Be respectful and curious when you are asking questions.
- Consider the impact cultural factors may have on the patient's ability to be open with you.
- Do you need an interpreter? Different cultures use varied language to describe interpersonal violence and it is our responsibility as healthcare professionals to ensure that we afford our patients access to interpreters in their first language.

But what do I say?

World Health Organization recommends the following suggestions for frontline support staff when responding to abuse:

- non-judgmental support and validation of the woman's account
- practical care that responds to the woman's concerns
- asking about the history of violence and carefully listening without pressure to talk
- assistance accessing information about resources including legal and other services
- assistance to increase safety
- provision or mobilisation of social support.

The type of questions and statements of validation may be used directly or more broadly depending on the situation at hand. Use your professional judgment around this.

Do not bombard the patient with an interrogation, let the natural flow of conversation guide you as to where you might ask/validate in your responses.

Examples of language may include:

- 'Can you tell me a little more about how your injury was caused?'
- 'When I see injuries like this I wonder if someone could have hurt you?'
- 'You seem very anxious—is there anything you want to talk about?'
- 'Violence in the home is very common. I ask a lot of my patients about abuse because everyone has a right to feel safe.'
- 'That must have been really frightening.'
- 'I'm so sorry this has happened.'
- 'You're not alone, this is a safe place.'
- 'Are you worried about the safety of your children?'
- 'It is unacceptable behaviour from your partner.'
- 'Is there a support person, friend or family member that I can call for you?'
- 'You're an important person and it takes a lot of courage to talk about this.'
- 'There is support available to help; I can assist you to connect with these services.'

At this point, best practice would be to refer to your social worker, whether they are on shift or via the after-hours service depending on your hospital's clinical delivery arrangements.

Social workers are highly skilled in providing in-depth psychosocial assessment, crisis intervention, risk assessment and safety planning, counselling, emotional and practical support. They can work with the individual to facilitate ongoing service coordination, mobilisation of social supports and refer to specialist domestic and family violence services.

In the absence of a social worker being available, your next step would be to conduct a basic risk assessment and safety plan.

RISK ASSESSMENT AND SAFETY PLANNING
Risk assessment

Risk assessments are used to identify those patients who may be in serious and imminent danger. Once you have established rapport with your patient and a supportive disclosure has occurred, it is necessary where possible to conduct a risk assessment. This is a means of identifying 'red flag' behaviours and planning for safety.

Below is an example list of commonly asked questions in various risk assessment frameworks to assess the level of threat to a woman and her children's safety in the context of DFV.

- Has the violence increased in frequency or severity over the past 6 months?
- Has he ever used a weapon or threatened you with a weapon?
- Do you believe he is capable of killing you?
- Does he choke you?
- Has he ever beaten you while you were pregnant?
- Does he stalk you?
- Does he have access to weapons?
- Has there been a recent or imminent plans for separation?

A 'yes' answer to one or more of these questions coupled with a disclosure of physical or emotional abuse would indicate need for a safety plan and for further referrals to occur as a part of your discharge plan.

Figure 35.1 can be used as a visual formula for 'best practice' aspects of risk assessment.

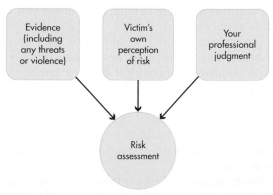

Figure 35.1 Risk assessment
Modified from Women's Legal Service NSW

Putting a woman's own sense of risk at the forefront of your assessment is integral to patient-centred care and effective intervention.

Safety planning

Your risk assessment (see previous section) will assist you to identify dangerous behaviours and help you give the patient the best resources on hand to access support and minimise further risk to the woman and her children's immediate safety. If you have access to a social worker, they can provide specialist psychosocial assessment and intervention in planning for safety in DFV presentations.

Elements of a safety plan may include:

- identifying protective behaviours—what is she already doing to keep herself and her children safe?
- who is already supporting her
- options to improve safety now
- if it escalates, what can she do
- using a public telephone or computer
- keeping a second phone
- GP documenting injuries
- keeping a bag hidden at home or at the local health/ community centre full of clothes and copies of important documents
- legal interventions with police such as Apprehended Domestic Violence Orders (language may change depending on state or territory) outlining special contact conditions between the victim and perpetrator may also be utilised in safety planning
- police domestic violence liaison officers may be involved for further safety planning in the community.

With the woman's consent, facilitate a phone call to the:

National Sexual Assault, Domestic Family Violence Counselling service (24 hours a day, 7 days a week): 1800 737 732

This will ensure that the woman has immediate and appropriate counselling support. This is your most useful resource and intervention!!!!

The MOST IMPORTANT thing above all else is that the woman leaves feeling VALIDATED, SUPPORTED and with ACTIVE FOLLOW-UP SERVICES in place.

Listed below in Table 35.1 are national organisations that may also be used for advice, consultation and referral. It also can be photocopied and provided as a resource; however, be mindful of whether it is safe for a patient to take resources with her. Sometimes entering important emergency phone numbers into her mobile phone under 'alias' or unsuspecting terminology is necessary to keep the woman safe while also allowing her quick access in an emergency.

Table 35.1 National referral services

	Contact Information	Description
Police	Dial 000 24 hours, 7 days	Immediate access to police and emergency services.
1800 RESPECT 1800 671 442 (TTY)	1800 737 732 24 hours, 7 days	24-hour telephone counselling service that offers support to people impacted by domestic and family violence, sexual assault and abuse; Aboriginal and Torres Strait Islander clients can access culturally specific services by state via 1800 RESPECT
Relationships Australia	1300 364 277	A leading provider of relationship support services for individuals, families and communities and respectful relationships
Kids Help Line	1800 551 800 24 hours, 7 days	Australia's only free, private and confidential, phone and online counselling service for young people aged 5 to 25
Lifeline	131 114 24 hours, 7 days	Telephone counselling service
Translating and interpreting	131 450	Access to telephone interpreting services

Table 35.1   National referral services (cont.)

	Contact Information	Description
WESNET	Wesnet.org.au	A national women's peak advocacy body which works on behalf of women and children who are experiencing or have experienced domestic or family violence
ACON	1800 063 060	Support and advocacy for LGBTIQ+ people and people with HIV
Another Closet	www.anothercloset.com.au	This website focuses on domestic and family violence issues for people in LGBTIQ+ relationships

CLINICAL DOCUMENTATION

It is possible that your clinical documentation may be requested by subpoena to be used as evidence in court. It may also require you to give evidence as a witness in court proceedings.

The following steps are guidelines for appropriate clinical documentation (modified from Women's Legal Service NSW).

• Include time, date, author's name and signature.
• Ensure that the entry is legible if you are handwriting your notes.
• Describe physical injuries—some EDs have health-approved body-mapping documentation which may be used in addition.
• Use only 'health-approved' symbols or abbreviations.
• Be objective and factual in your notes; what you saw, what you heard, what you did and relevant services contacted. For example:
  'The patient's hands were visibly shaking. She was crying throughout the conversation.'
• Use quotation marks when describing what the patient said; be specific.

CHILD PROTECTION AND MANDATORY REPORTING

Child safety is *our responsibility*. Whether you are a doctor, nurse or allied health professional, asking about 'caring responsibilities' and children in the home should be at the forefront of your clinical assessment especially when speaking with those who may be experiencing domestic and family violence. Witnessing domestic violence can have long-lasting psychological impacts on children and also put them at risk of physical harm.

Each state/territory and hospital will have varied policies, procedures and legal parameters for maintaining confidentiality and mandatory reporting to police around domestic and family violence.

- **Mandatory reporting does not stop with child protection: Check your hospital, state or territory policy and legislation about domestic violence in regards to reporting *serious injuries or high-risk perpetrator behaviour* to police.**

Be aware of limits to confidentiality for:

- child protection purposes
- reporting of serious injuries where a criminal offence may have been committed
- information sharing for the purpose of promoting client safety, where this is appropriate under state or territory laws or local memoranda of understanding.

If you have access to a social worker in your ED, they can provide subject matter expertise and guidance for screening around child protection and domestic violence issues.

Familiarising yourself with your relevant state or territory, mandatory reporting legislation and child protection phone numbers is paramount to making sure you are meeting your legal responsibilities as a health practitioner. (See Table 35.2.)

QUICKPOINT SURVIVAL GUIDE

If all else fails remember the following.

- It's never black and white; domestic and family violence is complex. 'Messy' is normal, especially in the chaos of an ED.
- You work in a team—there is always someone to ask.
- Safety first; be aware of your surroundings. Where is the perpetrator?

Table 35.2 Child protection mandatory reporting requirements across Australia by state

	ACT
Who is mandated to report?	A person who is: a doctor; a dentist; a nurse; an enrolled nurse; a midwife; a psychologist; a teacher at a school; a person authorised to inspect education programs, materials or other records used for home education of a child or young person under the *Education Act 2004*; a police officer; a person employed to counsel children or young people at a school; a person caring for a child at a child care centre; a person coordinating or monitoring home-based care for a family day care scheme proprietor; a public servant who, in the course of employment as a public servant, works with or provides services personally to children and young people or families; the public advocate; an official visitor; a person who, in the course of the person's employment, has contact with or provides services to children, young people and their families and is prescribed by regulation
What must be reported?	A belief, on reasonable grounds, that a child or young person has experienced or is experiencing sexual abuse or non-accidental physical injury; and the belief arises from information obtained by the person during the course of, or because of, the person's work (whether paid or unpaid)
Abuse and neglect types that must be reported	• Physical abuse • Sexual abuse
Legal provisions	Section 356 of the *Children and Young People Act 2008* (ACT)

	New South Wales
Who is mandated to report?	A person who, in the course of his or her professional work or other paid employment delivers health care, welfare, education, children's services, residential services or law enforcement, wholly or partly, to children. A person who holds a management position in an organisation, the duties of which include direct responsibility for, or direct supervision of, the provision of health care, welfare, education, children's services, residential services or law enforcement, wholly or partly, to children

Continued

New South Wales	
What must be reported?	Reasonable grounds to suspect that a child is at risk of significant harm; and those grounds arise during the course of or from the person's work
Abuse and neglect types that must be reported	• Physical abuse • Sexual abuse • Emotional/psychological abuse • Neglect • Exposure to domestic violence
Legal provisions	Sections 23 and 27 of the *Children and Young Persons (Care and Protection) Act 1998 (NSW)*

Northern Territory	
Who is mandated to report?	Any person	A health practitioner or someone who performs work of a kind that is prescribed by regulation
What must be reported?	A belief on reasonable grounds that a child has suffered or is likely to suffer harm or exploitation	Reasonable grounds to believe a child aged 14 or 15 years has been or is likely to be a victim of a sexual offence and the age difference between the child and offender is greater than 2 years
Abuse and neglect types that must be reported	• Physical abuse • Sexual abuse or other exploitation of the child • Emotional/psychological abuse • Neglect • Exposure to physical violence (e.g. a child witnessing violence between parents at home)	• Sexual abuse

Legal provisions	Sections 15, 16 and 26 of the *Care and Protection of Children Act 2007 (NT)*		Section 26(2) of the *Care and Protection of Children Act 2007 (NT)*
		Queensland	
Who is mandated to report?	An authorised officer, a public service employee employed in the department, a person employed in a departmental care service or licensed care service	Relevant persons: doctors; registered nurses; teachers; a police officer who, under a direction given by the commissioner of the police service under the *Police Service Administration Act 1990*, is responsible for reporting under this section; a person engaged to perform a child advocate function under the *Public Guardian Act 2014*; early childhood education and care professionals.	School staff
What must be reported?	Has a reasonable suspicion that a child in care (a child placed in the care of an entity conducting a departmental care service or a licensee) has suffered, is suffering or is at unacceptable risk of suffering, significant harm caused by physical or sexual abuse	Has a reasonable suspicion that a child has suffered, is suffering or is at an unacceptable risk of suffering, significant harm caused by physical or sexual abuse; and may not have a parent able and willing to protect the child from the harm	Awareness or reasonable suspicion that a child has been or is likely to be sexually abused; and the suspicion is formed in the course of the person's employment

Continued

	Queensland		
Abuse and neglect types that must be reported	• Physical abuse • Sexual abuse	• Physical abuse • Sexual abuse	• Sexual abuse
Legal provisions	Part 1AA, Section 13f of the *Child Protection Act 1999 (Qld)*	Part 1AA, Section 13e of the *Child Protection Act 1999 (Qld)*	Sections 364, 365, 365A, 366, 36EA of the *Education (General Provisions) Act 2006 (Qld)*

	South Australia
Who is mandated to report?	Medical practitioners; pharmacists; registered or enrolled nurses; dentists; psychologists; police officers; community corrections officers; social workers; a minister of religion, a person who is an employee of, or volunteer in, an organisation formed for religious or spiritual purposes (with the exception of disclosures made in the confessional); teachers in educational institutions including kindergartens; approved family day care providers; any other person who is an employee/volunteer in a government or non-government organisation that provides health, welfare, education, sporting or recreational, child care or residential services wholly or partly for children, being a person who is actively engaged in the delivery of those services to children or who holds a management position in the relevant organisation, the duties of which include direct responsibility for, or direct supervision of, the provision of those services to children
What must be reported?	Reasonable grounds to suspect that a child has been or is being abused or neglected; and the suspicion is formed in the course of the person's work (whether paid or voluntary) or carrying out official duties
Abuse and neglect types that must be reported	• Physical abuse • Sexual abuse • Emotional/psychological abuse • Neglect

Legal provisions	Sections 6, 10 and 11 of the *Children's Protection Act 1993* (SA)
	Tasmania
Who is mandated to report?	Medical practitioners; registered or enrolled nurses; persons registered under the Health Practitioner Regulation National Law (Tasmania) in the midwifery, dental (dentists, dental therapist, dental hygienist or oral health therapist) or psychology professions; police officers; probation officers; principals and teachers in any educational institution including kindergartens; persons who provide child care or a child care service for fee or reward; persons concerned in the management of an approved education and care service, within the meaning of the Education and Care Services National Law (Tasmania) or a child care service licensed under the *Child Care Act 2001*; any other person who is employed or engaged as an employee for, of, or in or who is a volunteer in, a government agency that provides health, welfare, education, child care or residential services wholly or partly for children, and an organisation that receives any funding from the Crown for the provision of such services; and any other person of a class determined by the Minister by notice in the Gazette to be prescribed persons
What must be reported?	A belief, or suspicion on reasonable grounds, or knowledge that: a child has been or is being abused or neglected or is an affected child within the meaning of the Family Violence Act 2004 (a child whose safety, psychological wellbeing or interests are affected or likely to be affected by family violence); there is a reasonable likelihood of a child being killed or abused or neglected by a person with whom the child resides; or while a woman is pregnant that there is reasonable likelihood that after the birth of the child the child will suffer abuse or neglect, or may be killed by a person with whom the child is likely to reside, or that the child will require medical treatment or other intervention as a result of the behaviour of the woman or another person with whom the woman resides or is likely to reside, before the birth of the child

Continued

	Tasmania
Abuse and neglect types that must be reported	• Physical abuse • Sexual abuse • Emotional/psychological abuse • Neglect • Exposure to family violence
Legal provisions	Sections 3, 4 and 14 of the *Children, Young Persons and Their Families Act 1997 (Tas.)*

	Victoria	
Who is mandated to report?	Registered medical practitioners, nurses, midwives, a person registered as a teacher or an early childhood teacher under the *Education and Training and Reform Act 2006* or teachers granted permission to teach under that Act; principals of government or non-government schools within the meaning of the *Education and Training Reform Act 2006*; and police officers.	Any adult
What must be reported?	Belief on reasonable grounds that a child is in need of protection on a ground referred to in Section 162(1)(c) or 162(1)(d), formed in the course of practising his or her profession or carrying out the duties of his or her office, position or employment as soon as practicable after forming the belief and after each occasion on which he or she becomes aware of any further reasonable grounds for the belief.	A reasonable belief that a sexual offence has been committed in Victoria against a child under the age of 16 years by another person of or over the age of 18 years must disclose that information to a police officer as soon as it is practicable to do so, unless the person has a reasonable excuse for not doing so. Failure to disclose the information to police is a criminal offence.
Abuse and neglect types that must be reported	• Physical injury • Sexual abuse	• Sexual offence

Legal provisions	Sections 182(1)(a)-(e), 184 and 162(c)-(d) of the *Children, Youth and Families Act 2005 (Vic.)*	Section 327 of the *Crimes Act 1958*
	Western Australia	
Who is mandated to report?	Doctors; nurses and midwives; teachers or boarding supervisors; and police officers	The Principal Registrar, a registrar or a deputy registrar; family counsellors; family consultants; family dispute resolution practitioners, arbitrators or legal practitioners independently representing the child's interests
What must be reported?	Belief on reasonable grounds that child sexual abuse has occurred or is occurring and forms this belief in the course of the person's work, whether paid or unpaid	Reasonable grounds for suspecting that a child has been: abused; or is at risk of being abused; ill-treated, or is at risk of being ill-treated; or exposed or subjected to behaviour that psychologically harms the child
Abuse and neglect types that must be reported	Sexual abuse	<ul><li>Physical abuse</li><li>Sexual abuse</li><li>Neglect</li></ul> Psychological harm including (but not limited to) harm caused by being subjected or exposed to family violence.
Legal provisions	Sections 124A and 124B of the *Children and Community Services Act 2004*	Sections 5, 160 of the *Family Court Act 1997 (WA)*

Commerford, J. 2017. *Mandatory reporting of childhood abuse and neglect—CFCA Resource Sheet* [Online]. Australian Institute of Family Studies. Available: https://aifs.gov.au/cfca/publications/mandatory-reporting-child-abuse-and-neglect [Accessed 2 January 2018].

- **Always ask about caring responsibilities:** Are there children in the home? Or with the patient currently?
- Know your hospital policy for responding to domestic violence in particular regarding confidentiality and reportable injuries to the police.
- Know your mandatory, legal responsibilities for responding to child protection (make this a priority).
- Be compassionate.
- Be empathetic.
- Speak and listen with non-judgment.
- Work together with a woman's own sense of risk and safety coupled with your professional judgment and assessment for the best plan moving forward.

And finally, if your instincts are telling you that a woman and her children are at imminent risk of significant harm, consult with your senior doctor and contact the police for further liaison.

Online resources

National Sexual Assault, Domestic & Family Violence Counselling service
www.1800respect.org.au
Women's Legal Service—GP Toolkit
http://itstimetotalk.net.au/gp-toolkit/
Reporting Child Abuse & Neglect—contact details for each state and territory
https://aifs.gov.au/cfca/publications/reporting-abuse-and-neglect

Further reading

NSW Health Sexual Assault Services Policy and Procedure Manual (Adult) https://www1.health.nsw.gov.au/pds/ActivePDSDocuments/PD2005_607.pdf
NSW Health Education Centre Against Violence (ECAV). Medical and Forensic Management of Adult Sexual Assault. 2016.
Al-Yaman F, Van Doeland M, Wallis M. 2006. Family violence among Aboriginal and Torres Strait Islander peoples, Australian Institute of Health and Welfare Canberra, Australia.

Australian Bureau of Statistics. 2013. Personal Safety, Australia, 2012 [Online]. Available: http://www.abs.gov.au/ausstats/abs@.nsf/Lookup/4906.0Chapter1002012 [Accessed 17 December 2017].

Commerford, J. 2017. Mandatory reporting of childhood abuse and neglect—CFCA Resource Sheet [Online]. Australian Institute of Family Studies. Available: https://aifs.gov.au/cfca/publications/mandatory-reporting-child-abuse-and-neglect [Accessed 2 January 2018].

Domestic Violence Resource Centre Victoria. 2004. Identifying and responding to domestic violence: a general guide for practitioners [Online]. Available: https://www.dvrcv.org.au/publications/books-and-reports/guide-for-general-practitioners [Accessed 21 January 2018].

Legal Aid NSW. 2017. *Legal Aid NSW* [Online]. Available: https://www.legalaid.nsw.gov.au [Accessed 15 January 2018].

National Sexual Assault Domestic Family Violence Counselling Service. 2016. *Risk* Assessment and Safety Planning [Online]. Available: https://www.1800respect.org.au/resources-and-tools/risk-assessment-frameworks-and-tools [Accessed 6 January 2018].

Spangaro J, Ruane J. 2014. Health Interventions for Domestic and Family Violence: A Literature Review [Online]. School of Social Sciences, University of New South Wales. Available: http://www.health.nsw.gov.au/kidsfamilies/protection/Documents/health-interventions-for-family-and-domestic-violence.pdf [Accessed 4 November 2017].

World Health Organization. 2013. Responding to Intimate Partner Violence and Sexual Violence Against Women: WHO Clinical and Policy Guidelines [Online]. World Health Organization. Available: http://apps.who.int/iris/bitstream/10665/85240/1/9789241548595_eng.pdf [Accessed 12 December 2017].

Acknowledgment

The author wishes to acknowledge the content used from the previous edition of *Emergency Medicine* which was provided by Dr Nicola Woods.

In 2016 just over 300 000 women gave birth in hospital in Australia, a small but significant number of those occurring within the ED.[1]

Most of these unexpected births were as a result of a precipitous labour, defined as an extremely rapid labour with delivery of the baby in less than 3 hours from the onset of regular contractions. A smaller number of births are due to undiagnosed or concealed pregnancy (teenage girls, patients with developmental delay or mental health conditions).

Although the delivery of a baby is not a routine part of Emergency Medicine medical staff need to know how to assist with delivery in this scenario as well as provide resuscitation to the neonate if necessary.

Preparation and assessment

- Call for help! Obstetrics and gynaecology (O&G), and if available, paediatrics.
- There are two patients in this scenario—the mother and the baby. Dedicated medical and nursing staff are required for each.
- Perform a focused obstetric assessment.
  - LMP/gestational age
  - Gravity, parity
  - Previous deliveries—vaginal or caesarean? Any complications?
  - Symptoms of labour
  - Pregnancy complications
  - Relevant previous medical history, medications, allergies

- Focused examination
  - Vital signs
  - Fundal height
  - Presentation/lie—use ultrasound if available
  - Cervix—dilation and effacement
  - Fetal heart rate
  - Contractions—frequency, duration, regularity
- Assess stage of labour
  - 1st stage: regular contractions causing cervical dilation
  - 2nd stage: presenting part descends, delivery of the baby
  - 3rd stage: delivery of the placenta
- Look out for signs of imminent delivery like a bloody show (mucus plug expelled from cervix), rupture of membranes, or a maternal sensation to push or defecate.

Management
- Obtain IV access (at least 18 gauge), send bloods for FBC, G&H
- Analgesia—nitrous, morphine
- Also depends on patient factors such as gestational age, stage of labour, estimated rate of progression

Transfer
If the mother does not feel an urge to push, and the baby's head is not crowning (visible at the perineum) and the mother is stable transfer to a delivery suite can be considered.
- This depends on the availability of obstetric services and options of transfer (safe transfer to delivery suite always preferable to delivery in ED).
- Also depends on patient factors such as gestational age, stage of labour and estimated rate of progression.
  If transfer is not possible, arrange to perform emergency delivery.

Emergency delivery
EQUIPMENT
- Warm water to wash perineum
- Gauze sponges
- Sterile gloves and gown
- 2 sterile clamps to clamp umbilical cord
- Umbilical cord clamp

- Sterile scissors to cut cord
- Clean towels and blanket to dry and wrap neonate
- Container for placenta
- Neonatal resuscitation equipment
- Oxytocin 10 units

PROCEDURE

1 Don't panic! Keep calm and reassure the patient.
2 Assist the patient to assume a comfortable position with knees flexed, ideally not flat on her back.
3 Wash your hands and put on gown and gloves.
4 Wash the patient's perineum with warm water.
5 Encourage the patient to push when she gets the urge to.
6 If the membranes have not ruptured and are bulging at the perineum break them open with your fingers.
7 Place one hand on the baby's head and apply gentle pressure to maintain it in a flexed position. Use the other hand to ease the perineum over the baby's face.
8 Feel for the umbilical cord around the baby's neck. If present, gently slip it over the baby's head.
9 With the next push guide the head downwards to deliver the anterior shoulder, then guide the head slightly upwards to deliver the posterior shoulder. Do NOT pull. The rest of the baby's body should follow immediately.
10 Place the baby on the mother's abdomen or chest, double-clamp the umbilical cord and cut in between, approximately 1–2 cm from the baby's abdomen.
11 Dry the baby and wrap in a blanket. Keep warm.
12 Resuscitate if necessary, as per neonatal resuscitation algorithm (Australian Resuscitation Council Guidelines; see Figure 1.4).
13 Assign Apgar scores at 1 and 5 minutes post-delivery (Table 36.1).
14 Administer 10 U intramuscular oxytocin to the mother.
15 Look for signs of placental separation—lengthening of the cord, gush of blood from the vagina, change in shape of uterus fundus from discoid to globular with elevation of fundal height. Apply traction on the cord, backwards and downwards with one hand, while the other is placed suprapubically to support the uterus.

Table 36.1   Apgar score for assessment of neonates

Sign	Score 0	Score 1	Score 2	'APGAR' acronym
Colour	Blue, pale all over	Body pink, extremities blue	Body and extremities pink	Appearance
Heart rate	Absent	Slow (< 100 bpm)	> 100 bpm	Pulse
Reflex irritability	No response	Crying, some motion	Vigorous cry/ pulls away	Grimace
Muscle tone	Flaccid	Some flexion of extremities	Active motion, good flexion	Activity
Breathing	Absent	Slow, irregular, hypoventilation	Strong, cries lustily	Respiration

16 Inspect the placenta to ensure it is complete.

17 Rub over the uterus to facilitate contraction and expulsion of clots.

18 Inspect the perineum for lacerations. Apply pressure until these can be repaired.

19 Check for an undiagnosed twin.

20 Finally, don't forget to record the time of birth!

DIFFICULT DELIVERY

It is important to remember that most births in the ED are relatively straightforward; however, it is vital that you know how to manage complications should they arise.

- **Shoulder dystocia** is difficulty in delivering the anterior or less commonly posterior shoulder of the fetus. Incidence is around 1 in 1000 births. May result in significant morbidity and mortality risks—maternal complications including postpartum haemorrhage and third- or fourth-degree tearing, and fetal complications such as hypoxic brain injury and brachial plexus injury. Risk factors include macrosomia, previous shoulder dystocia and diabetes. The McRoberts manoeuvre has a 90% success rate—lie the patient flat, hyperflex the legs and apply gentle axial traction to the head. Suprapubic pressure may increase chance of success.

- **Breech delivery diagnosed in labour** is a rare occurrence. Leave the membranes intact if they have not ruptured spontaneously. Avoid intervening until the fetus has been expelled to the level of the umbilicus, then place gentle suprapubic pressure to assist with descent of the head. Do NOT place traction on the trunk as this may result in shoulder dystocia. If there is difficulty delivering the shoulders, wrap the fetal legs and pelvis in a towel and gently rotate 180° and back to assist in delivering each shoulder. The head will usually follow; however, if there is a delay turn the fetus' body to face downwards and apply further suprapubic pressure.

MANAGEMENT OF POST-PARTUM HAEMORRHAGE

Post-partum haemorrhage (PPH) is a common complication affecting up to 15% deliveries where there is a blood loss of more than 500 mL. Causes include uterine atony and placenta praevia.

Management

- Get help! O&G If available.
- ABC approach to resuscitation.
- Apply monitoring—cardiac, pulse oximetry, BP.
- Obtain large-bore IV access.
- Send bloods for FBC, EUC, coagulation screen and G&H.
- Fluid resuscitation as required—consider early use of group O Rh negative blood and activation of the massive transfusion protocol.
- Keep the patient warm and give warm fluids where possible.
- Perform uterine massage, ensure the bladder is empty, inserting IDC if necessary.
- If this is unsuccessful give oxytocin 5 units IV followed by 40 units in an IV infusion over 4 hours.
- Ergometrine 0.25 mg IV repeated, up to 1 mg.
- PR misoprostol and prostaglandin analogues may also be used if ongoing bleeding.
- Assess perineum, vagina and cervix for source of bleeding.
- Inspect the placenta—is it intact?
- Tranexamic acid may be given—give 1 g IV stat followed by a second dose at 30 minutes if bleeding persists.
- Surgical exploration may be required—liaise with local O&G services.

When the baby has already arrived

Occasionally a mother might present to ED with a newborn having just given birth, perhaps in the car on the way!

Both the mother and the baby must be assessed to check their wellbeing before making arrangements for transfer to an obstetric facility.

ASSESSMENT OF THE MOTHER

* Vital signs.
* Bleeding—should be less than 1 pad in first hour, otherwise assess and manage for PPH.
* Fundal height and tone—should be at level of umbilicus.
* Bladder fullness—you should not be able to palpate the bladder. If you can, encourage her to void. If she is unable to, insert an IDC—a full bladder interferes with uterine contractility and may increase the bleeding.
* Perineum—apply pressure to any bleeding lacerations until they can be repaired; an ice pack can reduce swelling.

Checks should be performed every 15 minutes for the first hour and then hourly.

ASSESSMENT OF THE BABY

First impressions of the baby are important—does it appear vigorous? By that we mean it has a good cry, normal tone and a heart rate > 100. If no, needs rapid assessment of vital signs and newborn resuscitation as per Australian Resuscitation Council (ARC) guidelines.

Check the baby is dry and warm—can warm with towels or on a resuscitaire if available.

Assess Apgar score (see Table 36.1).

Resuscitation of the newborn
ANZCOR GUIDELINE 13.1—INTRODUCTION TO RESUSCITATION OF THE NEWBORN INFANT (AUGUST 2018)
Summary

Guidelines 13.1–13.10 and the Newborn Life Support algorithm are provided to assist in the resuscitation of newborn infants. Differences from the adult and paediatric guidelines reflect differences in the causes of cardiorespiratory arrest in, and anatomy and physiology of, newborns, older infants, children and adults. These guidelines draw from the consensus on resuscitation and treatment recommendations issued by the International Liaison Committee on Resuscitation (ILCOR), which included representation from ARC and NZRC. The 2015 American Heart Association Guidelines for Cardiopulmonary Resuscitation and Emergency Cardiovascular Care (Neonatal), the European Resuscitation Council Guidelines for Resuscitation 2015 and local practices have also been taken into account.

To whom do these guidelines apply?

The term 'newborn' refers to the infant in the first minutes to hours following birth. In contrast, the neonatal period is defined as the first 28 days of life. Infancy includes the neonatal period and extends through the first 12 months of life.

Guidelines 13.1–13.10 and the Newborn Life Support algorithm are specifically for the care of infants during the neonatal period, and particularly for newborn infants. The exact age at which paediatric techniques and, in particular, compression-ventilation ratios should replace neonatal methods is unknown, especially for very small premature infants. For term neonates beyond the newborn period, and particularly in those with known or suspected cardiac aetiology of their arrest, paediatric techniques may be used (see Paediatric Advanced Life Support Guidelines 12.1–12.7).

Who is this audience for these guidelines?

Guidelines 13.1–13.10 and the Newborn Life Support algorithm are for health professionals and those who provide healthcare in environments where equipment and drugs are available (such as a hospital). When parents are taught CPR for their infants who are being discharged from birth hospitals, the information in Basic Life Support Guidelines (Guidelines 1–8) is appropriate.

Recommendations

The Australian and New Zealand Resuscitation Committee on Resuscitation (ANZCOR) recommends that:

1 Newborn infants be assessed for the need for basic and advanced life support and receive care using the Newborn Life Support algorithm and according to these guidelines.

2 Healthcare providers implement policies and protocols that utilise this algorithm and these guidelines.

Guideline

1 Need for neonatal resuscitation

Approximately 85% of babies born at term will initiate spontaneous respirations within 10 to 30 seconds of birth. An additional 10% will respond during drying and stimulation, approximately 3% will initiate respirations following positive-pressure ventilation, 2% will be intubated to support respiratory function and 0.1% will require chest compressions and/or adrenaline (epinephrine) to achieve this transition. Resuscitation is defined as the preservation or restoration of life by the establishment and/or maintenance of airway, breathing and circulation, and related emergency care (ANZCOR Guideline 1.1). For most newborns, resuscitation manoeuvres are administered as part of a graded strategy to support their own physiological efforts to adapt after birth. Only a very few appear lifeless and require the full range of neonatal resuscitation interventions described in these guidelines.

Term infants who have had low or no risk factors for needing resuscitation, who are breathing or crying and who have good tone must be dried and kept warm. These actions can be provided on the mother's chest (skin-to-skin) and should not require separation of mother and baby.

Although the need for resuscitation of the newborn infant can often be anticipated, and the need for resuscitation in low-risk births may be 1% or less, there remain many occasions when it is unexpected. Therefore, a suitable place, equipment and personnel trained to resuscitate a newborn infant must be available at all times, and in all places, where infants are born.

2 Unique physiology of newborn infants

The transition from fetal to extrauterine life is characterised by a series of unique physiological events. Among these, the lungs change from liquid-filled to air-filled, pulmonary blood flow increases dramatically and intracardiac and extracardiac shunts cease.

During the normal onset of breathing, newborns exert negative pressure on the lung with each breath. For the first few breaths, these pressures are greater than those needed for subsequent breaths, due to the need to clear liquid from the airways and begin lung aeration. If the baby does not achieve this initial lung aeration and positive-pressure ventilation needs to be used, higher peak inspiratory pressures may be needed for the first inflations than subsequently.

The level of pressure will vary from baby to baby, depending on the maturity of the lungs and any lung disease that is present. (For this reason, the suggested starting pressures provided in Guideline 13.4 are only a guide, and pressures need to be individually adjusted according to the baby's response.)

The fetal lung liquid moves from the airways to the lung tissue, and then reabsorbs more slowly (over several hours) into the circulation. In babies who are preterm or who have difficulty breathing, lung liquid can move back from the lung tissue into the airways, whereupon it needs to be cleared again, perhaps repeatedly. Continuous positive end expiratory pressure can help prevent this.

Aeration of the lungs triggers a fall in pulmonary vascular resistance and increase in pulmonary blood flow, which rises 5- to 6-fold after birth. In healthy newborn infants, oxygen levels rise over several minutes, typically taking 5–10 minutes for oxygen saturation of haemoglobin to reach 90%. Uncompromised babies born at sea level have oxygen saturation levels of about 60% during labour. The 25th centile for oxygen saturation is approximately 80% at 5 minutes. Normal newborn infants have a heart rate within 3–4 minutes after birth varying between 110 and 160/min.

Adaptation to extrauterine life depends on many coordinated and interdependent physiological events, failure of any of which can impair successful transition. Inadequate lung aeration can cause respiratory failure and prevent the normal increase in pulmonary blood flow. If pulmonary vascular resistance does not fall, the consequence is persistent pulmonary hypertension, with inadequate blood flow through the lungs and hypoxaemia. Haemorrhage from the fetus before birth can cause neonatal hypovolaemia and hypotension. Acidosis and hypoxia before or during birth can depress respiratory drive and cardiac function.

In preterm infants there are additional considerations. Surfactant deficiency reduces lung compliance. Preterm infants also typically have weaker respiratory muscles, immature airway protective reflexes and a chest wall that deforms easily. Very premature infants and infants born by caesarean section, without the effect of labour, may not clear fetal lung liquid and therefore, may not aerate their lungs as easily as term babies born by vaginal delivery.

In advanced gestation, passage of meconium into the amniotic fluid becomes more common and, in some cases, it is associated with fetal compromise. If meconium is passed into the amniotic fluid it may be inhaled before or during delivery and lead to inflammation of the lungs and airway obstruction. Complications of meconium aspiration are more likely in infants who are small for their gestation, and those born after term or with significant perinatal compromise.

Perinatal infections and congenital anomalies are among other potential causes of impaired adaptation at birth.

3 Anticipating the need for resuscitation

3.1 Personnel

All personnel who attend births should be trained in neonatal resuscitation skills which include: basic measures to maintain an open airway, ventilation via a facemask / laryngeal mask and chest compressions. At least one person should be responsible for the care of each infant.

A person trained in advanced neonatal resuscitation (all of the above skills plus endotracheal intubation and ventilation, vascular cannulation and the use of drugs and fluids) may be needed even for low-risk births and should be in attendance for all births considered at high risk for needing neonatal resuscitation.

Guideline 13.2 lists examples of maternal, fetal and intrapartum circumstances that place the newborn infant at increased risk of needing resuscitation. If it is anticipated that the infant is at high risk of requiring advanced resuscitation more than one experienced person should be present.

3.2 Training

Organised programs to develop and maintain standards, skills and teamwork are required for newborn resuscitation and are essential for healthcare providers and institutions caring for mothers and infants at the time of birth.

3.3 Equipment

The need for resuscitation at birth cannot always be anticipated. Therefore, a complete set of resuscitation equipment and drugs should always be available for all births. This equipment should be regularly checked to ensure it is complete and operational. A list of suggested resuscitation equipment and drugs is provided at the end of this guideline.

3.4 Communication

Preparation for a high-risk birth requires communication between the people caring for the mother and those responsible for the infant. This should include any factors that may affect the resuscitation and management of the infant including:

- maternal conditions
- antenatal diagnoses
- assessments of fetal wellbeing.

4 Environment

4.1 Temperature

Newborns are at risk from hypothermia or hyperthermia so prevention of both heat loss and overheating is important. Hypothermia can increase oxygen consumption and impede effective resuscitation. The infant should be cared for in a warm, draught-free area. For term and near term infants, drying the infant and removing the wet linen reduce heat loss [Class A, expert consensus opinion]. When resuscitation is not required the mother's body can keep the infant warm, using her as a heat source by placing the infant skin-to-skin on her chest or abdomen in a position that maintains airway patency and covering both with a warm blanket or towel. If resuscitation is necessary, place the infant under a preheated radiant warmer or, if unavailable, an alternative heat source.

Non-asphyxiated babies of all gestations should be maintained with a temperature of between 36.5 and 37.5°C. [CoSTR 2015, strong recommendation, very low quality of evidence]

Admission temperatures to newborn units are predictors of outcome and should be recorded as a quality of care measure. [CoSTR 2015, strong recommendation, moderate quality of evidence] Hypothermia is associated with an increased risk of mortality.

There is evidence of a dose effect with mortality increasing by 28% for each degree below 36.5°C at admission.

Hypothermia on admission is also associated with worse respiratory outcomes and greater likelihood of hypoglycaemia, late onset sepsis and intraventricular haemorrhage.

For special considerations for preterm infants see Guideline 13.8.

4.2 Hyperthermia

No studies have examined the effects of hyperthermia after resuscitation of newborn infants. However, babies born to febrile mothers (temperature >38°C) have an increased risk of death, perinatal respiratory depression, neonatal seizures and cerebral palsy.

4.3 Induced hypothermia for hypoxic ischaemic encephalopathy

Inducing hypothermia in infants of 35 weeks gestation and above with evolving moderate to severe hypoxic ischaemic encephalopathy will reduce the degree of brain injury in some (see Guideline 13.9). The target during resuscitation and stabilisation should be to maintain normothermia (with care to avoid hyperthermia), until a decision has been made that the baby has signs of encephalopathy and meets criteria for induced hypothermia. Any infant who is considered a possible candidate for therapeutic hypothermia should be discussed as soon as possible after initial resuscitation with a neonatal intensive care specialist, and plans should be made for prompt admission to a neonatal intensive care unit. If indicated, whole body cooling can be initiated without specialised equipment. Local guidelines should be in place to ensure that infants that meet criteria for induced hypothermia are promptly recognised and referred. [Class A, expert consensus opinion]

5 Recommended equipment and drugs for resuscitation of the newborn infant

Resuscitation equipment and drugs should be readily available in the areas of hospitals where infants are born or receive neonatal care. Equipment should be checked regularly according to local policy and before any resuscitation to ensure it is complete and operational. A clear record documenting the checking procedure should be maintained for each set of resuscitation equipment and drugs.

Prior preparation of standardised kits containing the equipment needed for procedures such as umbilical catheterisation can save considerable time in emergencies [Class B, expert consensus opinion].

5.1 Recommended equipment and drugs
General
- Firm, horizontal, padded resuscitation surface
- Overhead warmer
- Light for the area
- Clock with timer in seconds
- Warmed towels or similar covering
- Polyethylene bag or sheet, big enough for a baby less than 1500 g birth weight
- Stethoscope, neonatal size preferred
- Pulse oximeter plus neonatal probe

Equipment for airway management
- Suction apparatus and suction catheters (6F, 8F and either 10F or 12F)
- Oropharyngeal airways (sizes 0 and 00)
- Intubation equipment:
  — Laryngoscopes with infant blades (00, 0, 1)
  — Spare bulbs and batteries
  — Endotracheal tubes (sizes 2.5, 3, 3.5 and 4 mm ID, uncuffed, no eye)
  — Endotracheal stylet or introducer
  — Supplies for fixing endotracheal tubes (e.g. scissors, tape)
- End-tidal carbon dioxide detector (to confirm intubation)
- Meconium suction device (to apply suction directly to endotracheal tube)
- Magill forceps, neonatal size (optional)
- Laryngeal Mask airway, size 1

Equipment for supporting breathing
- Face masks (range of sizes suitable for premature and term infants)

- Positive-pressure ventilation device, either:
  — T-piece device; or
  — Flow-inflating bag with a pressure safety valve and manometer; and
  — Self-inflating bag (approximately 240 mL) with a removable oxygen reservoir
- Medical gases:
  — Source of medical oxygen (reticulated and/or cylinder, allowing flow rate of up to 10 L/min) with flow meter and tubing
  — Source of medical air plus air/oxygen blender
- Feeding tubes for gastric decompression (e.g. size 6 and 8F)

Equipment for supporting the circulation
- Umbilical venous catheter (UVC) kit (including UVC size 5F)
- Peripheral IV cannulation kit
- Skin preparation solution suitable for newborn skin
- Tapes/devices to secure UVC/IV cannula
- Syringes and needles (assorted sizes)
- Intraosseous needles

Drugs and fluids
- Adrenaline (epinephrine): 1:10 000 concentration (0.1 mg/mL)
- Volume expanders
- Normal saline
- Blood suitable for emergency neonatal transfusion needs to be readily available for a profoundly anaemic baby

Documentation
- Resuscitation record sheet

6 Cord clamping
In both animal and human studies, deferring cord clamping for 30–60 seconds, when compared with immediate cord clamping, is associated with increased placental transfusion, increased cardiac output and higher and more stable neonatal blood pressure. There is good evidence from animal studies that among the benefits, placental transfusion can fill the expanding pulmonary vascular bed, obviating the need for it to fill by 'left to right' flow from the aorta

across the ductus arteriosus. However, there remains controversy about how long it is appropriate to delay clamping if the baby is perceived to require resuscitation.

For the uncomplicated term birth, a meta-analysis of studies comparing delaying cord clamping after birth for a time ranging from 30 seconds until the cord stops pulsating with immediate cord clamping (usually within 15 seconds) showed higher neonatal haemoglobin levels and improved iron status through early infancy, but a greater likelihood of needing phototherapy for jaundice.

For the uncomplicated preterm birth, delaying cord clamping for a minimum time of 30 seconds increases the infant's blood pressure during stabilisation and at 4 hours after birth, reduces risk of periventricular leukomalacia and intraventricular haemorrhage (although there is insufficient evidence to determine whether there is an effect on severe IVH), lowers the incidence of necrotising enterocolitis, increases blood volume and lowers the chance of needing a blood transfusion. Although this evidence is from randomised trials, it is very low quality, having been downgraded for imprecision and very high risk of bias. In preterm infants, there is also low quality evidence that delayed cord clamping increases peak bilirubin levels but without increasing the likelihood of needing phototherapy.

We suggest delayed umbilical cord clamping for preterm infants not requiring immediate resuscitation after birth. (CoSTR 2015, weak recommendation, very low quality of evidence)

Although on theoretical grounds, the depressed infant might receive greater benefit from deferred cord clamping, constriction of uterine arteries normally occurs immediately after birth. Therefore it is unclear whether the placenta can be relied upon to provide compensatory gas exchange in the infant who does not begin breathing soon after birth. Furthermore, a depressed newborn may have experienced impaired placental gas exchange even before birth. Small and sick infants who received immediate resuscitation were generally excluded from the randomised trials conducted to date. Therefore, there is insufficient evidence to recommend the optimal timing of cord clamping in the compromised newborn. The more severely compromised the infant, the more likely it is that resuscitation measures need to take priority over delayed cord clamping. It stands to reason that cardiac compressions will not improve the systemic and coronary perfusion if the cord remains unclamped and the low resistance placenta is still connected.

6.1 Cord milking

Milking of the umbilical cord from the placental side to the newborn has been studied as an alternative method to increase the newborn's intravascular blood volume.

We suggest against the routine use of cord milking because there is insufficient published human evidence of benefit (CoSTR 2015, weak recommendation, very low quality of evidence).

7 Checking resuscitation equipment

ANZCOR and ARC guidelines should be considered in conjunction with accepted National Standards and local policies. ANZCOR is aware of cases where equipment failure (e.g. oxygen pipes being incorrectly connected resulting in hypoxic gases being administered, and resuscitation bag valve devices incorrectly assembled) has led to adverse outcomes.

The checking and maintenance of hospital and resuscitation equipment is covered by National Standards and local policies. Practitioners involved in resuscitation should always be alert to errors of assembly or use, and have checking processes to minimise these risks before equipment is used. They should also respond to unexpected situations with further checking procedures, and in the case of unexplained hypoxia change gas supply and circuits, and include removing the patient from ventilators and gas supplies by using a self-inflating bag with room air. In this situation oxygen analysis of delivered gases should be considered and an oxygen analyser should be available.

Online resources

Australian Resuscitation Council (ARC) Guidelines
   www.resus.org.au
Australian Institute of Health and Welfare
   www.aihw.gov.au
Emergency Care Institute
   www.aci.health.nsw.gov.au

RANZCOG guidelines
www.ranzcog.edu.au
UpToDate
www.uptodate.com

Reference

1. Australian Institute of Health and Welfare 2018. Australia's mothers and babies 2016—in brief. Perinatal statistics series no. 34. Cat. no. PER 97. Canberra: AIHW.

Chapter 37
Hand injuries and care
Bill Croker

Hand injuries are common in EDs. Meticulous assessment and management is crucial because preservation of function is critical for livelihood and recreation. See also Chapter 29 Orthopaedic Emergencies.

Assessment
Document:
1 Handedness
2 Occupation
3 Special interests (guitar, piano, gaming, model making, etc.)
4 Mechanism of injury (cutting, crushing, industrial, high-pressure injection, burn, bite)
5 Contamination
6 Time of injury
7 Specific symptoms (tingling, numbness, weakness)
8 Treatment so far
9 Immunisation status.

Examination
Document:
1 Position of hand—noting variation of finger positions from usual 'rest' posture
2 Location of injury
   — name fingers (not number)
   — palmar (volar) or dorsal surface
   — radial or ulnar border
3 Perfusion
4 Nerve function (see below)
5 Tendon function (see below).

NERVE FUNCTION—SCREENING TESTS
Median nerve
- Motor: test abduction of the thumb from the plane of the palm while palpating the thenar eminence
- Sensory: volar surface—thumb, palm and radial 2½ fingers; dorsal surface—radial 2½ fingers distal to the proximal interphalangeal (PIP) joint.

Radial nerve
- Motor: wrist extension and extension of digits.
- Sensory: dorsal surface—radial 2½ fingers proximal to PIP joint and dorsum of hand.

Ulnar nerve
- Motor: adduction of fingers in extension (hold a piece of paper between the fingers).
- Sensory: ulnar 1½ fingers and hand on both volar and dorsal surfaces.

TENDON FUNCTION
Test each joint of the fingers and thumb in flexion and extension. This will detect complete laceration only. Warn the patient about the possibility of delayed rupture.

The exact posture of the injured part at the time of injury cannot be accurately known. Therefore, inspect the base of the wound through the full range of movement of the adjacent joints, watching for defects in visible tendons. Testing flexor digitorum profundus (FDP) at the distal interphalangeal (DIP) joint requires the joint more proximal to be held in extension during flexion of the joint being tested. Testing flexor digitorum superficialis (FDS) at the PIP joint requires all fingers except the one being tested to be held in extension to neutralise the mass flexor effect of FDP at the PIP joint.

Treatment
INITIAL TREATMENT
1 Analgesia:
   — digital block (avoid adrenaline)
   Always check sensation prior to application of local anaesthetic.

— wrist block
— IV narcotics.

2 X-ray the injured part if there is a possibility of bony injury or foreign body.
3 Check tetanus status.
4 Carefully clean open injuries and remove debris.
5 Antibiotics if extensive injury or compound fracture.
6 Elevate (pillow-case sling from an IV pole if being admitted).
7 Keep fasted and commence IV fluids if surgery a possibility.
8 Splint injured finger, especially if protracted delay to specialist review.

SPLINTING

The hand is splinted in a position to minimise the risk of stiffness after treatment: wrist extended (40°); metacarpophalangeal (MCP) joints flexed (90°) and fingers fully extended. This position keeps the collateral ligaments of the fingers at their maximal length.

Splint only those joints that need to be included for a particular injury. There are multiple commercially available splints. Discuss with your hand therapist.

Explain to the patient the importance of moving any joint not enclosed in the splint, to minimise stiffness.

HAND THERAPY

Follow-up that involves a hand therapist ensures optimal outcome.

Soft-tissue injuries
LACERATIONS

These require careful inspection through full range of movement following local anaesthetic. Document any sensory changes prior to anaesthetic.

Sutures, if required, should be 5/0 non-absorbable and are removed after 5–7 days—longer if over extensor joints, in the elderly or in patients on steroids.

PALMAR LACERATIONS

'No-man's land' is the zone from the mid-palm to the PIP joint where the tendons of the flexor superficialis and profundus are enclosed together in tendon sheaths. Great care in assessment is necessary. Palmar skin is thick and difficult to suture. Anaesthesia is difficult to achieve with local infiltration for similar reasons.

Request senior review.

FINGER LACERATIONS

Careful assessment for associated nerve and tendon injury. If present commence initial treatment as above, and specific treatment as described below and refer as appropriate. Otherwise, suture as indicated.

LACERATIONS OF THE EXTENSOR SURFACE OVERLYING THE PIP JOINT

Otherwise innocuous-looking lacerations of the extensor surface of the PIP joint can transect the central slip of the extensor mechanism with preservation of extensor function initially. However, a boutonnière deformity will subsequently develop if the tendon has been cut.

Refer to the hand/plastic/orthopaedic team as per your hospital's practice for exploration and repair. Commence initial treatment.

FINGERTIP INJURIES

Involve the pulp, the nail, the bone or any combination. While usually not large, these can be very painful.

SMALL SKIN LOSS WITHOUT BONE EXPOSED

(Small skin loss = area smaller than a 5-cent piece.)

1 Anaesthesia.
2 Clean.
3 Apply 'wet' dressing (membrane) or chloramphenicol (Chloromycetin) ointment.
4 Change every 2–3 days until healed (dressing clinic, LMO or home).
5 Elevate (hand above elbow) to reduce pain and swelling for first 2–3 days.
6 Refer to the hand/plastic/orthopaedic team according to your hospital's practice for outpatient follow-up.
7 Active and passive mobilisation to avoid stiffness after first 2–3 days.

8 Analgesia.

9 Review for infection (increasing pain, spreading redness, fever—a late manifestation).

LARGER DEFECT OR WITH BONE EXPOSED

Defects larger than 1 cm in diameter require skin graft. Refer to the hand/plastic/orthopaedic team according to your hospital's practice. Commence initial treatment.

Nails
NAIL BED LACERATIONS

Meticulous repair is critical. It is not just cosmetic; poor technique results in a permanently split or deformed nail. Refer to the hand/plastic/orthopaedic team according to your hospital's practice for repair of laceration.

Preserve the nail; it can be used as a splint.

Commence initial treatment.

SUBUNGUAL HAEMATOMA
With NO injury to nail or surrounding nail margin

Crush injury. X-ray to exclude fracture. If at least moderately painful, carefully clean the nail then drill through the nail in 2 or 3 spots with a 19-gauge needle spun between thumb and index finger to release the blood. The nail bed only needs to be examined if there is significant associated injury regardless of the size of the haematoma.

Dress, splint, analgesia, elevate for 48 hours.

Associated undisplaced fractures are considered 'open' and treated with oral antibiotics.

With injury to nail or surrounding nail margin

There is risk of nail bed laceration. X-ray and refer for review by the hand/plastic/orthopaedic team.

AVULSION

Nails take 3 months to grow from nail bed to tip, delayed by a month if the bed is injured.

If the nail is avulsed there is a risk of nail bed laceration. Refer for review by the hand/plastic/orthopaedic team.

Tendons
MALLET FINGER

A mallet finger is an avulsion of the extensor tendon at its insertion into the distal phalanx. The patient is unable to fully extend their distal phalanx. It occurs when there is a sudden forced flexion of an extended finger (hit by cricket ball, basketball, etc.).

Without fracture

Splint in gentle hyperextension for 6 weeks—commercially available splints recommended.

Refer to the hand/plastic/orthopaedic team according to your hospital's practice for outpatient follow-up.

With fracture

If there is a fracture involving more than 30% of the articular surface, this will need to be meticulously repaired. Refer to the hand/plastic/orthopaedic team according to your hospital's practice. Commence initial treatment.

Nerve injuries

The digital nerves and arteries run in a bundle along the line joining the flexion creases of a flexed finger. Beyond the distal flexion crease, the nerve breaks up into terminal branches which are not practical to repair. Some sensation will return eventually.

Lacerations proximal to the DIP joint causing sensory loss require exploration. Refer to the hand/plastic/orthopaedic team according to your hospital's practice. Commence initial treatment.

Nerves regrow at a rate of up to 1 mm a day. After repair, no guarantee can be given about return of function, which takes several months even when repair is successful. Commitment to physiotherapy is required to optimise outcome.

Vascular injuries

The ulnar artery is the dominant artery of the hand.
1 Control brisk bleeding with direct pressure—gauze and gloved fingers—to prevent exsanguination.
2 If bleeding persists when pressure removed, apply an arterial tourniquet (blood-pressure cuff inflated to 50 mmHg above systolic pressure for no longer than 20 minutes) prior to

exploration and definitive treatment. Tourniquets are very painful and carry the risk of tissue ischaemia if left inflated too long.

3 A history of pulsatile bleeding dictates exploration of the wound to tie off both ends of the artery, to prevent formation of a pseudoaneurysm.
4 Refer to the hand/plastic/orthopaedic team according to your hospital's practice.
5 Commence initial treatment.

Bony injuries
See also, Chapter 29 Orthopaedic Principles.

PHALANGES
Fractures with rotational deformities
1 Assess for the presence of any rotational deformation by getting the patient to touch their thenar eminence with all their fingers simultaneously. If the injured finger is twisted, then a rotational deformation is present.
2 Digital block.
3 Correct rotational deformation.
4 Buddy-strap finger (gauze between fingers to minimise rubbing).
5 Elevation, analgesia, active and passive movement of fingers to reduce stiffness.
6 Refer to the hand/plastic/orthopaedic team according to your hospital's practice for outpatient follow-up in about 1 week to ensure no delayed deformity.
7 If rotational deformation, or more than 10° of angulation, persists after reduction, refer to the hand/plastic/orthopaedic team according to your hospital's practice for accurate reduction and fixation.

Fractures without rotational deformities
If no rotational deformity is present, buddy-strap, elevate until acute pain settles and then use hand normally, provide analgesia and refer to LMO for review.

Any spiral fracture of digits or metacarpals is potentially unstable—refer to the hand/plastic/orthopaedic team according to your hospital's practice.

Fractures involving joint surfaces

Commence initial treatment.

Refer to the hand/plastic/orthopaedic team according to your hospital's practice for accurate reduction and fixation.

DISLOCATIONS

Position of fingers needs to be accurately documented by X-ray or photo prior to reduction.

1 Digital block.
2 Reduce dislocation, usually by gentle traction. If unsuccessful, try increasing the deformation (i.e. if dorsal dislocation, apply hyperextension before traction).
3 Buddy-strap finger (gauze between fingers to minimise rubbing).
4 Elevation, analgesia, active and passive movement of fingers to reduce stiffness.
5 Refer to the hand/plastic/orthopaedic team according to your hospital's practice for outpatient follow-up in about 1 week to assess for instability and continued hand therapy.

COMPOUND FRACTURES

Commence initial treatment.

Refer to the hand/plastic/orthopaedic team according to your hospital's practice for washout, reduction and closure.

FRACTURE OF THE FIFTH METACARPAL NECK

Provided angulation of this common 'punching' injury is less than 45°, a simple volar back slab for 3–4 weeks will usually provide sufficient support. Refer to LMO for review to ensure fracture does not slip.

Otherwise, refer to the hand/plastic/orthopaedic team according to your hospital's practice for reduction.

CARPAL BONES

Scaphoid fractures

The scaphoid is the keystone of the carpus, and non-union following fracture results in chronic pain and instability. Early CT or MRI will clarify the diagnosis. Management of definite fractures is controversial; conservative management in a scaphoid cast or open reduction internal fixation (ORIF) should be deferred to the appropriate specialist team (see also Chapter 29).

Emergency treatment for a suspected fracture is:
1 Wrist splint.
2 Elevate.
3 CT or MRI as rapidly as possible with referral if required.

Gamekeeper's thumb
Forced abduction of the thumb (as in skiing) results in rupture of the ulnar collateral ligament of the thumb.

Assess for tenderness over the ulnar border of the MCP joint. If present, treat with a scaphoid plaster or commercial splint and refer to the appropriate team for outpatient follow-up in about 1 week for reassessment and continued hand therapy.

Specific conditions
INFECTIONS
- Suspect foreign bodies.
- Pain on passive stretch suggests tendon sheath infection or compartment syndrome.
- If not septic and no suggestion of tendon sheath infection, foreign body or collection, commence oral antibiotics, splint, elevate and review in 24 hours (earlier if there is any sign of deterioration).
- If there is evidence of tenosynovitis, early referral for operative drainage of the tendon sheath under general anaesthetic is necessary. Refer to the hand/plastic/orthopaedic team according to your hospital's practice. Commence initial treatment, in particular early intravenous antibiotics.
  Specific infections are discussed below.

PARONYCHIA
Paronychia is infection of the tissues around the fingernail.
1 Digital block.
2 Soak the finger in warm water for about 10 minutes.
3 Blunt-dissect with fine scissors or number 11 scalpel under the skin fold to open the abscess.

751

4 Irrigate.
5 Pack.
6 Analgesia, elevate and review in 24 hours.
7 Antibiotics are only indicated if there is significant surrounding cellulitis. Oral cephalosporins are generally adequate, although non-multiresistant oxacillin-resistant *Staphylococcus aureus* (NORSA) strains, which are increasing in incidence, may respond to clindamycin. Refer to the Therapeutic Guidelines (www.ciap.health.nsw.gov.au/home.html).
8 Complications include subungual abscess, which requires the nail to be removed.

Chronic paronychia
Usually occupational from prolonged exposure of hands to water; involves bacterial and candidal infection.

Treatment involves drying hands with 70% alcohol and applying a topical antifungal cream such as clotrimazole 1%. The nail is removed only if the infection is intractable. Refer to hand surgery for marsupialisation and wedge resection of nail.

PYOGENIC GRANULOMA
These are collections of granulation tissue developing around a foreign body such as suture material. Treatment is by curette or formal surgical excision with histological examination of excised tissue.

FELON
A felon is an abscess of the pulp of the distal phalanx, which requires drainage. It usually presents with throbbing pain, swelling and tenderness without fluctuance.
1 Digital block.
2 Forearm tourniquet to provide a bloodless field.
3 A central longitudinal incision avoiding crossing the flexion crease protects the digital neurovascular bundle and flexor tendon sheath. Avoid incision of vertical pulp space fibres. Incision is made down to the bone avoiding FDP insertion.
4 Delay to treatment may result in osteomyelitis, pulp necrosis or loss of pinch function.

HERPETIC WHITLOW

Herpetic whitlow is most commonly seen in healthcare workers. It presents as a vesicle around the nail or finger pad and is intensely painful.

Swabs may be taken for herpes zoster polymerase chain reaction (PCR).

Topical aciclovir is used with variable success. Unlike bacterial infections, incision and drainage is not indicated.

BITES

Bites have a high rate of infection.

If the bite is **simple and superficial** (i.e. with no evidence of involvement of underlying structures, does not involve hands, feet or face), the patient is immunocompetent and seen in under 8 hours:

- irrigate copiously, clean carefully
- debride as necessary
- consider delayed primary closure
- elevate
- immobilise
- review at 24 hours to ensure no infection.

'Bites' or 'tooth penetration wounds' due to punching injuries should be X-rayed to ensure there are no tooth fragments in the wound. Oral flora inoculated into the MCP joint with clenched-fist injuries usually results in a septic joint. Operative drainage is required, splinting, elevation and broad-spectrum parenteral antibiotics (see Antibiotic Guidelines, www.ciap.health.nsw.gov. au/home.html).

For **all other injuries** (complex or deep lacerations, involvement of underlying structures or delayed presentation), refer to the hand/plastic/orthopaedic team according to your hospital's practice. Commence initial treatment.

CRUSH INJURIES

Crush injuries cause extensive soft-tissue damage, without necessarily causing any bony injury. Initial assessment may reveal minimal external evidence of injury. Contained bleeding and tissue oedema resulting from the crush injury can cause progressively increasing pressure resulting in tissue ischaemia—the compartment syndrome.

History should be extended to include mechanism of crush, duration of compression and areas included under the compressive forces.

Examine in particular for signs of the **compartment syndrome**: pain out of proportion to the injury, pain on passive stretch of the compartment, tense feel to the compartment and distal paraesthesia. Pulses are normal until very late in the evolution of the compartment syndrome.

Refer to the hand/plastic/orthopaedic team according to your hospital's practice for observation and possible fasciotomy. Commence initial treatment.

Treat associated injuries as appropriate (lacerations, fractures or dislocations, arterial injuries).

Commence strict elevation with hourly limb observations to detect early signs of compartment syndrome.

HIGH-PRESSURE INJECTION INJURIES

Industrial accidents involving injection (e.g. paint, grease, gas) into the hand are urgently referred to the hand/plastic/orthopaedic team according to your hospital's practice for observation and possible debridement of devitalised tissue or fasciotomy for decompression of ensuing compartment syndrome. Commence initial treatment.

BURNS

Burns of the hand represent a 'special area' injury and should be discussed with the regional burns injury unit. Commence initial treatment—adequate cooling (minimum of 20 minutes) at 15°C (range 8–25°C) within 3 hours of incident: generous analgesia.

Indications for referral to burns unit:

- Circumferential burns to hand or fingers
- Multiple digits or web spaces involved
- Burns involving joint surfaces
- Deep dermal burn or uncertain depth
- Electrical or chemical burn
- Crush injuries or other injuries or systemic illness
- Delayed healing > 1 week.

If transfer to burns unit is indicated, the wound area should be wrapped in plastic cling wrap after cooling is completed. Hand burns that do not require transfer should have paraffin gauze dressing.

Superficial partial-thickness dorsal surface burns (classically scalds or fat burns) should be reviewed at 24 hours to ensure correct initial assessment and then can be treated with analgesia, elevation and daily dressings by LMO or dressing clinic.

HYDROFLUORIC ACID BURNS

Hydrofluoric acid is an industrial cleaning agent which causes liquefactive necrosis resulting in deep-tissue damage and intense pain, often without much external sign of injury.

Specific treatment is calcium, which can be administered by a variety of routes. Calcium gluconate 2.5% gel (made by mixing 10% calcium gluconate solution with 3 times the volume of KY gel) can be used topically. For finger burns, the gel can be placed in a latex glove and the affected hand inserted into it for up to 45 minutes. This can be repeated 6-hourly for 24 hours until pain eases.

Intra-arterial calcium gluconate is effective second-line therapy for more severe and extensive hand burns. Infusion of 10–20 mL of 10% calcium gluconate in 200 mL 5% dextrose over 4 hours via a radial artery catheter is more effective than intravenous administration and safer than local infiltration, which risks compartment syndrome due to the volumes required.

Refer to the hand/plastic/orthopaedic team, according to your hospital's practice, for treatment.

ELECTRICAL INJURIES

Initial assessment can be misleading, as the full extent of injury may not be apparent at first.

Perform a very careful neurovascular examination.

Refer to the hand/plastic/orthopaedic team according to your hospital's practice.

AMPUTATIONS

Indications for replantation or revascularisation include thumb amputations, amputation of multiple digits, individual amputations distal to insertion of FDS and cold ischaemia time less than 24 hours.

Refer to the hand/plastic/orthopaedic team according to your hospital's practice for consideration of replantation. Commence initial treatment.

Care of the amputated part

No amputated part should be discarded until a formal plan of replantation has been discussed with surgeon and patient.

1 Carefully and gently clean the part.
2 Wrap in sterile saline-soaked gauze.
3 Place in a sealed plastic bag in an ice-water bath at 4°C.
4 X-ray both the stump and the amputated part.

CARPAL TUNNEL SYNDROME

Compression neuropathy of the median nerve as it traverses the wrist deep to the flexor retinaculum can be chronic or acute (suppurative infection, burn, haemorrhage, postoperative) and idiopathic or secondary to increase in carpal tunnel contents (tenosynovitis, haematoma, oedema) or decrease in size of tunnel (arthritis, fracture or dislocation of the lunate).

Indications for decompression include acute carpal tunnel syndrome with rapid onset and progression of median nerve impairment, persistent symptoms despite conservative measures, impaired sensation in radial 2½ fingers or thenar muscle palsy.

1 Conduct a thorough neurovascular and functional assessment.
2 Splint and elevate.
3 Refer to the hand/plastic/orthopaedic team according to your hospital's practice for endoscopic release or open carpal tunnel release.

Editorial Comment

Hand/finger injuries are very common, but require extra knowledge and care to avoid major functional problems that may affect livelihood, etc.

Chapter 38
Ophthalmic emergencies

Michael R Delaney and Gordian Fulde

Acknowledgment

The authors wish to acknowledge the content used from the previous edition of *Emergency Medicine* which was provided by Iromi Samarasinghe.

Principles of examination

1 All cases of suspected eye injuries need a good history and examination of:
   — visual acuity—visual loss sudden/gradual; central/peripheral; monocular/binocular
   — pupillary reactions
   — the fundus
   — ocular movement
   — fields to confrontation
   — lids and ocular adnexae.

2 Do not put pressure on the eye to examine it (especially if there is a possible penetrating injury).

3 Use a short-acting mydriatic (e.g. tropicamide 1%; duration of action 60 minutes), and only if essential.

4 Cycloplegics are not used when examining the eye due to their long duration of action. Only use a short-acting cycloplegic, if necessary for comfort (e.g. cyclopentolate 1% [effective for 4–8 hours] or homatropine 2% [effective for 8–12 hours]).

5 CT scan or X-ray the orbits in all cases of a suspected intraocular foreign body, especially if the patient was using a hammer on metal (e.g. a chisel). Request X-ray with eyes in up and down gazes.

Common Pitfalls

- Never use steroid drops in the ED in initial treatment. Refer for further assessment.
- Do not use atropine drops to dilate the pupil.
- Do not use mydriatics in cases where the ocular state and optic nerve function may need to be monitored.
- Eye swabs need to be plated out directly.
- Avoid contaminated diagnostic medications. Use only sterile drop solutions.
- Always pad an eye after instilling local anaesthetic.
- Never give local anaesthetic drops to the patient to take away and use.
- Do not apply ointment in cases of suspected penetrating injury.
- Do not persist in trying to remove a corneal foreign body if it is not easily removed—refer for ophthalmology review.
- Always provide adequate systemic analgesia in cases of corneal injury.
- When in doubt seek an ophthalmic consultation.

Use of the slit lamp

These remarks apply to the Haag-Streit slit lamp, but the principles apply to all slit lamps.

- The patient and the examining doctor must both be seated comfortably. In particular, the patient should not be straining to keep the chin on the chin rest, and the patient's forehead must rest comfortably against the forehead strap.
- The eye should be at the level of the black mark on the side of the two columns that hold the chin rest and forehead strap; this is achieved by adjusting the height of the chin rest. The slit lamp should then be adjusted so that it is in its mid-position, allowing a full range of vertical and horizontal movement. This position is adjusted by rotating the joystick which controls the height of the slit lamp (by rotating the handle alone) as well as the movement of the slit lamp in all directions, thereby controlling its focus.
- After the patient is positioned correctly, the eye can be examined. Turn power on at the base of the slit lamp table; adjust eye pieces to zero if no refractory error adjustments are required for the examiner; set magnification by adjusting the swing lever between eye pieces.

- On the bottom of the rotating light-source column of the slit lamp is a knob that controls the width of the slit beam; the knob on the left side can be adjusted with the examiner's left hand. Further up near the top of the light-source column, immediately under the globe-housing, is a control to adjust the intensity of the light; use the neutral-density filter (mid-position) to reduce discomfort for the patient from the brightness of the light. This same control also allows the insertion of a cobalt blue filter into the light, producing the characteristic blue light used to detect corneal ulcers with fluorescein dye. Below this control is another control knob that adjusts the height of the slit beam.

- Focus the slit beam on the eye before looking through the viewfinder. Move the joystick with one hand while looking through the viewfinder till the cornea comes into focus. Keep the other hand free for handling the eye.

- The slit lamp can be used in many ways.
  — The easiest is simply to use it as a high-powered illumination source with magnification using the broad beam; this is particularly useful to detect corneal ulceration after instilling fluorescein dye and using the cobalt blue filter.
  — To detect and assess iritis, a narrow slit beam can be shone through the anterior chamber; this will highlight any flare or cells.
  — A slit beam can be shone directly through the pupil to retro-illuminate the iris using the red reflex; this is also a useful way of assessing the clarity of the media.

- Intraocular pressures are measured using the application tonometer, which is either attached to the slit lamp on a swinging arm or is detached from the slit lamp and is placed on the platform immediately in front of the eye pieces.

Trauma
FOREIGN BODY (FB)
Conjunctiva
Carefully examine posterior lid surfaces and fornices by everting the upper lid. Remove FB with moist swabstick or fine forceps.

Cornea

- Remove FB with a sterile swab stick or sterile 25-gauge needle. Do not attempt to remove any rust ring. Apply antibiotic ointment and pad firmly.
- Topical antibiotic drops are often preferred to ointment by patients following the initial management.
- Patients with a residual rust ring and foreign body remnants must be referred to an ophthalmologist according to your hospital's practice.

Intraocular

- Always suspect FB if there has been an eye injury after using a metal hammer on metal, or where there have been high-velocity particles.
- There are often minimal signs. CT scan or X-ray of the orbit is mandatory.
- Treat as a penetrating injury (see later in this chapter) and organise urgent ophthalmic consultation.

CORNEAL ABRASIONS

- Examine the eye under cobalt blue light after instilling local anaesthetic drops (amethocaine 0.5%, also known as tetracaine) and fluorescein.
- Check for subtarsal FB.
- Treat with chloramphenicol 1% antibiotic ointment and firm pad for 24 hours and provide adequate analgesia.

LID LACERATIONS

- All lid lacerations must be carefully assessed to exclude penetrating eye injury.
- Lacerations nasal to the punctum on the upper or the lower eyelids should be referred to an ophthalmologist to exclude damage to the nasolacrimal drainage system.
- Inspect punctum and look for lacerations to the canaliculus, which require prompt repair.
- Lacerations through the lid margin need meticulous repair to prevent lid notching. Refer to ophthalmology service according to your hospital's practice.

BURNS
Chemical: acid or alkali

1 Immediate irrigation with copious amounts of water or saline solution for at least 30 minutes until the pH neutralises to 7.5. Use universal indicator paper (if available) to check corneal pH in the forniceal space after every litre of fluid irrigation.
2 If pain limits eye opening, instil local anaesthetic drops (amethocaine [tetracaine] 0.5%).
3 Alkali burns from lime, mortar and plaster are the most damaging of all chemical injuries. All particles of lime must be removed using a cotton bud or fine forceps. Evert lids to inspect fornices.
4 Acid burns commonly result from exposure to car battery fluid, toilet cleaners and pool cleaners.
5 All chemical burns should be referred to ophthalmology on the same day. Systemic analgesia is often required.

Thermal burns

Remove any obvious loose FBs after instilling anaesthetic drops. Start antibiotic drops and pad if possible.

Flash burns

• Symptoms appear hours after exposure to sunlamps or welding arcs without eye protection. These are intensely painful with blepharospasm, tearing and redness. Pain can start up to 6–12 hours after injury and last for 24 hours.
• Examination is only possible after topical anaesthesia. Slit lamp examination with fluorescein will show widespread epithelial defects bilaterally.

Management

1 Apply chloramphenicol 1% ointment and pad. Cycloplegics may be needed to minimise severe eye pain (homatropine 2% BD for 3 days). Systemic analgesia and sedation are usually needed.
2 Ophthalmic review in 24 hours.

BLUNT OCULAR TRAUMA

Severe injuries can be easily missed. The history is not always a good guide to the severity of the injuries.

Subconjunctival haemorrhage
◆ The appearance is alarming. No treatment is needed except reassurance.
◆ Examine the eye to exclude any other injuries.

Hyphaema
Blood in anterior chamber following blunt trauma involving punch or cricket/squash ball to eye. Consider lymphoma, leukaemia and child abuse if bleed is 'spontaneous'.

Management
1 Admit to hospital for bed rest, head elevation to 30–45° and limit eye movement with pad. Bed rest at home if circumstances are appropriate. Arrange for urgent ophthalmic consultation within 24 hours.
2 Rule out orbital fracture and ruptured globe with CT of orbits and facial bones.
3 Provide adequate analgesia, avoiding aspirin.
4 After ophthalmic consultation control intraocular pressure (IOP) with:
   — prostaglandin analogues (e.g. latanoprost 1 drop) AND/OR
   — daily beta-blockers (e.g. timolol 0.5% 1 drop BD) OR
   — acetazolamide 250–1000 mg/day OR
   — mannitol 20% in 500 mL IV in severe cases.
5 Complications include:
   — a more severe secondary haemorrhage in 30% of cases, 2–5 days after the initial bleed (especially in children)
   — secondary glaucoma due to outflow obstruction
   — raised IOP
   — missed blowout fractures of orbit.

Editorial Comment

To minimise side effects from naso-oral absorption of eyedrops ask patient to occlude nasolacrimal duct by finger pressure medially for a couple of minutes. It also decreases loss of drop fluid from eye.

Traumatic mydriasis and iridodialysis
No treatment is available. Often associated with hyphaema. Remember as a cause of abnormal pupillary reactions in cases with head and eye injuries.

Lens and retinal injuries
These need referral within 24 hours. See the section Retinal Detachment under Sudden Painless Monocular Visual Loss later in this chapter.

Ruptured globe
Occurs following blunt trauma with sufficient force, resulting in rupture at thinnest point of scleral wall, usually near corneal limbus.
- Examination may be significantly limited by oedema. Assess visual acuity and extraocular movements. Ophthalmoscopy may often reveal loss of red reflex due to vitreal haemorrhage.
- Urgent CT scan of orbits to exclude blowout fracture and referral to ophthalmologist, if otherwise stable from trauma point of view.
- Ensure eye is lightly padded and patient has adequate analgesia.

Traumatic vitreous haemorrhage and choroidal haemorrhage
Advise bed rest at home. Arrange ophthalmology referral within 24 hours to exclude retinal detachment. See the section Vitreous Haemorrhage under Sudden Painless Monocular Visual Loss later this chapter.

ORBITAL FRACTURES AND HAEMORRHAGE
Blowout fractures
Mechanism of injury involves punch or squash/cricket ball to orbit. Often associated with fractures of malar complex and of the middle third of the face.
- Pain on vertical eye movement and local tenderness along orbital margin. Suspect if there is restriction of extraocular movement, enophthalmos or the patient complains of double vision (restricted up and down gaze).

- Assess infraorbital nerve involvement by testing sensation on unilateral cheek and upper incisors. The eye must be examined during initial assessment.
- Investigations include CT scan of brain and orbital reconstructions (coronal views most useful).

Management

1 Admit if other injuries require treatment. Otherwise needs referral within 24 hours for evaluation of diplopia and enophthalmos.
2 Start oral antibiotics (cefalexin 500 mg QID).
3 Instruct patient not to blow nose and to avoid Valsalva manoeuvres in the first week. Nasal decongestants for 7–10 days.
4 Surgical repair is usually done after 7–14 days.

Orbital haemorrhage

- Often associated with orbital fractures.
- Can be sight-threatening. Needs urgent consultation if severe or the patient has reduced vision, non-reacting pupils or ophthalmoplegia (diplopia on up and down gaze) and proptosis.
- May need urgent orbital decompression.

Optic canal fractures

- Often cause total visual loss due to compression of the optic nerve. Diagnosed on CT scans of brain and orbits.
- Needs urgent referral to ophthalmic surgeon.

PENETRATING INJURIES

- Suspect from history, especially hammering on metal.
- Examine very gently. Do not put pressure on the eye. Check visual acuity; red reflex; slit lamp examination for anterior chamber and corneal disruptions should only be done if trauma is not obvious.

Management

1 Keep nil by mouth. Provide adequate parenteral narcotics with antiemetics. Check tetanus immunisation and update as

appropriate. Start systemic antibiotics (ceftriaxone 1 g daily) and local antibiotic drops (do not use ointment). Gently shield (do not pad) the eye.

2 Obtain X-ray or CT scan of the orbit if there is any possibility of intraocular FB.

3 Admit to hospital for bed rest or refer for urgent ophthalmology review according to your hospital's practice.

The painful red eye
ACUTE BLEPHARITIS
Localised eyelid inflammation. Can present as chalazion or stye.

• Treat with topical antibiotics and warm compresses. Routine referral to ophthalmologist.

CORNEAL FOREIGN BODY OR ABRASION
(Discussed earlier.)

ACUTE CONJUNCTIVITIS
Red inflamed eye, less congested towards the limbus. May be allergic, viral or bacterial. Often gritty with copious mucopurulent discharge in bacterial infections. Copious serous discharge in viral infections. Highly contagious.

Management
1 Observe strict hand hygiene.
2 Swab for culture and polymerase chain reaction (PCR).
3 Start broad-spectrum antibiotic drops every 1–2 hours (e.g. chloramphenicol 0.5% drops or ciprofloxacin drops in contact-lens wearers).
4 If viral conjunctivitis suspected, treat with antihistamine drops or another suitable over-the-counter (OTC) preparation to reduce chemosis and itching.
5 Patient should avoid wearing contact lenses for duration of treatment.
6 Does not need ophthalmic review unless photophobia is associated with decreased visual acuity, or protracted inflammation longer than 3 weeks, or swabs reveal *Chlamydia*.

ACUTE KERATITIS (HERPES SIMPLEX)

* Painful eye often with blurred vision, diffuse conjunctival injection and watery discharge.
* Look for dendrite using fluorescein stain and cobalt blue light of ophthalmoscope or slit lamp. Branching dendritic pattern of herpes simplex ulceration of cornea will appear green.

Management

* Herpes simplex ulceration is treated with aciclovir 3% ointment 5 times a day for 14 days plus antibiotic drops 4 times a day. Do not patch due to risk of *Pseudomonas* infection. Refer for ophthalmology review on following day.
* In non-herpetic keratitis, start antibiotic drops 4–6 times a day.
* Refer for urgent ophthalmology review if history of contact-lens use.

HERPES ZOSTER OPHTHALMICUS

* Shingles in trigeminal nerve distribution involving ophthalmic branch.
* Vesicular rash noted on forehead or upper eyelid. Hutchinson's sign is a vesicle on the tip of the nose.
* On corneal examination, 'pseudodendritic' ulcer may be seen.

Management

1 Treat with famciclovir 250 mg TDS or aciclovir 800 mg every 4 waking hours for 7 days.
2 Ophthalmology referral if visual acuity affected or eye is red.

ACUTE IRITIS (UVEITIS)

* Dull pain, photophobia and red eye; ciliary injection (more injected near the limbus).
* Sluggish small pupil and blurred vision.
* Hypopyon (collection of white cells in anterior chamber) may be seen in severe uveitis.
* Slit lamp examination essential: anterior chamber appears cloudy from cells and flare.
* Intraocular pressure is normal.

Management
1 Dilate pupil with short-acting cycloplegic drops (e.g. cyclopentolate 1% 3 times a day) and local steroid drops 4–6 times a day after consultation with ophthalmologist.
2 Analgesia and dark glasses may be required.

ACUTE NARROW-ANGLE (ANGLE-CLOSURE) GLAUCOMA
- Severe pain in unilateral red eye. Poor vision associated with headache, nausea and vomiting.
- Semi-dilated non-reacting pupil. Cornea appears hazy.
- Intraocular pressure is markedly raised. Eye is tender and tense to palpation.
- Headache, nausea and vomiting may be systemic features.
- The main differential diagnosis is acute iritis, which can cause secondary glaucoma.

Management
1 Urgent referral to ophthalmologist, as acute glaucoma is a sight-threatening condition.
2 Start miotic drops—pilocarpine 2% every 5 minutes for 1 hour; then hourly. In addition timolol 0.5% twice daily plus prednisolone 0.5% 4 times a day topical to affected eye.
3 Acetazolamide 500 mg IV, then 250 mg every 8 hours (orally if tolerated).
4 Narcotic analgesia for pain management (e.g. morphine 5–10 mg IM injection).
5 Admit under care of ophthalmologist.

PERIORBITAL CELLULITIS
Periocular superficial cellulitis involving pre-septal tissue. Eye not involved. Requires systemic antibiotics and observation. Usually due to *Staphylococcus aureus*, *Streptococcus pneumoniae* or *Haemophilus influenzae* (if unimmunised) in children with otitis media.
- Examination of the eye may be difficult due to marked swelling. In children, especially, may require examination under general anaesthetic to exclude eye involvement. CT of the orbits is an essential part of investigations.

- Consider admitting for intravenous flucloxacillin 12.5 mg/kg QID or cephazolin 12.5 mg/kg QID. Can usually be managed with oral antibiotics and good follow-up.

ORBITAL CELLULITIS

Potentially life-threatening eye infection.

- Oedema and swelling of eyelids and conjunctiva. Often with proptosis, restriction of eye movement, dull pain and fever. There may be altered pupillary response; reduced visual acuity is a late sign. Usually secondary to trauma or orbital extension of paranasal sinusitis.
- Commonly due to *Staphylococcus aureus*, *Haemophilus influenzae* or *Streptococcus pneumoniae*.

Management

1 Swab any wounds, start high-dose IV antibiotics: dicloxacillin 2 g QID plus ceftriaxone 2 g daily in adults.
2 CT scan of orbits and paranasal sinuses to exclude cavernous sinus thrombosis.
3 Admit to hospital and observe the vision and the eye. Urgent ophthalmology referral.

Sudden painless monocular visual loss
AMAUROSIS FUGAX

Sudden painless visual loss, usually partial and transient, due to embolic occlusion of retinal artery in transient ischaemic attack. Visual loss lasts minutes and returns to normal by the time of presentation to the ED.

- Fundoscopic examination essentially normal. Often not associated with history of dysphasia or hemiparesis.
- Requires timely referral to neurologist for appropriate investigations, including CT cerebral angiogram, echo, carotid duplex scans, cerebral perfusion scans and interventions in stroke management. Stroke pathway work-up is indicated if presenting within 4.5 hours of onset of symptoms.

CENTRAL RETINAL ARTERY OCCLUSION

- Sudden painless total or partial loss of vision, more often in the elderly. Visual acuity < 6/60.

- Fundoscopic findings: pale disc, retinal oedema, cherry red spot on the macula and narrowed arteries.
- This is an ophthalmological emergency—likely embolic cause.
- Consider differential diagnoses, especially giant cell arteritis (see below).

Initial treatment

If seen within 2 hours of onset of symptoms:

1 Lower IOP with digital massage and acetazolamide 500 mg IV.
2 Attempt to dilate blood vessels by breathing carbogen (95% O_2 and 5% CO_2) via mask, or re-breathing from a paper bag.
3 Continue treatment for at least 30 minutes.
4 Do urgent ESR and CRP to exclude giant cell arteritis.
5 Obtain urgent ophthalmology consultation for treatment options. Admit to hospital.

GIANT CELL ARTERITIS (TEMPORAL ARTERITIS)

- An ophthalmological emergency with similar presentation to central retinal artery occlusion (see above).
- Giant cell arteritis (GCA) is an ischaemic optic neuropathy characterised by blurred vision and temporal headache, generally in the elderly.
- GCA results in progressive blindness in both eyes if treatment is not instituted early.

Initial treatment of GCA

1 Attempt to reduce intraocular pressure and vasodilate.
 — Lower IOP with digital massage and acetazolamide 500 mg IV.
 — Attempt to dilate blood vessels by breathing carbogen (95% O_2 and 5% CO_2) via mask, or re-breathing from a paper bag.
 — Continue treatment for at least 30 minutes.
2 Do urgent ESR and CRP to assist diagnosis.
3 Obtain urgent ophthalmology consultation for treatment options and rheumatology consultation for diagnostic temporal artery biopsy.

4 Admit to hospital.

5 Commence high-dose steroids: methylprednisolone
1000 mg/day IV infusion over 1 hour or prednisone 1–2 mg/
kg/day (maximum 150 mg) PO. High-dose steroids should
commence on clinical suspicion prior to biopsy results
being available. GCA is associated with a high incidence of
blindness and the aim of steroids is to stop progression of
visual impairment in the affected eye and prevent blindness
in the other eye.

RETINAL VEIN OCCLUSION

Sudden and painless loss of vision that is usually incomplete and
variable. Commonly seen in the elderly, diabetics and hypertensives.

- Fundoscopy shows dilated retinal veins with multiple
  haemorrhages throughout the retina; optic disc often swollen.
  Referred to as 'blood and thunder' fundus if severe.
- Urgent ophthalmology consultation.
- No treatment.

OPTIC NEURITIS

Loss of vision over hours to days, usually painless but pain may
occur with eye movement.

- Common presenting feature of multiple sclerosis. Examine
  for other focal neurological defects.
- Variable visual loss, more frequently central field loss.
- Afferent pupillary defect and marked loss of red saturation
  (i.e. reduced visual acuity affecting colour and contrast vision).
- Urgent ophthalmology referral for investigation, including
  MRI.
- No initial or urgent treatment, but may respond to intravenous
  corticosteroids or immune modulators after appropriate
  consultation. There is no indication for oral steroids.

RETINAL DETACHMENT

- Painless visual loss with partial field loss, after a recent
  history of visual flashes and floaters. More common in
  myopic and aphakic (lens-extracted) patients; often occurs
  after blunt trauma.
- Grey, elevated veil-like retina seen. Red reflex is lost.

Management

1 If macula still not detached, admit to hospital for bed rest and urgent ophthalmic assessment.

2 If macula detached (visual acuity is reduced), refer for assessment within 24 hours.

VITREOUS HAEMORRHAGE

- Often preceded by large black floaters. Vision may vary up to complete visual loss.
- Advise bed rest at home. Needs referral within 24 hours to exclude retinal detachment.

Postoperative problems
VITREORETINAL SURGERY

Intraocular gases used in retinal surgery to tamponade and flatten the retina can create symptoms of a row of bubbles in the visual field, which the patient may mistake for a recurrent retinal detachment.

- Fundoscopy to exclude retinal detachment and visualise air bubbles on retina.
- Get patient to sit up and then lie on their side. The patient will note that the direction of the bubbles has changed, as the row of gas bubbles will always remain parallel to the floor.
- Reassure patient as the air bubbles will resorb in about 5 days postoperatively; other intraocular gases may take from 2–8 weeks to resorb.
- Flying is an absolute contraindication until gas bubbles are completely resorbed, as intraocular gas expansion can cause central retinal artery occlusion.
- Nitrous oxide anaesthetic is contraindicated as it can cause expansion of the gas bubbles with similar complications from rising IOP.
- Silicon oil, used instead of intraocular gases, can cause acute open-angle glaucoma; but cornea remains clear, unlike in glaucoma. Silicon oil may be seen in the anterior chamber or the vitreous cavity, on slit lamp examination. Treatment is as for open-angle glaucoma, but the pupil is dilated with cyclopentolate or homatropine to allow oil to move back into the vitreous cavity.

REFRACTIVE SURGERY

Dislocation of the corneal flap following laser eye surgery (Lasik) is a surgical emergency.

+ Blurred vision and a foreign body sensation following laser surgery.
+ Do not attempt to manipulate or reposition flap.
+ Instil local anaesthetic (tetracaine) to relieve pain and lid spasm. Cover eye with clear shield. Do not pad or apply any pressure to eye.
+ Refer for urgent ophthalmological consultation.

CATARACT SURGERY

Cataract surgery is one of the most common operations performed; patients present with symptoms of floaters and flashes and reduced vision.

+ Check visual acuity.
+ The pupil should be dilated prior to fundoscopy to look for retinal detachment or vitreous haemorrhage.
+ Urgent ophthalmological consultation if significant findings.

Ophthalmic conditions needing referral

+ **Acute dacryocystitis.** Treat with warm compresses and massage of tear sac. Start antibiotics.
+ **Squints in children.** Need to be seen by an ophthalmologist without delay. Perform cover test to diagnose.
+ **Chronic glaucoma.** Patient needs full assessment and institution of therapy. Refer without delay.
+ **Meibomian gland cyst/abscess.** Treat with hot compresses plus local antibiotic drops (oral antibiotics if severe). Refer.

Common ophthalmic medications

+ **Antibiotics.** Availability and use varies from country to country. A routine course of treatment would be 1 or 2 drops, 4–5 times a day for 4 days. Intensive treatment needs drops every 1 or 2 hours during waking hours with ointment at night. Antibiotics suitable for initial treatment: sulfacetamide 10%; chloramphenicol 0.5%; gentamicin 0.3%; tobramycin 0.3%, ciprofloxacin 3 mg/mL.

- **Antiviral agents.** Aciclovir 30 mg/g (3%) ophthalmic ointment.
- **Local anaesthetics.** Tetracaine hydrochloride 0.5% (available as Minims; also known as amethocaine); proxymetacaine hydrochloride 0.5%.
- **Mydriatics.** Fundal observation is best carried out using 1 drop of tropicamide 0.5% (Mydriacyl) and waiting about 15 minutes. Reverse with pilocarpine 2% drops.
- **Cycloplegics.** Use short-acting preparations (e.g. cyclopentolate 1% or homatropine 2%, 1–3 times a day). Do not use atropine.
- **Miotics.** Pilocarpine 2% is the most commonly used strength.
- **Glaucoma preparations.** Latanoprost; bimatoprost; brimonidine tartrate; apraclonidine HCl; pilocarpine HCl 1%, 2%, 4%; acetazolamide 250 mg PO.
- **Non-steroidal anti-inflammatory drugs (NSAIDs).** Diclofenac; ketorolac.
- **Steroids.** Fluorometholone 0.1%; prednisolone 0.5%, 1%; dexamethasone 0.1%.
- **Frequency of use.** Remember to tell the patient to wait 5 minutes between different drops.

Chapter 39
Ear, nose and throat (ENT) emergencies

Shalini Arunanthy

The care of these patients requires an organised approach and some basic equipment (see Box 39.1).

Ear emergencies
OTITIS EXTERNA
Clinical features
- Ear pain
- History of water exposure or trauma—commonly cotton tips
- Oedema of canal, with debris

Organisms
- *Pseudomonas*
- *Staphylococcus*
- Rarely fungal

Box 39.1   ENT equipment

- Head light
- Nasal speculum
- Ear speculum
- Jobson Horne curette
- Packing forceps
- Alligator forceps
- Magill's forceps
- Suction catheters—including fine metal sucker
- Co-phenylcaine spray (lignocaine 5% + phenylephrine 0.5%)
- Tampons (Merocel)—ear, nasal
- Rapid Rhino devices—anterior and posterior

Management
1 Analgesia.
2 Remove debris gently—suction catheter or cottonwool swab.
3 Insert a wick (Merocel tampon-ear) in severe cases.
4 Instil antibiotic/steroid drops (Otodex, Sofradex).
5 ENT admission and IV antibiotics if has spread outside ear canal. Otherwise outpatient ENT follow-up.

OTITIS MEDIA
Clinical features
- Common in children
- Earache +/− fever
- Pulling at pinna
- Injection of tympanic membrane with bulging of membrane
- Effusion behind membrane
- Purulent discharge if tympanic membrane ruptured

Organisms
- Viral
- *Streptococcus pneumoniae*
- *Haemophilus influenzae*
- *Moraxella catarrhalis*

Management
1 Analgesia.
2 Antibiotics if < 6 months old, if systemic features (fever, vomiting) or special patient populations (some Aboriginal and Torres Strait Islander patients).
3 Otherwise wait for 48 hours.
4 Review and start antibiotics if not improving.
5 Antibiotic of choice is amoxycillin.
Note: Antibiotics are no longer routinely recommended for children with acute otitis media. Adults are usually treated with antibiotics.

Complications
- Ruptured tympanic membrane usually heals spontaneously without complications within 2–3 weeks. Advise to keep dry and avoid instilling any drops.

- Recurrent infections/otitis media with effusion—outpatient ENT referral.
- Mastoiditis—see section below.
- Intracranial complications—epidural abscess, meningitis are rare.

MASTOIDITIS
Mastoiditis is a rare but significant complication of otitis media.

Clinical features of mastoiditis
- Symptoms of otitis media
- Pain over mastoid region
- Fever
- Erythematous, bulging ear drum
- Tenderness +/− swelling over mastoid
- Raised inflammatory markers
- CT scan shows changes of mastoiditis (mainly fluid in mastoid air cells)

Organisms
Similar to acute otitis media.

Management
1 IV antibiotics—usually ceftriaxone plus flucloxacillin
2 Analgesia
3 ENT referral for admission +/− surgery

PERICHONDRITIS
Becoming more common due to infected ear piercings involving cartilage (high piercings).

Clinical features
- Painful auricle
- Erythema and swelling of auricle
- Fever

Organisms
- *Pseudomonas aeruginosa*
- *Staphylococcus aureus*

• *Streptococcus pyogenes*

Management
1 Analgesia.
2 Remove ear piercing—use auricular block (see Figure 39.1 below), if embedded.
3 Antibiotics—flucloxacillin and gentamicin.
4 ENT referral for admission +/− drainage.
5 Explain risk of necrosis of cartilage with associated deformity.

RUPTURED TYMPANIC MEMBRANE
Caused by otitis media, blows to the ear, barotrauma or direct trauma (cotton tips).

Clinical features
• Hearing loss—conductive
• If associated with infection, acute pain; relieved once membrane has ruptured
• Discharge from ear if associated with infection
• Visible tear of membrane on otoscopy

Management
Most perforations, especially if central, do not require specific treatment and will heal spontaneously.
1 Keep ear dry—the most important instruction for the patient.
2 Oral antibiotics if associated with infection.
3 Hearing test.
4 Outpatient ENT follow-up.
5 Immediate ENT referral if associated tinnitus or vertigo (signifies inner ear injury).

AURICULAR HAEMATOMA
Clinical features
Patient presents with a swollen, painful pinna following blunt trauma.

Management
ENT referral for drainage and pressure dressing to prevent further bleeding.

Complication
Warn patient of high risk of cartilage necrosis leading to 'cauliflower ear'

AURICULAR LACERATIONS
Simple lacerations may be repaired in the ED. Complex wounds should be referred to the ENT or plastic surgeon for repair.

Refer the following wounds:

- loss of skin
- multiple lacerations
- exposed cartilage
- involvement of external auditory canal
- avulsion or near-avulsion of ear.

Warn patient of possible poor cosmetic result, including cauliflower ear.

Management of simple lacerations
1 Irrigate with saline (place gauze in canal to reduce amount of saline going into external ear).
2 Anaesthetise with a block (see Figure 39.1).
  — Insert needle just above the attachment of the ear to the head. Direct the needle first anteriorly towards the tragus and inject local anaesthetic, then withdraw to point of insertion and inject posteriorly behind ear.
  — Do the same at inferior attachment of ear.
  — DO NOT inject into pinna.
3 Repair perichondrium with 5/0 or 6/0 absorbable suture.
4 Repair skin with 5/0 or 6/0 non-absorbable suture.
5 Pressure dressing.
6 Remove sutures in 5 days.

TEMPORAL BONE FRACTURES
Temporal bone fractures are reported to be present in 15–20% of all skull fractures.

Low priority in the multi-trauma patient, but should not be forgotten. May be associated with an extradural haematoma.

Clinical features
- CSF or blood in ear canal
- Battle sign

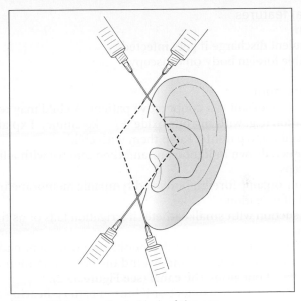

Figure 39.1 Anaesthetic block of the ear

- Facial nerve palsy
- Vertigo
- Deafness
- CT scan with fine cuts through temporal bone for evaluation

Management

1 Most important is to look for the injury in the secondary survey.
2 ENT/neurosurgery referral.
3 Most are managed conservatively.

FOREIGN BODIES: EAR

- Common in children. Usually beads, bits of toys, seeds, paper.
- In adults may be insects or cotton off the tip of a cotton bud.
- Embedded piercings in pinna becoming more common.

Clinical features
* Pain
* Purulent discharge if gets infected
* Visible foreign body on otoscopy

Management
1 Most important is a cooperative patient. A child may require sedation (e.g. with nitrous oxide $+/-$ ketamine). Explain procedure to parents. Keep them with child.
2 If insect, drown in lignocaine and then remove with alligator forceps.
3 If non-organic foreign body and tympanic membrane intact, trial of irrigation.
4 Try suction with small catheter if irrigation fails or as first choice.
5 If unsuccessful, use an angled hook, curette or bent end of paper clip to get above and behind the object and then move the object out along the canal (see Figure 39.2).
6 If unable to remove object or if button battery/hearing aid battery, refer to ENT immediately.
   Note: DO NOT try to grab a hard round object with forceps, as this is likely to push it further into the auditory canal.
7 Embedded piercings can be removed under an auricular block. Make skin incision posteriorly if required.

VERTIGO
Vertigo is the sensation of motion of self or surroundings. Causes may be central or peripheral.
   Peripheral causes are:
* labyrinthitis
* vestibular neuronitis
* Ménière's disease
* benign paroxysmal positional vertigo (BPPV).
This section will only deal with the peripheral causes of vertigo.

Clinical features
* Onset sudden and severe.
* May be paroxysmal and brought on by change in position of head in BPPV.

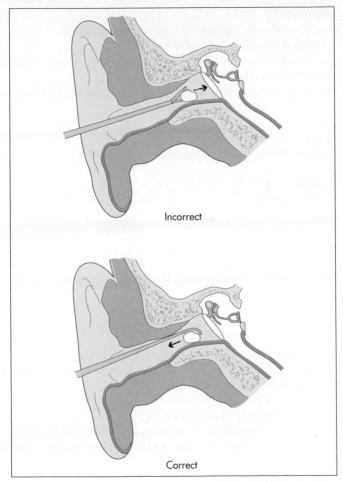

Figure 39.2 Incorrect and correct ways to remove a foreign body from the ear

- Associated with nausea and vomiting.
- Tinnitus and deafness, especially in Ménière's disease.
- Exclude central causes with a complete neurological examination.
- Examine the ears for infection/inflammation.

Management
1 Symptomatic: diazepam $+/-$ prochlorperazine.
2 IV fluids if vomiting/dehydrated.
3 Diagnose BPPV with Dix-Hallpike manoeuvre and use trial of Epley manoeuvre for treatment.
4 If peripheral cause and not settling admit to the ED short stay unit (ESSU) until symptoms settle.

Dix-Hallpike manoeuvre
To diagnose BPPV, use Dix-Hallpike manoeuvre.

Indications
Peripheral vertigo.

Contraindications
- Neck injury
- Cervical spondylosis
- Vertebrobasilar insufficiency, transient ischaemic attack, cerebrovascular accident
- Carotid bruits

Method
1 Warn patient this may provoke/worsen vertigo.
2 Sit patient up in bed so that, should they now lie down, their head would be off the end of the bed.
3 Turn patient's head 45° to one side.
4 Ask patient to keep the eyes open.
5 Lie patient flat rapidly with head over end of bed by 20°.
6 Look for nystagmus—rotatory nystagmus indicates a positive test on that side.
7 Sit the patient back up.
8 Repeat with head turned to other side.

Epley manoeuvre
Indications
BPPV with positive Dix-Hallpike test.

Contraindications
As for Dix-Hallpike, above.

Method
1 Warn patient this may worsen or provoke symptoms temporarily or may be ineffective.
2 Sit patient as for the Dix-Hallpike manoeuvre.
3 Turn the patient's head to the side that was positive on the Dix-Hallpike test.
4 Gently lower patient to lying position with head hanging over the end of the bed by around 20°.
5 Leave patient in each position for 1–2 minutes.
6 Turn patient's head 45° to opposite side.
7 Turn patient onto shoulder so that head faces a further 45° to that side.
8 Sit patient up with head in same position.
9 Return head to midline.

Nose emergencies
ACUTE SINUSITIS
Most cases are viral—approximately 90% of patients with upper respiratory tract infection (URTI) have involvement of the para-nasal sinuses.
Only 0.5–2% of these proceed to have bacterial infection.

Clinical features
• Symptoms of viral URTI not resolved after 10 days
• Purulent nasal discharge
• Facial or maxillary dental pain
• Fever
• Postnasal drip
• Tenderness over sinuses
• CT of sinuses confirms sinusitis

Organisms
• *Streptococcus pneumoniae*
• *Haemophilus influenzae*
• *Moraxella catarrhalis*

Management
1 Analgesia.

2 Antibiotics—amoxycillin or amoxycillin + clavulanate is recommended. A recent Cochrane review found minimal effect in patients with uncomplicated acute sinusitis.

3 Intranasal corticosteroids—limited evidence to support use as monotherapy or adjunct with antibiotics.

4 Intranasal saline douches/spray—little evidence to support use.

5 Oral steroids in combination with antibiotics may offer some added benefit.

Complications
- Periorbital/orbital cellulitis
- Meningitis
- Brain abscess

EPISTAXIS
One of the commonest ENT emergencies. Approximately 90% are anterior bleeds from Little's area. Posterior bleeds are harder to visualise, more difficult to treat and occur in older patients with co-existing cardiovascular disease.

Clinical features
- Bleeding from nostril
- Blood in the oropharynx
- Airway usually intact
- May be haemodynamically compromised

Management
1 Protect yourself with gloves, gown and goggles.
2 Assess and manage ABCs initially.
3 Large-bore IV cannula, blood for FBC, group-and-hold +/− coagulation studies.
4 Ask patient to blow nose then compress anterior nares between thumb and forefinger, applying constant pressure for 10–15 minutes.
5 Sit the patient up, leaning forwards; ask the patient to hold a kidney dish below the mouth and spit into this.
6 Inspect nose to identify bleeding point.
7 Apply cottonwool pledgets soaked in co-phenylcaine to visible bleeding spot or vessel.

8   If bleeding controlled and bleeding point identified, use silver nitrate stick to cauterise the area. Be careful not to apply to large area. Do not apply on both sides of septum—could lead to necrosis of the cartilage.

9   Observe patient for a few hours. If no further bleeding, discharge with outpatient ENT follow-up.

10 If bleeding is too heavy or posterior, spray with co-phenylcaine and then use a nasal (Merocel) tampon (see Box 39.2) or a Rapid Rhino device (inflatable balloon covered with hydrocolloid fabric; see Box 39.3).

11 If above not available, pack with gauze (see Figure 39.3).

12 Not often used are:
    — Epistat nasal balloon (see Box 39.4)
    — Foley catheter and Vaseline gauze pack (see Figure 39.4).

13 May need to pack both sides to stop bleeding.

14 Depending on hospital policy and if posterior bleed, patient may require admission (ENT or ESSU) if packing left in situ.

15 Consider prophylactic antibiotics if packing left in situ.

16 Consider tranexamic acid topically or orally if ongoing bleed and no contraindications.

Box 39.2   Insertion of Merocel nasal tampon

1   Anterior bleeds: shorter tampon; posterior bleeds: longer tampon.
2   Use co-phenylcaine spray.
3   Lubricate tampon tip with water-soluble gel (KY gel).
4   Advance as far as possible along floor of nasal cavity.
5   When soaked with blood, expands to fill nasal cavity.
6   Tape attached thread to side of face.
7   To remove soak with saline, remove tape and slide gently out.

Box 39.3   Insertion of Rapid Rhino device

1   Soak in sterile water for 30 seconds.
2   Get patient to blow nose to expel clots/blood.
3   Use co-phenylcaine spray.
4   Advance full length along floor of nasal cavity.
5   Inflate with air using syringe until pilot cuff firm. Device will expand to fit nasal cavity.
6   Tape pilot cuff to side of face.

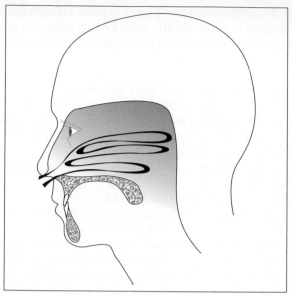

Figure 39.3 Correct placement of Vaseline gauze packing, with antibiotics commenced (possible bacteraemia in presence of nasal packing)

Box 39.4   Insertion of Epistat nasal balloon

1   Use co-phenylcaine spray.
2   Lubricate device and insert to full length.
3   Inflate posterior balloon with approximately 5 mL of air.
4   Pull forward gently till fits against posterior choana.
5   Fill anterior balloon till tamponade achieved.
6   Tape to side of face.

FOREIGN BODIES: NOSE

Usually seen in children. Maybe beads, parts of toys, paper, seeds, pebbles. Usually present soon after as child tells parent or parent/sibling witnesses the child putting something in the nose. If presentation delayed, may present with offensive unilateral nasal discharge.

Note: Button batteries should be removed as soon as possible as they may lead to a corrosive injury.

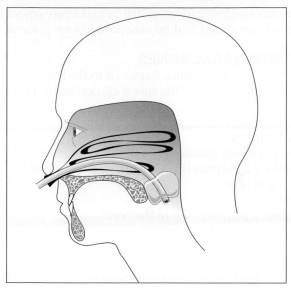

Figure 39.4 Foley's catheter used as postnasal balloon packing, with gauze anterior pack

Management

1 Ask the parent to blow hard into the child's mouth (or use bag–mask to give positive pressure over mouth only) while occluding the normal nostril—foreign body (FB) may be expelled by the positive pressure. Worth trying before other methods, especially for things like beads.
2 Spray co-phenylcaine into nostril.
3 Sedate child if required.
4 Get a good view using headlight (if available).
5 If hard, round object, use angled hook to get behind object and pull out.
6 If soft, irregular and can be grasped by forceps, use these.
7 Other methods described include using a Foley or Fogarty catheter to get behind the object, then blowing balloon up and pulling object out; or using a suction catheter to apply suction on object and bring it out.

8 Once removed, re-inspect nostril to make sure object is removed completely and no other objects are present.

FRACTURED NASAL BONES

One of the commonest bones fractured in the body.

Note: Diagnosis of nasal fracture is clinical and X-rays are rarely if ever indicated.

Clinical features
- History of direct trauma to nose
- Immediate deformity if fracture with displacement
- Swelling of nose
- Epistaxis
- May have a palpable step in the bone
- X-rays are difficult to interpret

Management
1 Treat any life-threatening injuries first.
2 Exclude other facial bone injuries.
3 Manage epistaxis if present with pressure or packing.
4 Inspect for septal haematoma—cherry-red swelling arising from septum. If present refer immediately to ENT for drainage. If left untreated, may lead to necrosis of cartilage and saddle nose deformity.
5 The fracture is left for a few days.
6 If deformity is present once swelling decreased, refer to ENT/ plastic surgeon for reduction.

Throat emergencies
PHARYNGITIS/TONSILLITIS
- More common in children.
- Most are viral.
- Difficult to differentiate clinically between bacterial and viral infections. However, it is important to try to differentiate between group A streptococcal infection and other causes of sore throat.

Aetiology of pharyngitis/tonsillitis
- Viral including Epstein–Barr virus (EBV)
- Group A *Streptococcus* (GAS)

- Other bacteria including other *Streptococci, Chlamydiae, Gonococcus*

Clinical features
- Sore throat
- Fever
- Odynophagia
- Associated runny nose, cough—more likely with viral infection
- Inflamed pharynx, enlarged tonsils with or without exudate/pus
- Cervical lymphadenopathy
- Hepatosplenomegaly usually indicates EBV
- Raised WCC, CRP
- Lymphocytosis with atypical lymphocytes—viral, especially EBV
- Abnormal liver function tests (LFTs)—EBV
- Throat swab for GAS
- Monospot, EBV serology
  Of the above, a combination of fever with temperatures $> 38°C$, tender cervical lymphadenopathy, tonsillar exudate and no cough is suggestive of GAS sore throat—Centor criteria.

Management
1 Analgesia.
2 IV fluids, as patients are often dehydrated.
3 Steroids are used to reduce symptoms, although the evidence is not strong. Dexamethasone 8 mg as a one-off dose.
4 Penicillin for GAS if there is a high index of clinical suspicion or confirmed on throat swab PCR or culture.
5 If uncomplicated, discharge patient after symptomatic treatment.

Complications
- Airway compromise—unusual if not complicated. Requires admission to high-dependency unit under ENT. Nasendoscopy performed by ENT to assess degree of swelling/obstruction. Rarely requires airway intervention.
- Peritonsillar abscess—see below.

- Non-suppurative complications of GAS—rheumatic fever, glomerulonephritis.

PERITONSILLAR ABSCESS (QUINSY)

Starts as pharyngitis or tonsillitis and progresses to form abscess. Common in young adults. Usually polymicrobial—mixture of aerobic and anaerobic organisms.

Clinical features

- Starts like a sore throat, but gets progressively worse.
- Difficulty swallowing and talking.
- Fever and systemic symptoms more marked.
- Examination reveals trismus and a unilateral swelling displacing the tonsil inferomedially.
- Uvula is displaced to the contralateral side.
- Enlarged cervical lymph nodes.

Management

1 Analgesia.
2 IV fluids.
3 Antibiotics—combination of penicillin and metronidazole.
4 Clindamycin may be used instead of metronidazole.
5 Anaesthetise with co-phenylcaine spray.
6 Needle aspiration (see Box 39.5) is generally curative, and incision and drainage is rarely indicated.
7 ENT referral for 24-hour admission or for follow-up if discharged from ED.
8 Use of steroids is controversial.

Box 39.5   Needle aspiration of quinsy
1   Have patient sitting up with kidney dish under chin.
2   Use a large-bore needle on a 10 mL syringe and insert at area of maximal pointing while applying continuous negative pressure. You will feel a 'give' when you enter the abscess cavity.
3   Aspirate pus and send for culture.

Epiglottitis

Inflammation of the supraglottic region, including epiglottis, should be called supraglottitis.

Epiglottitis used to be a disease of childhood. After immunisation against *H. influenzae* B was started, it is now usually seen in adults.

Clinical features

- Sore throat—pain is lower than in tonsillitis
- Muffled voice
- Difficulty swallowing
- Fever
- Acute onset in children, may have prodromal URTI symptoms in adults
- Examination reveals a toxic-looking patient
- Drooling of saliva in children
- Cervical lymphadenopathy may be present
- Stridor is a late sign
- Lateral soft-tissue X-ray of neck may show classic 'thumb print'

Organisms

- *H. influenzae*, type B
- *Streptococcus pneumoniae*
- *Streptococcus pyogenes*
- *Staphylococcus aureus* and Gram-negatives are less common

Management of epiglottitis

1 If respiratory distress with stridor, consult anaesthetics and ENT and organise urgent transfer to operating theatre for gaseous induction and intubation.
2 If intubation fails, cricothyroidotomy or tracheostomy will need to be performed.
3 Children should be kept with parent with minimal intervention until taken to OT.
4 Adults who are not in respiratory distress, refer to ENT for nasendoscopy.
5 Airway intervention is rarely required in adults.
6 Ceftriaxone is the antibiotic of choice.

7 Steroids may be used to reduce swelling.
8 Admit to high-dependency unit or ICU for close observation and airway intervention if required.
9 If patient has a respiratory arrest, commence bag–valve–mask ventilation and then intubation should be attempted. If this fails, proceed to a cricothyroidotomy.

FOREIGN BODIES: OROPHARYNGEAL

Usually an adult who has eaten chicken or fish and has a bone stuck in the pharynx.

Note: Swallowed button battery is an emergency. ENT service should be called immediately.

Clinical features and examination
- Feeling of FB stuck in throat.
- Examine neck for surgical emphysema.
- Inspect pharynx with headlight to visualise object if able.
- X-ray lateral soft tissue of neck, looking for FB and retropharyngeal air.

Management
1 If FB visible with headlight and tongue depressor, anaesthetise with lignocaine spray and remove with Magill's forceps.
2 If not visualised but visible on X-ray, refer to ENT for endoscopic removal.
3 If not visualised on inspection and not visible on X-ray, a FB may still be present or the patient may feel a scratch on the mucosa as a FB. These patients will also require endoscopy if the feeling of FB is persistent.

Complications
If left unattended, may perforate and lead to retropharyngeal infection and mediastinitis.

FOREIGN BODIES: OESOPHAGEAL

Depending on the hospital policy, these may be dealt with by ENT or gastroenterology. Upper oesophageal objects are commonly dealt with by ENT. In adults usually a food bolus and in children a coin are the commonest objects. Beware of button batteries in children, as this is an emergency to prevent perforation of the oesophagus.

Clinical features
* Sensation of FB
* Inability to swallow—varying degrees depending on degree of obstruction
* Drooling in complete obstruction
* Chest X-ray +/− lateral soft tissue of neck, depending on level of obstruction

Note: Coin in oesophagus appears in coronal plane (front on) on X-ray. Coin in airway appears in sagittal plane (side on) due to incomplete tracheal rings posteriorly.

Management
1 Trial of glucagon 1–2 mg IV +/− carbonated beverage if FB is food bolus or coin. Do not attempt if sharp object or button battery.
2 If above method unsuccessful or sharp object/button battery, requires urgent ENT referral for endoscopic removal.
3 Keep patient nil by mouth (NBM).
4 Pre-anaesthetic work-up if indicated.

Complications
Oesophageal perforation and mediastinitis.

FOREIGN BODIES: AIRWAY
Common in children and the very elderly. Usually aspirated and lodged in right main or lower lobe bronchus. Complete airway obstruction is a life-threatening emergency and should be treated with back blows and chest thrusts.

Clinical features
* History of choking, coughing, gagging.
* If aspirated, child may be minimally symptomatic initially and only have a cough or wheeze, especially unilateral wheeze.
* Stridor.

- Respiratory distress if causing upper airway obstruction.
- Chest X-ray may reveal FB if radio-opaque or unilateral hypertranslucency, atelectasis or consolidation.

Management

1 Supportive therapy till endoscopic removal—oxygen, IV access and monitoring.
2 Urgent ENT referral for endoscopy.
3 If patient has complete obstruction and respiratory arrest, intubate and push tube as far as possible, thus pushing object into one bronchus. Then withdraw the tube to normal position to ventilate until endoscopic removal is organised.

POST-TONSILLECTOMY BLEED

Secondary haemorrhage may occur after 24 hours, but commonly between 5 and 10 days. Can be fatal from airway obstruction or haemorrhagic shock.

Management

1 Keep patient seated upright with kidney dish to spit into.
2 Continuous monitoring.
3 NBM.
4 Large-bore IV access, blood for FBC, group-and-hold +/− coagulation studies.
5 Resuscitate as required including airway protection if necessary. Prepare to perform surgical airway if unable to intubate.
6 Notify ENT team immediately. May require OT.
7 Commence IV penicillin and metronidazole.
8 Hydrogen peroxide gargles are prescribed, but there is no evidence to support their use.
9 Tranexamic acid IV.
10 Attempt pressure with adrenaline-soaked gauze held in Magill's forceps—not always possible.

References

Antibiotic guidelines eTG complete [Internet]. Melbourne: Therapeutic Guidelines Limited; 2017.

Dix-Hallpike Manoeuvre from BMJ Learning https://www.youtube.com/watch?v=8RYB2QlO1N4

Lemiengre MB, van Driel ML, Merenstein D, et al. Antibiotics for clinically diagnosed acute rhinosinusitis in adults. Cochrane Database of Systematic Reviews 2012, Issue 10. Art. No.: CD006089. DOI: 10.1002/14651858.CD006089.pub4.

Ozbek C, Aygenc E, Tuna EU et al. Use of steroids in the treatment of peritonsillar abscess. J Laryngol Otol 2004;118(6):439–42.

Sadeghirad B, Siemieniuk RA, Brignardello-Petersen R, et al. Corticosteroids for treatment of sore throat: a systematic review and meta-analysis of randomised trials. BMJ 2017;358:j3887.

Venekamp RP, Sanders SL, Glasziou PP, et al. Antibiotics for acute otitis media in children. Cochrane Database of Systematic Reviews 2015, Issue 6. Art. No.: CD000219. DOI: 10.1002/14651858.CD000219.pub4

Venekamp RP, Thompson MJ, Hayward G, et al. Systemic corticosteroids for acute sinusitis. Cochrane Database of Systematic Reviews 2014, Issue 3. Art. No.: CD008115. DOI: 10.1002/14651858.CD008115.pub3.

Zahed R, Moharamzadeh P, Alizadeharasi S, et al. 2013. A new and rapid method for epistaxis treatment using injectable form of tranexamic acid topically: a randomized controlled trial. The American Journal of Emergency Medicine, no. 9 (July 30). doi:10.1016/j.ajem.2013.06.043. http://www.ncbi.nlm.nih.gov/pubmed/23911102.

Zalmanovici Trestioreanu A, Yaphe J. Intranasal steroids for acute sinusitis. Cochrane Database of Systematic Reviews 2013, Issue 12. Art. No.: CD005149. DOI: 10.1002/14651858.CD005149.pub4.

Chapter 40
Management of dental emergencies

Peter Foltyn

There are many kinds of dental emergencies, some of which can be extremely subjective. Whereas a small carious lesion or infected extraction socket may cause excruciating pain for one person, a fractured jaw may be asymptomatic and only discovered as an incidental finding after routine X-rays. EDs in teaching hospitals will nearly always have an accredited on-call dentist or in rural settings may refer all dental emergencies to a local dental emergency service or individual dentist. As dental emergencies are rarely life-threatening, commonsense measures such as antibiotics, sedatives and analgesics where appropriate should get the patient through the night or weekend until an appointment can be arranged for the next working day.

It would be an inappropriate utilisation of resources to ask an on-call dentist to personally attend all cases of dental or oral pain. Many dental problems are the result of dental neglect, which would have initially presented many days or weeks earlier.

If the patient is to be admitted, or there is doubt about management, contact the on-call dentist. Always have any relevant medical history at hand and try to establish a history for the dental problem. The dental history should include duration and nature of any pain or swelling and any measures taken to counter the problem by the patient's own doctor, dentist or by themselves.

Toothache
In the majority of instances toothache can be narrowed down to a specific tooth, which may be tender to touch and is often a direct result of tooth decay. However, pain can be referred to adjacent teeth, the opposing jaw, facial areas or the neck but does

not generally extend across the midline except when the origin is the anterior teeth. As ED imaging may be limited to taking ortho-pantomogram (OPG) X-rays or standard views of facial bones the source of the toothache may not be immediately evident. Clinical examination by ED staff may prove unrewarding without some training in oral examination. A strong light source, dental mirror and probe and an air source are required (wall outlet medical air or oxygen or cylinder gases and tubing would normally be available in all EDs).

1 Dental caries may be minor or extensive and may undermine an existing dental restoration or artificial crown.
Response/advice:
Provide adequate analgesia until the next working day.

2 Erosion or abrasion areas at the tooth/gum junction may produce extreme hypersensitivity.
Response/advice:
Provide adequate analgesia until the next working day and suggest an anti-hypersensitivity toothpaste such as Sensodyne or Colgate Gel-Kam.

3 Dental pulp (nerve) involvement is often an extension of decay in the body or branches of the dental pulp. Invasion by microorganisms into the dental pulp often leads to an initial acute pulpitis which may settle and return as a chronic, more diffuse pain many weeks or even months or years later. The microorganisms, which invaded the dental pulp, may now extend beyond the tooth apex and be responsible for dental abscess formation (also refer to the section Facial Swellings later in this chapter).
Response/advice:
Provide adequate analgesia until the next working day; however, antibiotics may also be required if there is established lymphadenopathy, pyrexia or visible dental abscess formation on X-ray. Advise the patient to attend a dentist as a matter of urgency.

4 Fractured or split teeth may be as a result of trauma or a heavily filled tooth giving way. In some instances intact teeth may fracture as a result of an anatomical irregularity in their formation or as a result of an occlusal or bite discrepancy.

Response/advice:
Provide adequate analgesia until the next working day. Advise the patient to attend a dentist as soon as possible.

Infected gums

Poor oral health may lead initially to marginal gingivitis, progressing over many years to moderate or severe periodontitis and associated problems with the bone surrounding the teeth. Advanced periodontal disease may lead to tooth mobility, bad breath, oral bleeding, periodontal abscess formation, extrusion, drifting or exfoliation of teeth and generalised mouth pain. Periodontal disease may be an early clinical clue for systemic diseases such as HIV infection and diabetes or following treatment in the case of graft-versus-host disease (GVHD) in bone marrow transplantation and radiation therapy of the head and neck.

Response/advice:
Provide adequate analgesia until the next working day; however, antibiotics may also be required. A chlorhexidine mouth rinse, preferably alcohol-free (Colgate—PerioGard), will reduce microorganism numbers. Advise the patient to attend a dentist as soon as possible.

Acute necrotising ulcerative gingivitis (ANUG) is a severe gingival infection often characterised by severe pain, pyrexia and bad breath with punched out and ulcerated interdental papillae. ANUG can be found in otherwise healthy mouths and is often associated with stress. ANUG is not uncommon around exam time or in times of partnership breakdown.

Response/advice:
Provide adequate analgesia until the next working day and prescribe metronidazole (Flagyl) or tinidazole (Fasigyn). A chlorhexidine mouth rinse, preferably alcohol-free (Colgate—PerioGard), will reduce microorganism numbers. Advise the patient to attend a dentist as soon as possible.

Impacted teeth

The usual age for eruption of wisdom teeth or third molars is 17–22 years; however, eruption can occur as early as 15. In the past, when oral health was poor and fluoridation of water supplies had not commenced, it was common for young adults to have had a number of teeth removed due to tooth decay before the end of their teenage years. Today most young adults born and raised in communities with fluoridated water are rarely missing any teeth and also have had a minimal number of teeth restored. A consequence of having good teeth is that for many there is little room for their orderly eruption. This has now led to a significant increase in not only impaction of wisdom teeth but occasionally other teeth as well, especially when there is a discrepancy between tooth and mouth size.

Impacted teeth can cause pain for numerous reasons. In most instances the cause of pain is a result of local infection which often leads to regional lymphadenopathy. Carious breakdown with acute pulpitis and pressure on an adjacent tooth can also cause severe pain.

Response/advice:
Provide adequate analgesia until the next working day; however, antibiotics may also be required if there is established lymphadenopathy or pyrexia. Advise the patient to attend a dentist or a specialist oral surgeon as soon as possible.

Mouth sores and ulceration

Oral ulceration and mouth sores may be the result of a myriad of precipitating factors including stress, acidic foods and even specific foods. Sodium lauryl sulfate (SLS), a detergent commonly found in toothpastes, has also been implicated. Random aphthous and traumatic ulceration is not uncommon; however, ulceration as an oral manifestation of a systemic disease can also occur. Severe mouth sores also occur in GVHD following bone marrow transplantation and canker sores during head and neck irradiation. Nutritional deficiencies in the aged and unwell may also lead to oral ulceration. Denture wearers who have lost 5–10 kg or more since the dentures were initially fabricated may have experienced shrinkage of alveolar ridges and other changes within their mouths altering the once good fit of their dentures. As shrinkage of oral tissues is not uniform, the denture may impinge or dig in at various locations.

Response/advice:
Good oral hygiene and reducing stress is a starting point for limiting the recurrence of oral ulceration. Rinsing or topical application

of Xylocaine viscous with a cotton bud to a specific ulcer may help. Chlorhexidine mouth rinse and topical steroids, such as Kenalog in Orabase, should be prescribed until the patient can get to their dentist. Thalidomide has been shown to reduce pain in large intractable ulcers found in immune-compromised patients as has nicotine-containing gum (Nicorette) in non-smokers suffering random aphthous ulceration.

Neoplasia

The average age of a person with an oral cancer in Australia is 64; however, young people are regularly being diagnosed with oral-based malignancies. An area of induration, leucoplakia or erythroplasia, which has progressed in size or has been managed topically or systemically without resolution, requires urgent attention.

Long-term immune suppression is closely linked to a higher risk for a neoplasm. Any lumps and bumps in and around the mouth for a person who has been HIV-positive for 10 or more years should be carefully assessed. Unusual and aggressive lymphomas are appearing in this cohort. Similarly any person who has received solid organ transplantation should have any unusual swellings quickly assessed.

Response/advice:

As the consequences of delay in providing a definitive diagnosis of an oral cancer may compromise the patient in many ways, biopsy of the suspect lesion should be carried out as soon as possible. Punch biopsy or excisional biopsy can be carried out by a surgical or plastics registrar or on-call dentist.

Facial swellings

The most common cause of facial swellings is dental abscess formation. A dental abscess is an infection around the root of a tooth or in the gum which causes an accumulation of pus. At this stage there is often associated pain but not necessarily swelling. If the infection is left unchecked, the accumulated pus attempts to drain and will track via the path of least resistance and accumulate further as an intra or extra oral swelling which may not necessarily be overlying the abscessed tooth. Local lymphadenopathy is common with marked facial swellings caused by dental abscess formation.

Response/advice:
Provide adequate analgesia until the next working day together with antibiotics if the swelling is slight and there is no concern for airway obstruction or progression to cellulitis. Have the patient rinse their mouth with warm salty water every hour or as needed to ease the pain. If the patient is able, they can cover the handle of a teaspoon with cotton wool and immerse in hot salty water and press on the swelling. This may help to establish drainage. Using ice packs or frozen peas, 20 minutes on and 10 off, over the affected area may also help to relieve the pain. The patient should be advised to return to the ED should there be increased swelling in their face, jaw, cheek or eye, or if swelling spreads to their neck or chest or there are any symptoms of airway obstruction or the pain becomes worse or they develop pyrexia.

Should the swelling be significant or has spread to the eye, neck or chest, or there is concern for potential airway obstruction (Ludwig's angina) the patient should be admitted and commenced immediately on IV antibiotics such as benzylpenicillin 1.2 g 6-hourly. In the more severe or unresponsive cases, add Metronidazole. For patients hypersensitive to penicillin, clindamycin 300 mg 8-hourly or lincomycin 600 mg 8-hourly. IV fluids should also be considered. Contact the on-call dentist; however, if the swelling is significant and CT X-rays are available fine-cut views in the area of the swelling will help determine if there is an accumulation of pus and if incision and drainage is required.

Heart disease and dental care

The following recommendations from the St Vincent's Hospital Dental Department are based on guidelines and antibiotic regimens which have been endorsed by all Australian state, territory and Commonwealth health departments, the Cardiac Society of Australia and New Zealand and the Australian Dental Association.

Several heart conditions require the patient and dentist to take special precautions. These recommendations are especially important for:

• people with artificial heart valves (aortic, mitral)
• people with a previous history of heart valve infection; and

- people born with or who acquire heart problems such as:
  — most at-birth heart malformations
  — damaged heart valves
  — thickened heart muscle
- cardiac transplantation recipients with cardiac valvular disease.

  Someone with a heart problem has three responsibilities:
- First, they need to establish and maintain a clean and healthy mouth. That means practising good oral hygiene and visiting their dentist regularly.
- Second, they need to make sure that they know that they have a heart problem.
- Thirdly, they must carefully follow both their doctor's and their dentist's instructions when prescribed any medications and in particular antibiotics.

ANTIBIOTIC GUIDELINES FOR DENTAL PROCEDURES IN HIGH-RISK PATIENTS[1]

Amoxycillin 2 g (children: 50 mg/kg up to 2 g) orally as a single dose 1 hour before the procedure. (*Note:* The Australian Guidelines are 2 g not 3 g.)

For patients hypersensitive to penicillin, on long-term penicillin therapy or having taken penicillin or a related β-lactam antibiotic more than once in the previous month, use: clindamycin 600 mg not erythromycin or tetracycline (children: 10 mg/kg up to 600 mg) orally, as a single dose, 1 hour before the procedure commences.

Post-extraction instructions

Often teeth need to be removed due to excessive dental decay or formation of a dental abscess. Immediately following a tooth extraction the patient should be advised to keep biting on the rolled gauze, which has been placed in their mouth for at least 20–30 minutes. If they are still bleeding provide extra gauze.

Response/advice:

General:
- Do not smoke or rinse the mouth vigorously.
- Do not spit or continually wipe away blood.
- Do not drink through a straw for 24 hours.
- Do not suck on the extraction site.

These activities may disturb the healing blood clot. Immediately after a tooth is extracted, the patient may experience discomfort and notice some swelling. This is normal. The initial healing period typically takes from 1–2 weeks, and some swelling and residual bleeding should be expected in the 24 hours following an extraction. It is important not to dislodge the blood clot that forms on the wound. Occasionally, this clot can break down leaving what is known as a dry socket. This can cause temporary pain and discomfort that will subside as the socket heals through a secondary healing process.

Response/advice:

To limit swelling:

- Place ice packs or frozen peas on the area of the face overlying the extraction site—20 minutes on and 10 minutes off for 2–3 hours.
- Should there still be bleeding after 2–3 hours place a tea bag on the extraction site and bite down on it firmly but without rupturing the bag.
- Reduce strenuous activity for 24 hours.
- Drink plenty of fluids and maintain as normal a diet as possible, which may be limited to soft foods for the first few days.
- Avoid alcoholic beverages and hot liquids.
- Brush and floss as normal being extra careful around the extraction area.
- On the following day gently rinse the mouth with warm salt water (½ tsp in one glass of water).
- Medication may be prescribed to help control pain and infection.

Dry socket

Alveolar osteitis or dry socket is often a severe pain following a recent extraction. It is the result of disintegration of the blood clot formed in the socket after the extraction and may not be relieved by over-the-counter analgesics. The pain may radiate to the ear and is often accompanied by fetor oris or bad breath. When the usual process of healing is disturbed the blood clot may be dislodged leaving bone within the socket exposed to saliva, food and other mouth debris rather than surrounded by an organising blood clot.

If a dry socket occurs it usually does so immediately following the extraction, although breakdown of the blood clot occasionally occurs after several days of uneventful healing.

Response/advice:

Provide adequate analgesia, which may include the addition of an NSAID, until the next working day; however, antibiotics may also be required if there is established lymphadenopathy or pyrexia. Advise the patient to attend a dentist as soon as possible to have the dry socket irrigated and dressed.

Oral bleeding

Generally warfarin, the newer oral anticoagulants or antiplatelet medications need not be ceased prior to dental extractions or deep cleaning; however, appropriate local measures should be adopted in addition to checking with the patient's cardiologist, in the case of an underlying cardiovascular disease, or haematologist if the concern is due to a blood dyscrasia. Most patients can be managed in an outpatient or general dental practice setting and do not need to be admitted to hospital. St Vincent's Hospital has adopted as the basis for new prescribing and formulary guidelines dental recommendations from the Scottish Dental Effectiveness Programme.[2]

Patients being treated with oral anticoagulant medication who have an international normalisation ratio (INR) below 4.0 may have dental extractions without interruption to their treatment. Local measures, which include suturing and packing the extraction site with absorbable gelatine sponge, are generally sufficient to prevent post-extraction bleeding. Excessive post-extraction or oral bleeding for other reasons may still however occur. The most common cause of post-extraction bleeding for the patient with no known systemic problems is failure to follow instructions from the dentist.

Generally, warfarin or antiplatelet medications need not be ceased prior to dental extractions or deep cleaning; however, appropriate local measures should be adopted in addition to checking with the patient's cardiologist. Most patients can be managed in an outpatient setting.

If bleeding persists in spite of repeating local measures as described in the St Vincent's Hospital Dental Department 'Mouth

Care after Tooth Extraction' information sheet or if a bleeding disorder or dyscrasia is suspected follow the department's protocol for local anti-fibrinolytic treatment as follows.

Outpatient

- Cyklokapron (tranexamic acid) may be used as a mouth rinse; however, it will need to be prepared by a pharmacy as it is only available in tablet form and must be dissolved for local use.
- In patients with established coagulopathies 25 mg/kg of Cyklokapron may be given 2 hours before the procedure as well as factor VIII and factor IX.
- After the procedure Cyklokapron 25 mg/kg 3–4 times a day for 6–8 days should be provided.

Inpatient

- In an emergency, tranexamic acid may be available as a made-up ampoule or IV solution from an ED or general theatres.

Response/advice:

If bleeding persists in spite of repeating local measures as described in the above section or if a bleeding disorder or dyscrasia is suspected, follow the St Vincent's Hospital Dental Department Protocol for local anti-fibrinolytic treatment as follows.

General

- Wet but do not saturate a sterile gauze square in tranexamic acid.
- Fold or roll the gauze so that it can be placed on the extraction site.
- Ensure that the gauze is exerting pressure on the site.
- Repeat after half an hour or as required.
- If being discharged give patient the remaining tranexamic acid and additional bite pads to repeat at home if required.
- Have the patient use an alcohol/phenol free mouthwash twice daily commencing after 24 hours.

Traumatic injuries to teeth

Traumatic injuries to teeth can be divided into several categories. The Ellis classification is one that has been universally accepted (Figure 40.1).

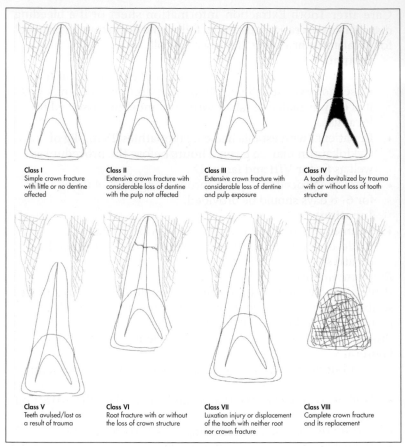

Figure 40.1 Ellis classification of teeth trauma

Response/advice:
If the traumatic injury is the result of a minor accident, provide analgesia if required until the next working day. However, if the injury is the result of a motor vehicle crash, assault or other significant incident, a periapical dental X-ray or OPG (if available) should be taken. Often undisplaced and asymptomatic fractures of the body of the mandible, ramus, condylar head or coronoid

process may be detected with an OPG. With grade 1–4 fractures when there are no other bodily injuries present other than minor local lacerations, provide analgesia until the next working day. Should the patient be admitted or require observation in the ED for any length of time, contact the on-call dentist.

WARNING

A tooth with a comminuted fracture may look simple to extract; however, microfractures may be present resulting in attached labial crest of bone coming away with the tooth which in turn may preclude implant placement with a bone grafting.

Response/advice:

Consider a pulpal dressing and temporary restoration for 6–8 weeks before extraction if uncertain about the integrity of the bone surrounding the tooth.

LUXATION: ELLIS GRADE VII

A tooth is considered luxated when it has been moved, often occupying a position other than its original one. Luxated teeth can be:

- concussed—trauma to a tooth without eliciting a positional change
- subluxation—overt loosening without demonstrable clinical or radiographic change to its position
- extrusive luxation—partial displacement or avulsion which is evident radiographically
- lateral luxation—eccentric displacement of the tooth within the socket which may involve a fracture within the socket itself
- intrusive luxation—pushed intraorally, often associated with intrasocket fractures.

Response/advice:

Except for a concussion or subluxation injury, always contact the on-call dentist as soon as possible. If there are no other bodily injuries precluding dental management, repositioning and splinting of the loosened teeth will generally be required.

AVULSION

Evidence suggests that avulsed or knocked out teeth that have been reimplanted within 30–45 minutes have a reasonable chance of long-term retention; however, after 2 hours out of the mouth the prospects are diminished. Correct handling, transportation and storage of the knocked-out tooth is critical.

Response/advice·

Ideally, the patient should be encouraged to push the tooth back into the socket, even if it is out of alignment and loose. If this is too painful or not possible, holding the tooth in the floor of the mouth will keep the root bathed in the patient's own saliva. Should other injuries or the patient's mental state preclude the above, immediate storage in UHT milk is preferred to whole milk or water. Only handle avulsed teeth by the enamel and do not rinse in any disinfectant solution. Always contact the on-call dentist as soon as possible as implantation, repositioning and splinting of an avulsed tooth will be required.

Should the dentist be unavailable immediately, small rectangular strips of ConvaTec Stomahesive wafer can be used to provisionally hold the tooth. This will provide additional working time for the dentist and could save the patient many thousands of dollars.

- Only hold the tooth by the crown.
- Try not to touch the root.
- Remove visible debris by gently washing with saline.
- Replace back in dental socket ASAP.
- Use a single rectangular piece of ConvaTec Stomahesive.
- Wetting the wafer first can help.
- It may take 10–15 minutes for the wafer to feel secure.
- When in place, the wafer can last several hours.

The case below was jointly managed by both the St Vincent's Hospital Emergency Department and the Dental Department (Figures 40.2 to 40.4).

Trismus and temporomandibular joint (TMJ) dysfunction

Many people have pain or discomfort in and around the TMJ at some time during their lives. The symptoms may include pain, tenderness, spasm, clicking or crepitus as well as direct or referred pain in the muscles of the face, neck, shoulder and ears. TMJ dysfunction may lead to loss of jaw function with the pain ranging from a mild discomfort in the morning to a chronic debilitating

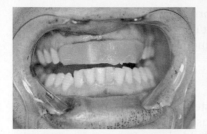

Figure 40.2 Upper central incisor teeth were avulsed following an assault. They were placed back in their sockets and secured using ConvaTec Stomahesive wafer.

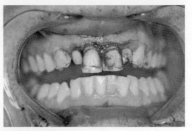

Figure 40.3 Upper central incisor teeth were avulsed following an assault. They were placed back in their sockets and secured using ConvaTec Stomahesive wafer.

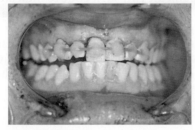

Figure 40.4 The upper central incisor teeth were splinted using flexible nylon and flowable composite resin.

pain rendering the patient unable to open their mouth by the afternoon.

Conservative treatment (NSAIDs plus alternating hot and cold packs or compresses and rest) may prove effective following acute trauma to the jaw after a motor vehicle crash, fall or bashing. Direct trauma to the TMJ area or either jaw may also cause chronic or latent damage which may eventually contribute to a TMJ problem, often years later.

Bruxism is a non-functional clenching or grinding of the teeth. Some people will brux during waking hours; however, bruxing is generally carried out subconsciously while asleep. Although bruxing while asleep is extremely common and can lead to enamel wear, pathological bruxing can lead to significant TMJ damage over time especially when the dentition is less than optimal in the first place. Dentists can fabricate a variety of splints which the patient will generally wear at night and help in either alleviating the symptoms of TMJ dysfunction or in the retraining of the facial musculature.

Dental nomenclature

The international numbering system of teeth (Fédération Dentaire Internationale [FDI]) should be used in any written or verbal communication. The mouth can be divided into four quadrants. In the adult dentition the maxillary right is quadrant 1, the maxillary left quadrant 2, the mandibular left quadrant 3 and the mandibular right quadrant 4. The individual teeth are numbered from the central incisor outwards to the third molar. This provides an easy-to-use and communicate two-digit code to indicate the tooth or region of concern. Deciduous or baby teeth follow a similar pattern. The maxillary right is quadrant 5, the maxillary left quadrant 6, the mandibular left quadrant 7 and the mandibular right quadrant 8. The complete deciduous dentition has only five teeth in each quadrant as opposed to eight teeth in each quadrant in the adult dentition (Figure 40.5).

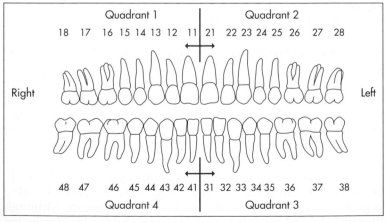

Figure 40.5 Adult dental nomenclature

Copies of information sheets referred to are available from: Dr Peter Foltyn, Consultant Dentist, Dental Department, St Vincent's Hospital, peter.foltyn

References

1 Daly CG. Antibiotic prophylaxis for dental procedures. Aust Prescr 2017;40:184–8. 3 October. Retrieved from: https://www. nps.org.au/australian-prescriber/articles/antibiotic-prophylaxis-for-dental-procedures

2 Scottish Dental Clinical Effectiveness Programme. Management of patients taking anticoagulants or antiplatelet drugs. Quick Reference Guide. August 2015. Retrieved from: http://www.sdcep. org.uk/wp-content/uploads/2015/09/SDCEP-Anticoagulants-Quick-Reference-Guide.pdf

Chapter 41
Psychiatric, mental health presentations

Jackie Huber and Tad Tietze

Acknowledgment

The authors wish to acknowledge the content used from the previous edition of *Emergency Medicine* which was provided by Dr Paul Preisz and Beaver Hudson.

Working in the emergency setting
OVERVIEW

Psychiatric presentations to the ED are increasingly common in the wake of deinstitutionalisation and 'mainstreaming', where a closer focus has been placed on community-based care. Additional pressure on EDs has occurred due to the redirection of intoxicated or behaviourally disturbed patients from police custody, as well as increasing public awareness of mental illness. All these trends make it increasingly important for EDs to be able to manage mental health presentations safely and efficiently.

Editorial Comment

As mental health is now being mainstreamed through EDs, increasingly with better-designed flow paths and areas in the ED (e.g. 'PANDA' psychiatric and non-prescription drug assessment), it has become easier but no less important to ensure that the patient does not have an organic illness/cause contributing to their behaviour (i.e. a delirium). Also, the patient must be assessed for any risk that their therapy may present. Medical clearance is a clumsy term; the modern approach is for mental health and emergency doctors to simultaneously and collaboratively assess the patient.

Hospitals have responded to these developments with a variety of models, from providing in-reach from community mental health services to consultation-liaison input to having their own in-house mental health team. These different service models will guide how much of the emergency mental health assessment is carried out by ED clinicians and how much is carried out by specialist mental health clinicians. Regardless of the model, cooperation between ED and mental health teams is imperative to ensure they collaborate fully, with a good understanding of the different skills offered, and to ensure that mental health patients are not discriminated against with respect to their physical care.

HOW MENTAL HEALTH PATIENTS PRESENT

Patients with mental health problems present to the ED with undifferentiated clusters of symptoms, which reflect a complex interplay of biological, psychological and social factors. Symptoms and signs can overlap in a way that obscures diagnosis, requiring the ED doctor to take the role of 'bio-psycho-social detective'.

Optimal outcomes and maximum safety are achieved when there is a holistic assessment of the patient's physical and mental health in their social context, on the background of their unique personal history. After briefly reviewing the types of presentations that can be expected, this chapter describes the general assessment of mental health patients in the ED, from triage to disposition. The chapter then focuses on more specific details about some of the most common mental health presentations.

COMMON PSYCHIATRIC EMERGENCIES

The most common mental health symptom clusters presenting to EDs include:
- behavioural disturbance (including agitation and violence)
- suicidality and self-harm
- acute severe behavioural disturbance
- acute psychosis and mania
- confusion and delirium
- anxiety

- iatrogenic emergencies: neuroleptic malignant syndrome and serotonin syndrome
- factitious presentations.

NON-PSYCHIATRIC REFERRALS THAT MAY BE SEEN AS 'MENTAL HEALTH PROBLEMS'

- Malingering
- Repeat attenders
- Domestic violence
- Rape
- Child abuse and children at risk
- Elder abuse
- Homelessness

TREATMENT GOALS IN EMERGENCY PSYCHIATRY[1]

- Exclude medical aetiologies for symptoms.
- Rapid stabilisation of acute crisis.
- Avoid coercion.
- Treat in the least restrictive setting.
- Form a therapeutic alliance.
- Organise appropriate disposition and aftercare plan.

The ED mental health assessment
GOALS OF EMERGENCY CLINICIAN INVOLVEMENT

- Ensure a safe environment.
- Triage.
- Assessment.
    - End-of-the-bed inspection and address emergencies and immediate barriers to assessment.
    - Identify likely trigger to presentation (Why now?).
    - Specific questions for specific symptom clusters (e.g. psychosis, mood, anxiety).
    - Exclude emergency medical issues and medical causes of psychiatric symptoms.
- Do a basic risk assessment.
- Establish a hypothesis.
- Manage immediate psychiatric emergency.
- Ensure least restrictive care, using appropriate legal instruments.
- Appropriate referral/disposition.

ENVIRONMENT
- Quiet, non-threatening.
- If the patient is aggressive or suicidal: remove sharp objects and cords from immediate vicinity, ensure patient can be seen easily from nursing station or consider 1:1 nursing if environment requires it.
- If aggressive also: remove personal items that present a threat and ensure furniture cannot be thrown.
- Ensure staffing is appropriate: where necessary, bring with you staff skilled at verbal de-escalation; if restraint is required, ensure staff are experienced and ideally minimum six staff members.
- Remember that EDs contain more potential hazards than psychiatric units, and so special care must be taken to ensure patient and staff safety.

TRIAGE
Most locations will have a mental health-specific triage system in place to ensure that serious and potentially life-threatening psychiatric emergencies are triaged appropriately even when physical injuries or illness are not present.[2]

HISTORY
The history should start with the presenting complaint.
- **History of presenting complaint:** see individual sections for presentation-specific questions.
- **Past psychiatric history:** diagnoses, admissions, previous suicide attempts and severity, past and current therapists and treatments.
- **Substance use history:** illicit, prescribed, alcohol, cigarettes, how much, when, episodes of abstinence, admissions to rehabilitation or detoxification centres, history of withdrawal.
- **Forensic history:** type of offence, when, incarcerations.
- **Medications:** current, past, side effects and allergies.
- **Past medical history:** include illnesses that may have psychiatric sequelae and metabolic syndrome.
- **Current social situation:** living situation, supports, employment status/income source, gambling.
- **Family history:** psychiatric illness, suicide.

- **Developmental history:** family tree, relationship with parents, obvious episodes of trauma, jobs, romantic relationships.

COLLATERAL INFORMATION

'**Trust but verify**': It is imperative to obtain information from past psychiatric encounters, and from those who know the patient, to ascertain patient insight and judgment, aid diagnostic clarity and assess risk. Include past hospital inpatient notes, community mental health notes, ED notes and information from GP, family, partner and friends.

STRATEGIES FOR A SUCCESSFUL INTERVIEW

1 **Listen:** give the patient some time to speak uninterrupted for around 2–3 minutes initially.
2 **Validate:** comment that the patient's emotional response is understandable.
3 **Normalise:** comment that the patient's reaction is common.
4 **Demonstrate empathy:** try to sit in the patient's experience, and demonstrate understanding of their emotional plight.
5 **Address our own intense emotional reactions:** do not let strong negative *or* positive emotions obstruct rapport.
6 **Avoid the concept of the 'bad patient':** do not allow apparent 'bad behaviour' lead to blaming, and thus punishing the patient for their emotional predicament.

PHYSICAL EXAMINATION AND INVESTIGATIONS

When the presentation is primarily psychiatric, it is essential to exclude urgent medical issues and medical causes of psychiatric symptoms. Aim for medical stability, identify emergency medical issues and start investigations.

- Focused physical examination
  — Be guided by any physical symptoms but remember that some mentally ill patients have problems expressing these and especially consider possible causes of delirium and neurological symptoms.
- Investigations
  — FBCs, EUCs, LFTs, CMP.
  — Blood alcohol level (BAL; see Box 41.1), urine drug screen (UDS).

Box 41.1   Blood alcohol level (BAL)

- The only reliable way to identify whether someone is alcohol intoxicated and the level of their intoxication is to take a BAL.
- It is important to take BAL for safety reasons in the ED (risk of oversedation, alcohol withdrawal, behavioural dysregulation), to ensure reliability of assessment (because intoxication deranges mental state and behaviour) and to ensure appropriate, safe disposition once sober.

— More specialised tests: TFTs, CRP, B_{12}, folate, Fe panel, syphilis, CT, EEG.
— Subspecialised tests will depend on hypothesis (e.g. lumbar puncture, MRI).
- 'Mimics' of psychiatric illness
  — Many organic illnesses can mimic psychiatric illness, most commonly anxiety and psychosis. Investigate where necessary for the following.
    ○ Anxiety: medications or substances (stimulants, hallucinogens, sympathomimetics, xanthines, anticholinergics, steroids); withdrawal (alcohol, opioids, benzodiazepines); cardiovascular or respiratory distress (CCF, hypertension [HTN], pulmonary fibrosis, infectious cause); endocrine disorders (hyperthyroidism, Cushing's syndrome); neurological disorders (stroke, pain, epilepsy, migraine).
    ○ Organic psychotic disorders: intoxication (stimulants, hallucinogens); withdrawal (alcohol, benzodiazepines); delirium; dementia; neurological disorders (encephalopathy, stroke, traumatic brain injury [TBI], multiple sclerosis, vasculitis, meningitis, normal pressure hydrocephalus [NPH]), endocrine disorders (hyper/hypothyroidism, diabetic ketoacidosis [DKA], hypoglycaemia).

ESTABLISHING A HYPOTHESIS

Once history, physical examination and investigations have occurred, for each patient the goal is to establish a hypothesis. In order to establish a hypothesis, further assessment needs to be directed at the patient's particular presentation (see Box 41.2).

> ### Box 41.2 Psychiatric hypothesis: formulating the problem
>
> • What is the patient's predicament/trigger to presentation?
> • What are the precipitants?
> • Why is the patient predisposed to reacting in this way?
> • What protective factors will help them recover?

REMEMBER: In the emergency setting a working hypothesis is more useful than a definitive diagnosis.

RISK ASSESSMENT

Risk assessment involves the consideration of static, dynamic and current factors. The main purpose of risk assessment is to identify risk factors which can be mitigated through appropriate interventions, in order to prevent undesirable outcomes. On the other hand, structured risk assessments designed to stratify overall level of risk have low predictive validity[3] and therefore are of limited utility in emergency psychiatry settings. Risk factors to be considered are set out in Table 41.1.

LEGAL ISSUES

Each location will have its own rules regarding the use of Mental Health Act and Guardianship legislation. Familiarise yourself with the local rules so that patients may always be treated in a least restrictive environment that still provides safety for the patient and others.

IMMEDIATE MANAGEMENT

While definitive psychiatric, medical or surgical care is beyond the scope of the ED, patients presenting with psychiatric emergencies often need immediate treatment in the department. This can include:

• management of acute severe behavioural disturbance (ASBD)
• stabilisation and initial treatment of self-injury such as self-poisoning, lacerations, fractures, self-strangulation/hanging, etc.
• stabilisation and immediate management of comorbid physical health conditions, including those causing mental health symptoms (e.g. delirium).

Table 41.1   Risk factors in mental health presentations

	Static factors	Dynamic factors	Factors specific to this presentation
Suicidality	• Male gender • Older age • Low SES/ education • Family history of suicide and mental health problems • Mental health diagnosis • Past suicide attempts or suicidal ideation	• Unemployed • Living alone • Single • Substance abuse • Physical health problems • Level of distress may correlate • Unwilling to engage with interventions	• Adverse life event • Anniversary • Recent discharge from mental health service • Access to lethal means • Preparation for self-harm
Aggression	• History of aggression • Forensic history	• Violent event prior to presenting to ED • Substance use in the past 6–12 months	• Threats in ED • Intent and plan • Adverse life event • Agitation • Persecutory ideation • Delusions or hallucinations with violent content • Intoxication

Mental Health and Drug and Alcohol Office, Mental Health for Emergency Departments—A reference guide. NSW Ministry of Health. Amended March 2015.

APPROPRIATE REFERRAL/DISPOSITION

♦ In most cases, the main referral pathway will be to the relevant mental health team serving the ED, either for discharge planning or inpatient admission.
  — Not all aspects of the ED assessment need to be complete prior to referral being made. For example, pending investigations where there is low suspicion of physical health problems should not delay referral.
  — A suggested form of words for the referral/handover is presented in Box 41.3.

> **Box 41.3 How to summarise a case for referral to the mental health team**
>
> 'Mr/s [name] is an [age] year old woman/man, who is single/in a relationship, [sexuality], living in [living situation], and supporting her/himself by [main source of income]. S/he presented to the ED via [method of arriving in ED], [voluntarily/under the Mental Health Act], complaining of [presenting complaint].
>
> 'I believe they are suffering from [mental health complaint] in the context of [precipitants to presentation]. This occurs on the background of [relevant mental health and medical history, including serious suicide attempts and violence]. Her/his history is notable for the following: [relevant features of history].'

- In a proportion of cases the ED may be able to assess and manage a psychiatric emergency and discharge the patient from hospital for appropriate follow-up (by mental health or other appropriate services).
- Where physical health problems play the major part in the patient's current problems, referral to the appropriate medical or surgical inpatient team with consultation-liaison psychiatry input may be the best option.

Suicidality and self-harm

Suicidality (i.e. suicidal ideation and/or behaviour) and deliberate self-harm are potentially life-threatening emergencies, regardless of the patient's motivation or intent. Emergency assessment and management are directed towards ensuring immediate safety, addressing any physical injuries and delineating the predicament that led the patient to this situation, with a view to providing an intervention that addresses those factors.

SPECIFIC ASPECTS OF ASSESSMENT AND MANAGEMENT

- End-of-the-bed inspection: address medical emergencies and obvious barriers to psychiatric assessment first:
  — medical and surgical sequelae of and deliberate self-harm
  — altered sensorium (e.g. intoxication/delirium/withdrawal)
  — extremely upset and requiring de-escalation or sedation (see sedation pathway).

- Identify the trigger to the presentation (Why now?):
  - engage in empathic listening
  - psychosocial trigger—job loss, homelessness, loss of relationship, financial difficulties, physical illness, interpersonal disharmony
  - evidence of 'biological' trigger: depression, mania, psychosis or substance-induced mood changes.
- Specific information:
  - identify intention to suicide or self-harm
  - identify means and access (e.g. access to firearms? medications? rope?)
  - recent overdose or suicide attempt—did the patient seek medical attention?
  - identify protective factors (e.g. job, family, friends, pets, religion, professional psychiatric involvement)
  - enquire as to past history and seriousness of past attempts
  - assess risk of absconding
  - if no longer suicidal, identify what has changed
  - if no longer suicidal, identify specific future plans for community support and treatment
  - important special tests: BAL, paracetamol level, UDS.
- Collateral information:
  - previous suicide attempts and seriousness
  - recent mental state and mood
  - recent triggers.
- Focused physical examination:
  - look especially for physical consequences of known or possible self-harm
  - paracetamol level should be mandatory.
- Establish a hypothesis (see Box 41.2).
- Consider use of local Mental Health Act.
- Refer appropriately:
  - medical/surgical teams for any serious self-injury
  - psychiatric team for further assessment and management of causes of suicidality.
    - Not all patients who present with suicidality need to have a formal psychiatric review, but it is generally advisable to at least ask for advice from the local

mental health team and document. Especially any danger to self and others.

Acute severe behavioural disturbance (ASBD)
ASSESSMENT
- End-of-the-bed inspection and address immediate barriers to assessment.
- Ensure adequate staff for safety and control if possible before patient arrives, once in ED.
- Consider as a continuum, from agitation to aggression.

MANAGE AGITATION AS A PRIORITY
- Aim intervention at level of patient agitation.
- Consider use of Mental Health Act.
- The best treatment for aggression/agitation is prevention:
  — verbal de-escalation; establish rapport[4]
  — take note of one's own body language, tone of voice, word choice, facial expression
  — listen
  — identify patient requests and feelings
  — don't provoke
  — don't argue but agree to disagree
  — validate/provide empathic responses
  — bargain/offer choices where possible
  — set clear limits in a flexible way
  — be empathically clear about consequences.
- Pharmacotherapy:
  — the choice of medication and route of administration will depend on the patient's clinical state and cooperativeness
  — local areas have their own protocols, based on current evidence and factors present in their specific patient populations
  — recent evidence suggests that droperidol is a safe and effective parenteral agent for highly agitated patients in the emergency setting; Box 41.4 sets out the sedation algorithm used where the authors of this chapter practice.

Box 41.4 St Vincent's Hospital Sydney algorithm for sedation in ASBD in the ED

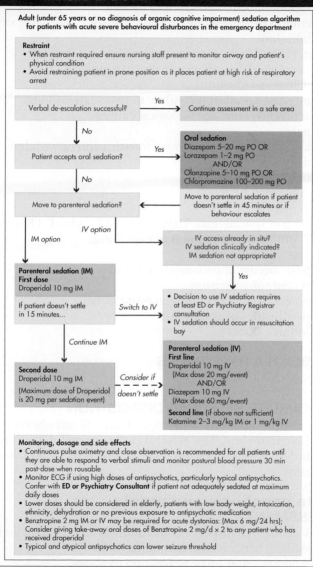

Adult (under 65 years or no diagnosis of organic cognitive impairment) sedation algorithm for patients with acute severe behavioural disturbances in the emergency department

Restraint
- When restraint required ensure nursing staff present to monitor airway and patient's physical condition
- Avoid restraining patient in prone position as it places patient at high risk of respiratory arrest

Verbal de-escalation successful? — Yes → Continue assessment in a safe area

↓ No

Patient accepts oral sedation? — Yes → **Oral sedation**
Diazepam 5–20 mg PO OR
Lorazepam 1–2 mg PO
AND/OR
Olanzapine 5–10 mg PO OR
Chlorpromazine 100–200 mg PO

↓ No

Move to parenteral sedation? ← Move to parenteral sedation if patient doesn't settle in 45 minutes or if behaviour escalates

IM option | IV option →

IV access already in situ?
IV sedation clinically indicated?
IM sedation not appropriate?

↓ Yes

Parenteral sedation (IM)
First dose
Droperidol 10 mg IM

If patient doesn't settle in 15 minutes... — Switch to IV →
- Decision to use IV sedation requires at least ED or Psychiatry Registrar consultation
- IV sedation should occur in resuscitation bay

↓ Continue IM

Second dose
Droperidol 10 mg IM
(Maximum dose of Droperidol is 20 mg per sedation event)

— Consider if doesn't settle - - →

Parenteral sedation (IV)
First line
Droperidol 10 mg IV
(Max dose 20 mg/event)
AND/OR
Diazepam 10 mg IV
(Max dose 60 mg/event)

Second line (if above not sufficient)
Ketamine 2–3 mg/kg IM or 1 mg/kg IV

Monitoring, dosage and side effects
- Continuous pulse oximetry and close observation is recommended for all patients until they are able to respond to verbal stimuli and monitor postural blood pressure 30 min post-dose when rousable
- Monitor ECG if using high doses of antipsychotics, particularly typical antipsychotics. Confer with **ED or Psychiatry Consultant** if patient not adequately sedated at maximum daily doses
- Lower doses should be considered in elderly, patients with low body weight, intoxication, ethnicity, dehydration or no previous exposure to antipsychotic medication
- Benztropine 2 mg IM or IV may be required for acute dystonias: (Max 6 mg/24 hrs); Consider giving take-away oral doses of Benztropine 2 mg/d × 2 to any patient who has received droperidol
- Typical and atypical antipsychotics can lower seizure threshold

CONSIDER CAUSES OF ASBD

- Consider psychological and psychiatric causes:
  - lack of information given to patient
  - emotional distress due to recent stressor OR pending stressor
  - boredom
  - perceived lack of understanding by hospital staff
  - perceptual disturbance (hallucinations)
  - delusional ideation
  - internal agitation secondary to psychiatric illness.
- Concurrently consider biological causes:
  - pain
  - alcohol/substance/nicotine intoxication or withdrawal
  - drug reaction
  - neurological
  - delirium
  - dementia.
- Important special tests: UDS, BAL, TFTs, plus CTB or MRI, EEG and LP if aggression is unexplained.
- Collateral information:
  - past successful treatment of aggression in the ED
  - recent substance use
  - recent behaviours and aggressive acts
  - past history of aggression
  - forensic history.

ESTABLISH A HYPOTHESIS

See Box 41.2.

APPROPRIATE REFERRAL/DISPOSITION

A patient with behavioural dysregulation will not always require a psychiatric review. The referral pathway will depend on the likely underlying cause for aggression, which will arise from your hypothesis.

Acute psychosis and mania
ASSESSMENT

- End-of-the-bed inspection and address emergencies and immediate barriers to assessment.
  - Address agitation or aggression as above.

- — Abnormal movements: parkinsonian symptoms, chorea, posturing, tics.
- — Affect: incongruent to mood or thought content, labile, fatuous, perplexed, blunt.
- — Poverty of speech or thought content.
• Identify likely trigger to presentation.
- — Pharmacological: sudden cessation or reduction in medication, medication change.
- — Substance use/withdrawal: stimulants, alcohol, benzodiazepines.
- — Emotional trigger.
- — New organic illness.
• Specific information.
- — Does the patient have perceptual abnormalities (auditory, visual or tactile hallucinations)?
- — Does the patient have delusional ideation (persecutory, delusions of reference, thought insertion or removal, thought broadcasting) or overvalued ideas?
- — Does the patient have an attentional deficit (required for a diagnosis of delirium)?
- — What is the patient's premorbid mental status?
- — What has been the timeframe of the development of symptoms and signs?
- — Has the patient taken risks lately that are out of character?
- — Important special tests: UDS, BAL, TFTs, CTB or MRI, EEG and LP if psychosis is unexplained.
• Collateral information.
- — History of psychosis or bipolar disorder.
  - ○ Previous diagnoses and treatment.

ESTABLISH A HYPOTHESIS
See Box 41.2.

Consider the following diagnostic possibilities throughout the assessment:
• functional psychosis (schizophrenia, delusional disorder, drug induced psychosis, brief reactive psychosis)
• affective psychosis—mania, psychotic depression
• delirium
• organic psychosis.

APPROPRIATE REFERRAL/DISPOSITION

• Consider using local mental health legislation.
• A patient with new onset psychosis will generally require a psychiatric assessment in the ED, except where delirium or organic psychosis are suspected. A psychiatric referral should be made if behaviour management advice is required.
• In the case of a chronically psychotic patient, the reason for presentation to the ED may not be mental health related.

Drugs and their consequences

See Chapter 18 Poisoning and Overdose and Chapter 19 Drugs and Alcohol.

Confusion and delirium

Confusion is common in presentations in the elderly, but less common in those under 65. A thorough search for an organic cause is always warranted.

ASSESSMENT

• End-of-the-bed inspection and address immediate barriers to assessment:
  — ensure sensory impairments corrected (hearing aids, glasses)
  — address severe agitation as above, pain or other obvious physical concerns
  — gestures that might indicate pain
  — inattention
  — affect—emotional incontinence, perplexity
  — disorganised thought form
  — fluctuating sensorium
  — agitation.

MANAGE AGITATION AS A PRIORITY

Behavioural interventions

• Interventions listed earlier in the ASBD section apply.
• Additional behavioural management of the confused patient:
  — if sensory deficits, speak loudly (don't shout), slowly, clearly
  — use simple language—rephrase if patient does not understand

— use positive nonverbal cues (warm smile, eye contact)
— use visual aids (demonstrate, point)
— give simple choices
— avoid arguments—agree then distract, using activities where possible that are tailored to the patient's interests
— encourage phone call or face-to-face contact with spouse, family or friends.

Pharmacological interventions

◆ Avoid benzodiazepines.
◆ In the elderly, if there is behavioural disturbance that does not respond solely to behavioural intervention, consider risperidone 0.25–0.5 mg BD PRN. In Australia, olanzapine is the only antipsychotic approved for parenteral use in the context of behavioural and psychological symptoms of dementia. Consider olanzapine 2.5–5 mg IM in cases of severe behavioural disturbance.[5]
◆ In younger adults, follow the sedation pathway outlined in Box 41.4.

CONSIDER THE CAUSES OF CONFUSION

◆ Identify the trigger to presentation (why now)
— Thoroughly investigate organic triggers:
  ○ metabolic derangements
  ○ infection
  ○ meningitis/encephalitides
  ○ cerebral haemorrhage.
— Medication change/withdrawal or polypharmacy.
— Substance use/withdrawal.
— Consider acute trigger on the background of dementia.
◆ Specific information
— BAL, UDS, M&S, CXR, ECG, CTB
— All other investigations should depend on the patient's medical history.
◆ Collateral information
— History of delirium or dementia.
— Recent level of function.
— Timeframe of deterioration.

ESTABLISH A HYPOTHESIS
See Box 41.2.

APPROPRIATE MANAGEMENT, REFERRAL/ DISPOSITION

- Behavioural and psychological symptoms: see 'agitation'.
- Confused patients should be referred to the appropriate medical team. If over 65, it is often appropriate to refer to the geriatrics team. Psychiatric team can be involved for behaviour management advice.

Anxiety
ASSESSMENT

- End-of-the-bed inspection and address immediate barriers to assessment:
  — address agitation and restlessness
  — treat severe withdrawal
  — panic attack—palpitations, sweating, tremor, shortness of breath, choking, chest pain, nausea, dizziness, derealisation, fear of dying or losing control, paraesthesia, chills or hot flushes
  — hypervigilance and easily startled.
- Identify the trigger to presentation (why now):
  — organic causes (e.g. thyroid dysfunction)
  — substance or medication withdrawal (alcohol, benzodiazepines, opioids, antidepressants) or medication change/increase (antidepressants, anticholinergics)
  — akathisia (from antipsychotics, antidepressants and stimulants)
  — emotional stressor
  — panic attack (if there is new onset panic after the age of 45, strongly consider an organic cause[6]).
- Specific information
  — Is anxiety accompanied by panic, agoraphobia, obsessional symptoms?
  — Is anxiety associated with social situations?
  — Special tests: UDS, BAL, TFTs, ECG.

ESTABLISH A HYPOTHESIS
See Box 41.2.

APPROPRIATE MANAGEMENT, REFERRAL AND DISPOSITION

- Almost always, anxiety can be treated as an outpatient.
- Cognitive behavioural therapy is effective (in person or via several internet treatment providers).
- SSRIs are efficacious, have few side effects and are preferred over benzodiazepines in the long term.[6]
- If the anxiety is so catastrophic or crippling that the patient is unable to care for him/herself or has suicidal ideation, a psychiatric review is warranted in the ED.

Iatrogenic emergencies

Psychotropic medications can sometimes produce iatrogenic emergencies, the clinical presentation of which can closely mimic the symptoms and signs of other medical and psychiatric emergencies. The two most common are neuroleptic malignant syndrome and serotonin syndrome. See Table 41.2 for details on assessment, differential diagnosis and treatment.

Table 41.2   Neuroleptic malignant (NMS) and serotonin syndrome

	NMS	Serotonin syndrome
Description	Life-threatening reaction to dopamine blockade that usually occurs in response to initiating dopamine antagonists (e.g. antipsychotics) or ceasing dopamine agonists	Excessive stimulation of 5-HT_2 receptors, in cases where serotonin agonists are administered with other serotonin agonists including SSRIs, SNRIs, MAOIs, TCAs and antipsychotics
Risk factors	High-potency antipsychotics, rapid dose increase or reduction, agitation, dehydration, psychosis, alcoholism, Parkinson's disease, hyperthyroidism, organic brain disease	Recent change of serotonin agonist dose, several agonists at once, use with illicit serotonin agonists (e.g. MDMA)

Continued

Table 41.2 Neuroleptic malignant (NMS) and serotonin syndrome (cont.)

	NMS	Serotonin syndrome
Common symptoms and signs	• Altered mental state, muscular rigidity, autonomic dysfunction (blood pressure fluctuations or severe hypertension, tachycardia, diaphoresis, sialorrhoea, urinary incontinence), hyperpyrexia • Symptoms evolve over 24–72 hours; can take up to 3 weeks to resolve	• Deep tendon hyporreflexia, inducible or spontaneous muscle clonus, muscle rigidity, hyperthermia, agitation, ocular clonus, dilated pupils, tremor, akathisia, bilateral Babinski signs, diaphoresis, nausea, vomiting, diarrhoea) • Symptoms evolve over 24-hour timeframe,[7] and resolve quickly depending on half-life of cause
Investigations	• Elevated CK 3700–5000 units/L • WCC often elevated • Severe dehydration can affect electrolytes • Serial renal function panels • ECG	• Leucocytosis • Elevated CK but not as high as NMS • Elevated hepatic transaminases • Metabolic acidosis
	• Consider CT/MRI, EEG, lumbar puncture to exclude infection • Also consider toxicology screen, lithium levels, coagulation studies, arterial blood gases	
Differential diagnosis	NMS, serotonin syndrome, catatonia, malignant hyperthermia, neuroleptic heat stroke, parkinsonism-hyperpyrexia syndrome (medication withdrawal), drug withdrawal/intoxication, infection, autoimmune, metabolic derangement	
Acute management	• IV fluids and supportive measures • Discontinue antipsychotic agents and lithium • Continue dopamine agonists if they are currently in use (cessation may worsen NMS)	• Discontinue all serotonergic agents • IV fluids, oxygen administration, cardiac monitoring • Sedation with parenteral benzodiazepines • Avoid using antipsychotics

Table 41.2 **Neuroleptic malignant (NMS) and serotonin syndrome (cont.)**

NMS	Serotonin syndrome
• Manage agitation with benzodiazepines • If severe hypertension, use short-acting anti-hypertensive (e.g. nifedipine) • If respiratory failure then oxygen mask or intubation and mechanical ventilation • There is some evidence that bromocriptine may reduce response time (2.5 mg BD or TDS, titrate by up to 7.5 mg/d, max 40 mg/d)[8–10] • Second line: amantadine or dantrolene • Syndrome can take up to 3 weeks to resolve	• If symptoms continue, consider cyproheptadine 12 mg PO plus 2 mg PR every 2 hours until symptoms improve (*note:* further evidence is required)[11] • Syndrome usually resolves within 24 hours, depending on half-life of serotonergic agents

Malingering and factitious presentations

Sometimes patients manufacture symptoms and other signs of illness, either to obtain psychological satisfaction by coming into medical care (i.e. primary gain in factitious disorder) or to obtain a material benefit such as medication, accommodation or avoidance of court appearance (i.e. secondary gain in malingering). Such patients can often present with apparent psychiatric symptoms which need to be explored in such a way that the real motivation becomes clear. Collateral information is extremely important in these cases, to triangulate the patient's presentation with other known information about them. The patient should always be evaluated and organic causes be considered before such a diagnosis is made.

ASSESSMENT

- End-of-the-bed inspection and address immediate barriers to assessment
    - Serious physical trauma or other medical emergency that requires treatment (e.g. overdose, poisoning, infection, laceration)
    — Sudden changes in affect or behaviour on clinician's approach
    — Multiple scars
    — Atypical or inconsistent examination
- Identify the trigger to presentation (Why now?)
    — Recent loss of accommodation
    — Withdrawal from benzodiazepines or opiates
    — Upcoming court case
    — Loss of funds (e.g. from gambling or theft)
    — Under external threat
- Specific information
    — Signs of possible malingering include:
        ° resistant to allow physician to talk to friends or family
        ° requesting specific medication, usually drug of dependence
        ° vague, unverifiable history
        ° refusing tests
        ° presenting out of regular hours
        ° evidence of 'doctor-shopping'.
    — Signs of possible factitious disorder:
        ° no objections to invasive tests
        ° failure to respond to typical treatments
        ° normal investigations
        ° presenting out of regular hours.
- Collateral information:
    — multiple hospital admissions
    — lack of verifiable history
    — failure to respond to typical treatments in the past.

ESTABLISH A HYPOTHESIS
See Box 41.2.

APPROPRIATE MANAGEMENT, REFERRAL/DISPOSITION

- Often it will not be 100% certain whether the presentation is that of malingering or factitious disorder, and a psychiatric assessment may complement the ED assessment. If the past history indicates a high likelihood of risky behaviour, a psychiatric referral is appropriate.
- Avoid invasive procedures where possible.
- Empathically set appropriate limits.
- There is debate as to whether 'calling the patient out' or giving a 'face-saving' way out is the best management approach, but in every case the decision as to how to approach them should be decided by consensus between all teams involved.
- Patients tend not to benefit from admission unless the goal of admission is very clear, and boundaries of admission are stated early (e.g. acute treatment of any self-injury in factitious presentations or to provide appropriate and limited social assistance if a malingering patient is willing to engage around this), and maintained throughout admission.
- Document findings clearly and in detail.

Frequent attenders

- Advance management planning for these patients can give the ED physician a quickly accessible document that includes usual presentations and triggers, management interventions that work, and clinicians involved in that patient's care so that follow-up options are clear.
- The group writing the document should include emergency physician and psychiatrist who know patient well, as well as members of team that manage comorbid illness (e.g. drug and alcohol team, toxicology/clinical pharmacology).
- See the proforma in Figure 41.1 for an example of a useful structure.

Name:	**Identifier:**	**Date of birth:**
Address:		

Brief description:
Include a summary of diagnoses, risk factors, salient features of the patient's background including significant or particularly dangerous episodes of self-harm, and whether the patient has a substitute decision-maker.

Usual presentation:
Include the usual manner of presenting to hospital, presenting complaints, extent of usual self-harm or outcome of harm to others, usual response to intervention in the ED, interventions that are helpful or unhelpful, use of local mental health legislation.

List of clinicians and carers involved in the patient's care:
Include names of phone numbers of family members, GP, specialist physician, psychologist, social worker, non-government organisations.

Current management:
Include all regular and PRN medications and significant side effects, psychological interventions.

Management plan:
Include specifics of HOW to de-escalate the patient, medications that should and should not be prescribed, certain phrases that are helpful, distraction strategies, team members with whom the patient has particularly good rapport, specific circumstances under which the patient should be admitted, discharged or referred to the mental health team, boundaries that should be set and how they should be ensured.

Specific risk items:
Outline specific risks within the ED and how to best manage them.

Plan written by:
Names of those who wrote the plan.

Review date:
The review date should be within 1 year of writing the initial plan.

Figure 41.1 Frequent attender pro forma

Recommended readings

Mental Health and Drug and Alcohol Office, Mental Health for Emergency Departments—A reference guide. NSW Ministry of Health. Amended March 2015.

Behavioural Emergencies for the Emergency Physician, Ed Zun LS, Chepenik LG, Mallory MNS, Cambridge University Press, UK, 2013.

Emergency Psychiatry, Ed Chanmugam A, Triplett P, Kelen G, Cambridge University Press, UK, 2013.

References

1. Zeller SL. Treatment of psychiatric patients in emergency settings. Primary Psychiatry. 2010 Jun 1;17(6):35–41.

2. Mental Health and Drug and Alcohol Office, Mental Health for Emergency Departments – A reference guide. NSW Ministry of Health. Amended March 2015

3. NICE Guideline No 10, Violence and Aggression: Short-term management in mental health, health and community settings: Updated edition. National Collaborating Centre for Mental Health (UK), London: British Psychological Society; 2015

4. Beauford JE, McNiel DE, Binder RL. Utility of the initial therapeutic alliance in evaluating psychiatric patients' risk of violence. Am J Psychiatry 1997;154;1272–6.

5. RANZCP Professional Practice Guideline 10: Antipsychotic medications as a treatment of behavioural and psychological symptoms of dementia. August 2016.

6. Australian and New Zealand clinical practice guidelines for the treatment of panic disorder and agoraphobia, RANZCP Clinical Practice Guidelines Team for Panic Disorder and Agoraphobia, Australian and New Zealand Journal of Psychiatry 2003;37:641–56.

7. Boyer EW, Shannon M, The serotonin syndrome, N Engl J Med. 2005;352(11):1112.

8. Pelonero AL, Levenson JL, Pandurangi AK. Neuroleptic malignant syndrome: a review. Psychiatr Serv. 1998;49(9):1163–72.

9. Rosenberg MR, Green M. Neuroleptic malignant syndrome. Review of response to therapy. Arch Intern Med. 1989;149(9): 1927–31.

10. Adityanjee PA et al. Case report: neuroleptic malignant syndrome in an elderly patient: problems in management. Int J Geriatr Psychiatry. 1992;7(11):843–6.

11. Kapur S, Zipursky RB, Jones C, et al. Cyproheptadine: a potent in vivo serotonin antagonist. Am J Psychiatry 1997 Jun;154(6):884.

Chapter 42
Dermatological emergencies

Kevin Phan, Alicia O'Connor and Deshan Sebaratnam

Acknowledgment

The authors wish to acknowledge the content used from the previous edition of *Emergency Medicine* which was provided by John Sullivan, Veronica Preda and Margot Whitfield.

Dermatological presentations to the ED are common as patients are acutely aware of any change to their skin. The vast majority of skin disease exerts minimal threat to mortality though there are exceptions. This chapter outlines an approach to the patient with an acute dermatological presentation.

General approach to acute dermatological presentations
HISTORY

- Preceding infectious exposures
- Preceding drug exposures (review up to 12 weeks antecedent to presentation and include PRN medications, stat doses, alternative medications and illicit drugs)
- Onset and evolution
- Symptoms: itch, pain, systemic symptoms (fevers, arthralgias etc.)
- Previous investigations (specifically swabs, skin scraping or biopsy) as well as treatments trialled and their effect
- Personal and family history of skin disease
- Any other family members/colleagues/school friends affected

EXAMINATION

- Morphology
- Distribution: symmetrical, dermatomal, photosensitive etc.
- Hair, nail, oral or genital changes
- Lymphadenopathy

MORPHOLOGY

An appreciation of the morphology of a patient's skin problem is essential for diagnosis and communication between health professionals. The terminology of skin lesions in presented in Table 42.1 and approach to determining the morphology of a skin lesion is presented in Figure 42.1.

An approach to acute dermatological presentations is outlined based on the morphology of the skin problem: 1. erythema; 2. papulosquamous; 3. urticated; 4. blistering; 5. purpuric; 6. papular; and 7. deep nodules.

BIOPSY

The skin is a unique organ in that tissue diagnosis is readily accessible through biopsy. For inflammatory skin conditions; however,

Table 42.1 Terminology of skin lesions

Lesion	Description
Bulla(e)	Fluid-filled lesion ≥ 1 cm
Erosion	Broken skin with partial loss of epidermis
Erythema	Abnormal redness of the skin
Macule	Small flat skin lesion
Nodule	Solid mass ≥ 1 cm
Papule	Small bump < 1 cm
Papulosquamous	Raised and scaly lesions
Patch	Large flat skin lesion
Petechiae	Non-blanching lesion ≥ 1 cm
Plaque	Solid plateau-like lesion > 1 cm
Purpura	Non-blanching lesion ≥ 1 cm
Pustule	Turbid fluid-filled lesion < 1 cm
Ulcer	Break in skin with full loss of epidermis
Urticaria	Raised lumps which characteristically change over 24 hours
Vesicle	Clear fluid-filled lesion < 1 cm

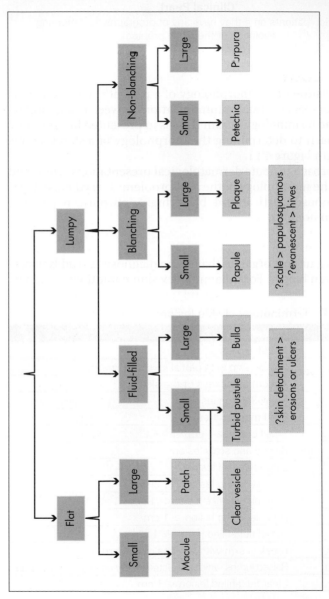

Figure 42.1 Morphology of skin disease

clinicopathological correlation is vital as several different skin diseases can look identical under the microscope. Always consider dermatology input prior to biopsy.

Generally biopsies will be of highest yield in newer lesions compared to older ones. If multiple morphologies are present, multiple biopsies may be indicated. Where possible, select a biopsy site where the cosmetic burden of the scar can be minimised.

There are several different ways of completing a biopsy, but the punch biopsy is the most frequently employed. A 3 mm punch biopsy sent in formalin is the workhorse of most skin biopsies. An incision biopsy using a scalpel may be indicated to encompass fat and medium-sized vessels. In some settings, skin biopsies should be sent in saline for immunofluorescence or microbial culture.

PHOTOGRAPHY IN THE ED

The advent of the smartphone has revolutionised communication between health professionals. Photography is a helpful adjunctive tool when communicating between colleagues, particularly because dermatology is neglected by most medical curriculums, and a picture often tells a thousand words.

Unfortunately, health policy lags behind and there is wide variation between hospitals with regards to patient photography. It is prudent to know your hospital's policy before taking a photograph of a patient. Before approaching a patient for photography, consider the purpose of the photo. Explain to the patient the reasons for taking the clinical image, how it will be used and who will be able to see the image. Document the consent process and obtain written consent where possible. Where possible, only send images via secure means such as encrypted email.

Dermatological diseases by morphology
ERYTHEMA

Increased redness of the skin without significant elevation or surface change.

Sunburn
Clinical features

Ultraviolet radiation leads to a phototoxic effect commonly known as sunburn. Sunburn presents with confluent erythema in exposed areas which may be painful or blister. It is a clinical diagnosis.

Differential diagnosis
Phototoxic drug reactions, cutaneous lupus.

Treatment
Emulsifying ointment, potent topical corticosteroids or systemic prednisolone, analgesia.

Cellulitis and erysipelas
Clinical features
Hot, swollen, tender erythematous skin. Patient may have lymphadenopathy, lymphangitis, be systemically unwell and have a leucocytosis and raised inflammatory markers. Cellulitis may be caused by *Streptococcus* or *Staphylococcus*. In erysipelas, the infection is within the superficial dermis and there is a sharp demarcation between affected and normal skin. It is usually caused by *Streptococcus*.

Differential diagnosis
Irritant contact dermatitis, panniculitis, venous thrombosis, lipodermatosclerosis if bilateral (bilateral cellulitis is rare).

Treatment
- Flucloxacillin 500 mg QID (12.5 mg/kg QID in children) for 5–10 days
- Clindamycin 450 mg TDS for 5–10 days in setting of allergy
- Analgesia

RED AND SCALY (PAPULOSQUAMOUS)
Erythematous scaly plaques
Atopic dermatitis
Clinical features
One in 5 Australian children have eczema and there may be a personal or family history of atopy. Dry, red, pruritic plaques typically involving the flexures. Assess the patient for secondary impetiginisation or herpes infection.

Differential diagnosis
Scabies, irritant contact dermatitis, allergic contact dermatitis, tinea, psoriasis, infective exanthem, cutaneous lupus.

Investigation
Consider the need for bacterial swabs or HSV PCR.

Treatment
- Bland emollient (e.g. emulsifying ointment or Dermeze) TDS.
- Methylprednisolone (Advantan fatty) ointment daily to facial lesions.
- Betamethasone dipropionate (Diprosone) ointment daily to the body applied liberally.
- If there is evidence of impetiginisation, consider the need for antibiotic cover (e.g. flucloxacillin 500 mg [12.5 mg/kg in children] QID for 5–10 days). If there is evidence of herpes simplex infection, consider valaciclovir 1 g BD for 7 days or aciclovir 400 mg (10 mg/kg in children) 5 times daily for 7 days.
- Consider dermatology review for patients with severe disease who might benefit from systemic immunosuppressants, phototherapy or dupilumab.

SCABIES
Clinical features
Infection by the mite *Sarcoptes scabiei*. Acute-onset global pruritus with pustules and scale classically involving the interdigital web spaces, wrists, cubital fossa, axillae, nipples and genitals. The mite may be visualised using a dermatoscope. Assess for secondary bacterial infection; in Aboriginal and Torres Strait Islander populations, this can lead to rheumatic fever and glomerulonephritis.

Differential diagnosis
Eczema, tinea, psoriasis

Treatment
- Permethrin (Lyclear) is applied from the neck down (including the head in children) overnight and washed off the next day. All family members, even those who are not itchy, should follow this regimen. Clothing and bedding should

either be hot-washed or tied in plastic bags for 72 hours. The entire process is repeated a week later.

- Where ineffective or impossible, ivermectin 200 microg/kg PO can be used instead of permethrin.
- Consider a topical corticosteroid such as methylprednisolone (Advantan fatty) ointment for symptomatic relief and inform patients the pruritus can persist for up to 6 weeks after eradication of the mite.
- Where *Streptococcus* has been identified, consider need for surveillance for glomerulonephritis.

ERYTHRODERMA
Clinical features
Erythroderma refers to erythema affecting $> 80\%$ of the body surface area. It is not a diagnosis, but rather a clinical presentation. In some patients, the pathological redistribution of blood into the skin mimics shock and they may be at risk of cardiovascular collapse.

The most common causes of erythroderma are eczema, psoriasis, drug reactions, pityriasis rubra pilaris and cutaneous lymphoma, though there are several others.

Management depends on the underlying cause.

URTICARIAL
Swollen, plaques with minimal surface change (no scale).

Acute urticaria
Clinical features
Acute urticaria is characterised by dermal plaques, which characteristically come and go and migrate to different sites over a 24-hour period. The associated pruritus can be disabling. It is imperative that patients be assessed for symptoms of angio-oedema. Patients should also be assessed for physical triggers: sun, water, pressure, vibration, heat, cold, sweating.

Differential diagnosis
Erythema multiforme, urticarial vasculitis, insect bites

Investigation
If the urticaria is of < 6 weeks duration, no investigation is necessary; only exclusion of differential diagnoses.

Treatment
- Methylprednisolone (Advantan fatty) ointment daily to facial lesions.
- Betamethasone dipropionate (Diprosone) ointment daily to the body applied liberally.
- Loratadine 10 mg QID (up to 4 times the standard dosing may be required).
- Consider adding ranitidine, montelukast or doxepin in recalcitrant cases.
- Organise dermatology review for patients with symptoms > 6 weeks who may require phototherapy, cyclosporin, omalizumab.

Angio-oedema
Clinical features
Acute oedema of the subcutaneous tissues. It may occur in isolation or with urticaria and anaphylaxis. Treat as anaphylaxis if there is concern about cardiovascular, respiratory or gastrointestinal involvement. Consider drug causes (NSAID, ACE inhibitors) and in the setting of angio-oedema without urticaria the need for testing C4 and C1 inhibitor levels to exclude hereditary angio-oedema.

Treatment
Prednisolone 25–50 mg (0.5–1 mg/kg in children) daily for 3 days

Urticarial vasculitis
Clinical features
Small to medium vessel vasculitis can present with urticated plaques initially. There is also a distinct disease known as urticarial vasculitis characterised by purpura within urticated plaques. This can be associated with systemic lupus erythematosus.

Investigation
C1q, C3, C4 levels: markers for systemic involvement

Treatment
Varies according to the degree of systemic involvement, with systemic corticosteroids the cornerstone of treatment.

Erythema multiforme
Clinical features
Classic lesions are urticated papules with a concentric red-white-red 'target' morphology. Erythema multiforme major is characterised by mucosal involvement while in erythema multiforme minor, the mucosa is spared. It is usually triggered by an infective agent—most commonly herpes simplex virus or *Mycoplasma*—or drug.

Differential diagnosis
Stevens-Johnson syndrome (SJS)

Treatment
- Usually self-resolving over 2 weeks. Address the underlying cause: treat any infective precipitant and substitute any culprit drug.
- Methylprednisolone (Advantan fatty) ointment daily to facial lesions.
- Betamethasone dipropionate (Diprosone) ointment daily to the body applied liberally.
- Consider systemic prednisolone 25–50 mg (0.5–1 mg/kg in children) daily for 7 days if severe and infection contained.

Polymorphic eruption of pregnancy
Clinical features
Previously known as pruritic urticarial papules and plaques of pregnancy (PUPPP), this usually begins in the third trimester or immediate postpartum period. Erythematous papules and plaques, usually urticated, erupt over a few days. It starts over the abdomen in areas of striae gravidarum, spreads to the buttocks, back and proximal thighs, but spares the face, palms and soles. The immediate periumbilical area is spared.

Differential diagnosis
Pemphigoid gestationis, scabies, atopic eruption of pregnancy, pustular psoriasis

Investigations
Clinical diagnosis. Skin biopsy is not diagnostic.

Treatment
- Dexchlorpheniramine (category A)
- Betamethasone dipropionate (Diprosone) ointment daily to the body applied liberally (category A)
- Dermatology and obstetrics consult

Pemphigoid gestationis
Clinical features
Acute-onset urticated plaques which evolve to tense blisters. Usually occurs in late pregnancy with involvement of the abdomen and umbilicus. There is a risk of passive transfer of autoantibodies to newborn causing neonatal blistering.

Differential diagnosis
Polymorphic eruption of pregnancy, pustular psoriasis, scabies, bullous pemphigoid

Investigation
Biopsy for histology and direct immunofluorescence, serum ELISA and indirect immunofluorescence

Treatment
- Dexchlorpheniramine (category A)
- Betamethasone dipropionate (Diprosone) ointment daily to the body applied liberally (category A)
- Dermatology and obstetrics consultation with view to prednisolone 0.5 mg/kg daily

BLISTERS
Fluid-filled lesions which may be small (vesicles), large (bullae) or contain pus (pustules) Where blisters rupture, the patient may present with erosions and exfoliative changes.

Herpes simplex
Primary gingivostomatitis: scallop-shaped blisters and erosions, which may coalesce on lips and oral mucosa. Local recurrence is common. Genital lesions have a similar morphology.

Differential diagnosis
Erythema multiforme, varicella, enterovirus

Investigation
- Clinical diagnosis usually
- Tzanck smear of vesicle base looking for multinucleated giant cells
- HSV PCR +/− varicella PCR

Treatment
- Topical aciclovir
- Oral aciclovir 400 mg TDS for 5 days or valaciclovir 500 mg BD for 5 days
- If recurrent (> 6 episodes per year) consider prophylactic antiviral therapy

Varicella zoster
Clinical features
Erythematous macules evolving to papules then vesicles with surrounding erythema. Characteristically patients have a rash with three morphologies concomitantly. It has centripetal distribution, usually starting on the trunk, oral mucosa, scalp.

Differential diagnosis
Herpes simplex virus, hand-foot-mouth disease, impetigo, eczema herpeticum

Investigation
- Clinical diagnosis usually
- PCR for varicella zoster virus (VZV) +/− HSV
- Tzanck smear, VZV IgM/IgG

Treatment
- Antihistamines for pruritus.
- Consider aciclovir 800 mg 5 times daily for 7 days to reduce the course of the disease.
- Consider intravenous aciclovir in severe cases or immunosuppression.

- Non-immune pregnant females require varicella zoster immunoglobulin for post-exposure prophylaxis within 10 days of exposure.
- Antibiotics (topical or systemic) for secondary infections.

Impetigo
Clinical features
Cutaneous bacterial infection characterised by honey yellow crusts and superficial pustules; due to *Streptococcus* or *Staphylococcus* infection.

Differential diagnosis
Scabies, tinea, arthropod bites

Investigation
Bacterial swab M/C/S

Treatment
Mupirocin ointment daily.
- If widespread:
  — Dicloxacillin 250 mg QID for 1 week or
  — Cephalexin 250 mg QID for 1 week.
- If MRSA:
  — Clindamycin 300–400 mg QID for 1 week.
- Avoid contact with other children, avoid shared towels/clothing.

Irritant contact dermatitis
Clinical features
Exposure to a noxious stimulus leads to inflammation within the epidermis, which when severe can lead to frank blistering. It will usually have sharp demarcation lines corresponding to exposed areas. Phytophotodermatitis is a specific type of irritant dermatitis caused by exposure to photosensitising compounds in plant matter and often has a linear appearance.

Differential diagnosis
Allergic contact dermatitis, dermatitis artefacta

Treatment
- Avoid further exposure to irritant.
- Methylprednisolone (Advantan fatty) ointment daily to facial lesions applied liberally.
- Betamethasone dipropionate (Diprosone) ointment daily to the body applied liberally.

Autoimmune bullous disease
Clinical features
A spectrum of diseases including bullous pemphigoid, pemphigus vulgaris, pemphigus foliaceus, pemphigoid gestationis, bullous lupus erythematosus, epidermolysis bullosa acquisita and linear IgA bullous dermatosis. Morphology varies according to the location of the target epitope within the skin. Where the target is epidermal, patients have flaccid blisters, which easily rupture often presenting as erosions. Where the target is the dermoepidermal junction, patients present with tense blisters. A detailed drug history is important as is detailed physical examination. Clinical features of note include distribution of bullae, presence of milia and ophthalmological, oral, genital and anal involvement.

Differential diagnosis
Bullous drug eruption, Stevens-Johnson syndrome, porphyria

Investigation
Skin biopsy for histopathology (encompassing the blister and normal skin) and immunofluorescence (of perilesional skin) for diagnosis.

Treatment
Prednisolone 0.5–1 mg/kg daily

Acute generalised exanthematous pustulosis
Clinical features
Typically drug induced, commencing within a week of exposure to the culprit drug. Widespread pustulation and superficial erosion, often with flexural accentuation.

Differential diagnosis
Pustular psoriasis, impetigo, tinea, Sweet syndrome

Investigation
FBC, LFT, EUC, fungal and bacterial studies, skin biopsy

Treatment
Withhold culprit drug and substitute as indicated:
- methylprednisolone (Advantan fatty) ointment daily to facial lesions
- betamethasone dipropionate (Diprosone) ointment daily to the body applied liberally.

Admission and systemic prednisolone can be considered in severe cases.

Porphyria
Clinical features
A spectrum of diseases reflecting defects in the haem synthesis pathway. Porphyrias presenting with bullae include variegate porphyria (VP), porphyria cutanea tarda (PCT) and pseudoporphyria. Patients will present with skin fragility, tense bullae and milia. Less commonly hypertrichosis and waxy scarring may be observed. Patients should be questioned on family history and symptoms of acute attacks as seen in VP, drug causes of pseudoporphyria and risk factors for PCT; haemochromatosis, HBV/HCV, HIV, alcohol intake, oestrogen.

Differential diagnosis
Epidermolysis bullosa acquisita and other autoimmune bullous disease, Stevens-Johnson syndrome

Investigation
FBC, LFT, serum and urine, and stool porphyrin studies

Treatment
Therapy depends on type of porphyria

Staphylococcal scalded skin syndrome (SSSS)
Clinical features
Widespread flaccid blisters and superficial erosions caused by a *Staphylococcus* toxin producing cleavage of the epidermis. Classically accentuated around eyes and mouth and causes a 'wrinkled' look to skin. Usually has a prodrome of malaise and fevers,

without a necessary infective focus. Typically occurs in young children; it is rare in adults outside of immunosuppressed or renally impaired setting.

Differential diagnosis
Bullous impetigo (localised SSSS), Stevens-Johnson syndrome

Investigation
Usually a clinical diagnosis but biopsy may be helpful in excluding differential diagnoses

Treatment
- Admission
- Analgesia
- Emulsifying ointment and non-stick dressings (e.g. Mepitel, DuoDERM)
- Fluid resuscitation as indicated (significant oral disease can encumber oral intake)
- Flucloxacillin 500 mg QID (12.5 mg/kg QID in children) for 5–10 days. Clindamycin 450 mg TDS for 5–10 days in setting of allergy
- Consider need for vancomycin in patients with risk factors for MRSA
- Generally gets worse before it gets better but resolves within a week of antibiotic therapy

Stevens-Johnson syndrome / toxic epidermal necrolysis (SJS/TEN)
Clinical features
Usually triggered by drugs, less commonly by infection. Coryzal prodrome is followed by dusky grey-purple erythema evolving to blisters, erosion and denuding. Patients may have ophthalmological, oral and anogenital involvement. A spectrum ranging from SJS (< 10% body surface area involvement), SJS/TEN overlap (10–30% BSA involvement) and TEN (> 30% BSA involvement).

Differential diagnosis
Autoimmune bullous disease, Staphylococcal scalded skin syndrome, porphyria

Investigation
- Skin biopsy: frozen sections yield satisfactory pathological confirmation within minutes if needed. Formal review of tissue fixed in formalin is still recommended.
- FBC, LFT, EUC, CMP.

Treatment
- Cease drug or treat infection
- Transfer to a burns unit or intensive care unit
- IVIg 2 g/kg (usually over 72 hours) can be accessed through the Red Cross once diagnosis confirmed by dermatology
- Consider consults with ophthalmology, urology, otolaryngology, pain, gynaecology
- Maintain barrier function with emollient (e.g. emulsifying ointment) and non-stick dressings (e.g. Acticoat)
- Minimise handling and avoid adhesives, tapes and electrodes
- Monitor fluid balance, electrolytes, temperature, nutrition and for infection
- Analgesia

NON-BLANCHING

Vascular damage causing extravasation of erythrocytes into the dermis. Pressure on the skin will not suspend erythema. Causes of purpura are wide (Figure 42.2) and beyond the scope of this chapter.

Investigations directed according to clinical presentation might include:
- FBC + film, INR/APTT, EUC, LFT
- +/− haemolysis screen—D-dimer, LDH, fibrinogen, unconjugated bilirubin, haptoglobin, Coombs
- +/− septic screen—CXR, blood culture, urine M/C/S, lumbar puncture
- +/− vasculitis screen—antinuclear antibody (ANA), antineutrophil cytoplasmic antibody (ANCA), urine microscopy for casts/dysmorphic RBCs, ESR
- +/− thrombophilia screen—protein C, protein S, antithrombin III, prothrombin gene mutation, Factor V Leiden, homocysteine, anti-cardiolipin, lupus anticoagulant, anti-β2-glycoprotein.

Purpura

Vasculitis
- Cutaneous small vessel vasculitis
- Henoch Schönlein
- Urticarial vasculitis
- Polyarteritis nodosa
- Granulomatosis with polyangiitis (formerly Wegner's)
- Microscopic polyangiitis
- Eosinophilic granulomatosis with polyangiitis (formerly Churg-Strauss)

Altered blood constituents
- Reticulocytes
- Polycythaemia rubra vera
- Intravascular lymphoma
- Paraprotenaemia

Altered platelets
- HITTS
- Early TIP/HUS
- DIC
- Essential thrombocytosis
- PNH

Decreased clotting factors
- Protein C/S (warfarin, vasculitis)
- Antithrombin III
- Prothrombin gene mutation
- Factor V Leiden
- Homocysteine
- Cardiolipin/ β2 glycoprotein / lupus anticoagulant

Cold-related
- Cryoglobulins
- Cryofibrinogens
- Cold agglutinins

Septic occlusion
- Bacteria
- Fungal
- Strongyloides

Inorganic occlusion
- Thrombi (infective endocarditis, aortic dissection, atrial myxoma)
- Cholesterol
- Calcium
- Oxalate
- Fat

Figure 42.2 Differential diagnoses for purpura

Vasculitis
Clinical features
These vary according to the target blood vessel affected. Cutaneous signs include livedo reticularis, livedo racemosa, stellate ulceration or purpura or deep painful nodules. Patients may present with

neurological, otolaryngology, respiratory, cardiac or renal signs depending on degree of systemic involvement.

Differential diagnosis
Thrombophilia, sepsis

Investigation
* Incisional skin biopsy to fat for histopathology. Consider need for immunofluorescence and microbial studies.
* Consider FBC, EUC, LFT, ANA, ANCA, urine microscopy and further investigations according to clinical presentation.

Treatment
Varies according to time of vasculitis, but systemic corticosteroids are the cornerstone of treatment in most cases

Meningococcaemia
Clinical features
Neisseria meningitides infection may be asymptomatic, present with a mild upper respiratory tract infection (URTI), meningitis or frank meningococcaemia. Meningococcaemia begins with fevers and coryzal symptoms, evolving to papular or petechial rash with neurological symptoms potentially culminating in DIC, shock or death. The petechial rash can progress to ecchymoses and bullous haemorrhage. Patients may also show signs of meningism: photophobia, nuchal rigidity, positive Brudzinski or Kernig sign.

Differential diagnosis
Viral exanthem, sepsis, purpuric enterovirus exanthem, *Rickettsiae*

Investigations
* Blood cultures
* Lumbar puncture for CSF MCS, assays, glucose
* FBC: leucocytosis, thrombocytopenia, altered PT/APTT if DIC
* Skin biopsy may be of some diagnostic assistance

Management
* Admission
* Antibiotic therapy should not be delayed by lumbar puncture

- Ceftriaxone IV 2 g BD for 2 weeks
- Dexamethasone 10 mg (child 0.15 mg/kg up to 10 mg) IV stat with first dose of antibiotic, then QID for 4 days

Necrotising fasciitis
Clinical features
Deep bacterial infection that tracks along fascial planes. Early on there is erythema and oedema typical of cellulitis, with extreme pain out of proportion to skin changes, with or without fever. Oedema can progress; bullae and cyanosis can develop and lead to gangrene. Crepitus may be present. Systemic symptoms include fever, delirium, renal failure, hypotension and tachycardia. Type I necrotising fasciitis is caused by mixed anaerobes, Gram-negative aerobic bacilli and enterococci; type II is Group A *Streptococci*. Risk factors are diabetes mellitus, peripheral vascular disease, immunosuppression.

Diagnosis
- Diagnosis is clinical.
- Small exploratory incision at site of suspicion may show thin brown exudate with undermining of surrounding tissue; dissect easily with blunt instrument or gloved finger.
- Blood culture.
- Tissue culture.
- CT/MRI imaging: oedema tracking along fascial planes.

Differentials
- Pyoderma gangrenosum, cellulitis, calciphylaxis, ecthyma gangrenosum, erysipelas, purpura fulminans

Management
- Urgent surgical consult with view to debridement
- Consider ICU admission
- Fluid resuscitation
- IV antibiotics: broad spectrum then switch based on sensitivities
- IV piperacillin-tazobactam + IV vancomycin OR IV meropenem 1 g TDS
- Surgical debridement and drainage

PAPULES (NON-SPECIFIC BUMPS)
Elevated papules and plaques with minimal surface change (no scale).

Infective exanthems
Clinical features
Non-specific bilateral symmetrical eruption of macules and papules. Identification of underlying pathogen can be difficult (see Table 42.2).

Differential diagnosis
Infective exanthem, exclude acute generalised exanthematic pustulosis (AGEP), drug reaction/rash with eosinophilia and systemic symptoms (DRESS), Stevens–Johnson syndrome / toxic epidermal necrolysis (SJS/TEN)

Investigation
• Directed according to suspected focus of infection
• Limited role for skin biopsy as pathological findings are non-specific

Treatment
• Treat underlying infection.
• Methylprednisolone (Advantan fatty) ointment daily to facial lesions.
• Betamethasone dipropionate (Diprosone) ointment daily to the body applied liberally.
• Consider prednisolone 0.5–1 mg/kg daily.

Drug exanthem
Clinical features
Non-specific bilateral symmetrical eruption of macules and papules

Differential diagnosis
Infective exanthem, exclude serious drug reactions (e.g. AGEP, DRESS, SJS-TEN).

Investigation
• FBC + film, EUC, LFT
• Limited role for skin biopsy as pathological findings are non-specific

Table 42.2   Features and management of common viral exanthems in paediatric patients

Disease/virus	Signs/symptoms	Management
Enterovirus	Commonly respiratory or gastroenterology presentations +/− exanthem or urticaria	Presentation-dependent
Varicella—chicken pox/varicella zoster virus (VZV) Reactivation → herpes zoster (HZ)	Incubation 10–21 days Mid-prodrome—pruritic vesicles that break and crust, starts centrally or facially and spreads to the extremities New lesions appear 3–5 days, typically take 3 days to crust Contagious for 24 hours prior to rash onset and until lesions crust	Immunocompromised children with VZV are given VZ immunoglobulin (VZIG) within 96 hours of exposure Aciclovir for immunocompromised children with disseminated VZ or HZ
Measles (rubeola)/ paramyxovirus	Prodrome fever, malaise, coryza, conjunctivitis, cough; then erythematous maculopapular rash on face, trunk, legs, buccal mucosal lesions, Koplik spots Incubation 8–12 days	Symptomatic management, contact considerations, vaccinations
Rubella (German measles)/RNA togavirus	No prodrome during incubation 14–21 days	Symptomatic, consider contacts including pregnant contacts
Roseola infantum/ HHV-6	Infants 6–8 months—high fever, relatively well; multiple pale pink macules/papules as fever breaks	Supportive
Erythema infectiosum (fifth disease)/ parvovirus B19 'slapped cheeks'	Sore throat, cough, headache, nausea, fever with rash, slapped-cheek appearance followed by lace-like erythema on the extremities and buttocks	Supportive but consider concurrent haematological disease or exposure of pregnant contacts

Scarlet fever/toxins from *Streptococcus pyogenes*	Child 4–8 years—high fever, sore throat, headache, vomiting Exanthem 1–2 days post—small papules with diffuse erythema Skin may feel rough, like sandpaper Linear petechiae = Pastia's lines in the axillae and groin Desquamation 7–10 days post, hand and feet worse Strawberry tongue; lips normal; tonsils/pharynx usual site of infection +/− surgical wounds Investigations include anti-DNase B, anti-streptolysin O titre	If suspected treat with penicillin, (clindamycin or erythromycin if allergic) Management is to avoid complications (e.g. rheumatic heart disease)
Mumps	Morbilliform rash with lymphadenopathy, an issue in young males with potential infertility	Despite vaccination consider occurrence
Mycoplasma pneumoniae	Mainly in school children, cough, coryza Non-specific rash observed in 10% of children with mycoplasma Swab throat—polymerase chain reaction	Antimicrobial therapy for *Mycoplasma* (e.g. rifampicin)
Hand-foot-and-mouth disease/enterovirus, coxsackievirus	Generally mild clinical course Usually in children < 10 years, can affect adults Hands, feet and buttocks involved; 2–10 mm erythematous macules, with central grey oval vesicle Skin lesions asymptomatic, resolve in 3–7 days Mucosal oral ulcers are painful Associated fever, malaise, diarrhoea, systemic involvement can progress to myocarditis, pneumonia, meningoencephalitis	Symptomatic management Note: Can be serious, especially in the immunosuppressed population

Treatment
- Cease culprit drug and substitute as needed.
- Methylprednisolone (Advantan fatty) ointment daily to facial lesions.
- Betamethasone dipropionate (Diprosone) ointment daily to the body applied liberally.
- Consider prednisolone 0.5–1 mg/kg daily.
- Drug rash eosinophilia systemic symptoms.

Clinical features
Rash of any morphology usually commences 2–12 weeks following exposure to the drug. It is characteristically associated with facial oedema, lymphadenopathy, myocarditis, pneumonitis, hepatitis and nephritis. Other organ systems may be involved. The mortality rate is 10–20%.

Differential diagnosis
Depends according to the morphology of a rash

Investigation
- Biopsy will generally show histology compatible with morphology of lesion with variable eosinophils.
- FBC + film, LFT, EUC, lipase, ECG, CXR, urine protein:creatinine ratio.

Treatment
- Cease drug and substitute as needed
- Admission under dermatology
- Prednisolone 1 mg/kg daily
- Sweet syndrome (acute febrile neutrophilic dermatosis)

Clinical features
Variably tender, non-pruritic plaques which appear almost bullous. Common triggers include haematological malignancy, pregnancy, irritable bowel syndrome, cancer, infection and medications including frusemide and minocycline. Fevers and leucocytosis are commonly seen, but systemic involvement is otherwise rare.

Differential diagnosis
Well's, pseudolymphoma, urticarial vasculitis

Investigation
- FBC, skin biopsy, CRP, ESR
- Consider EUC, LFT, CMP, electrophoretogram (EPG), immune EPG (IEPG), Bence Jones protein and malignancy screening as directed according to clinical findings
- G6PD with view to dapsone

Treatment
Treat underlying precipitant:
- methylprednisolone (Advantan fatty) ointment daily to facial lesions
- betamethasone dipropionate (Diprosone) ointment daily to the body applied liberally
- prednisolone 0.5–1 mg/kg daily.

Kawasaki
Clinical features
Usually in children < 5 years old. Inflammation of medium-sized muscular arteries. Fever for 5 days (without an alternative cause) with polymorphic rash, conjunctivitis, mucositis, lymphadenopathy and brawny induration and inflammation of the peripheries. Coronary artery aneurysms develop after a week of illness presenting with tachycardia, muffled heart sounds, gallop rhythms.

Differential diagnosis
Depends according to the morphology of a rash

Investigation
- FBC, EUC, LFT, lipid, ESR, CRP, urine microscopy
- Echocardiogram, ECG, CXR
- There is only limited role for skin biopsy as pathological findings are non-specific.

Treatment
- Admission at tertiary paediatric centre with close cardiology input
- IVIg 2 g/kg as a single infusion over 12 hours

- Aspirin 16–20 mg QID until fever abates for 48 hours, then 3–5 mg/kg daily for 8 weeks or once inflammatory markers settle

DEEP NODULES
Swollen plaques with minimal surface change (no scale)

Erythema nodosum
Clinical features
Inflammation of fat presenting as deep erythematous nodules; multiple causes including *Streptococcus*, pregnancy, tuberculosis, sarcoidosis, inflammatory bowel disease and drugs among others.

Differential diagnosis
Vasculitis, venothrombosis, panniculitis

Investigation
- Incisional biopsy to fat
- Consider ASOT, beta-hCG, QuantiFERON gold, CXR, calcium

Treatment
- Treat underlying cause
- Rest, elevation, compression, ice
- Ibuprofen 400 mg TDS (caution if IBD considered)
- Prednisolone 0.5 mg/kg daily

Online resources
DermNet NZ: https://www.dermnetnz.org/
A to Z of Skin: https://www.dermcoll.edu.au/a-to-z-of-skin/

Chapter 43
Drowning

Kent Robinson

Introduction

- Every year across the globe, there are approximately 450 000 deaths each year from drowning. Most of these deaths are accidental and occur in low- and middle-income countries.
- In 2017, 291 people drowned in Australian waterways and 685 non-fatal drownings have required hospitalisation.
- The age distribution is bimodal with the first peak occurring in children less than 5 years of age, and the second peak in males between the ages of 15 and 25 years.
- Men were involved in a drowning incident 74% of the time and the top three activities associated with drowning were swimming, falls into water and boating accidents.
- The most common place to drown was in an inland waterway.
- Alcohol was implicated in 41% of all drowning incidents.
- Indigenous Australians are four times more likely to drown than other Australians.
- In the paediatric age group, females accounted for 52% of all drownings and the most common site was a swimming pool.

Editorial Comments

There are few events as distressing to parents, family and ED staff as a child drowning. Recognise this early. Mobilise resources for support. If set up for it, having the parent(s) present with a dedicated staff member during resuscitation can be very beneficial in both the short and the long term. It has been shown also to improve staff satisfaction.

Pathophysiology

- The Utstein guidelines recommend that terms such as near-drowning, secondary drowning and wet and dry drowning should not be used and that the all-embracing term of drowning be used to describe the syndrome that patients present with.

- During an episode of drowning, the patient becomes unable to keep fluid out of their airway. This results in a breath hold that may last for up to a minute. When the respiratory drive becomes too much, a small amount of fluid is aspirated into the airway and coughing occurs. Sometimes laryngospasm can occur, but it is usually rapidly terminated by the onset of brain hypoxia. Aspiration of water continues with continued submersion followed by hypoxaemia and apnoea.

- The sequence of cardiac activity is a sinus tachycardia, followed by bradycardia, pulseless electrical activity and then asystole.

- If the patient is resuscitated, they will have evidence of an acute lung injury with water in the alveoli causing surfactant dysfunction, disruption of the cell membrane integrity and fluid and electrolyte shifts. This results in very low lung compliance, poor ventilation to perfusion ratios in the lungs, atelectasis and bronchospasm.

- Hypothermia is more commonly seen in paediatric drownings due to their large surface-area-to-body-mass ratio. Hypothermia can be associated with a better outcome in drowning, particularly if the ambient water temperature is very cold and the rate of cooling is rapid. There are many case reports of patients surviving a submersive arrest in cold water for prolonged periods of up to 66 minutes.

- Delayed respiratory failure may develop from surfactant dysfunction, intrapulmonary shunting and atelectasis. There may also be aspiration of organic matter or vomitus resulting in airway occlusion, damage to the airways, abscess formation and pneumonia.

Precipitating events

- Sometimes, a drowning event can be precipitated by an injury or a medical event.
- In younger patients think of precipitants such as hypoglycaemia, seizures, drugs or alcohol and arrhythmias.
- In the elderly population, they may have suffered a cardiac arrest or a stroke.

- If there has been a traumatic injury, think about a closed head injury and concussion.
- It is also important to recognise the potential for suicide.

Pre-hospital

- Most drowning victims are able to rescue themselves or are rescued by professional lifeguards or bystanders. The majority of them do not require hospital evaluation and treatment and only 0.5% of all drownings require CPR.
- If the patient is conscious, they should be brought to shore as soon as possible. If the patient is unresponsive, an attempt at rescue breaths can be made while still in the water; however, CPR is ineffective and the patient should be brought to land promptly.
- On retrieval of the patient to land, they should be laid supine with the head and body at the same level. If the airway is obstructed with fluid or particulate matter, then the patient should be rolled on their side to allow this to drain with the aid of gravity.
- Cervical spine injury is uncommon in drowning victims. Unless there are clinical signs of injury or a mechanism of injury (dive into shallow water), routine cervical spine immobilisation can interfere with airway management and is not recommended.
- The Heimlich manoeuvre and other postural drainage techniques have not been shown to be of benefit in removing water from the lungs.
- The European Resuscitation Council and Australian Resuscitation Council guidelines recommend five rescue breaths at the onset of resuscitation. This is in recognition of the fact that water in the airway impairs effective alveolar expansion, and the initial ventilation can be difficult to achieve.
- The most common complication of drowning is aspiration which occurs in 65–86% of those patients who require rescue breathing.
- Management of the drowning patient is dependent on the severity of the symptoms. Drowning severity can be classified into six grades based on the clinical examination.
  1 Alert, normal lung auscultation, normal oxygenation
  2 Alert, occasional rales on auscultation, normal oxygenation

3 Alert, widespread rales, normal blood pressure
4 Alert, widespread rales, hypotension
5 Unresponsive, pulse present
6 Unresponsive, pulse absent, down time less than 1 hour, does not appear dead

- Patients with respiratory symptoms and mild respiratory distress should be treated with high-flow oxygen.
- Those patients with moderate to severe respiratory distress should be intubated and mechanically ventilated. Positive end expiratory pressure (PEEP) should be applied to improve oxygenation.
- There may be significant amounts of pulmonary oedema fluid in the airway following intubation. Try to limit the amount of suctioning in this instance as it may impede oxygenation.
- Compression-only CPR is not recommended as the usual cause of arrest is from a lack of breathing and this does not address the precipitant. It should only be used if there is no mask ventilation and the rescuer is unwilling to provide mouth-to-mouth ventilation.
- Delivery of drugs should be via the vascular or intraosseous route. Endotracheal administration of resuscitation drugs in the drowning patient is not recommended.
- Hypotension should be treated with administration of a crystalloid solution regardless of whether the immersion was in fresh or salt water.
- If the patient is in cardiac arrest, commence cardiopulmonary resuscitation (CPR) with a compression to ventilation ratio of 30:2. Early defibrillation should be undertaken for shockable rhythms and reversible causes for the arrest should be identified (hypothermia and hypoxia are the two most common causes in drowning). Adrenaline should be administered every 3–5 minutes.

Emergency department
- The majority of drowning patients aspirate only small amounts of fluid and will usually recover spontaneously. Only 6% of patients who are rescued by lifesavers require assessment and management in a hospital.

- Examination of the patient should follow a systematic course and the assessment of the patient should be tailored to include work-up for potential medical causes for the patient's presentation. A detailed assessment should be made to exclude any injuries sustained during the drowning.

- Investigations performed should be directed by the clinical condition of the patient. The two most useful tests to order are a chest radiograph and an arterial blood gas. Routine biochemistry and haematology tests are frequently normal in the drowning patient and while commonly ordered they are considered unnecessary tests.

- Metabolic acidosis is commonly seen following a drowning—this usually resolves with appropriate oxygenation and increased minute ventilation from the patient. If the patient is intubated and mechanically ventilated, you may have to set a higher minute ventilation to improve the acidosis. Routine administration of sodium bicarbonate to treat the acidosis is not recommended.

- Patients with no respiratory symptoms and normal oxygenation levels can be safely discharged from the ED. Grade 2–6 drownings should be admitted to hospital.

- Grade 2 drowning warrants a short admission to hospital for high-flow oxygen therapy. If the patient remains stable at 6–8 hours, they can be safely discharged.

- The airway should be assessed for particulate matter and suction performed under direct vision. Basic airway manoeuvres may be required to open the airway—the jaw thrust should be applied in anyone with a history of trauma to ensure a neutral alignment of the cervical spine.

- If PEEP is required and the airway needs to be secured, intubation with a cuffed tube is preferable. There is an increased risk of gastric aspiration with supraglottic airways; however, there are laryngeal masks with a gastric port for tube decompression, which may facilitate safer airway management.

- Adequate oxygenation and ventilation are required to reverse the effects of hypoxia and acidosis. If the patient is conscious and has a patent airway, then high-flow oxygen therapy should be delivered at 15 L/min via a non-rebreathing mask.

- Unconscious patients with a definitive airway in place should be initially given 100% oxygen therapy.
- Awake patients with chest signs and respiratory distress may benefit from the use of non-invasive ventilation (NIV). This can be delivered as continuous positive airway pressure (CPAP) or bi-level positive airway pressure (BiPAP). The use of NIV has been shown to reduce rates of intubation.
- The use of diuretics in patients with non-cardiogenic pulmonary oedema has not been shown to reduce morbidity and mortality and is not recommended.
- Current indications for rapid sequence induction (RSI) and intubation in drowning patients include:
  — decreased level of consciousness and inability to protect the airway.
  — significant hypoxia (PaO_2 60 mmHg, or saturations > 90% on high-flow oxygen therapy)
  — respiratory failure (clinical deterioration, increased work of breathing with associated hypercapnia).
- The use of a venous blood gas is a good screening tool for respiratory failure; however, the venous PCO_2 is usually approximately 5 mmHg higher than the arterial PCO_2. A better way to monitor respiratory failure is with serial samples, particularly in the deteriorating patient. In the mechanically ventilated patient arterial samples are preferred and should be taken from an indwelling arterial catheter.
- Intubated patients should have a gastric tube placed to decompress the stomach of air, fluid and particulate matter.
- Think of tension pneumothorax particularly in the patient with hypotension resistant to fluid resuscitation. This can be rapidly excluded with the use of bedside ultrasonography. Small pneumothoraces can be managed expectantly; however, in the mechanically ventilated patient, have a low threshold for decompression with a formal intercostal catheter.
- Cardiac arrhythmias are usually caused by hypoxia, acidosis and hypothermia and will usually resolve when these problems are corrected.

- Patients are frequently hypothermic and rewarming is essential. In the first instance, wet clothing should be removed, the skin should be dried and the patient wrapped in warm blankets or a warming sheet. Intravenous fluids should be warmed to 40°C and ventilator circuits should contain a humidifier or warmer.
- In severe hypothermia and cardiac arrest, only three attempts at defibrillation should be made and resuscitation drugs should be withheld until the core temperature reaches 30°C.
- Patients should be fully exposed to assess for potential injuries or causative problems. An indwelling temperature probe should be inserted as well as a urinary catheter. Patients should be log-rolled to exclude any posterior injuries and the cervical spine should be immobilised until the cervical spine has been imaged.

Inpatient management

- In drowning victims, the pattern of acute lung injury is similar to patients who suffer from acute respiratory distress syndrome (ARDS) and they should be ventilated in a similar fashion. Patients tend to recover faster than those with true ARDS.
- Patients should be ventilated for at least 24 hours following normalisation of gas exchange as the lung injury sustained may necessitate the need to re-intubate the patient.
- Only 12% of patients will progress to develop pneumonia. Prophylactic antibiotics are not indicated and should only be given when there is fever, leucocytosis and new infiltrate on the chest radiograph. Pneumonia is usually caused by nosocomial agents and broad spectrum antibiotics to cover the usual pathogens should be used while waiting for definitive diagnosis from sputum and blood cultures.
- Bronchoscopy can be performed to diagnose pneumonia and is also used to clear the airway of mucus plugs and particulate matter.
- Patients with refractory respiratory failure may need to be placed on extracorporeal membrane oxygenation (ECMO).
- The use of artificial surfactant, nitric oxide and partial liquid ventilation is still undergoing research and cannot be recommended to be used routinely.

- Hypotension usually resolves following correction of hypoxia, hypothermia and acidosis. It may require the administration of crystalloids. Refractory hypotension should prompt one to think of cardiac dysfunction and an early ECG should be attained to guide the use of appropriate inotropic and vasopressor support.
- In patients with severe hypothermia from cold ambient temperatures who are in arrest, the use of ECMO has been shown to improve the outcomes in a select group of patients.
- Sepsis and disseminated intravascular coagulation (DIC) have been reported within the first 72 hours following resuscitation. Renal failure is unusual, but can be precipitated by shock and hypoxia.
- In the setting of a neurological injury, ensure that there is no evidence of a secondary brain injury—avoid hypoxia and hypotension as they significantly increase the mortality.
- Elevate the head of the bed to 30°.
- Aggressively treat seizures, as they will increase cerebral oxygen consumption.
- Maintain euglycaemia, as extremes in the blood glucose may be harmful to the brain.

Outcome

- Commonest cause of death is hypoxic encephalopathy. Other common causes include ARDS, multi-organ dysfunction syndrome (MODS) or sepsis.
- Judging prognosis after drowning can be difficult. Factors associated with a poor prognosis include:
  — prolonged submersion ($>$ 5 minutes)
  — delay to basic life support ($>$ 10 minutes)
  — prolonged resuscitation ($>$ 25 minutes)
  — age $>$ 14 years
  — Glasgow Coma Scale score $<$ 5
  — ongoing CPR in the ED
  — arterial pH $<$ 7.1 on presentation.
- Age has no independent association with outcome.

Further readings

Handley AJ (2014) Drowning, BMJ 348:bmj.g1734

Royal Life Saving National Drowning Report 2017. Online. Available: www.royallifesaving.com.au

Szpilman D, Joost JL et al. (2012) Drowning, NEJM 366:2102–10.

Soar J, Perkins GD, Abbas G et al. (2010) European Resuscitation Council Guidelines for Resuscitation 2010. Section 8. Cardiac arrest in special circumstances: electrolyte abnormalities, poisoning, drowning, accidental hypothermia, hyperthermia, asthma, anaphylaxis, cardiac surgery, trauma, pregnancy, electrocution. Resuscitation 81:1400–33.

Van Berkel M, Bierens JJ et al. (1996) Pulmonary oedema, pneumonia and mortality in submersions victims: a retrospective study in 125 patients. Intensive Care Med 22:101–7.

Chapter 44
Envenomation

Andrew Orr

Acknowledgement

The author wishes to acknowledge the content used from the previous edition of *Emergency Medicine* which was provided by Shane Curran and Thomas McDonagh.

Introduction

Australia is home to many venomous creatures. Australian animals that are important in causing envenoming in humans include snakes, spiders, octopuses, fish and other marine creatures. The distribution of venomous creatures is wide, and each region has its own pattern of envenomation. Local knowledge is very important and local expert knowledge can be invaluable.

Resources that are available to you include the local emergency doctor or the on-call toxinologist, who can be contacted via the Poisons Information Centre (nationwide telephone **13 11 26**). They are available to discuss management of patients with possible or definite envenomation.

Snakebite

Australia is home to a number of the most venomous snakes in the world. Snake venom is a complex mixture of substances. Australian snakes produce venoms that have a range of clinical effects, including neurotoxic (presenting as progressive paralysis), myotoxic (causing rhabdomyolysis and subsequent renal failure) and coagulopathic (causing severe coagulation disturbances) (Table 44.1).

Snakebite is a medical emergency. Patients presenting following possible snakebite should receive urgent assessment and management. Patients who have significant envenomation may initially appear well.

Table 44.1 Clinical effects of Australian snake venom

	Defibrination coagulopathy	Anticoagulation	Paralysis	Myolysis	Renal failure
	Low fibrinogen Raised FDP/XDP	Normal fibrinogen Normal FDP/XDP			ATN
Brown snake	+++				+
Tiger snake	+++		++ Presynaptic	+++	+
Taipan	+++		+++ Presynaptic	+++	+++
Mulga snake (king brown)		++	++	+++	+
Sea snake				+++	
Death adder		+	Postsynaptic		
Red-bellied black snake	Venom is low in potency and small in volume—no major complications				

ATN = acute tubular necrosis; FDP/XDP = fibrin degradation products

Potential early life threats include paralysis and respiratory failure or haemorrhage due to coagulopathy. Look for evidence of ptosis, diplopia, dysarthria or dysphagia, or haemorrhage from skin, gums, needle puncture sites, gastrointestinal tract or intracranial.

The majority of snakebites will not result in significant envenoming, and so will not require antivenom. This is because many snakebites are 'dry bites' where no venom is injected. The amount of venom injected by a snake depends on snake maturity, fang length, venom yield, snake temperament, the number of bites and the time since the snake's last meal. Overall, fewer than 1 in 4 patients with a snakebite requires antivenom.

Editorial Comment

Check up-to-date guidelines as to antivenom use and doses, as this is constantly changing—for example, in many cases less is now given due to current research and evidence.

FIRST AID: THE PRESSURE–IMMOBILISATION TECHNIQUE

Snake venom spreads via the lymphatics, and its spread is increased by muscle contraction or activity. The pressure–immobilisation method of first aid prevents spread of the venom via the lymphatics and can prevent clinical envenomation. See Table 44.2 for when to use the technique.

- It involves applying a firm broad bandage, commencing at the site of the bite and then applying the bandage over the entire limb, extending both proximally and distally. The pressure is the same as that used for a sprained ankle. A splint (it is possible to use a stick) is then applied to the limb, to immobilise the limb and reduce muscle contraction. The patient is then kept as still as possible and transported to hospital.
- The pressure–immobilisation technique can prevent clinical envenomation if applied early and correctly. Both the limb and the patient should be immobilised. The bandages are kept in place until facilities are available to treat clinical envenomation in a hospital with a supply of antivenom.

**Table 44.2   Use of the pressure–immobilisation technique
of first aid**

Pressure–immobilisation is recommended for:	Do not use pressure–immobilisation first aid for:
All Australian venomous snake bites, including sea snake bites	
Funnel web-spider bites	Redback spider bites Other spider bites, including mouse spiders, white-tailed spiders
Bee, wasp and ant stings in allergic individuals	Bee and wasp stings in non-allergic individuals
Blue-ringed octopus bites Cone snail (cone shell) stings	Bluebottle jellyfish stings Box jellyfish and other jellyfish stings Stonefish and other fish stings
	Bites or stings by scorpions, centipedes, beetles

Adapted with permission of the Australian Venom Research Unit.

+ It is important not to wash the site of the bite, as it may contain traces of venom that are important for identifying the snake type.
+ If a patient arrives following a possible snakebite and has had no first aid but is well and there are no signs of envenoming, there is no need to apply the pressure–immobilisation technique.
+ If deterioration occurs when the bandages are removed, the bandages should be reapplied.
+ The pressure–immobilisation first aid is not removed until the patient has been assessed and there is no clinical or laboratory evidence of envenoming or, in the envenomed patient, the antivenom has been commenced. The bandage can be removed halfway through the antivenom infusion.

VENOM DETECTION KIT
The venom detection kit (VDK) developed by Commonwealth Serum Laboratories (CSL) has been important in the management of the patient with snakebite. The VDK can detect minute amounts of snake venom if present, and has been used to determine what family of snake that venom came from.

- The VDK does not indicate that a patient has been envenomed. It also does not determine whether a patient should be given antivenom.
- It has a high false positive rate, particularly in the brown snake well.
- The VDK may assist in regions where the range of possible snakes is too broad to allow the use of monovalent antivenoms. The decision to give antivenom is a clinical decision based on geography, symptoms, signs and pathology testing.
- A swab of the bite site is best, as this is where venom is present in the highest quantities. A small window can be cut in the bandages overlying the bite site. When the swab has been taken, the bandage is reapplied.
- Urine is the second best for venom detection, as Australian snake venoms are excreted in the urine. False-positive results are higher in urine testing with the VDK, so care is needed in interpretation in the non-envenomed patient. A positive urine result is not an indication for antivenom.
- Blood or serum is not used.

The venom detection kit can be used by trained laboratory staff and takes at least 20 minutes to complete.

ANTIVENOM

- Antivenom exists for all major terrestrial snake types in Australia, and a multi-valent antivenom is available for sea snakes.
- Antivenom is the definitive treatment for a patient with systemic envenomation. The administration of antivenom can reverse the clinical effects of envenomation. The treatment of envenomation following snakebite involves the administration of adequate quantities of the appropriate antivenom.
- Antivenom is produced by CSL from antibodies harvested from horses that have been injected with subclinical doses of snake-venom toxins. As the antibodies are obtained from horse serum there is the risk of anaphylaxis, allergic reaction or delayed serum sickness. Prior to administration, therefore, preparations should be made to treat a possible anaphylactic reaction. Currently, premedication with adrenaline is not recommended.

- Monovalent antivenom is indicated if the type of snake is known, when the VDK determines the type of antivenom to be given or in geographical areas where the occurrence of snakes is limited to specific snake types such as in Tasmania (tiger snake). Monovalent antivenom is preferred as it is less expensive, is a smaller load of foreign protein and has fewer side-effects.
- Polyvalent antivenom contains antibodies to the venom of all groups of land snakes. It consists of a large volume and is expensive. It may be used when a patient presents with significant envenoming on arrival as the determination of snake type with the VDK will take too long.
- When the snake identification remains unclear, two monovalent antivenoms (e.g. brown snake and tiger snake antivenom) that cover possible snakes or a polyvalent antivenom can be used.
- The dose of antivenom is dependent on the dose of venom injected by the snake, *not* patient size, so children require the same amount of antivenom as adults do.
- Antivenom is always given intravenously. One vial of the relevant antivenom is sufficient to bind all circulating venom. However, recovery may be delayed as clinical and laboratory effects can take time to reverse. The antivenom is diluted 1:10 in saline or Hartmann's solution. The volume of fluid (but not the dose of antivenom) may need to be modified in children.
- Premedication with adrenaline, antihistamines or steroids is not recommended.

LABORATORY TESTING

Laboratory tests are vital to assessing the patient possibly bitten by a snake, as patients may remain asymptomatic for some time. A patient with suspected snakebite needs to be managed in a hospital with laboratory facilities and this may require patient transfer.

Patients with possible snakebite should have **blood** taken for:
- coagulation—activated partial thromboplastin time (APTT), prothrombin time (PT), fibrinogen level, D-dimer/fibrinogen degradation products (XDP), platelet count
- creatine kinase
- renal function
- electrolytes.

Urine should be tested for myoglobin and blood.

If there is no access to a laboratory, a whole-blood clotting time can be performed to determine the presence of coagulopathy. To perform a whole-blood clotting time, 5–10 mL of blood is placed in a clean plain-glass test tube and allowed to stand. The time to clotting is measured and is normally less than 10 minutes. A time prolonged more than 20 minutes indicates coagulopathy.

Laboratory tests may be normal initially and need to be repeated. If all tests are normal, then the first-aid bandages should be removed and pathology tests repeated after 1 hour. As onset of coagulopathy may be delayed, blood tests should be repeated at 6 hours and 12 hours. The D-dimer may be elevated for days and so serial levels are not helpful.

SIGNS AND SYMPTOMS

- Local signs of snakebite may vary from obvious bite marks, with local pain and swelling, to a trivial puncture or scratch. The absence of bite marks does not exclude significant snakebite, as no visible bite mark is quite common.
- General symptoms may be non-specific, such as nausea, headache, abdominal pain and collapse.
- Specific symptoms may include muscle pain, external or internal bleeding and muscle weakness.

In an emergency, it may be possible to determine the snake from the clinical and laboratory effects. It is advisable to seek expert advice prior to administering antivenom.

DISPOSITION

- Admit and observe all cases of possible snakebite. Patients should be checked frequently for signs of envenomation, and blood tests should be repeated, even if normal initially. Urine should be tested again for blood and myoglobin. The patient should be observed for early signs of paralysis, e.g. ptosis, diplopia and dysarthria, as small muscles are paralysed first.
- Patients who receive multiple doses of antivenom should also be given doses of steroids to prevent serum sickness.
- All patients with brown snake bite should be admitted for 24 hours.

Spider bites
REDBACK SPIDER (*LATRODECTUS HASSELTI*)
Redback spiders are common throughout Australia. They are common in urban areas, in and around houses, gardens, sheds, rubbish piles and discarded objects. It is the female spider that is responsible for envenoming. The bite of the redback can become very painful but envenoming is not normally life-threatening.

- Only one-fifth of bites will result in significant envenoming. Only people with significant envenoming receive antivenom.
- The redback bite is usually felt as an initial mild sting, with no signs of a bite at the site. Between 10 and 60 minutes later, the bite site may become painful, with local sweating and piloerection. The pain can become severe and extend up the limb to the regional lymph nodes. In a minority of patients, there may be systemic autonomic features including hypertension, tachycardia and diaphoresis.
- Redback spider bite has been mistaken for acute surgical abdomen in children or myocardial infarction in adults.
- The triad of local pain, sweating and piloerection around the bite site increasing in the hour after a bite is diagnostic.
- Profuse sweating and pain in both arms or both legs following a bite is characteristic of systemic envenoming.
- The use of redback antivenom is controversial. It has been used historically to treat moderate–severe pain and systemic symptoms; however, recent studies suggest there is no benefit over standard analgesia and supportive care. There is, however, anecdotal opinion that it does have some benefit.
  — If redback antivenom is given, there is no difference between the IM and IV route, and the dose is 2 vials. No premedication is required, but facilities to treat anaphylaxis should be at hand.
  — Redback antivenom may be useful for relief of symptoms up to days after the initial bite.

FUNNEL-WEB SPIDER (*ATRAX* SPP.)
There are at least 40 species of funnel-web spiders, but only one is known to cause death in humans. It is the Sydney funnel-web

(*Atrax robustus*), which has a restricted range that includes the Sydney, Gosford and Wollongong regions. Other types are found over a wider range along the eastern seaboard of Australia.

• Following a bite from the Sydney funnel-web, death can occur within 1 hour. The effects are a bite that is usually painful, followed by perioral tingling, fasciculation of the tongue, profuse sweating, lacrimation and salivation, then skeletal muscle fasciculation and spasms. Hypertension and tachycardia usually occur and there may be rapid onset of pulmonary oedema.

• First aid is with the pressure–immobilisation technique. Definitive treatment is with Sydney funnel-web antivenom. Multiple vials of antivenom, usually 2–4, may be required. Resuscitation with airway control and ventilation may be necessary. Atropine may help reduce secretions.

• All Sydney funnel-web spider bites should be admitted for close observation.

The Sydney funnel-web spider appears similar to a number of non-venomous big black spiders (e.g. mouse spiders, trapdoor spiders). It is therefore important to have an approach to the management of the patient who presents with a *big black spider* bite if you practise within the distribution of Sydney funnel-web spiders. The unknown *big black spider* bite in these areas should be managed with pressure–immobilisation first aid, transport to a facility with antivenom and close observation for signs of envenoming.

WHITE-TAILED SPIDER (*LAMPONA CYLINDRATA*)

The white-tailed spider is a common hunting spider that is often found in houses. Definite bites from this spider may cause some local pain and inflammation, but are usually only mild or moderate. The evidence linking the white-tailed spider to necrotic ulcers is limited, and research has failed to show that its venom causes significant skin damage.

• The patient who presents with a white-tailed spider bite usually only requires reassurance.

• There is an extensive list of causes of skin ulcers or necrotic skin lesions. Patients presenting with these may need referral to their GP or dermatologist.

NECROTIC ARACHNIDISM

Many spiders can cause a bite that may be painful and mildly inflamed locally. In some patients the skin may ulcerate. These small ulcers usually heal without specific treatment.

The development of lesions that ulcerate and develop necrosis is usually only tenuously linked to a spider bite. Patients with skin lesions often presume it was a spider bite, even though no spider has been sighted.

A number of overseas spiders not found in Australia, such as the recluse and fiddleback spiders, are implicated in causing necrotic skin ulceration and systemic illness.

There is little evidence to suggest that any single species of Australian spider is the cause of necrotic skin damage. In many cases, the cause of the tissue damage is a secondary bacterial infection.

Management includes adequate debridement of the wound, microbiological specimens and antibiotics if required. They may need investigation for other causes.

Marine envenomation
BOX JELLYFISH OR SEA WASP (*CHIRONEX FLECKERI*)

The box jellyfish is one of the most venomous creatures in the world. It is found in the tropical waters of northern Australia, and is most commonly encountered in the summer months.

- The venom of the box jellyfish contains cardiotoxic, neurotoxic and dermatotoxic compounds. Its tentacles contain stinging cells called nematocysts that contain the venom, and a spring-loaded harpoon. On contact with a victim the nematocyst releases the coiled harpoon, which pierces the skin and releases the stored venom. Victims may further discharge nematocysts as they attempt to remove the tentacles that still contain intact stinging cells.
- Clinically, there is severe localised pain, and local skin changes range from painful erythema to full-thickness skin necrosis. Typically, there are linear red welts that may go on to blister and ulcerate. Confusion, agitation and collapse with respiratory or cardiac arrest can occur.
- Rarely, envenomation may be very rapid and death can occur in 5 minutes, probably due to direct cardiotoxicity.

Immediate and prolonged CPR is indicated in the event of cardiovascular collapse.

- The extent of envenoming is dependent on the area of skin suffering tentacle contact. An area of tentacle contact of 10% of the total body surface area is potentially lethal. One metre of tentacle-to-skin contact in a child, or several metres in the adult, can result in severe envenoming.

- Immediate first aid is vital. First, do not try to remove the tentacles. Any undischarged nematocysts can be inactivated by applying large volumes of household vinegar (dilute acetic acid). A pressure bandage is not applied as it can increase toxin load.

- Antivenom is available and is given by IV injection. IM injection of antivenom is no longer recommended as it will not be effective in the case of cardiovascular collapse. Early administration of antivenom may result in reduced pain and reduces skin necrosis and scarring.

- Severe envenoming is rare and most box jellyfish stings require only first aid.

IRUKANDJI (*CARUKIA BARNESI*)

The irukandji is a small jellyfish, about 2 cm in diameter, found in the coastal waters of northern Australia.

- The sting of the irukandji is moderately painful, with little skin damage, but within 30 minutes onset of systemic envenoming may occur, with severe abdominal and back pain, nausea and vomiting, and muscle or joint pain. Autonomic features may occur due to catecholamine release including tachycardia, hypertension, sweating and agitation. Rarely pulmonary oedema may develop.

- Treatment includes opiate analgesia, and antihypertensive treatment may be required, in which case alpha-blocking drugs (phentolamine) may be used. Treatment of pulmonary oedema includes non-invasive ventilation and GTN infusion.

- No antivenom is available to treat irukandji envenomation.

PORTUGUESE MAN-O'-WAR OR BLUEBOTTLE (*PHYSALIA* SPP.)

The Portuguese man-o'-war, or bluebottle, occurs throughout Australian coastal waters, where it is often found washed up on beaches. It has a typical bright blue appearance, an air-filled flotation sac and long tentacles.

- The bluebottle causes a painful sting with localised discrete wheals and surrounding erythema. A line of redness with raised wheals or blisters is typical. Systemic symptoms are uncommon, but comprise nausea, vomiting, headache and abdominal pains. Deaths have not been reported following bluebottle sting in Australia.
- First aid involves washing the sting site with sea water, and removing the tentacles with forceps. Vinegar is not recommended.
- Treatment consists of hot-water immersion at 45°C for 20 minutes. Analgesia is indicated, as is local anaesthesia.

BLUE-RINGED OCTOPUS (*HAPALOCHLAENA* SPP.)

The blue-ringed octopus is found in coastal waters around Australia. They are small, only a few centimetres in size, and exhibit electric-blue rings when aroused.

- A bite from the blue-ringed octopus may be painless and difficult to see, and so may go unnoticed. The bites usually occur when the octopus is handled. The victim, often a child, will usually report playing with a small octopus in or around a coastal rock pool.
- The saliva of the blue-ringed octopus contains a potent neurotoxin, tetrodotoxin, which causes a rapidly progressive flaccid paralysis, followed by respiratory failure and hypotension.
- First aid involves applying a pressure–immobilisation bandage.
- There is no antivenom, and treatment is based on maintaining supportive measures. Respiratory support with ventilation may be required for a few days, until the effects of the toxin wear off.

SEA SNAKES

Sea snakes are found predominantly in the tropical waters of northern Australia. There are more than 30 species found in Australian waters. They are inquisitive and rarely aggressive. All are potentially dangerous to humans, but very few sea snake bites of significance occur. Bites may occur when a sea snake is being handled or removed from the nets of a fishing trawler.

- Sea snake venoms contain postsynaptic neurotoxins and myolysins. Victims may therefore develop paralysis, with ptosis and diplopia, or muscle pain, weakness and myoglobinuria and hyperkalaemia, and renal failure may occur secondary to muscle breakdown. Coagulopathy is not a feature of sea snake bite.
- Treatment is with the pressure–immobilisation technique of first aid.
- Sea snake antivenom is available and is used for neutralising venoms of all species of sea snakes. Sea snake venoms are not reliably detected by the VDK.

STONEFISH

The stonefish is responsible for a painful sting that usually occurs when waders step on the fish in shallow waters around reefs and rock pools. They are well camouflaged and their spines may pierce the sole of a wader's shoe.

- When the fish is stepped on, the spines inject venom, which causes instant and severe pain. Local swelling, which may be marked, follows. Dizziness, nausea, hypotension and pulmonary oedema may rarely occur.
- As some components of the venom are denatured by heat, first aid involves immersing the limb in hot water. The water should not be hot enough to cause a scald.
- Analgesics are usually required. Local or regional anaesthesia may help in providing analgesia.
- Antivenom is available if there is significant envenoming, and is indicated if there is severe local pain. The number of ampoules given relates to the number of puncture wounds from the venomous spines.
- A remnant of the spine may remain embedded in the foot and removal of the remnant is necessary. Imaging with X-ray or ultrasound may be indicated.
- The role of prophylactic antibiotics is unclear. However, wound irrigation, debridement and removal of foreign debris is paramount.
- Secondary infection is the major complication and may be from marine or aquatic organisms.

STINGRAYS

Stingrays of all sizes are prevalent in Australian waters. They are not aggressive unless provoked, commonly by being accidentally trodden on.

- The tail of a stingray has a barb or stinger on the dorsal surface some 2/3 distally. This is its main defence.
- This barb is sharp and common injuries seen include lacerations around the foot and ankle. If deep enough, tendons can be injured.
- Envenomation also occurs from toxins which cause pain as well as some cardiotoxicity.
- Like most marine toxins, they are inactivated by heat (e.g. put foot in hot water).
- ECG, troponins ordered as clinically indicated.
- Wound standard care, but remember marine bacterial infections, if indicated, require different antibiotics (e.g. tetracyclines).

Tick bites

- Ticks most commonly cause a local skin reaction, consisting of irritation and pruritus as the tick attaches and sucks blood from the host. Multiple bites may cause a rash.
- There are many species of tick and the most dangerous are those that cause paralysis, belonging to the *Ixodes* group. The *Ixodes* paralysis tick is found along the eastern coastal strip of Australia.
  — Paralysis occurs due to a neuromuscular-junction toxin that occurs in the saliva of the *Ixodes* ticks. The toxin causes a progressive flaccid paralysis. Paralysis may take a few days to develop.
  — Tick paralysis is rare, and usually occurs in children less than 3 years old and presents as an ataxic gait with drowsiness, malaise and unsteadiness or leg weakness. The weakness may progress slowly, and even up to 48 hours after removal of the ticks. Clinicians should keep a broad differential when assessing a child with weakness, including snakebite envenomation, infant botulism and Guillain-Barré syndrome.

- A thorough search should be conducted to find ticks, which may be multiple, including scalp, ear canals, axillae, natal cleft and genitals. Ticks are removed by using tweezers on either side of the embedded mouthparts. Care is taken not to squeeze the body of the tick, or more toxin can be injected. Care is also taken not to break off the mouthparts that may remain embedded in the skin.
- Paralysis is treated with appropriate supportive care. Tick antivenom is no longer available.
- A local reaction to the tick bite that may last a number of weeks is common, especially if the tick has been incompletely removed.

Centipedes and scorpions

None of the species of centipedes or scorpions found in Australia are dangerous to humans. In other parts of the world they may be responsible for life-threatening envenomation.

Scorpions sting with their tail, not with their paired pincers. They may cause a painful bite, but the pain does not usually last long. Systemic symptoms are unusual and are not usually severe.

Additional resources

- Many hospitals have their own policies for management of potential bites.
- Many smaller hospitals have a clinical relationship with a larger hospital, and a local or regional emergency doctor will be available on the end of a phone. (Use them!)

Pearls and Pitfalls

- The most common pitfall is not relying on the history that is provided to you or underestimating the potential for envenomation.
- Unexplained coagulopathy, muscle pain or weakness should include envenomation as a differential diagnosis.
- Children with unexplained irritability, pain or sweating or boys with unexplained groin pain should have redback spider bites as part of the differential diagnosis.
- Gloves and forceps are used to remove marine tentacles from patients, as undischarged nematocysts can injure the first aider.

- Failure to apply, or removal of, a pressure–immobilisation bandage in snake or funnel-web envenomation may cause worsening symptoms; a pressure bandage should be applied and left in situ until no longer necessary.
- The decision to administer antivenom when clinically indicated should not be delayed.
- Adequate antivenom should be used as indicated on either clinical or laboratory grounds.
- Being bitten does not automatically indicate the need for antivenom administration. Many definite bites do not result in envenoming.
- A positive result for a VDK does not indicate the need for antivenom administration. There may be venom on the skin without systemic envenoming.
- The VDK tells us which antivenom to give, but not whether we should give it.
- Toxinologists who are on call do not regard any question as silly if it relates to a patient or presentation you do not fully understand. They are available through the Poisons Information Centre, telephone 13 11 26, Australia-wide.
- Ask for advice, and ask early. There are no stupid questions, only stupid people who don't ask questions.

Online resources

Australian Venom Research Unit
    www.avru.org/general/general_main.html
Clinical Toxinology Resources
    www.toxinology.com
Emergency Therapeutic Guidelines, toxinology
    http://proxy9.use.hcn.com.au

Chapter 45
Electrical injuries

Chris Mobbs and Gordian Fulde

Overview

In Australia, people come to emergency departments as the result of an electrical injury, including by lightning. Some 15–20% are aged 0–14 years.

Each year there are preventable deaths attributable to electrical injury (> 90% are male). Many deaths from lightning strikes (mostly male) could have been avoided.

Electrical injuries are more common in males, and mostly occur in the young adult and adult years. The most common locations for injury are, in order, the home (often children < 6 years old) and the workplace.

The **source of an electrical injury** may be divided into three broad subgroups, with important differences in assessment and management of patients relevant to each. For example, cardiac arrest, as provoked by an electrical current, will more commonly be asystole from a lightning strike and ventricular fibrillation (VF) from a household AC current. The three subgroups, therefore, are:

1 lightning injury
2 high-voltage (> 1000 V) electrical injury
3 low-voltage (< 1000 V) electrical injury.

Low-voltage electrical injury may be further subdivided into patients *with* or *without* cardiac and/or respiratory arrest.

PATHOPHYSIOLOGY

Electricity may cause injury via three broad mechanisms.

1 Electricity causing direct tissue damage, altering cell membrane resting potential and eliciting muscle tetany, cardiac arrests and arrhythmias (thus better results from prolonged CPR).

2 Conversion of electrical energy into thermal energy (heat), causing tissue destruction and coagulative necrosis.

3 Traumatic injury resulting from falls or violent muscle contractions.

The site of either direct tissue or thermal energy damage depends on the pathway of current flow. Skin wound inspection alone will miss and underdiagnose damage to deep and distant structures.

PHYSICS

Electricity is the flow of electrons from higher to lower potential. Direct current (DC), from sources such as car batteries or defibrillators, flows in one direction. Domestic alternating current (AC) switches to and fro at 50–60 cycles per second (hertz), as this confers advantages in terms of current generation and transmission. Ironically, human muscular tissue is sensitive to frequencies in this range, with tetany of peripheral muscles and VF arrest of cardiac muscles a risk during contact with household electricity. Domestic voltage in Australia is 230 V.

Lightning contains around 10×10^6 volts and a current of 10 000–200 000 amperes. However, as the result of the incredibly brief time (microseconds to milliseconds) involved in a lightning strike, the final amount of current is much less than expected.

It is the electrical current that is important in terms of human morbidity and mortality, and thus basic electrical injury potential rests with two laws.

• Ohm's law:

$$\text{resistance (ohms)} = \frac{\text{voltage (volts)}}{\text{current (amperes)}}$$

• Joule's law:

$$\text{heat generated} = \text{current}^2 \propto \text{resistance}$$

So, while dry, thick, calloused skin may be more resistant to injury by virtue of its very high resistance (up to 100 000 ohms), the resistance of moist skin is only 1000 ohms. It is therefore of vital importance to preach **good electrical safety**, especially in the home and workplace, and especially relating to moisture and electrical appliances and the installation of circuit-breakers, as well as ensuring circuits have a functioning earth.

Similarly, it is the role of all health professionals to educate the public about **safety during electrical storms**. Those who enjoy outdoor recreation, such as golfers and hikers, are the major group of people affected by lightning strike. Solo people who are struck make up 70% of the recorded mortality. Most fatalities (about 70%) are recorded between midday and 6 pm. Deaths occur five times more frequently in the country than in urban areas. The summer storm season is associated with the highest mortality rate. The annual mortality rate is decreasing in all recording countries.

Three major predictors of mortality are: cardiac arrest at the time of injury, cranial burns (5 times increased) and leg burns.

In order to **avoid lightning** there are some simple measures which should be followed.

- Stay indoors during a storm, or seek shelter in a building or car (not a convertible).
- Avoid contact with any metal such as golf clubs, umbrellas, tent poles, gates, roofs or hair clips.
- Do not stand next to or under the tallest object in sight, such as a tree, pole or haystack.
- Avoid being in a group—split up so that someone can call for help if necessary; give CPR (fixed dilated pupils can be an electrical brain injury which responds to CPR).
- Do not stand with your feet apart, as this increases your stride potential and can result in major burns.
- If caught alone, the correct procedure is to curl up on the ground, preferably in a ditch, well away from higher objects.
- It is important to note that, contrary to popular belief, lightning does strike twice or more in the same spot.

Wideband magnetic direction finders are increasingly used to warn of incoming lightning storms. Lightning injuries can be markedly decreased by taking measures to prevent oneself becoming a conductor, and by not being near an obvious one. Piloerection during an electrical storm can mean that a lightning strike is imminent, and immediate evasive measures along the lines of those described above should be taken.

Low- and high-voltage electrical injury

- The type and amount of current can be inferred from the nature of the source. Electricians and other tradespeople may be able to give accurate information as to strength of power source and current type. However, within appliances, conversions from the more dangerous AC to DC, and to a different voltage, are possible.
- Entry and exit wounds may be visible, but their absence does not rule out serious injury and they may give no indication as to severity of underlying organ damage. The current between any such wounds does not necessarily travel in straight lines.
- Electrical flash burns, often seen in tradespeople, may occur where a short-circuit causes an explosion (e.g. on a switchboard). It is likely that patients have had very little actual current pass through them, and dermal and corneal burns and sequelae of any blunt trauma may dominate the clinical picture.
- If a patient was 'frozen' to the circuit, due to muscle tetany with AC, a life-threatening injury may have occurred, with multi-organ and limb damage.
- Significant electrical injury resembles more closely a crush injury than a burn. Necrosis of deep soft tissues and organs has both immediate (e.g. cardiac arrest) and long-term (e.g. rhabdomyolysis and renal failure) adverse sequelae. Tissues and organs distant to the site of electrical injury may be affected, as large- and small-vessel arterial and venous thrombosis occurs.
- Infants and young children are prone to sustaining oral electrical injuries from electrical appliances. Mucous membranes have less resistance than skin and the current is therefore higher. These injuries may lead to eventual scarring and deformity of the face in later years. If the current travels close to the eyes, cataracts may form.
- Injuries, burns and complications are frequently under-diagnosed and poorly documented. Because litigation can ensue, good clinical recording is mandatory—as with all instances of burns and trauma in the ED. Diagrams are essential, photography desirable.

MANAGEMENT

Pre-hospital

The most important initial consideration is the safety of the rescuer and other bystanders. No more electrocutions should be allowed to occur. All wires and appliances should be considered live, as should any patients still in contact with them. Power should be shut down and/or the victim should be removed from the current with a non-conductive substance—for example a rubber car mat. Any water or moisture should be regarded as electrically live and the potential source of more electrical injury.

An electrocuted patient must then continue to be treated along standard life support guidelines. Nowadays, with automated and semi-automated external defibrillators (AEDs/SAEDs) available in many public areas, these devices should be utilised as rapidly as is safely possible, as early defibrillation from VF gives the greatest chance of survival. CPR has higher success rates with electrical injuries.

Hospital

- The standard approach to an *unconscious or critically ill patient* must always be employed. This includes neck immobilisation where necessary and exclusion of other causes of altered conscious state such as hypoglycaemia, overdose, cerebrovascular accident or trauma. This approach is particularly important in view of the fact that the prime treatment modality for the electrically injured is support of systems while waiting for recovery, and attempting to avoid complications.
- The majority of survivors presenting to the ED after an electrical injury are relatively well. A high level of suspicion for secondary traumatic injuries needs to be maintained, however, if there is a possibility of a fall, having been thrown or a violent muscle contraction. Emergency doctors should think of 'worst-case scenarios', as electrical injuries can affect multiple systems and may well be covert. It is essential to keep an open mind as to causation, and to carefully explore the possibility of serious concomitant disease.
- A thorough ABC reassessment and then a meticulous whole-body examination (primary then secondary surveys)

with aggressive early management of any injuries must occur. Fractures may be present; fasciotomies of digits and limbs may need to be done in the ED. An ECG should be performed.

- A good urine flow (1 mL/kg/h) in the face of myoglobinuria (urine dipstick positive for blood) or shock is essential, as with standard treatment of rhabdomyolysis. Urinary alkalinisation and use of mannitol and/or frusemide may be indicated and late renal failure with acidosis must be anticipated.
- A check of tetanus immunisation status is mandatory.
- Cardiac monitoring and admission for observation is indicated in high-voltage (> 1000 V) injury, following seizures or loss of consciousness, raised cardiac markers and with ECG changes including arrhythmias. Arrhythmias will usually settle spontaneously and without sinister sequelae. Admission may also be required as dictated by traumatic injury, exacerbation of preexisting chronic illness or in the elderly.
- Thus patients with 'low-voltage' injuries not meeting the adverse criteria detailed above may be discharged home with simple analgesia as required, following a normal ECG. No blood tests are necessary. An exception to this rule is in the case of the pregnant female; the fetus, situated within amniotic fluid within a hyperaemic uterus, is at great risk, even with apparently 'minor' exposures having no noticeable effect on the mother. An urgent obstetric ultrasound and consultation should be sought.
- Adequate follow-up, both physical and psychological, must be arranged, as a high proportion of patients have some long-term effects following a significant electrical injury. Neurological damage has an especially poor prognosis. Electrical burns should be referred to a specialist burns centre.
- Many electrical injuries may involve workers' compensation or insurance claims, so good documentation is useful.

LIGHTNING INJURIES
Physics
Lightning occurs when particles moving up and down during a thunderstorm create static electricity. A massive negative charge builds up on the underside of a cloud until the charge difference between it and the positively charged ground is enough to

cause electrical discharge. This lightning strike may last between 1 and 100 milliseconds. It differs from 'high-voltage' electrocution in additional ways—the energy level is many tens of millions of volts, it is a direct current (DC), it may cause a shock wave and may demonstrate the 'flashover' phenomenon, where the current passes over and around, rather than through, the patient.

Lightning is also associated with asystolic cardiac arrest, rather than ventricular fibrillation. Good CPR rather than early defibrillation is of paramount importance as, although return to sinus rhythm may spontaneously occur, there is a risk of secondary hypoxic arrest if resuscitation is delayed.

Some 30% of victims who are struck die, and up to 75% can have serious complications.

MECHANISMS OF STRIKE

1 **Direct strike**
   a Current passes through patient.
   b Current passes over surface of patient (flashover), often via wet clothes, which can explode or burn.

2 **Side flash**

The patient becomes part of the main conductor. This occurs for example when standing under a tree which is struck by lightning. The current can pass as in a direct strike.

3 **Direct contact**

The patient is in physical contact with the main conductor.

4 **Stride potential**

This arises when current from a lightning strike travels along the ground near a person who has his/her legs separated. The current takes the path of lesser resistance up a leg, across the body and down the other leg, rather than along the high-resistance ground. This process is associated with a significant mortality.

PATHOPHYSIOLOGY

As the injuries sustained are both multisystemic and multifactorial in aetiology (from diverse sources such as electricity, heat, blunt trauma and anoxia), the clinical possibilities are vast. Certain injuries and their sequelae are typical or may even be diagnostic (see Table 44.1).

- Cardiac—asystolic arrest.
- Neurological—loss of consciousness, paraplegia, hemiplegia, amnesia, seizure, tinnitus, autonomic nervous system dysfunction including fixed dilated pupils.
- Vascular—keraunoparalysis; vascular spasm with absent pulses, mottled limbs. Usually resolves over a period of hours.
- Skin—'Lichtenberg flowers'; may look severe but fade within hours.
- Severe burns with their sequelae of renal failure, anaemia and tissue damage are very uncommon.

As a generalisation, patients who survive the initial strike will usually have no major problems. Clinical expertise, including a high index of suspicion, must be used to rule out potential complications to the eyes, ears, heart and nervous system.

MANAGEMENT
Pre-hospital
- Rescuer safety is vital. A very special aspect of lightning victims is that they require aggressive resuscitation even in the light of asystole, apparent fixed dilated pupils or pulseless limbs, for the reasons detailed earlier.
- This is also the reason for a group caught by a storm splitting up—CPR can be administered to the victim by those not affected.
- A particular pitfall to avoid is withholding CPR to the victim of a lightning strike in the mistaken assumption that they remain charged by electricity.
- Paradoxically to usual disaster responses, if several people are struck by lightning at once, the care must go to the sickest (arrested) first, as the walking and talking wounded will survive whereas the arrested patient has only a brief opportunity to be salvaged.
- The diagnosis itself may be challenging, as the strike may be unwitnessed. Again, a high index of suspicion must be maintained and clues such as multiple unconscious people, exploded clothes and Lichtenberg flowers may point to the cause.

Hospital

- Patients may arrive arrested, unconscious, amnesic, as a trauma patient or as one that has very few clinical problems.
- A standard approach (e.g. advanced cardiac life support [ACLS], advanced trauma life support [ATLS]) is indicated with simultaneous assessment and management systematically by an organised team.
- The clinical picture dictates the management. It is essential that other possible causes and concomitant illness be sought and excluded as part of the patient's management.
- As always, the ABCs are secured. Lightning-strike patients rarely need fluid loading. Hypothermia due to exposure is common. If there is any loss of consciousness, arrhythmia or rise in cardiac markers, cardiac monitoring for 24 hours is indicated. MRI is useful for subtle lesions of the brain and spinal cord. Usually the surviving victim needs mainly supportive treatment.
- Special attention should be paid to the ear and eye examinations, for tympanic rupture and corneal defects respectively. Other ocular pathology will also need to be excluded, most easily when the patient is alert and able to cooperate with full eye examination. Basal visual acuity should be recorded if possible.
- Disposition is guided by the same considerations that govern other electrical injuries. A period of observation in hospital is warranted for changes in neurological or cardiological status and for other organ-specific pathology.

Tasers

- Invented and named by a NASA researcher, Jack Cover, in the early 1970s with reference to Tom Swift and His Electric Rifle, these 'less than lethal' or 'less lethal' (as opposed to the previous 'non-lethal' designation) are now utilised, with varying restrictions, by all Australian and New Zealand police forces.
- The overall intention is to avoid more serious injury to a person who is putting themselves or others at significant risk by their behaviour than might be caused by discharge of a

firearm. Much of the data available regarding discharges of the device and medical sequelae is from the United States but law enforcement agencies in more than 100 countries utilise Tasers and there have been approximately 5 million discharges over the last two decades.

- A knowledge of the physics utilised by the device and possible sequelae resulting from their discharge is therefore important for doctors in the emergency department.
- There are various taser models but all are designed to cause temporary neuromuscular incapacitation (by involuntary strong muscle contractions) of an individual via an electric current delivered by two small darts fired utilising gas propulsion approximately 10 metres while remaining connected to the handheld device and its inbuilt battery. The device can also be utilised, after discharge of the darts, as a 'stun' device via direct contact of the remaining electrical terminals with the target individual.
- While a peak voltage of approximately 50 000 V is generated, this is substantially less (approximately 1200 V) by the time it reaches the body. At any rate, it is the current (measured in amperes) which is of importance in terms of danger to humans. By way of an example, a small Van de Graaff generator (beloved of schoolchildren everywhere for its ability to make one's hair stand on end) routinely produces more than 1 million volts. In terms of energy, the joules delivered per pulse is 0.07 J (compared to 50 J or more for the standard initial electrical dose used in synchronised cardioversion in the ED).
- A taser will produce approximately 0.0021 amperes. A household kettle, by comparison, will run off about 13 amps. While there are many articles in the popular press describing taser-related deaths, there is considerable debate regarding their accuracy. Many instances of mortality are rather related to associated trauma (e.g. falls while incapacitated) or co-ingested illicit substances.
- A sensible approach, therefore, to a patient brought in for assessment after a taser incapacitation is a careful history and examination focusing on secondary trauma. In addition, a standard 12-lead ECG should be taken.

- For the 'successful' delivery of the electrical current, both barbs, attached to the wires that attach to the handheld unit, must lodge either in the skin or clothing (up to 2 inches combined distance from the skin). Emergency department staff may therefore be called on to remove these barbs and an analogy to fishhook removal is appropriate.
- Importantly, there is no residual electric current in either barbs or wire once discharged and therefore no risk to staff from electrical injury. The same cannot be said for the sharp barbs and all care should be taken when handling either these or the patient where they remain attached.
- Remember tetanus prophylaxis.

Pearls and Pitfalls

- Do not become a victim of electrical injury—ensure self and bystander safety before attending patient.
- Early CPR is potentially life-saving.
- The victim of lightning strike does not remain electrically charged.
- Even apparently 'harmless' electrical injury may have fatal consequences for the intrauterine fetus.
- Asymptomatic patients following a low-voltage electrical injury may be safely discharged from the ED following a normal ECG.
- Preach prevention, especially to golfers.

Online resources

Cushing TA, Wright RK. Electrical injuries in emergency medicine. E-medicine. April 2013. Retrieved from: http://emedicine. medscape.com/article/770179-overview

UpToDate; search on 'electrical injuries'
www.uptodate.com

City of London Police, Taser
www.cityoflondon.police.uk

Chapter 46
Hypothermia and hyperthermia

Gordian Fulde

Acknowledgment

The author wishes to acknowledge the content used from the previous edition of *Emergency Medicine* which was provided by David Lewis-Driver.

Although Canadians write more about hypothermia and Saudis write more about hyperthermia, in fact neither condition is rare in Australia. Heat waves and fun-runs occur every year in every Australian city; at the opposite end of the spectrum, hypothermia is a regular accompaniment to injury and disease throughout the year, and can occur in summer; for example, when nursing-home patients are left scantily clothed under an air conditioner to cool them. It is important, too, to remember that the average multiple-trauma patient in any country will become hypothermic unless specific preventive steps are taken.

Physiology

Temperature control requires a functioning hypothalamic centre, adequate cardiovascular function to be able to dissipate or conserve heat, adequate muscle bulk to generate heat, intact skin and sweat glands and sufficient common sense and mobility to escape the heat or cold. All of these may be affected by disease, trauma or environmental factors.

In both hyperthermia and hypothermia, skin circulation is a problem. Overheating cold skin induces vasodilation, which feels good but may overwhelm the pumping capacity of a cold heart, resulting in 'rewarming shock'. Ice on hot skin induces vasoconstriction, which may limit heat transfer.

Hypothermia

This condition is defined as a core temperature of $< 35°C$. It is classified as shown in Table 46.1.

PHYSIOLOGY

The body responds to a fall in temperature by attempting to seek warmth and by shivering. If these efforts fail because of environmental factors or drugs, injury or disease and the temperature continues to fall, an initial rise in respiration, heart rate and blood pressure is followed by a gradual slowing of all body systems, with death due to cardiovascular failure. Central nervous system (CNS) slowing results in apathy and confusion, and cardiovascular system slowing proceeds to death in asystole, unless an irritable heart is jolted into ventricular fibrillation (VF).

In general, slow warming and gentle handling are appropriate. Vigorous attempts at external rewarming can result in skin burns or death from 'rewarming shock', an ill-understood phenomenon that can best be considered as shunting of needed blood to the surface while the core is still too cold to cope with the demand. Also the trunk should be rewarmed before very cold limbs. Core temperature lags behind surface temperature during rewarming, and healthy volunteers start to feel better when rewarmed while their core temperature is still falling due to continued cold penetration. An 'undressing phenomenon' is also well described,

Table 46.1 Stages of hypothermia

Stage	Clinical	Core temperature
1 Mild	Normal mental state with shivering	35–32°C
2 Moderate	Altered mental state without shivering	32–28°C
3 Severe	Unconscious	28–24°C
4 Profound	Apparent death—resuscitation may be possible	24–14°C
5 Dead	Definite death—resuscitation not possible	< 14°C

Modified from The International Commission for Mountain Emergency Medicine

where failure of skin vasoconstriction as a terminal event allows return of skin circulation and leads to a sensation of warmth so that victims are found to have undressed themselves as a last act before death.

DIAGNOSIS AND DIFFERENTIAL DIAGNOSIS

If temperature is not a routine observation on every patient, ensure it is taken in those patients who are potential hypothermia candidates, as outlined in Box 46.1.

If the temperature is < 36°C on a standard instrument, use a low-reading thermometer. The tympanic thermometers commonly used in EDs will generally read down to 26°C and are thus adequate to suggest the diagnosis. However, they are not accurate enough to guide treatment. Use an electronic probe—rectal in an awake patient and oesophageal in an intubated patient.

Box 46.1   Conditions associated with hypothermia
Conditions associated with accidental hypothermia Trauma that limits protective mechanisms (e.g. neck of femur [NOF]) Overdose Alcoholism
Conditions that may cause hypothermia Sepsis Myxoedema or adrenal insufficiency Parkinsonism (failure to shiver) Wernicke's encephalopathy Drugs (e.g. phenothiazines, beta-blockers, clozapine, sedatives) Hypoglycaemia; diabetic ketoacidosis (affects the body's 'thermostat') Pancreatitis Myocardial infarction or other cause of low cardiac output Malnutrition/anorexia Burns; extensive skin rashes (excessive heat loss)
Conditions that hypothermia may be mistaken for Cerebrovascular accident (CVA) Dementia; confusion in the elderly; delirium Hypoglycaemia Myocardial ischaemia Drunk and disorderly patient Myxoedema

INVESTIGATIONS AND MANAGEMENT
Mild hypothermia (35–32°C)

1 **Stop further heat loss.** The most powerful way to prevent heat loss in any ED patient is to stem conduction and radiation loss (i.e. remove wet clothes and provide a blanket or space blanket). This is also called passive external rewarming, because prevention of heat loss allows the patient's own metabolism to raise body temperature.

2 **Treat the underlying cause** (Box 46.1). The ability to shiver is very important.

3 **Monitor temperature.** A rise of > 0.5°C per hour is acceptable, but do not exceed a rise of 2°C per hour with a Bair Hugger (see below).

4 **Apply a Bair Hugger**, if available. This method of active external warming using hot air is commonly available and is unlikely to cause rewarming shock or burns. Active warming, however, is not vital unless the patient is incapable of generating heat (e.g. shivering) because of systemic disease or a condition (e.g. CVA) that has reset the temperature centre. If a Bair Hugger is used, do not exceed a rise of 2°C per hour. It is probably better to leave the arms exposed, because the main risk is that sequestered cold blood will be restored to the circulating pool by skin vasodilation, causing an afterdrop in the core temperature. This risk is less from the trunk than the limbs.

5 **Give oxygen and monitor oxygen saturation.** If the saturation monitor will not read because of vasoconstriction, warm the finger or even do a digital block to overcome vasospasm.

6 **Set up IV access and take blood** for the following.
   — Blood sugar level (BSL). Physiologically, hypothermia causes first a rise in BSL due to catecholamine-induced glycogenolysis, then reduced insulin secretion. Finally (below 30°C), insulin stops working. However, there is a strong association with hypoglycaemia in alcoholics, and elderly or malnourished patients may have exhausted glycogen stores by the increased metabolism of shivering. Treat hypoglycaemia but not hyperglycaemia. If rewarming does not correct

hyperglycaemia, exclude haemorrhagic pancreatitis (a complication of hypothermia) or diabetic ketoacidosis (a cause of hypothermia).

— Urea and electrolytes. Fluid shifts and renal dysfunction mean that sodium and potassium can go in either direction. Minor changes in the initial results do not require treatment and can simply be observed during rewarming. Significant changes should be treated and may be a clue to the underlying cause of the hypothermia.

— Lipase. Pancreatitis is both a cause and a result of hypothermia.

— Full blood count (FBC). Expect the haematocrit to be high (due to cold diuresis—an attempt to compensate for central fluid overload due to peripheral vasoconstriction) and the white cell count (WCC) and platelets to be normal or low (due to sequestration). A normal Hb/Hct (haemoglobin/haematocrit) may indicate anaemia and a normal WCC does not rule out infection. Thus the main reason for doing the tests is that a high WCC increases suspicion of an underlying disease process.

— Troponin. Patients who become hypothermic during surgery have a higher incidence of myocardial events. Subendocardial infarctions have been found at autopsy in the absence of ECG changes. In elderly patients, repeat troponin after rewarming.

— Creatine kinase (CK). May be a clue to rhabdomyolysis in overdose or injury.

— Not coagulation screens. Hypothermic patients bleed more after surgery and trauma, and this is generally attributed to failure of one or more of the enzymes in the coagulation cascade and qualitative platelet dysfunction. However, coagulation screens will generally be normal because these tests are done in the lab at room temperature. Rewarming is the best treatment. It is not generally possible either to get the lab to re-do the tests at the patient's temperature or to make fresh frozen plasma (FFP) work while the patient is still cold.

— CRP may help find a diagnosis (e.g. sepsis).

7 **Give fluid.**
   — Give 500–1000 mL of dextrose/saline or normal saline (warmed!)
   — Hartmann's solution is contraindicated because the cold liver cannot metabolise the lactate.
   — Assume that the patient is dehydrated due to 3rd-space shifts and cold diuresis. Some fluid is required to compensate for the return of skin flow during rewarming, but when the patient is warmer the 3rd-space fluid will return.
   — Elderly patients require cautious fluid replacement but younger patients can have the full litre fairly quickly.

8 **Do an ECG.** Hypothermia increases conduction times and often causes a slow atrial fibrillation which reverses with rewarming. The classical ECG change is the appearance of a J wave between the QRS complex and the T wave. Some computerised ECG programs interpret this wave incorrectly as myocardial infarction.

9 **Institute cardiac monitoring.** VF is the terminal event in a significant number of hypothermia deaths, and is commonly thought to be provoked by jostling or rescue or treatment procedures. It is unlikely above 29°C, however.

10 **Monitor blood pressure (BP).** If it drops, turn off the Bair Hugger if it is being used (rewarming shock due to skin vasodilation).

11 **Take an ABG** (arterial blood gas) and use the result, which is uncorrected for temperature. Expect hypoxia (due to ventilation/perfusion defects plus shift in oxyhaemoglobin curve plus increased haematocrit) and a lactic acidosis due to shivering. Below 32°C a respiratory acidosis due to slowed respiration will be added. Try to keep the uncorrected pH close to normal, but only by warming and ventilation. Bicarbonate (HCO_3^-) level is not indicated.

12 **Measure urine output.** Use an indwelling catheter (IDC) if required. None of heart rate (HR), BP or urine output will be *reliable* indicators of hydration status, but urine output will be the best of the three.

13 **Keep nil by mouth** until 35°C is reached (poor gut motility).

14 **Consider central venous pressure (CVP).** This may be the only way to measure fluid replacement requirements

in the elderly, but the risk of coagulopathy is a strong disincentive. If a CVP catheter is introduced, it should stop well above the right atrium to avoid an arrhythmia in the irritable heart. Thoracic ultrasound may show venous and ventricular status.

15 **Do a chest X-ray (CXR).** Cold induces bronchorrhoea and reduces ciliary activity and resistance to infection, making bronchopneumonia more likely.

16 **Give thiamine to alcoholic or malnourished patients**, because of the association between Wernicke's encephalopathy and hypothermia.

17 Confirm that the patient can protect the airway, cooperate with treatment, maintain a satisfactory partial oxygen pressure (pO₂) on oxygen, and has a fairly stable HR, BP and cardiac rhythm. If not, proceed to the more aggressive measures in the next section.

Moderate hypothermia (32–28°C)

Treatment should not be based on temperature alone, particularly since core temperature may not initially reflect the rewarming that has been commenced. BP, HR, oxygen saturations and ability to protect the airway all influence treatment decisions. Because VF is a frequent complication in this temperature range, patients with frequent ventricular ectopic beats (VEBs) merit vigorous rewarming.

In addition to the measures above, most moderately hypothermic patients will need the following.

1 **Intubation.** The patient will be hypoventilating and having problems dealing with copious bronchial secretions.
   — Use standard drugs and dosages. Pharmacokinetics and pharmacodynamics are altered by hypothermia, but there is no specific information to guide dosing. Below 30°C, most drugs do not work at all, and 'cold' intubation may be required. At higher temperatures, if the drugs work, they will generally have a longer half-life.
   — Insert a heat–moisture exchanger into the circuit. 70% of respiratory heat loss goes into humidifying expired air. Most EDs do not have mechanisms for heating inspired air, and this additional effort brings marginal benefit.

2 **Nasogastric tube (NGT).** Cold reduces gastric motility and distension is likely.

3 **Active external rewarming.** If a Bair Hugger is not available, put hands and feet in warm water or use radiant heat or hot-water bottles. Be careful of burning poorly vascularised and insensitive skin.

Severe hypothermia (< 28°C)

1 Most of these patients will need active core rewarming and ICU admission. Heated gastric lavage and/or bladder irrigation through the NGT and IDC are non-invasive but not as effective as peritoneal lavage (one or two catheters) or thoracic lavage (two catheters). The most effective rewarming procedure is extracorporeal rewarming using cardiopulmonary bypass or haemodialysis machines.

2 Give broad-spectrum antibiotic prophylaxis because of the high incidence of sepsis due to impaired resistance.

If there is no cardiac output

Death from hypothermia will be preceded by slow HR and respirations, so more care than usual in seeking signs of life is indicated. Unfortunately, the muscular rigidity associated with severe hypothermia is similar to rigor mortis, so the clinical diagnosis of death is difficult without an ECG. But there are also cases of cold asystolic people recovering or being resuscitated, so the axiom 'no one is dead until they are warm and dead' creates a dilemma in the ED, particularly if CPR has been started pre-hospital.

Some guidelines are as follows.

• Temperature < 15°C or potassium > 12 mmol/L is unsalvageable.

• A reasonable level to achieve is 32°C. Once it has been reached, if resuscitation has not already been successful, it probably will not be.

• With temperatures < 32°C, if cardiopulmonary bypass is available, use it. If it is not available, use warmed fluids through two intercostal catheters while CPR continues. VF may not respond to either drugs or defibrillation if temperature is < 32°C.

PRE-HOSPITAL CARE

Shivering is a very effective method of heat production, so simply rescuing and drying the patient is a good start. A warm carbohydrate drink provides core rewarming and energy for more shivering. Warm blankets stop shivering but are now considered to do no harm and they make the patient feel better.

Jostling a severely hypothermic patient (including unnecessary CPR) may precipitate VF. This makes the decision about whether to commence CPR very difficult. If the victim has no pulse or respirations, bag them with oxygen for a few minutes. This may improve output enough for a carotid pulse to be detected. (Wait at least 60 seconds before declaring it absent.) If there is still no pulse, CPR will not make things any worse. Start CPR unless:

- it will endanger rescuers by evacuation delays
- there are obvious lethal injuries
- airway is blocked with ice
- chest is too rigid to be compressed.

Hyperthermia

Hyperthermia is technically different to fever. It is an increased body temperature due to failure of the temperature regulation systems. Unlike hypothermia, it is not possible to say that the diagnosis is defined by temperature. However, it is reasonable to say that below 40°C urgent treatment is unlikely to be needed. Above 42°C, cellular damage is likely whatever the cause—fever or hyperthermia.

DEFINITIONS

- In **fever**, the body's temperature regulation is reset to a new level. Resetting the temperature control with antipyretics may help.
- **Heat stress** is a sense of discomfort in a hot environment.
- **Heat exhaustion** is thirst, weakness, dizziness, etc., plus a normal or mildly elevated temperature due to water or salt depletion.
- **Heat stroke** is a medical emergency; described below.

HEAT STROKE

This is defined as collapse plus CNS abnormalities plus temperature > 40°C occurring once temperature regulation is overwhelmed. In athletes it occurs despite sweating (exertional heat stroke), but in sedentary elderly or frail people (classical heat stroke) it usually occurs after sweating stops. There is a risk of multi-organ failure from the combination of hyperthermia and an exaggerated acute-phase response. Once this response has started, temperature correction may not be enough to avert death.

Key clinical features are:

- CNS disturbances, including altered behaviour, delirium, convulsions
- dry skin (when sweating eventually fails)
- hypotension
- muscle rigidity, rhabdomyolysis
- coagulopathy, petechiae
- renal failure.

Diagnosis

Diagnosis is easy if a patient has been exercising in hot conditions, but the presentation may be more subtle. Refer to Table 46.2 for a list of situations that predispose to hyperthermia.

As with hypothermia, surface temperature may not reflect core temperature. Tympanic infrared thermometers are technically capable of detecting high temperatures, but results may be unreliable due to technique. As with hypothermia, the diagnosis should be confirmed with a rectal probe if suspected.

Table 46.2 Conditions predisposing to hyperthermia

Condition	Reason
Advanced age	Impaired adaptation/mobility
Infancy	Immature sweating
Cardiac disease/drugs	Unable to increase cardiac output
Dehydration/diuretics	Less circulating fluid
Anticholinergics/skin disease	Reduced sweating
High humidity	Reduced evaporative cooling
Hyperthyroidism/stimulant drugs	Increased heat production

Differential diagnosis

Temperature of > 40°C plus CNS dysfunction equals heat stroke unless an alternative diagnosis is evident. The most obvious alternative diagnosis is a febrile illness, particularly CNS infection. A more detailed list of differential diagnoses is found in Box 46.2.

Investigations

- FBE—WCC usually high
- BSL—usually high but give glucose if low
- Electrolytes
- Liver function tests (LFTs)
- CK to check for rhabdomyolysis
- CRP
- Urine analysis to check for myoglobinuria
- Coagulation studies
- ECG
- CXR to check for aspiration, acute respiratory distress syndrome (ARDS)
- ABG

Management

Heat stroke is a medical emergency. If the diagnosis is suspected, commence treatment immediately.

1 **Cool the patient.** Remove clothing as far as modesty permits, place a fan at each end of the bed, and continuously spray the patient with water at room temperature (or warmer) using a misting device. This evaporative cooling is the most effective cooling mechanism. If the temptation to use ice is irresistible, try to confine it to strategic areas (groin and axilla). Aim to reduce the temperature to 39°C within 30 minutes. Stop cooling when 39°C is reached.

Box 46.2 Differential diagnosis of heat stroke
Meningitis/encephalitis
Cerebral malaria
Thyroid storm
Anticholinergic poisoning
Delirium tremens
Neuroleptic malignant syndrome

2 **Give oxygen.**

3 **Intubate** if hypoxic or unable to protect the airway.

4 **Give normal saline.** Marathon runners can have 1 L stat and 1 L in the first hour. Other patients should have half this. If BP and urine output are not restored, use CVP to monitor further replacement. Pulmonary oedema is a risk because of renal failure and cardiovascular compromise.

5 **Insert an IDC.** Monitor urine output. If myoglobinuria is present, alkalinise the urine with HCO_3^- and give mannitol.

6 Consider sedation. Use a benzodiazepine to sedate the patient if agitated or confused and to control seizures.

7 Do not use aspirin or paracetamol. In theory they will not work: aspirin will exacerbate bleeding and paracetamol will require metabolising by a deranged liver. In fact, pyrogenic cytokines have been implicated in heat stress, but there have been no controlled trials of antipyretics.

8 Consider chlorpromazine 25 mg IV injection if shivering is impeding cooling, but do not use it routinely because it may lower BP and impair sweating.

9 Use FFP and platelets if bleeding is a problem. Disseminated intravascular coagulation (DIC) may be present, but treatment with heparin is controversial. Coagulation defects should correct with time and cooling.

If symptoms and blood abnormalities do not correct with cooling, ICU admission will be required. Heat stroke has a significant mortality rate.

Pre-hospital considerations

Cooling, rest and fluids are the cornerstones of pre-hospital care. Fans and evaporative cooling are preferred for the frail elderly. Fun-runners and athletes can be put into an ice-slurry bath. Despite inducing vasoconstriction and shivering, this is effective and has been shown to be safe in young people.

MALIGNANT HYPERTHERMIA

This is a rare complication of anaesthesia that usually occurs soon after anaesthesia, but may be delayed up to 11 hours. Most anaesthetic agents (including suxamethonium/succinylcholine) can cause it. Temperature is 41–45°C. Treatment is similar to heat stroke but with the addition of dantrolene 2–3 mg/kg/day.

NEUROLEPTIC MALIGNANT SYNDROME

This is an idiosyncratic reaction occurring in about 0.2% of patients given neuroleptics. Haloperidol is the commonest offender. Dopamine receptor blockade leads to skeletal muscle spasticity (generating heat) and impaired hypothalamic regulation (interfering with response). The patient has a temperature of > 41°C plus muscle rigidity plus altered consciousness plus autonomic instability. Treatment is as for heat stroke. Both dantrolene and bromocriptine are thought to be helpful, although there have been no controlled trials.

Controversies

Will intubation precipitate ventricular fibrillation in the cold heart? There are isolated reports, but a multicentre study that collected 117 intubated hypothermic patients (Ann Emerg Med 1987;16:1042–55) showed no problems.[1]

Online resources

Practical recommendations for heatstroke management: Bouchama, A, Dehbi, M, Chaves-Carballo, E. Cooling and hemodynamic management in heatstroke: practical recommendations. Critical Care 11, Article number R54, 2007. Retrieved from: http://ccforum. com/content/11/3/R54

UpToDate. Accidental hypothermia in adults
    https://www.uptodate.com.acs.hcn.com.au/contents/accidental-
        hypothermia-in-adults?search=accidental%20hypothermia%20
        in%20adults&source=search_result&selectedTitle=1~150&
        usage_type=default&display_rank=1

UpToDate. Severe nonexertional hyperthermia (classic heat stroke) in adults
    https://www.uptodate.com.acs.hcn.com.au/contents/severe-
        nonexertional-hyperthermia-classic-heat-stroke-in-adults?
        search=severe%20nonexertional&source=search_result&
        selectedTitle=1~150&usage_type=default&display_rank=1

UpToDate. Exertional heat illness in adolescents and adults: Management and prevention
https://www.uptodate.com.acs.hcn.com.au/contents/exertional-heat-illness-in-adolescents-and-adults-management-and-prevention?search=exertional%20heat%20illness&source=search_result&selectedTitle=1~45&usage_type=default&display_rank=1

Reference

1 Danzl DF, et al. Multicenter hypothermia survey. Ann Emerg Med. 1987 Sep;16(9):1042–55.

Chapter 47
Mass-casualty incidents, chemical, biological and radiological hazard contingencies

Iromi Samarasinghe

Introduction *(By Jeff Wassertheil)*

Incidents involving mass casualties are infrequent. However, they have the potential to overwhelm usual health resources with very little notice. It is therefore important that contingencies are developed, tested and ready for immediate implementation. Such contingencies outline the responsibilities for overall medical control, coordination and effective casualty management in major emergencies and disaster situations. They include the procedures for triage, first aid and resuscitation, some of which require modification when resource availability needs to be rationed. Response plans must provide a framework for coordination of transporting injured or incident-affected individuals to appropriate treatment sites. Plans must incorporate procedures to enable the presence of medical, nursing and first-aid providers, as well as other welfare personnel and psychological carers, to provide care at the scene of a mass-casualty incident (MCI).

At a hospital level, plans need to be developed, implemented, rehearsed and evaluated. This enables hospitals that are often full to manage a large number of patients in excess of usual workloads or capacities and, in certain circumstances, victims with special or specific management needs.

Incorporation of public health resources and interventions is integral to providing guidance and procedures where hygiene, sanitation, communicable disease or biological hazards potentially exist. Contingencies must provide an interface for concurrent activation of recovery plans. Access to appropriate and timely psychological support for victims and care providers is included in both early and ongoing recovery phases. The overall objective is to mitigate disasters by participation in event planning and medical and emergency service activation and training.

This chapter focuses on the health service response to an MCI, as it is not within the scope of this book to describe other emergency services frameworks.

Phases of a disaster

The phases of disaster management are prevention, preparedness, response and recovery.

PREVENTION

The prevention phase concentrates on strategies that minimise the severity of an incident. It aims to cushion the severity, reduce the effects, minimise adversity and contain the impact of a disaster. Prevention strategies also include incorporation of lessons learned from previous experiences. Legislation ensures plans are in readiness for such eventualities.

PREPAREDNESS

Effort in optimal preparedness promotes effective and optimal resource allocation and consumption. This phase occurs with an expectation that the plan will at some time need to be activated. Preparedness occurs from within and external to the health service.

Planning includes providers from both within and stakeholders from outside the health service that would be expected to respond in accordance with emergency management contingency plans. Local community stakeholders—such as the police, ambulance and the fire department—as well as public health and recovery agencies should be included in health service planning committees. Likewise, health service representation should be included in local council, shire or regional planning committees.

As highlighted under prevention, the recommendations from previous operational debriefings, adverse incidents or experience are woven into response plans.

Preparedness of medical services involves training and accreditation processes for each facility to work in conjunction with other agencies. Exercises to coordinate resources within and across agencies are aimed at improving the preparation phase.

RESPONSE
This involves the activation of a pre-determined and well-rehearsed emergency plan to respond to multicasualty external disasters resulting in the rapid mobilisation of personnel and other resources to manage the surge of patients.

RECOVERY
Recovery contingencies are implemented and provide for both short- and long-term recovery of the community (victims and helpers) affected by the disaster. This includes the health service staff and the repair and reinstatement of physical resources, consumables and services. A coordinated organisational approach is required to rebuild the infrastructure and economic, social and emotional needs of the affected community.

Administrative and legislative mandates
A national legislative framework for emergency management provides for counter-disaster planning for response to and recovery from emergency situations that take place throughout Australia, and provides a blueprint for state or territory response plans.

MANAGEMENT STRUCTURE
National
At the Commonwealth level, Emergency Management Australia (EMA) is responsible for guidance and support of disaster-management procedures within each of the states and territories.

- EMA will fund any nationally coordinated response, especially any international deployments. A national response is triggered when: an affected state is overwhelmed by a disaster and asks for assistance; there is a political interest in the response involving international aspects, media or border regions; or there is a terrorist threat and the National Counter-Terrorism Committee is required to respond.
- The Commonwealth can also engage defence forces if a civilian disaster requires defence assistance. This commonly

involves transportation, whether in the form of trucks for carrying equipment or aircraft for transporting casualties back to Australian shores. Highly trained medical teams may also be available if not engaged in areas of conflict.

- The Commonwealth can provide expertise in emergency management and assistance with political and media management.
- The Commonwealth can coordinate state assets such as aeromedical capability and medical teams. Although these medical teams are state-based and designed for intrastate deployment, if a state is overwhelmed other medical teams can be coordinated for interstate deployment.
- In addition, the Commonwealth can coordinate any foreign offers of help.
- COMDISPLAN has been established to coordinate the provision of Australian government assistance in the form of physical assets by funding the interstate deployment of medical teams and resources to the state in crisis.
- AUSTRAUMAPLAN allows the Commonwealth to become involved in a local incident if it is of national significance.
- OSMASSCASPLAN is a national overseas MCI response plan to deal with repatriation of Australian citizens, victims and nationals of other countries involved in an MCI in a foreign land.
- AUSASSISTPLAN involves Commonwealth funding, through the Department of Foreign Affairs and Trade (DFAT), for an MCI response in a foreign land. It differs from Australian Aid, which involves financial support from DFAT provided to a developing nation affected by a disaster.

States and territories

Separate state and territory emergency response plans, designed to provide long-term assistance to people and communities, are activated during the response phase of an incident to provide early commitment of resources. The principal role of the state/territory health department is to deal with matters associated with the general health of the community and to provide health and medical services required as a result of a major emergency or disaster. Specific specialty plans for events such as shore retrieval, major burns management and terrorism and chemical, biological and radiation (CBR) incidents have been developed in order to harness a coordinated and cooperative multi-city response.

Very broadly, these legislative frameworks provide for:

- disaster planning and response coordination of activities throughout the state/territory to be enacted by the chief commissioner for police or nominated deputies
- roles and responsibilities of emergency services and support organisations for various types of emergencies or disasters
- state/territory health departments to coordinate agencies involved in providing recovery actions in communities following major incidents and disasters.

The state/territory health department ensures coordination of:

- provision of hospital and medical services to an incident
- provision of transport and hospitalisation for the injured or sick
- supply of medical and first-aid teams
- setting up of medical centres and casualty clearing stations
- provision of disease control and other scientific and pathological services required
- health and scientific survey teams
- public health information, advice and warnings, to control and support agencies and for release to the affected communities.

The state/territory health department has direct responsibilities as the control agency for:

- infectious disease outbreaks
- contaminated foodstuffs and water
- CBR substance releases
- nuclear incidents.

State/territory emergency management plans involve cooperation between all combat agencies, usually led by police, to develop appropriate non-medical responses for all incidents. The state/territory health departments have statutory responsibility to provide the necessary planning and response required to deal with matters associated with the general health of the community and to provide medical and hospital services required as a result of a major emergency or disaster.

Local health districts

Individual local health districts will develop detailed plans specific to that local area. Local emergency management committees, which include key stakeholders, ensure that the local community will be prepared and able to commit local resources.

Hospitals and departments within health facilities

In compliance with state/territory health plans, all hospitals and health facilities are required to have emergency response plans, including disaster plans, referred to as external emergency response plans. Each hospital will have a command structure for effective communication and coordinate deployment of essential resources.

'All hazards' approach

This approach to disaster planning ensures that contingencies are in place to respond to a variety of incidents involving a large number of victims. The plans must be flexible to respond to a wide scope of scenarios. For instance, a disaster plan should be able to respond to a natural disaster such as a cyclone with some forewarning or a man-made disaster such as a terrorist attack which is a sudden-impact disaster without preparation time.

'All agencies' approach

This approach to disaster response helps to build a resilient community where all emergency service key stakeholders are prepared, trained and capable of responding to an MCI situation. It requires a clearly defined command structure in order to coordinate and control the chaos that would otherwise ensue in a major incident.

Medical emergency response plans and agencies

A medical response plan (health plan) is a support plan for the state/territory DISPLAN. It provides for a clinical care organisational framework that outlines the roles and responsibilities of the various participating medical and healthcare responders, and provides the necessary integrated procedures for altering and mobilising medical and healthcare personnel, for establishing on-site medical control and for definitive treatment of casualties.

The concept is that all arrangements and procedures made within the medical response can be applied from the smallest to the largest incident with a build-up of medical coordination and medical and health resources as necessary, following the general pattern of normal daily operational procedures wherever possible. This extends to contingency planning and has a presence at major events where potential public threat is perceived to exist.

The state/territory DISPLAN is further divided into district and local emergency response committees, to ensure that an integrated effective response can be provided in times of emergency.

EMERGENCY SERVICE ORGANISATIONS

Also referred to as combat agencies, and include:
- Police Service
- Fire Brigade
- Rural Fire Service
- Ambulance Service
- State Emergency Service
- Volunteer Rescue Associations such as Marine Search & Rescue, Ski Patrol, Cave Rescue Squad

EMERGENCY OPERATION CENTRE (EOC)

These operation centres are in a centralised location where the heads of all combat agencies can meet to communicate, share information and achieve command and control of an incident. EOCs will be activated when a major incident is declared and a coordinated support effort is required to assist with on-site medical care and transport of injured victims to appropriate hospitals for further treatment. For longer-term recovery assistance, EOCs are essential to coordinate the physical, medical, mental health and public health issues of victims and to assist with ongoing needs of communities. EOCs have representatives from all essential emergency service organisations. EOCs are activated at all levels of government, including receiving hospitals.

HEALTH SERVICE COMMAND AND CONTROL

This is determined by the state/territory DISPLAN and is coordinated by the state/territory health service's functional area coordinator (HSFAC) who controls the mobilisation of all healthcare personnel and resources to the scene of any emergency when the plan is activated. This includes:

- the mobilisation of resources to the incident site, and initiation of triage and treatment
- establishing 24-hour operational communications to initiate and instigate the necessary mobilisation of site medical commanders, medical response teams and notify casualty receiving hospitals in major emergencies
- the initial setting up of a casualty clearing station by the first ambulance team for triage and treatment on-site until a joint medical command post is established
- coordination of first aid with the ambulance service until the establishment of adequate medical response teams on-site
- coordination with ambulance command for transportation of casualties to appropriate hospitals
- coordination with HazMat and fire services for assistance with on-site decontamination of people exposed to toxic or microbiological hazards deploying the expertise of public health officers in emergencies where public health is threatened; all work within the framework of the health department public health sector for preventing and controlling outbreaks of communicable diseases, and for the preservation of acceptable standards for safe drinking water and foodstuffs.

HEALTH SERVICES FUNCTIONAL AREA COORDINATOR (HSFAC)

This senior medical advisor manages the internal administrative functions of the medical response plan and is responsible for activating a health response in a disaster, allocating resources and coordinating the initial recovery operations. All health personnel involved must be appropriately trained in emergency management and understand the command and control structure of disaster response.

Although specific contingencies and structures vary throughout Australia, the senior medical advisor generally manages the EOC when activated in support of the medical response system. The HSFAC also assists with the distribution of mass casualties to hospitals and, in times of major emergencies, will provide briefings via the health department to the appropriate minister and the media.

Pre-hospital medical coordination and disaster scene control

Although titles, role delineations, responsibilities, definitions and plans may vary among the states, the following principles are generic. The descriptions outline the events and actions that are required for proficient on-site disaster medicine management.

INCIDENT CONTROL

The disaster-site medical procedures in place for establishing early medical control for the proper triage, treatment and transportation of casualties are initially provided by officers of the first responding ambulance vehicle. As an ambulance commander arrives on-site, further assessments will be made and an incident command centre (ICC) established. The ICC is the location for commanders from each of the emergency services. These officers take command of their own agency and communicate across agencies to control the incident and allocate resources. All incoming medical responders report to the command post.

The medical services provided on-site will be limited initially, and will use the principle of packaging for safe transport to definitive care, thereby doing as little as possible, as simply as possible, as quickly as possible and to as many as possible.

Life-saving procedures, such as airway management, immediate decompression of tension pneumothorax, arrest of haemorrhage, fracture stabilisation and relief of pain where necessary, may be the limit of medical assistance where medical resources are few. Effective triage prioritisation of casualties by a triage officer, usually an ambulance officer from the first responding team, is essential to determine number and type of casualty in the MCI. Early, accurate communication to the ICC and further up the chain of command to the HSFAC will enable effective delivery of personnel and resources to the scene.

INCIDENT MEDICAL COMMANDER

The medical commander (MC) at the scene directs medical aspects of treatment which occurs primarily in the casualty clearing station. The MC coordinates medical teams on-site and is the top of the chain of command for medical response. Hence, all requests for resupply, resources and personnel pass through the MC. The MC determines the need for specialist teams, which include mental health and public health officers depending on the particular incident. As the MC oversees several medical response teams, coordinates transport and prioritises resource allocation, it is imperative that they do not get involved in medical care of individual patients. The MC is usually located in the ICC.

The MC is responsible for:

- liaising with the ambulance commander to coordinate the health response at the scene
- establishing a casualty clearing station (CCS)
- ensuring an ambulance circuit with suitable access and egress routes is established to transport casualties from the CCS to hospital
- establishing clear liaison with the police commander and other emergency services
- providing a frequent and accurate manifest to HSFAC detailing numbers and triage priorities of MCI victims following assessment of the scene
- allocating roles for health personnel in the CCS and determining the need for health personnel to be deployed to the scene of the incident (hot zone)
- assessing the requirement for relief of health response teams or for further medical teams at the scene, including specialist surgical services for amputation and extrication for further first-aid support and whether psychological services may be needed.

The MC's role is to:

- initiate and arrange distribution of casualties to appropriate hospital facilities, in conjunction with an ambulance commander—the concept is to distribute casualties to as many hospitals as practicable to avoid facility overload
- alert HSFAC to mobilise medical response teams and other medical and healthcare responders to the disaster scene
- liaise and request activation of health department emergency operation centres at state, territory and national level if necessary, and provide situation reports at frequent intervals to EOC and to request further assistance

- instigate stand-down of the various medical and health responders after consultation with the on-site ambulance commander and other emergency service authorities
- participate in regular media updates and community notifications as instructed by the HSFAC.

CASUALTY CLEARING STATION (CCS)

This is initially established by the ambulance service and eventually managed by the medical response teams deployed to the scene. The primary requirement is that the CCS must be located in a safe place. When establishing a CCS, it should be a safe distance away from the 'hot zone', as sheltered as possible from elements such as sun, rain and wind and of an adequate size to safely manage casualties delivered from the scene. It serves as a point for secondary triage by the medical response teams and for provision of essential treatments to safely package the casualties for transport to hospital for definitive care. The CCS must be accessible to ambulances and other vehicles to transport casualties away from the scene.

The CCS is coordinated by the casualty clearing officer (CCO). The CCO reports up to the incident medical commander. The role of the CCO is to assess the number and types of casualties, to commence secondary triage of casualties and to determine which casualties are packaged and ready for transport. The CCO must ensure the area selected as the CCS is appropriate and suited to treating casualties.

HEALTH RESPONSE TEAMS (HRTs)

State/territory health plans have designated hospitals with capacity to deploy disaster response teams in the event of a major incident. The selection and dispatch of HRTs is the responsibility of the HSFAC. HRTs are generally deployed from local health districts (LHDs) away from the incident, so as not to deplete staff from receiving hospitals. Each team consists of 2 senior doctors and 4 resuscitation nurses. In Australia, all team members must be appropriately trained and accredited to work in the pre-hospital environment using the Major Incident Medical Management Support (MIMMS) structure. All team members are registered on arrival at the site and need to be in appropriate pre-hospital uniforms, including regulation hats and footwear. Each team deployed to the incident site carries regulation disaster packs containing essential equipment. In NSW, this is coordinated by the Health Emergency Management Unit (HEMU).

These teams provide treatment to injured victims based on disaster triage priorities (SMART triage, discussed later in this chapter). Working in austere conditions with minimal resources, these teams provide essential treatment to allow safe passage of critically injured victims to hospitals for definitive care.

HRTs have a critical role in minimising surge impact on hospitals by sorting victims based on their triage priority and stabilising them to allow safe transport to the most appropriate hospitals both within and outside the immediate network. Those not needing in-hospital or ED management can be referred to outpatient and community-based resources, in keeping with regional or state/territory plans.

Triage

Triage generally implies direction of clinical resources to the most seriously ill or injured by a trieur or triage officer, in order to get the right casualty to the right place at the right time. In a mass-casualty situation, demand may exceed resource availability. It is neither ethical nor practical to classify clearly non-salvageable victims as top priorities. (See Table 47.1.)

TRIAGE SIEVE AND SORT

The triaging system in an MCI must be quick, simple, safe and reproducible. Triage performed by emergency personnel at the disaster site must be a 'quick look' and is referred to as *triage sieve*; this is followed by a more detailed reassessment in the treatment area of the CCS, referred to as *triage sort*. This process enables pre-hospital personnel to prioritise medical care and transport victims to definitive care in hospital in an organised and rational way.

Triage is a dynamic process that is repeated at each reassessment to ensure refinement of urgency stratification and to respond appropriately to the ongoing evolution of a casualty's injury complex and consequent physiology.

In Australia, disaster triage follows the international standardised processes of Major Incident Management Support, a tested and validated tool for pre-hospital triage in a mass-casualty situation, where the number of casualties exceeds available resources.

Table 47.1 Triage priorities and criteria for MCI victims

Priority	Colour	Description	Criteria
1	Red	Immediate	• Severely injured • Immediate resuscitation, life-saving procedures and transportation required
2	Yellow	Urgent	• Significant injuries • Intervention required within 4–6 hours
3	Green	Delayed	• Casualty ambulant—'walking wounded' • Has less-serious injuries, can await delayed treatment • Uninjured psychologically disturbed victims are included in this category
4	Blue	Expectant	• Injuries so severe will require extensive medical care which will compromise the treatment of large numbers of other casualties
Dead	Black	Deceased	• Medical officer is required to certify death on triage card • Body becomes the responsibility of police/coroner's office • Body not to be moved without police in attendance; then body is stored in mortuary on/near incident site

Sieve

This initial casualty assessment is based on the findings of a primary survey.

- If casualties are ambulant, they are initially regarded as 'walking wounded' and are directed or escorted to a separate area of the CCS. These casualties are given a **priority 3** and will await delayed treatment and transport. Ambulant casualties are also referred to as 'green' patients.
- If casualties are not ambulant, a triaging primary survey is performed (see Figure 47.1). This looks at the airway,

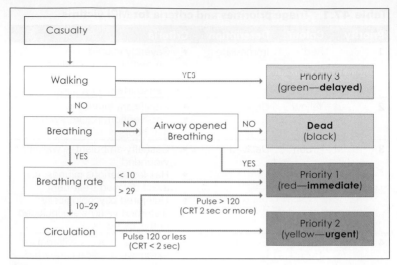

Figure 47.1 Triage sieve protocol

respiratory rate and capillary refill time. If there is haemodynamic instability, the casualty will be given a **priority 1** triage category to be moved to the CCS for commencement of immediate life-saving interventions. They are also referred to by colour code as 'red' patients.

- Non-ambulant casualties who are stable on primary ABC survey are given a **priority 2**. These second-priority patients may have significant injuries, but at the time of initial triage there is no evidence of airway compromise and they have normal respiratory and perfusion status assessments. These constitute most of the injuries that are time-critical on a pattern of blast injury. The implication of being stratified as a priority 2 ('yellow') patient is that treatment should be provided in a hospital within 4–6 hours.

- The operation of **priority 4** ('blue' patients) assignment is declared by the incident commander if the number of critically ill casualties far outweighs the resources available to treat at the scene or to transport to definitive care in hospitals. In normal circumstances these patients would be given a priority 1 for immediate intervention to treat life-threatening

TRIAGE REVISED TRAUMA SCORE (TRTS)	
SYSTOLIC BP	CODED VALUE
> 89	4
76–89	3
50–75	2
1–49	1
0	0

RESPIRATORY RATE	CODED VALUE
10–29	4
> 29	3
6–9	2
1–51	1
0	0

GLASGOW COMA SCALE SCORE	CODED VALUE
13–15	4
9–12	3
6–8	2
4–5	1
3	0

Immediate priority 1 Score = 1–10	Urgent priority 2 Score = 11	Delayed priority 3 Score = 12–15

Figure 47.2 Triage Revised Trauma Score system to sort casualty priority

injuries, but in the resource-poor and austere conditions of an MCI the aim is to do the best for the most, and it may be deemed inappropriate to direct several personnel and much resources to provide treatment at the scene for a single victim in an MCI of great magnitude (Figure 47.2).

Treatment

Treatment at the scene is limited to the institution of simple life-saving primary survey manoeuvres. These are:

- airway clearance by manual or other available methods
- decompression of a tension pneumothorax by needle thoracotomy

- control of external haemorrhage by compression bandage, tourniquets or splinting open-limb fractures
- appropriate positioning of unconscious patients or patients with head, chest, abdominal, pelvic or spinal injuries.

SMART tags

Standardised triage tags are currently used across NSW Health and most other states and territories. These nationally accepted triage tags are waterproof, carry personal details of the victim, allow documentation of injuries, allow serial assessment of the Triage Revised Trauma Score (TRTS; see below) and can be used to document treatment instituted at the scene. They become part of the patient's medical record in the incident. Casualties must be re-triaged on the basis of response to simple first aid, injury pattern and likely prognosis.

- Priority 1 patients based on triage sieve assessment will be tagged with the red side of the SMART tag showing. These patients require immediate medical attention and are moved to the CCS as first priority, to commence treatment and transport to definitive care.
- Priority 2 patients will have the yellow side of the SMART tag visible.
- The walking wounded, priority 3 patients, have the green side showing. If the casualty's triage priority changes, the SMART tag is easily changed to reflect this.
- Those casualties that die at the scene have a separate black 'Deceased' SMART tag attached to them. All personal belongings of these deceased victims must remain with the body as forensic evidence.
- In the event of a MCI involving a CBR agent, an alternative SMART tag is available which can be included in the plastic bag along with the standard triage tag.
- Priority 4: If critically injured or ill patients are unresponsive to these measures and unlikely to survive, they become second-priority casualties. This is sometimes known as reverse triage. In current MCI parlance, this is the priority 4/Blue/Expectant category. If use of priority 4 is declared at the MCI, a corner of the red triage tag is folded over to show a blue triangular patch. These casualties are critically

ill and will require significant resources to treat. The incident commander must declare the operation of this priority 4 triage category at the commencement of the emergency response, based on information regarding casualty numbers and availability of resources. A senior doctor or a senior nurse may be allocated at the scene to the care of extremely severely injured patients with a low probability of survival. Intensive efforts to resuscitate these patients may jeopardise the survival of large numbers of other casualties because of an excessive drain on resources. Supportive and palliative care only should be given until resources are available to commence more vigorous resuscitation, if appropriate.

Sort

This triage method is the more formal risk stratification that identifies time-critical patients and assists in scheduling optimal allocation of available resources. It is commonly used by emergency medical personnel on admission of patients to casualty clearing stations or field hospitals.

This method of triage is based on the Revised Trauma Score (RTS) and is consistent with the Australasian Triage Scale and triage practices taught in emergency management of severe trauma (EMST), emergency life support (ELS), advanced paediatric life support (APLS) and Major Incident Medical Management and Support (MIMMS) courses. It is a repeated process that is dependent on traditional ongoing patient observation.

Triage sort is generally implemented in the field utilising the RTS in order to rank physiological embarrassment and allocating an ordinal score using respiratory rate, systolic blood pressure and Glasgow Coma Scale scores. This assists with re-prioritisation or risk stratification of casualties.

Further refinement of triage can be assisted by attention to pattern of injuries or mechanism of injuries. However, in a trauma-related MCI, a considerable number of patients may be classified as time-critical on mechanism of injury alone (Table 47.2). Although these patients are of lesser priority owing to normal physiological parameters or the absence of an identified pattern of injury, they are victims of major trauma, have sustained major forces and are at risk of significant and occult internal injury (Figure 47.3).

Table 47.2 Features suggestive of severe trauma or time-critical casualties

Pattern of injury	All penetrating injuries: head/neck/chest/abdomen/pelvis/axilla/groin
	Blunt injuries: • patients with a significant injury to a single region—head/neck/chest/abdomen/axilla/groin • patients with injuries involving 2 or more of the above body regions
	Specific injuries: • limb amputations/limb-threatening injuries • suspected spinal cord injury • burns > 20% of body surface area or suspected respiratory tract involvement • crush injuries where pressure is maintained for > 1 hour • major compound fracture or open dislocation • fracture to 2 or more proximal long bones • fractured pelvis
Mechanism of injury	• Car occupants involved in high-speed motor vehicle crash (e.g. impact speed > 60 km/h with major vehicle damage) • Pedestrians or cyclists hit by vehicles travelling at > 30 km/h • Patients ejected from a vehicle • Patients in a car that has rolled over • Patients in a motor vehicle crash where there is a death of another or same vehicle occupant • Patients who have fallen from a height > 3 m • Patients hit by an object that has fallen from > 3 m • Motorcyclists, cyclists • Explosion victims • Patients who are trapped and likely to remain so for > 30 min
Age and concurrent medical problems	Age > 55 years or < 5 years Pregnancy Significant underlying medical condition

Triage officers

It is preferable for the triage role to be undertaken by a senior doctor or resuscitation nurse, experienced and accredited in the sort and sieve methods of disaster triage.

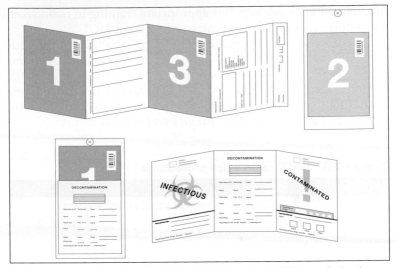

Figure 47.3 Triage cards—SMART tags (above) and CBR tags (below)

FIRST-AID SERVICES

First-aid services can be provided by several different organisations; primarily St John Ambulance Australia and the Australian Red Cross. These may be complemented by other first-aid providers such as the Australian Ski Patrol Association, the Royal Life Saving Society or Surf Life Saving Australia, depending on the circumstances. First-aid agencies are often activated by the ambulance service. The principal role of first-aid organisations is to assist with minor injuries where the setting up of separate treatment centres is necessary to cope with walking wounded. First-aid teams generally work under the direction of a site MC or ambulance commander in casualty collecting stations or in field hospitals.

Communication

Good communication is essential to the effective functioning and coordination of an MCI operation. Breakdown in communication has been cited as one of the commonest failures of major incident management. Various methods of communication are used in MCI management, including landlines, mobile phones, megaphones and television broadcasts, but appropriate training in radio voice procedures is essential for those working in an MCI.

There are several advantages of radio communication through a specific network for the MCI, especially in remote areas and when mobile networks are jammed. All members of a health response team must be trained in NATO radio voice procedures, including use of standardised phrases (Table 47.3), phonetic alphabet (Table 47.4), clarity, brevity and accuracy.

Table 47.3 NATO radio voice procedures

Word/phrase	Meaning
THIS IS	When calling, say the call sign that you want followed by your call sign. For example: ALPHA THIS IS BRAVO.
OVER	I have finished speaking and it is your turn to reply.
OUT	I have finished talking to you.
RADIO CHECK	Can you hear me? If you can, then how well? Ideally it will be LOUD and CLEAR. If it isn't then describe it, such as WEAK BUT READABLE, etc. Reply in numerical/alphabetical order.
OK/ROGER	Use either word to show that you have received and understood the message. Note: 'COPY THAT' is just another, non-standard way of saying OK or ROGER but can be confusing if you really want them to copy it!
MESSAGE	I have a message for you—are you ready to receive it?
SEND	I am ready to receive your message.
MORE TO FOLLOW	The message isn't finished—but have you got it all so far?
SAY AGAIN	This can be SAY AGAIN ALL BEFORE or ALL AFTER or NUMBER or anything else that you didn't get down.
ACKNOWLEDGE	Please tell me that you have received the message. If you have, then respond as ROGER (or OK)—you do not have to read it all back.
WAIT	Give me 10 seconds to find a pencil or whatever.
WAIT OUT	I'll get back to you.
I SPELL	Say the word followed by I SPELL, then spell the word phonetically. If there is more than one word then say FIRST WORD—*say the word*—I SPELL … etc.

Table 47.4   NATO alphabet and numbers for radio communication in an MCI situation

Letter	Word	Letter	Word
A	Alpha	T	Tango
B	Bravo	U	Uniform
C	Charlie	V	Victor
D	Delta	W	Whisky
E	Echo	X	X-ray
F	Foxtrot	Y	Yankee
G	Golf	Z	Zulu
H	Hotel	**Numbers**	
I	India	1	Wun
J	Juliet	2	Too
K	Kilo	3	Th-ree
L	Lima	4	For-wer
M	Mike	5	Fi-yiv
N	November	6	Six
O	Oscar	7	Sev-en
P	Papa	8	Ate
Q	Quebec	9	Niner
R	Romeo	0	Zero
S	Sierra		

From the Advanced Life Support Group Australia (MIMMS), September 2003; updated 3rd Edition December 2012.

Code Brown: hospital external disaster or emergency response plan

All public hospitals are required to have external emergency response (EER) plans to cope with mass casualties directed to hospital facilities for treatment. In keeping with national standards for colour-coding emergency responses, an external emergency, which includes disasters and MCIs, is referred to as a Code Brown.

Public hospitals are required to develop, implement and test contingencies for the reception of an influx of casualties from a major incident. This is a requirement both of legislature and of the Australian Council on Healthcare Standards. During a health emergency, hospitals will have to convert quickly from their standard care capacity to surge capacity. This is achieved through re-prioritisation of healthcare needs to provide essential services to mass casualties. This would include cancellation of elective surgeries, early discharge of hospitalised patients and diversion of patients with minor complaints to alternative healthcare providers such as local GPs and medical centres. However, all public hospitals throughout the state/territory are expected to maintain core functions during a Code Brown.

Some private hospitals participate in counter-disaster planning activities, especially if they are affiliated with or in close proximity to a large general hospital. Their Code Brown plans work side-by-side with the main receiving hospital, and a memorandum of understanding exists between the hospital management and the local health district or state/territory HSFAC. They may be required to provide sheltered accommodation for casualties from an incident or ongoing care of admitted patients being decanted from a local public hospital for it to receive casualties.

Code Brown (EER) plans may also include procedures for providing a trained and equipped medical team for casualty treatment at a disaster site. These teams are referred to as HRTs. The provision of such medical teams may reduce the ED's effectiveness. The state/territory HSFAC will give consideration to replacing or providing a team from another facility if the responding hospital is to continue to be a major casualty receiving hospital. Some base hospitals in rural regions also have the capability to provide such teams, with smaller hospitals having a reduced capability.

Certain first-aid organisations such as St John Ambulance are also able to provide medical teams on request through the state/territory HSFAC to the Commissioner of St John Ambulance Australia. The Royal Flying Doctor Service (RFDS) of Australia has the capacity to provide medical teams for deployment to a MCI site within or outside its normal area of operation. The coordination of these resources is through the state/territory HSFAC and the chief medical controller of RFDS as well as the director of the aeromedical retrieval service.

PLANNING, EXERCISES AND REVIEW OF PLANS
All participating agencies integral to a medical DISPLAN response have sub-plans to ensure that effective response is available when

required. Integrated medical response planning with other emergency services takes place at all levels, addressing various hazards that exist. The exercising and testing of plans takes place at frequent intervals, both within and between agencies, as necessary following planning reviews.

HEALTHCARE FACILITY EMERGENCY MANAGEMENT PLANS

The role of a healthcare facility in responding to external incidents will depend on the size and scope of healthcare services usually offered. Healthcare facilities that offer acute, subacute, long-term care and community outreach healthcare have a greater capacity to manage demand and overflows. The Code Brown plan of such large facilities will include arrangements for the reception of large numbers of casualties and will include designated treatment areas, security arrangements and the control of vehicular and pedestrian traffic to facilitate ambulance turnaround. Smaller hospitals can contribute by providing care to patients or casualties not requiring intensive resources or by assisting in decanting convalescing patients from other acute services, thus freeing resources to receive disaster victims.

EMERGENCY OPERATIONS CENTRE

A designated area is established within each healthcare facility to function as the EOC in the event of a major incident impacting the operation of the hospital. The EOC is equipped with computers providing data relating to the Code Brown, televisions available for following media alerts, adequate phone lines, radio communications and fax machines. The EOC is staffed by the hospital incident commander and the disaster coordinator as well as media relations officers and other essential executive officers. It becomes responsible for the management of all aspects of the incident as it affects the hospital. In addition to overseeing clinical operations in a Code Brown situation, the EOC manages planning, logistics and finance duties.

Stages of response

In general, the phases of an external disaster emergency management plan are as follows.

Alert: a disaster situation is possible

Begin preparations

Develop contingency for potential escalation in required response

Standby: a disaster situation is probable

Complete preparations

Ensure readiness to receive casualties

Prepare to receive: a disaster situation exists

Activation of Code Brown EER plan

Prepare to receive casualties

Stand down: a disaster situation is contained

Cancellation of response

Replacement of equipment

All personnel resume normal duties

STAGES OF THE EXTERNAL EMERGENCY RESPONSE PLAN

Alert

Notification

A hospital may become aware of a possible disaster by one of several ways:

- advised by one of the emergency services
- media enquiry
- member of the public
- ambulant victims presenting to the ED for treatment prior to any other notification
- several patients presenting with similar symptoms or clinical syndromes over a short time suggesting a CBR incident
- HSFAC notification of an incident which will impact on the health service.

All notifications or alerts should be validated before activation of an EER plan.

Incident response team

Each healthcare facility should have an incident response team (IRT) which can assess the situation and validate the alert. The IRT should consist of at least the hospital's disaster coordinator and incident commander. When the alert has been validated, the hospital incident commander or similarly authorised person will activate the EER plan.

Standby
Standby advises the health service of the presence of an external incident that may impact on hospital resources and services. During this phase, designated officers assess resources. Current staffing levels, any imminent shift changes and any extra staff that would be required in such a situation are noted. Bed availability is estimated.

The designated EOC is established. Staff must access action cards or documents and become familiar with their roles during the various stages of an EER. Staff not covered by specific action cards must follow instructions from their line manager or continue normal duties.

The operations chief will determine which staff are to be called in for duty and at what stage in the EER this should occur. If a protracted response is anticipated, staff may be required to come in several hours later. Notification is dependent on the nature of the incident. For example, for a Code Brown involving a chemical hazard it may be decided not to advise the senior surgical staff. In addition, the time of day may determine extent of notification within the healthcare facility. For example, an MCI occurring out of hours would be limited to the ED, ICU and operating theatres and might not include areas such as ambulatory care and other outpatient facilities which would not be staffed out of hours.

It is a priority for the operations chief to decant the ED in order for the treating teams to receive casualties from the incident.

Activation (Prepare to receive)
Access to hospital beds
The following are principles to guide creation of bed capacity. It is desirable to accommodate all the disaster victims in one area or receiving ward. The following groups of patients are considered for discharge or transfer to less-acute facilities:
• electives with non-life-threatening conditions
• patients for routine investigation
• stable postnatal patients

- stable patients undergoing long-term treatment
- stable postoperative patients
- patients able to be accommodated by a 'hospital in the home' program.

Emergency department response

Aim

The aim of care in the ED is to rapidly assess and stabilise patients and then clear them from the department as soon as possible to enable offloading of ambulances. If the external disaster is limited with no possibility of further casualties, a full patient assessment could be completed in the ED in keeping with usual practices. Most priority 1 casualties would require emergency operative management of open wounds and fractured limbs, and as such have no place in the ED on arrival from the scene. Other priority 1 casualties with airway compromise or significant blunt trauma would require ICU admission and the hospital's Code Brown plan should allow for direct or rapid admission of such patients to its ICU.

Staff deployment and call-in notifications

Key clinical staff, clinical departments and management staff placed on standby are advised of the escalation. Departmental managers should call staff in individually. Clinical staff called in must be briefed and allocated roles by the hospital in charge (HIC). Resources are initially directed to the ED to manage the surge of casualties. Ward staff may be required to assist with early discharges of existing patients to decant essential wards.

Triage officers

An appropriately trained senior medical officer and senior nurse would be allocated to perform secondary or tertiary triage on arriving casualties. The triage officers should be assisted by a clerical officer to document details on arrival. The triage officers should be in close communication with the ED team leader regarding numbers and acuity of casualties arriving from the scene. This is usually done via hand-held radio, as other modalities of communication can be unreliable in an MCI. There may be a need for more than one triage officer if the influx of casualties is high.

There is also an ongoing obligation to continue triage of non-disaster patients. It may be elected to simply use the Australasian Triage Scale with reverse triage of expectant cases designated as urgent.

Resuscitation team leader

This role is allocated to an appropriately trained senior medical officer who may need to manage all the resuscitation rooms simultaneously. All available clinical support is directed to the critically ill casualties arriving from the scene. Close communication with both the surgical team leader and the ICU is essential for the safe and rapid disposition of these casualties.

Acute care team leader

A senior medical officer with appropriate training will oversee the care of patients with triage priority 2. Many of these patients may have significant occult injuries and may ideally need to be managed in resuscitation areas. Thorough clinical assessment and close monitoring is essential to avoid missing significant occult injuries.

Clinical records

Currently, most hospitals do not have electronic medical record (EMR) capabilities to operate in a major incident. Hence, casualties from a MCI will need clinical notes to be documented on paper. However, progress is being made to use existing electronic medical records during such incidents. Previously compiled standard clinical records containing progress notes, medication charts, pathology and medical imaging request forms should be utilised for all MCI victims. Each MCI victim should be allocated an MCI medical record number for ease of tracking. The SMART triage tags should be retained within the clinical records.

Clinical zones

In order to coordinate clinical care, and depending on the size of the department and the anticipated workload, the ED can be divided into different zones with separate teams of clinical staff. Other clinical areas, such as outpatients, could be set up as satellite EDs to manage overflow ambulatory care patients.

Medical staff

During the standby stage of a Code Brown response, the emergency team leader should brief all medical and nursing staff on the expectations during the ensuing hours. It is preferable for ED doctors to be allocated to work in specific zones. Their roles should be clearly defined in their action cards. They should be appropriately dressed in personal protective equipment (PPE) and wear tabards showing their designation.

Additional medical officers may be requested through the EOC. It is imperative that staff follow their chain of command for all requests. All staff should work within their scope of practice and preferably in clinical areas in which they are familiar in order to reduce risk of mishaps.

In trauma incidents, a surgeon should remain in the ED for immediate referrals and assessments. That surgeon is responsible for prioritising patients for theatre.

An anaesthetist will assist with urgent airway intervention, referrals and preoperative assessments as required.

Junior medical staff may be utilised to manage ambulatory patients in designated satellite areas. Similarly, medical and nursing students may be utilised appropriately in clinical areas.

Nursing staff

ED nursing staff roles generally parallel those of the medical staff, as treating teams are allocated to specific areas. Their role focuses on the nursing aspects of patient care and the management of the designated ED zones or other designated areas. Nurses receive and assess patients and assist with the examination and treatment of patients.

Senior nursing staff allocate nurses and clerical support staff to the designated areas and assist the triage officer in resource allocation.

Other

A particular focus is the availability of extra equipment, sterile stock and medications. All requests for resupply must be escalated through the team leader to ensure that requests are not duplicated nor missed in the potentially chaotic working environment associated with a Code Brown response.

> **Box 47.1 Hospital-wide services necessary for external disaster plan**
>
> **Departments and services contributing to Code Brown external disaster responses:**
> - Executive management
> - Emergency department
> - Intensive care unit and high-dependency unit
> - Operating theatres and recovery units
> - Receiving and non-receiving wards
> - Outpatients department for managing ambulatory victims with minor injuries or psychological complaints
> - Medical imaging
> - Laboratory services
> - Pharmacy services
> - Supply and materials department
> - Central sterilising supply department
> - Environmental services
> - Wardspersons and porters
> - Linen and waste services
> - Food services
> - Engineering and facilities department
> - Security
> - Traffic control
> - Mortuary services
> - Social work department for management of worried-well victims and families of disaster victims
> - Community relations and media management
> - Volunteers

In-hospital responses

The detailed management of in-hospital responses and executive management issues are beyond the scope of this chapter.

Stand down

The cessation of the EER and return to usual operations is initiated by the hospital incident commander via the EOC. The response may conclude on advice from the disaster site or the area HSFAC. However, the response plan may require ongoing activation until pressure on the health service or hospital resources has subsided and normal activities can be resumed.

The stand-down mechanism may be total or progressive. Progressive stand-down can be initiated when certain areas are no longer required to function under response plan conditions.

Debriefing

There are two types of debriefing: operational debriefing and psychological debriefing. The latter has two components: immediate debriefing is a defusing of staff; formal counselling is offered for ongoing symptoms.

Operational debrief

A formal operational debrief, involving key participants and heads of departments, should be conducted within 1 week. This debriefing examines the incident and the organisational response. Reports are prepared for the emergency response committee and health department as required. Recommendations in this report will form the basis of revisions to the healthcare facility's EER plan.

Defusing

Defusing is the immediate attention to the psychological needs of staff. This provides staff with an opportunity to express their feelings and thoughts about the episode.

Counselling

Counselling aims to assist staff with long-term distress suffered as a consequence of the disaster response. These services are generally provided by employee assistance programs or may be accessed through the various health departments.

Chemical, biological and radiological (CBR) hazards

The approach to CBR exposures is similar in principle to multi-casualty trauma incidents whether exposed victims are single casualties, several or within the context of mass casualties. The prime difference is the need to prevent contamination and/or infection of rescuers, healthcare providers and the community. The approach aims to provide optimum care while maintaining safety for other patients and staff. A second broad aim is to effectively decontaminate patients prior to entering the ED. It focuses on a sequence of actions and interventions that admits decontaminated casualties to EDs. A further aim is the expedient identification of causal agents that may enable specific treatment.

Acute recovery incorporates the restoration of areas used for decontamination to usual functions. It includes management of contaminated items for cleaning and inspection by hazard management or public health agencies. Where applicable, non-disposable medical equipment is cleaned and returned to regular use. Some contingency plans include specific equipment kits reserved for use in CBR incidents.

In the field, the sequence begins with identification of casualties and proceeds to isolation, decontamination, triage, treatment and transport to hospital. ED contingencies are similar. However, treatment may need to commence before or concurrently with decontamination. The main risk for hospitals is the arrival of contaminated or infected individuals prior to recognition or advice of a CBR incident, with consequent contamination of the ED and, potentially, the whole healthcare facility.

FEATURES OF CBR AND NUCLEAR HAZARDS

CBR and nuclear substances potentially cause harm to human health. Incidents involving these substances often generate vapours, fumes, dusts and mists. Hazardous wastes can pollute waste streams, causing a threat to public health, safety or to the environment. They can also be invisible.

CBR hazards can be infectious, toxic, mutagenic, carcinogenic, teratogenic, explosive, flammable, corrosive, oxidising and radioactive and may cause immediate and/or long-term health effects. Exposure may result in poisoning, irritation, chemical burns, sensitisation, cancer, birth defects or organ disease of the skin, lungs, liver, kidneys and nervous system. The severity of the illness or disease depends on the nature of the substance and the dose absorbed.

Detailed information on all the hazards, their properties, effects and treatments is beyond the scope of this discussion. The following is provided as a broad overview.

MODE OF PRESENTATION

Education of all staff in recognising a contaminated or CBR-hazard-exposed person is necessary in order to minimise the risk of ED exposure and contamination. Self-presentation prior to notification by emergency services agencies is common in chemical incidents. Occasionally, emergency services may be unaware of the incident. In this situation the health service has a system-initiation function. In biological incidents, there is often a trickle followed by an epidemic flood of patients. Radiological incidents may involve burns, the consequences of initial radiation illness or the management of ongoing radioactivity.

Impact on the ED is compounded by an uninformed public, presentations of the worried well and a lack of knowledge by community-based doctors and healthcare providers. It has been estimated that the ratio of worried well to affected victims is 10:1.

CHEMICAL AGENTS

Nerve agents

Nerve agents are organophosphates that act by irreversibly bonding with acetylcholine esterase and inhibiting its action at the neuromuscular junction, causing a cholinergic crisis of glandular hypersecretion, vomiting, diarrhoea, incontinence and flaccid paralysis of skeletal muscles. Examples include Tabun (GA), sarin (GB), soman (GD), VX and most recently Novichok used in the United Kingdom.

Blistering agents

These irritate the epithelial surfaces by direct contact. The skin and mucosal surfaces are the target tissues. The mustard agents and lewisite are examples of this group.

Incapacitating agents

This group causes short-term disabling physical and/or mental effects by affecting higher cortical function. The group includes central nervous system depressants, stimulants and hallucinogens. To qualify for membership of this group, agents must be potent, last hours to days, not be potentially lethal at effective doses and have no long-term adverse sequelae. Lysergic acid diethylamide (LSD) and 3-quinuclidinyl benzilate (BZ) are examples of incapacitating agents. BZ is an anticholinergic agent.

Blood agents: the cyanides
These agents impair cellular function by uncoupling oxidative phosphorylation.

Pulmonary/choking agents
Choking agents impair the respiratory system by irritating the respiratory tract mucosa and alveolar epithelium. These can produce a spectrum of illness from minor irritation to acute respiratory distress syndrome. Examples include chlorine and phosgene.

BIOLOGICAL HAZARDS
These are varied. Illness is usually of insidious onset. Because early symptoms may be non-specific, especially when patients may have a prodrome, early recognition can be difficult. Once the community is aware, workload is increased. Patient load will include those with non-specific symptoms, worried patients with usual clinical features of a non-exposure-related illness and those with unusual symptoms or clinical signs needing diagnostic refinement.

Patients exposed to microbiological agents may be recognised when a number of patients present with unusual similar symptoms or clinical signs. Alternatively an influx of patients with similar symptoms may present, with diagnostic refinement identifying a common broad illness such as pneumonia with isolation of an unusual causal agent.

Other dilemmas include when to immunise and when to definitively treat. These decisions must be made in conjunction with infectious disease doctors and public health agencies. Rationalisation of available therapeutic substances is a logistical problem. The principles of managing this issue are no different to those of disaster triage and reverse triage. However, within this context, development of inclusion and exclusion criteria is more relevant.

The impact of the exposure on hospitals is likely to increase the workload of laboratory facilities in initial identification and ongoing examinations for isolation of infective agents or bacterial endotoxins and exotoxins.

RADIOLOGICAL HAZARDS

There are two broad considerations in radiological exposure.

- Has the patient been irradiated?
- Is the patient radioactive?

Irradiation alone can cause life-threatening illness. The latter additionally poses a risk to rescuers and their ongoing careers.

All forms of ionising radiation can cause illness.

- Alpha particles generally have poor tissue penetration. They are of significance if ingested, inhaled or have contacted open wounds.
- Gamma rays penetrate tissues, directly affecting cells.
- Neutrons cause effects indirectly.
- Beta particles can penetrate deeper tissue, but human tissue provides some resistance, thus decreasing their impact and causing only tissue damage when they have penetrated cells.

Bone marrow and gastrointestinal mucosa are the tissues at most risk. Injuries may be caused by a single radiation exposure, exposure to high levels of fallout and repeated exposures.

Acute radiation syndrome involves four phases: prodrome, latent period, manifest illness and death or recovery.

Prodrome

Initial symptoms often appear within 6 hours of exposure. Symptoms include nausea, vomiting, anorexia and general malaise. Treatment is largely symptomatic and supportive. A 48-hour lymphocyte count and chromosomal analysis of lymphocytes for dicentric fragments are predictors of likely bone marrow suppression and haemopoietic syndrome (see Figure 47.4).

Latent period

This phase is a variable symptom-free period of hours to weeks.

Manifest illness

In this, definitive radiation illness and its complications become evident. Four clinical syndromes are described: gastrointestinal, haemopoietic, vascular and cerebral.

- The symptoms of the gastrointestinal syndrome are similar to those of the prodrome phase with additional problems of diarrhoea, fever and gastrointestinal haemorrhage. Bowel

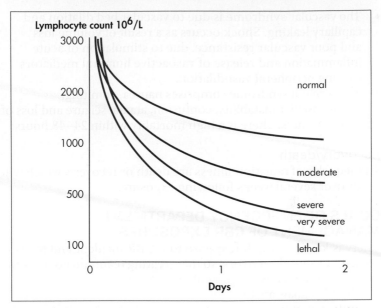

Figure 47.4 Lymphocyte count as a guide to severity of haemopoietic syndrome
Reproduced with permission from Emergency management practice manual 3: health aspects of chemical, biological and radiological hazards. Provisional edn. Australian emergency manuals series, part 3. Emergency Management Australia; 1999.

perforation and septicaemia are complications of severe illness. Treatment is supportive with intravenous fluid resuscitation, dehydration and parenteral nutrition.

• The haemopoietic syndrome is the effect of bone marrow suppression with increased susceptibility to infection, haemorrhage and occasionally anaemia. Treatment is generally supportive. Platelet transfusion may be necessary for thrombocytopenia-associated haemorrhage or if surgical intervention is required. Sepsis must be energetically treated. Wounds should be closed as soon as possible. Infected or devitalised tissue should be excised. Early skin grafting of burns prevents opportunistic infection. Other blood products to enhance immunocompetence may be considered as clinically indicated.

- The vascular syndrome is due to vascular bed dilation and capillary leaking. Shock occurs as a result of volume loss and poor vascular resistance, due to stimulation of acute inflammation and release of vasoactive humoral mediators causing peripheral vasodilation.
- The cerebral syndrome comprises nausea, vomiting, cardiovascular instability, confusion, ataxia, seizure and loss of consciousness. There is a high mortality within 24–48 hours.

Recovery/death

The sequelae of radiation illness are death or recovery, which will occur over several weeks following exposure.

GOALS OF EMERGENCY DEPARTMENT MANAGEMENT OF CBR EXPOSURES

Safety is key in a health response to a CBR incident and focus is on 'self, scene and survivors', so that treating teams do not become victims of the incident.

The ED's goals are to:
- protect staff from toxic exposure
- decontaminate
- rapidly assess and treat immediately life-threatening problems
- determine the identity of the hazardous materials or chemical agents and provide specific treatment as indicated
- prevent cross-contamination of staff, visitors and other patients. lockdown of affected area and isolation of victim to minimise exposure to others
- restore the clinical environment to normal functions following the incident.

Personal protective equipment (PPE)

The use of PPE by staff treating contaminated patients is the single most important line of defence against airborne agents. It prevents cross-contamination and provides a physical barrier and respiratory protection.

There are various safety standards of PPE. Hospitals generally require safety standard C equipment. The suggested contents of a level C PPE kit are outlined in Box 47.2.

Box 47.2	**Suggested contents of a level C PPE Kit**

- Chemically-resistant splash suit with hood, storm flap and sealed seams
- Waterproof boots
- Butyl gloves—1 pair
- Nitrile gloves—6 pairs
- Full-face respirator with disposable filters—3
- Filter shower covers—3
- Chemically resistant tape—1 roll

Isolation areas

CBR plans must include the availability of an isolation area. In some instances, this may be a physical structure that has been developed in keeping with appropriate standards that have been incorporated into new or renovated facilities. In other circumstances, the isolation area may be makeshift or portable. Decontamination takes place within or immediately adjacent to the isolation area. Many facilities will depend on preexisting arrangements with fire services and HazMat services for setting up these units.

Hot zone

The hot zone is an area of contamination. For practical purposes, this is an isolation area for dealing with contaminated casualties. In selecting an appropriate area for the hot zone, consideration needs to be given to wind direction, slope for run-off, access to water and drainage, ability to provide screening for privacy, traffic management and proximity to the ED. The hot zone should be set up in conjunction with guidance from fire services. They are the lead agency in managing such incidents in the pre-hospital setting and have most training in this sphere.

Warm zone

The warm zone is a buffer area between hot and cold zones to minimise cross-contamination. This may not be practicable within a hospital. Once a contaminated casualty has entered the ED, that area becomes part of the hot zone and every attempt should be made to cordon and control flow with separate entry and exits for such casualties.

Cold zone

This is a clean, non-contaminated area. Most treatment will occur in this area.

Decontamination corridor

The decontamination corridor traverses the warm zone. The decontamination process is functionally a one-way sequence and process. Contaminated casualties enter the hot zone, pass through the decontamination process and exit into the cold zone, prior to definitive treatment within the ED.

Contaminated-area and hot-zone issues

All staff working in the hot zone must be appropriately trained to do so, specifically able to don and doff PPE safely and operate respirators as required.

Life-saving equipment required in this area will be out of service until decontaminated. Specialist cleaning may be required.

All patient clothing and personal belongings are bagged and labelled. Contaminated waste and patient belongings are double-bagged, a red ('dirty') label is attached and the bag is placed in a yellow contaminated waste bin. Extreme care should be taken with patient clothing and valuables. These must be clearly labelled, as they may be the only form of patient identification and may be required for forensic evidence.

Decontamination requires the availability of showering facilities. Screening is necessary for patient privacy. The area must be well ventilated. If necessary, ventilation may need to be enhanced using portable industrial exhaust fans.

Decontamination

Decontamination is the first step in treatment as it aims to remove the noxious substance and stop ongoing exposure. Decontamination requires the removal of clothing and showering with copious amounts of water. If there is any doubt about contamination, then the person must be decontaminated prior to entering the cold zone. This also applies to emergency services personnel.

For safety reasons, only those staff designated as members of the decontamination team and wearing full PPE are permitted to decontaminate patients. If protective respiratory equipment is required, only appropriately trained staff in PPE use are to be deployed.

The following points serve as a guide to effective patient decontamination.

1 It is preferred that males and females be segregated.
2 The patient stands on a plastic sheet and removes clothing and personal belongings. These are wrapped in the sheet and placed in a bag. The bag is placed in a second bag. Identification and red 'contaminated' labels are attached.
3 Patients proceed to decontamination showers. Copious amounts of water and soap are used. Liquid, flour and disposable wipes and tissues may be required to remove thick liquid before showering.
4 Following decontamination, patients move through the warm zone or decontamination corridor to a 'clean area' or cold zone. The patient is dried and clothed in a standard examination gown. Once externally decontaminated, the patient must have an 'external decontamination' tag or armband applied and is moved to the triage area.

Editorial Comment

When a patient removes clothing, it should not be over their head. Consider cutting clothing off to avoid contamination of the face/airways.

Specific decontamination issues
- A contaminated appendage can be washed without wetting the whole body.
- Skin is washed down for 5 minutes with copious amounts of soap and water.
- Open wounds require gentle scrubbing or irrigation of wound for 5–10 minutes with lukewarm water.
- Eye exposures require irrigation of eyes with sterile normal saline for 15–30 minutes.
- Contaminated facial and nose hair and ear canals are to be gently irrigated, with frequent suctioning to ensure removal of contaminants.

Substance identification

Substance identification is necessary for correct decontamination and for providing medical treatment specific to the substance.

Chemical substances may be identified using:

- HazMat or product advice sheets
- computerised databases (e.g. POISINDEX)
- dangerous goods guide
- Poisons Information Centre—phone number 13 11 26 (Australia-wide).

A biological agent may have been identified and advised by the state/territory public health agency. If a biological agent is suspected, identification strategies should be planned in conjunction with health service clinical microbiologists or infectious disease doctors. Forewarning of and close liaison with laboratory medicine is required.

Radiation hazard identification may have already been advised by the relevant public health and environment protection agencies. However, local nuclear medicine departments, especially those associated with radiotherapy treatment centres, may initially be of assistance. It is preferable that a radiation physicist assist with on-site assessment of patients and the local environment for radioactive contamination.

Staff roles

It is essential that all staff members are familiar with their roles in a chemical, biological or radiation incident/disaster. The roles are similar to those identified for response to traumatically injured mass casualties.

- The triage nurse or officer remains 'clean', adjacent to the triage station.
- The senior doctor in charge remains in the cold zone and allocates medical personnel to specific duties and areas, such as to isolation and decontamination. The doctor in charge endeavours to determine substance identification and specific treatment.
- Doctors allocated to the hot zone must be familiar with the PPE, equipment and procedures for decontamination and treatment. The role of the nurse in charge of managing nursing and clerical resources parallels that of the senior

doctor. A specific responsibility is to ensure that the decontamination area is screened off for patient privacy, clearly marked, signposted and isolated to prevent cross-contamination.

Decontamination teams

A decontamination unit consists of 2 teams, each with a minimum of 3 staff: doctor, nurse and patient services assistant. One team triages using either sieve or sort methods, and where appropriate clinically manages time-critical patients in need of emergency care. The second team concentrates on decontamination procedures.

Men with full beards will not be able to obtain an accurate seal from the respirator and thus cannot participate in a medical decontamination team.

Clean-up and decontamination of hot zone equipment

Hot zone equipment may be separated into two groups—a chemical/disaster box and supplementary equipment—as outlined in Box 47.3.

Non-disposable hot zone equipment requires cleaning. Specialist cleaning may be necessary. These items should be doubled-bagged and labelled with a red 'contaminated' label.

Disposal of consumables, cleaning of equipment and restoration of decontamination areas to normal activities will vary among hospitals depending on the set-up. Issues include the following.

- Chemical disposal of any contaminated wastewater.
- Cleaning or disposal of contaminated clothing and contaminated disposable protective clothing.
- Cleaning of the shower and hot zone areas. Cleaning staff may need access to PPE.
- Cleaning of contaminated equipment.
- ED staff may be able to clean equipment if this can be achieved safely. If not, specialist cleaning may be required.
- Disposable equipment will need to be replaced. This includes PPE equipment such as suits, gloves, overshoes and respirator hoods.
- Government agencies responsible for environment protection are notified if hazardous chemicals have entered the sewers or stormwater drainage system.

Box 47.3   Suggested equipment lists for decontamination areas

Chemical disaster box equipment
- Personal protective equipment—disposable barrier suit, overshoes, nitrile gloves and respirator with disposable filter and air hose
- CBR procedure manual
- Liquid soap, flour, disposable wipes or tissues
- Clear bags for double-bagging of contaminated clothing and linen/ black pen to write on contents of bag (e.g. linen, patient clothing, disposable equipment)
- Plastic sheet
- Red CONTAMINATED tags and green DECONTAMINATED tags
- Red CONTAMINATED patient labels and green DECONTAMINATED patient labels
- Special specimen-carrying container for contaminated specimens
- Nozzle for hose
- Hazard signs and tape to identify isolation zone

Other equipment
- Hoses to connect to external outlets (depending on decontamination zone design)
- Dressing trolley for laying out resuscitation equipment
- Patient trolley(s)
- Portable oxygen and suction
- Transport resuscitation bag—adult and paediatric
- Defibrillator
- Portable BP cuff and sphygmomanometer
- Portable otoscope
- Towels, gowns to use after decontamination shower, warm blankets
- Clean trolleys for decontaminated patients
- Dirty linen skip

- Particulate matter removed from radiation exposure victims may need to be stored in lead-lined bags or sealed containers.

Staff decontamination

Staff should only remove and dispose of PPE and clothing when contaminated 'dirty' area clothing and linen has been double-bagged and trolleys and other equipment used in this area have been decontaminated.

Clinical and related wastes

The underlying principles for the treatment and disposal of clinical and related wastes are the health and safety of personnel and the public as well as minimisation of overall environmental impact.

Clinical wastes include sharp items and human tissue wastes. Related wastes include cytotoxic, pharmaceutical, chemical and radioactive wastes. Ultimate disposal of wastes will depend on their nature and on national, state, territory or local regulations governing the disposal of hazardous substances.

Wastes need to be segregated according to their category, bagged, packaged or containerised. Plastic bags are used for the collection and storage of clinical and related wastes, other than sharps. They need to be of sufficient strength to safely contain the waste class they are designated to hold. They need to conform to colour coding and marking. If moist sterilisation is to be used for decontamination, bags must be suitable for that purpose. Bags may only be filled to a maximum of two-thirds of their capacity or to a maximum weight of 6 kg. This allows for secure final closure and unlikely tearing of the bag. Rigid-walled containers are used for collection of sharp items. Containers such as mobile garbage bins should be resistant to leakage, impact rupture and corrosion. These containers should be inspected after each use to ascertain that they are clean, intact and without leaks. These containers must be appropriately colour-coded and securely closed, but not necessarily locked, during transport.

The key consideration for clinical and related wastes storage is their safe containment in a vermin-proof, clean and tidy area. Storage requirements will depend on the volume and type of clinical and related wastes to be contained and the mode of waste treatment to be employed. Procedures will also be dictated by the logistics of waste treatment methods and the requirements of disposal facilities.

Waste segregation is maintained during the movement and handling of wastes. If waste is mixed or loses identification during movement, it must be treated at the highest level of contamination. Movement of wastes through patient care areas should be avoided. Industrial trolleys should be used to move clinical wastes contained in plastic bags or non-mobile rigid-walled containers.

Chemical exposure register

A chemical exposure register may be managed by the fire service or an appropriate HazMat management agency. However, hospital staff may be required to manage this.

All staff, including visiting emergency service personnel, and patients involved in contaminated areas must be listed on the register. The minimum details required in the register include name, hospital record number, designation and injuries sustained. Contact details of involved staff are recorded to ensure timely access if additional follow-up is required.

A SMART triage tag for CBR exposures should be attached to the patient's wrist or included in clinical notes.

Online resources

South Australian Metropolitan Fire Service
  www.mfs.sa.gov.au
Victorian Metropolitan Fire and Emergency Services Board (MFB)
  www.mfb.vic.gov.au

References

NSW Health Services Functional Area Supporting Plan, NSW HEALTHPLAN, Emergency Management Arrangements of NSW, January 2016.
Decontamination Guidance for Hospitals. Dept of Human Services, Victoria, Australia.
Australian Clinical Guidelines for Acute Exposure to Chemical Agents of Health Concern; Australian Govt.

Further reading

Mackway-Jones K, Advanced Life Support Group (ALSG). Major incident management and support: the practical approach at the scene. Wiley-Blackwell. 3rd edn. December 2011.

Tribute

I wish to acknowledge the life and contribution to emergency medicine of Associate Professor Jeff Wassertheil who passed away on 22 September 2008. He will remain a highly esteemed emergency medicine specialist, researcher, teacher, colleague and friend who, in spite of being in hospital, put the finishing touches into a previous MCI chapter of this book.
Gordian Fulde

Chapter 48
Diagnostic imaging in emergency patients

E S Seelan

The aim of this chapter is to explain briefly the need and usefulness of diagnostic imaging services in emergency situations. Many of these emergencies arise 'after hours', and staff in most emergency departments have no immediate access to radiologists. The chapter also outlines the various diagnostic imaging modalities available, the basic principles involved in each modality and some clues to interpreting some of the most obvious lesions.

Editorial Comment

Although long, this chapter contains a wealth of practical information. Very few emergency patients escape diagnostic tests. Always, if there is any doubt, talk to the radiographers/radiologists about any study. Always arrange for follow-up of the formal report, as emergency doctors are not radiologists. Even if the images and reconstructions look easy—you are not an expert and are simply giving the patients an impression.

Imaging modalities
PLAIN X-RAYS

Plain X-rays are a commonly used modality. An X-ray beam is passed through the body.

Different tissues of the body absorb different amounts of X-rays. Unabsorbed X-rays are recorded on a film placed on the opposite side. Bone absorbs the most, hence it looks white on film. Air absorbs almost none, hence it looks black on film. Other tissues are demonstrated in shades between black and white.

Plain X-rays are performed as the first line of emergency investigations in many instances, as in fractures and abdominal or chest pain.

ULTRASOUND

Transducers used in this examination pass ultrasound into the body and also receive the echoes. The intensity of the echoes depends on the degree of absorption of sound waves by various tissues. On the image, echogenic areas appear white and sonolucent areas (that transmit sound, e.g. fluid) appear black.

Immediate and instant demonstration of organs by real-time ultrasound imaging and the fact that it is non-invasive and harmless (no radiation) have made this tool very popular. It is used in the following.

- To find out whether a lesion or lump is solid or cystic.
- Abdominal and pelvic organs: liver, gall bladder, bile ducts, pancreas, spleen, kidneys, aorta, inferior vena cava (IVC), bladder, prostate, uterus and ovaries, renal stones, gall stones, aortic aneurysm, traumatic and other haematomas—abscess and abnormal fluid collections can be demonstrated.
- To examine small parts (thyroid, testes and breast) and neonatal heads for ventricular size, etc.
- For obstetrical work-up, including study of fetus for early detection of abnormalities, and for emergencies like ectopic pregnancy, vaginal ultrasound is extremely useful.
- Ultrasound-guided biopsy and interventional procedures.
- Musculoskeletal investigations (e.g. shoulder, knee, muscle and tendon injuries and acute tenosynovitis).
- Duplex and colour Doppler ultrasound.
  — With the advent of duplex and colour-flow Doppler it is now easy to identify arteries and veins non-invasively. This modality should be the first line of imaging for the detection of deep vein thrombosis (DVT) in the limbs. (This study can be difficult in extremely swollen, oedematous lower legs.) In difficult cases venography can be performed. It should be remembered that ultrasound is non-invasive and can be performed repeatedly even in pregnant patients with suspected DVT.

— Duplex ultrasound is useful in identifying superficial thrombophlebitis.
— While excluding thrombosis, ultrasound study can also diagnose other causes of a swollen, tender calf such as ruptured Baker's cyst, haematoma in calf muscle (e.g. a gastrocnemius tear), mass in groin, axilla.
— Doppler ultrasound is useful in detecting and localising acute arterial occlusion in the limbs and in the investigation of peripheral vascular disease and carotid arterial disease.
— It is also useful in assessing renal artery stenosis and renal parenchymal vascular disease in the investigation of hypertension.

COMPUTED TOMOGRAPHY (CT)

The same principles are applied in CT as in plain X-rays, but there are two main modifications.

1 The X-ray tube is rotated around the body in an axial plane.
2 Instead of an X-ray film, detectors are used on the opposite side. Multiple fixed detectors are placed around the body to pick up the signals as the X-ray tube rotates around the body. Signals from the detectors are digitalised and the computer builds up an image which can be seen on a TV monitor or recorded on a film.

The resulting images are transverse sections of the part examined. Using the stored information of consecutive thin transverse sections, the images can be reconstructed in sagittal, coronal and oblique planes. CT is now a proven diagnostic tool which delivers valuable information to help in the early diagnosis of many lesions and diseases. Its use is greatly appreciated in many emergencies such as head injuries and some chest and abdominal emergencies. It is also useful in demonstrating fractures that are not shown by plain X-rays.

Helical CT scanning

Helical or spiral CT scanning is an improvement that allows very quick scanning of a patient (shorter scanning time than conventional CT) with increased accuracy of lesion detection resulting from volumetric data acquisition. In conventional CT, X-ray exposure and patient movement through the gantry alternate; whereas in helical CT, X-ray exposure and patient movement take place simultaneously giving a 'spiral impression'.

Advantages

- Greater length of the patient's body can be scanned with one 'breath-hold' thus producing contiguous images without interruption (e.g. a 30-second scan can cover most of the chest).
- Eliminates respiratory artefacts and reduces partial volume effect, peristaltic and other movement artefacts.
- Produces overlapping images without extra radiation exposures.
- Using a window workstation the acquired images can be reconstructed in multiplanes and three-dimensional images with excellent clarity.

Multislice CT scans

This is a further advancement whereby the speed of scanning and resolutions are considerably improved by using more-efficient detectors and obtaining thinner slices per rotation of the X-ray tube as the patient passes through the gantry.

Scanners are available to obtain 4, 8, 16, 32 or 64 slices (per rotation) of up to 0.5 mm thickness. A few 300-slice scanners are also available in Australia. These are faster than a heartbeat.

Advantages and uses

- Speed: some scanners can complete a body scan in 20 seconds; useful in the ICU and in paediatric, elderly, trauma and postoperative patients, where a shorter breath-hold and quick scanning are required.
- High resolution and fewer artefacts.
- Less IV contrast usage by allowing the scanning to start when the contrast reaches the area of interest (contrast detection system).
- Multi-plane reconstruction without loss of resolution.
- Three-dimensional reconstruction useful for surgical planning.
- CT angiography (including pulmonary angiography to detect pulmonary embolism) and cholangiography.

- CT fluoroscopy: useful in interventional work (e.g. placement of needle for biopsy, facet joint injection).
- Virtual endoscopy: enables a bronchoscopic view or colonoscopic view to be obtained.
- Coronary angiography: multislice, high-resolution low-dose CT is now being used for cardiac and coronary assessment without the need for conventional catheterisation.

MAGNETIC RESONANCE IMAGING (MRI)

In the past 20 years MRI has gradually become the technique of first choice in the investigation of many diseases. The physics involved in MRI is more complex than for any other radiological technique. However, the basic principles are indicated by the original terminology, nuclear magnetic resonance (NMR).

Nuclear

Unlike X-ray images, which are produced by attenuation of X-ray photons by the outer orbital electrons in the atoms of the elements in the body tissue, the MRI signal arises from the centre of the atom—the nucleus. The nuclei used in MRI are those of hydrogen atoms.

Hydrogen is selected because:

- it makes up about 80% of the human body
- its nucleus has only 1 proton, which has magnetic properties
- the solitary proton gives it a larger magnetic field (or moment).

Magnetic

The hydrogen ion, or proton, is a small, positively charged particle with associated angular momentum or spin. This situation represents a current loop and results in the formation of a magnetic field with north and south poles (dipoles). In other words, the protons behave as tiny magnets within the tissues. All nuclei used in MRI must have this property.

In the absence of influence from any external magnetic fields, the protons tend to orientate randomly in all directions. However, when a strong static external magnetic field is applied, these dipolar protons tend to align parallel to the direction of the external magnetic field (longitudinal plane).

The strong external magnetic field must be homogeneous over a volume large enough to contain the human body. This explains why the magnet tunnel is much longer than the CT gantry.

Resonance

This is a phenomenon whereby an object is exposed to an external oscillating disturbance that has a frequency similar to its own frequency of oscillation. Therefore, when a hydrogen proton is exposed to an external disturbance with a similar frequency to its own, the proton gains energy from the external disturbance. This is called resonance. This can happen only if the external disturbance is applied at 90° to the magnetic field of the proton. The oscillation frequency of the hydrogen proton in a static magnetic field of the strength used in clinical MRI corresponds to the radiofrequency band (RF) in the electromagnetic spectrum.

Therefore, for resonance of hydrogen to take place, an RF pulse at the same frequency as the oscillation of the hydrogen proton must be applied at 90° to the magnetic field of the proton. The application of the RF pulse that causes resonance is called excitation, as it results in the nuclei gaining energy. This energy causes the magnetic field of the protons to change direction. Enough RF pulse energy is given to the proton to change the direction from the longitudinal to the transverse plane (flip angle of 90°). Now the protons are rotating in the transverse plane. According to the laws of electromagnetism, if a receiver coil is placed in the transverse plane, the transverse magnetisation will produce a voltage in the coil. This voltage constitutes the MR signal.

When the RF pulse is turned off, the hydrogen protons return to their original orientations in the longitudinal plane. This is called relaxation.

There are two main types of relaxation (T1 and T2). T1 is the return of net magnetisation to the longitudinal plane. T2 is the decay of magnetisation in the transverse plane. These two relaxations and their time variances are used to create imaging sequences. All relaxation times are based on fat and water. This is where most of the body's hydrogen protons are.

- T1 images are known for their anatomical details. In T1 images, fluid appears black and fat appears white.

- T2 images are known for their contrast. In these images, fluid appears white and fat appears grey.
- Proton density images are a combination of T1 and T2. These images specifically look at the concentration of hydrogen protons.

This is a simple explanation of the basics, but more complex physics is involved in the formation of MR images which is beyond the scope of this chapter.

Summary

MRI involves the use of:

- a large magnet to produce a static magnetic field
- an RF generator to produce RF pulses
- hydrogen nuclei—different tissues have characteristic differences in hydrogen proton concentrations, therefore the MR signal and hence the image obtained basically represent the different distributions of hydrogen protons in the body
- a computer to convert the signals into images in various anatomical planes.

Advantages of MRI

- No ionising radiation.
- Free of artefacts from adjacent bones and gas. Therefore it is excellent to demonstrate soft tissues adjacent to bones (e.g. base of brain and spinal cord).
- Excellent resolution: even without contrast enhancement, MR is much more sensitive than CT in detecting contrast differences between various tissues. This is due to the intrinsic differences in hydrogen proton density as well as T1 and T2 relaxation, magnetic susceptibility and motion in various tissues.

Uses of MRI

Brain

- Stroke: MRI can diagnose acute infarction within hours of onset when the CT scan is still normal. This is done by using diffusion imaging, which tracks the motion of water that becomes acutely restricted in the area of infarction. Once infarction has been diagnosed, an intravenous MR angiogram can be performed at the same time to assess the calibre of the neck arteries.

- Haematoma: subdural and parenchymal haematoma and dural sinus thrombosis.
- Aneurysm and other vascular malformations: MR angiography is very sensitive in finding small aneurysms up to about 2 mm and can also give some idea of the degree of any associated vasospasm.
- Intracranial mass: MRI can accurately stage both primary and metastatic tumours. It is more sensitive than CT for metastases. Some masses like abscess and epidermoid can be differentiated from other tumours with certainty, as they have restricted water diffusion. In certain cases spectroscopy can also help in the differential diagnosis. MRI is also superior to CT in detecting lesions closer to the skull base, such as acoustic neuroma and pituitary tumour.
- Other uses: demyelination, congenital abnormality, meningeal disease and investigation of epilepsy.

Spine

MRI is the modality of choice for assessing cord contusion and haematoma in the acute stage, especially when there is an associated spinal fracture and neurological signs. It is also excellent in demonstrating cord compression, infarction, tumour, neuromas, metastases, myelopathy, radiculopathy and brachial plexus avulsion. It is also useful in post-laminectomy complications such as haematoma or infection as well as investigation of infective spondylodiscitis where early changes, such as fluid in the disc, paraspinal collections and end-plate erosions, are seen.

Musculoskeletal

MRI has the ability to simultaneously characterise soft tissues (muscles, ligaments, tendons and cartilage) as well as bone marrow. It is very useful in the investigation of musculotendinous injury and pathology, joint injury and pathology (e.g. rotator cuff injury in shoulder, meniscal and ligamentous injury in knee) and fractures not detected by X-ray (e.g. fracture in the neck of femur) as well as bone infection, avascular necrosis, marrow disorders and bone and soft-tissue tumours.

Chest
Constrictive pericarditis, aortic and great vessel dissection, congenital cardiac and great vessel abnormality, lung cancers closer to the chest wall and apex (e.g. Pancoast's tumour).

Abdomen
Adrenal mass using chemical shift imaging, cholangiography, etc.

Pelvis
Uterine and cervical tumours and abnormalities, differentiation of adenomyosis from fibroids, endometriosis assessment, bladder tumour, etc.

Contrast-enhanced MRI
In spite of the excellent tissue contrast definition without use of intravenous contrast, contrast-enhanced MRI (gadolinium) provides even better imaging sensitivity and specificity.

The enhanced contrast shows subtle parenchymal lesions as well as leptomeningeal lesions not otherwise visible (e.g. very small metastatic lesions, acoustic neuromas of 2–3 mm), pituitary microadenomas, differentiation of the actual size of tumour from the surrounding oedema and differentiation of more-malignant areas from less-malignant areas. These are helpful for the purpose of treatment and to select the exact site for biopsy.

Ongoing research into the development of new contrast agents targeted at specific organs, disease processes, cells or gene type is likely to result in considerable expansion of the use of MRI.

MR angiography (MRA)
Protons in flowing blood (moving protons) produce a high signal against the background of little or no signal from the surrounding stationary tissues—hence the development of the MR angiogram with no display of the background soft tissue.

Contraindications to MRI
Cardiac pacemakers, ferromagnetic intracranial aneurysm clips (except where MR-compatible clips have been used), cochlear implants, intravascular stainless steel stents inserted less than 6 weeks previously, surgical clips in chest and abdomen inserted

less than 1 week previously, metalworkers with metallic foreign body in the eye.

Disadvantages of MRI

Because of the length of the magnet (tunnel), some patients may experience claustrophobia. This can mostly be overcome by sedation. Scanners are now available with open gantry which will alleviate claustrophobia, but these scanners are dedicated and are used mainly for musculoskeletal and spinal work-up.

CONTRAST STUDY

The main limitation in the use of plain X-rays is the superimposition of the shadows of various organs. In many instances this can be overcome by introducing contrast.

- Barium to demonstrate the gastrointestinal (GI) tract.
- Intravenous pyelogram (IVP): IV contrast demonstrates kidneys, collecting system and bladder. Helpful to assess function (excretion) and to detect stones, obstruction, space-occupying lesion, deformities of renal tract, etc.
- Micturating cystourethrogram (MCU): to demonstrate urethra, bladder and vesicoureteral reflux.
- Arthrography: (e.g. shoulder, to detect rotator cuff tears). Sometimes this is combined with a CT scan, which helps to identify glenoid labral injury, etc. (Arthrograms may not be required if there is access to high-resolution ultrasound and MRI scan.)
- Herniography: contrast injected into the peritoneal cavity to detect clinically undetectable inguinal or femoral hernia that is producing symptoms.
- Myelography: contrast injected via lumbar puncture demonstrates the subarachnoid space around the spinal cord and nerve roots. With the advent of CT and MRI, the need for this examination is almost nil.
- Cholangiography: in the past, oral cholangiograms were performed, but this is now replaced by CT cholangiography. This examination requires slow infusion of contrast (which is excreted by bile) followed by helical CT scan and 3D reconstruction of the biliary tree.

- Sialography: contrast injected into the salivary ducts (parotid or submandibular) to identify stones, strictures, sialectasis and lesions in the glands.
- Hysterosalpingogram: contrast injected into the uterine cavity to demonstrate the uterine cavity, fallopian tubes and to detect patency of the tube in the investigation of infertility.
- Sinogram and fistulogram: contrast injection shows the cavities and communications.
- Venography: could detect clots, incompetent perforators and varicose veins (current trend is to do Doppler and colour Doppler ultrasound examination).
- Arteriography: contrast injected into various arteries using catheters demonstrates the arteries in various organs. It is used to demonstrate occlusions, narrowing of arteries, aneurysms, bleeding points, AV malformation and tumours. Digital subtraction angiography (DSA) has replaced the conventional angiograms. In this technique, the X-ray images are digitalised and stored and manipulated by computer. The image signal of an area or organ obtained before the injection of contrast is subtracted, by the computer, from the image signal obtained after injection of contrast into the vessels.

Advantages

The resulting image will demonstrate the vessels and branches without superimposition of bones and other soft-tissue shadows.

Owing to the fact that the image signals can be intensified by the computer, contrast media of low concentration and volume can be used with thinner catheters.

INTERVENTIONAL RADIOLOGY

Radiologists are able to perform certain therapeutic and interventional diagnostic procedures using various types of imaging equipment (fluoroscopy, ultrasound, CT and MRI), needles, catheters and guide wires.

- Dilation of narrowed arteries: transluminal angioplasty, insertion of vascular stents.
- Embolisation: of bleeding vessels, preoperative tumour embolisation to assist surgery by reducing blood loss and

reducing the duration of surgery, palliative embolisation of tumours, embolisation of some vascular abnormalities.

* Thrombolysis: using local low-dose intra-arterial injection of thrombolytic agents to relieve thromboembolism in certain vessels such as coronary artery and peripheral arteries.
* IVC filter insertion to prevent pulmonary embolism caused by clots arising from pelvis and lower limbs.
* Percutaneous insertion of stents to relieve biliary or ureteric obstruction.
* Percutaneous drainage of cysts, abscesses, pleural effusion, etc.
* Percutaneous removal of renal or biliary stones when other methods are contraindicated.
* Biopsy of deep and superficial lesions: lesions in liver, pancreas, kidneys, other abdominal masses, chest lesions, breast, thyroid, lymph node and other superficial and deep lesions.
* Clot extraction: cerebral strokes.

Intravenous contrast reaction

Even though the incidence of fatality is much lower than in street accidents, reaction to IV contrast is a great worry to doctors. Some statistics show that about 1 in 80 000 patients developed severe or fatal reaction when ionic contrast was used. Incidence of mild reaction is probably about 5–15%, moderate reaction about 1–2% and severe reaction is probably about 0.2%. However, with the use of non-ionic contrast and taking good precautions, the incidence of reaction is said to have reduced to about one-third to one-quarter of the frequency.

Usually patients who develop severe reaction have some other aggravating disease as well.

The exact pathogenesis of the reaction is not very clear. However, the following are possible mechanisms:

* chemotoxic effect
* hyperosmolar reactions causing erythrocyte or endothelial damage, blood–brain barrier damage and vasodilation
* vasomotor reactions with release of vasoactive substances such as histamine, serotonin and bradykinin
* vasovagal reaction with inhibition of enzymes such as cholinesterase.

Symptoms and signs

Most reactions occur within minutes of injection. However, delayed reactions have also been reported.

- **Mild reactions**—hot flush, burning sensation, arm pain, dizziness, nausea, vomiting, headache and urticaria—are thought to be due to systemic effects as a result of histamine liberation. Usually reassurance and restoration of the patient's confidence is all that is required, but sometimes oral antihistamine for urticaria, mild analgesics and sometimes tranquillisers for anxiety (5 mg diazepam) may also be helpful.
- **Moderate reactions** involve a slightly more serious manifestation of the above symptoms, with or without a moderate degree of hypotension and bronchospasm. They usually respond to reassurance and antihistamine (IM or IV), diazepam 5 mg, salbutamol inhalation for bronchospasm, hydrocortisone (100–500 mg IM or IV) and occasionally adrenaline 0.3–1 mL of 1/1000 IM. Oxygen by mask is administered.
- **Severe reaction** can be life-threatening and involve a severe form of the above reactions plus convulsion, unconsciousness, laryngeal oedema, bronchospasm, pulmonary oedema, arrhythmia, hypotension, cardiac arrest, anaphylactic shock. Severe reactions require urgent treatment (see treatment of anaphylaxis in Chapter 42 Dermatological Emergencies).
- **Predisposing factors**: in the presence of these, the incidence of reaction can be about 2–10 times as severe.
  - Previous adverse reaction to contrast.
  - Significant allergic history including iodides.
  - Asthma.
  - Cardiac disease.
  - Dehydration: all patients should be adequately hydrated as dehydration is dangerous, especially in patients with diabetes, renal impairment and multiple myeloma.
  - Haematological and metabolic conditions such as sickle-cell anaemia, patients with known phaeochromocytoma.
  - Renal disease: patients with preexisting renal disease, especially patients with diabetes, have an increased risk of reaction as well as of renal failure. Metformin, an oral

967

antidiabetic drug, is excreted by the kidneys and in patients with renal impairment this has been known to cause lactic acidosis and lead to acute alteration of renal function. In view of this, all diabetic patients treated with metformin drugs must have serum urea and creatinine levels reviewed before the IV contrast injection (serum urea must be less than 6.7 mmol/L and serum creatinine must be less than 0.1 mmol/L). The metformin drugs should be discontinued from 48 hours before until 48 hours after the injection, and should be recommenced only after checking the serum urea and creatinine. If required, another hypoglycaemic agent may be used during this period.

PREVENTION AND PRECAUTIONS

1 Always try to use non-ionic contrast.
2 Like other drugs, contrast agents should be used only if indicated and should be used in the smallest possible dose and concentration that will result in adequate imaging.
3 Weigh the possible advantages of using contrast against the possible risk. In patients with a strong family history of reaction, contrast should be avoided. In many cases the contrast study may be replaced by another examination such as ultrasound, CT or MRI.
4 A test dose may not help. However, some authors advise a small test dose of about 1 mL IV in high-risk patients who definitely require contrast for diagnosis.
5 In some patients (e.g. asthmatic and allergic patients), premedication with oral corticosteroid and possibly antihistamines could be given during the 24 hours preceding the test. The patient should also be adequately hydrated.

Imaging of the head

Common emergencies are trauma, severe headaches, collapse, syncope, seizures and stroke.

TRAUMA
Plain X-rays of skull
Indications
(Uncommon as CT is investigation of choice.)

- History of unconsciousness
- Palpable or visible depression on skull
- Laceration or penetrating wound
- Cerebrospinal fluid (CSF) or blood discharge from ear or nose
- Fits
- Presence of neurological signs

Views
- Include anteroposterior, lateral, Towne's and basal views.
- 'Shoot through' lateral (patient in supine position and X-ray beam horizontal) is useful to demonstrate air–fluid levels, especially in sinuses.

Interpretation
Every doctor working in the accident and emergency department should try to be familiar with the appearance of normal skull X-rays. The best way to detect abnormality is to know the normal. (This applies to every modality of imaging.)
- One should be familiar with the skull sutures, vascular markings, venous lakes along the inner table of the skull vault, appearance of normal sinuses and normal intracranial calcifications (e.g. pineal body, choroid plexus).
- Fracture of the skull can be an undepressed crack fracture or a depressed fracture.
- Do not misinterpret sutures and vascular markings as fractures. You can avoid this by knowing the normal positions of sutures and vascular markings. Sutures are usually serrated. Fracture lines are usually 'blacker' than the vascular markings.
- Beware of metopic sutures—in some patients such a suture may persist throughout life and may look like a fracture.
- In depressed fractures, one or more fragments may be depressed. In some cases, oblique or tangential views may be needed to demonstrate depression.
- If pineal calcification is present, look for shift. This indicates a space-occupying lesion such as a haematoma. (Towne's view is ideal for this.)
- Look for air–fluid level in sinuses or air in ventricles in the horizontal beam lateral view.

Plain X-rays of the face

Most facial injuries can be evaluated clinically. However, X-rays are performed for:

* confirmation
* assessment of the degree of displacement or depression of fragments
* detecting fractures in the presence of extreme facial swelling which makes palpation difficult.

In some cases facial fractures are associated with other serious emergencies, such as intracranial, neck or chest injuries, which may require emergency management such as maintenance of airway. In these patients, X-rays of the face can be postponed to the latter part of the management and may even be deferred for a few days.

Views

* Routine facial views: posteroanterior (PA), occipitomental (OM) and lateral
* Special views: nose (anteroposterior (AP), lateral and axial), zygoma (Towne's or modified basal view for the arch), orbital, mandible (PA, lateral, oblique and sometimes orthopantomogram (OPG) and occlusal view for symphysis menti)

Classification

For convenience, facial fractures can be divided into three types: upper third, middle third and lower third.

1 **Upper third.** The upper third, which is above the superior orbital margin, includes the superior orbital margin, the frontal sinuses and the adjacent frontal bone.
   — Fracture of superior orbital margin appears as interrupted cortical margin with or without depression, either craniocaudally or posteriorly.
   — Fracture of the frontal sinuses may involve anterior wall or both anterior and posterior walls.
   — Fracture may be linear or comminuted, depressed or undisplaced.
   — Fracture of sinus may extend into orbit; therefore, look for orbital emphysema.

— Fractures causing laceration of mucosa in sinus or fractures communicating with skin laceration are compound fractures.

2 **Middle third.** This includes the nose, zygoma, orbit (floor, lateral and medial walls) and maxillae (midfacial bones).

— *Nose.* Nasal fracture and deviations are easily detectable clinically, but X-rays are needed in patients with severe swelling or for confirmation of the degree of damage. Fractures of nasal bones are better seen in lateral view (soft-tissue exposure). Deviation is seen in axial view. PA view may demonstrate fracture of frontal process of maxilla and also deviation of fracture of the bony part of the nasal septum. Associated fractures in severe cases are bony nasal septum, cribriform plate, frontal process of maxilla, anterior nasal spine of maxilla.

— *Zygoma.* Fracture of the arch usually involves three sites causing depression of the arch. A commonly seen severe form of fracture is of the zygomaticomaxillary complex. One fracture line extends from the zygomaticofrontal suture across the orbital process of the zygoma (lateral wall of orbit) up to the lateral aspect of the inferior orbital fissure. Another fracture extends from the lateral wall of the maxilla to the inferior orbital margin (near the inferior orbital foramen) and extends along the floor of the orbit to the lateral aspect of the inferior orbital fissure, thus completing a circle. This fracture can cause separation of the zygomatic bone from the maxilla and orbit. (This fracture can be well understood if the reader takes a dry skull and follows the line of the fracture described above).

— *Orbit:* blowout fracture. The orbital margin is stronger than the floor and medial wall of the orbit. The posterior half of the orbital floor is formed by the thin orbital plate of the maxilla. The medial wall is formed by the orbital plate of the ethmoid. These two orbital plates are very weak. Sometimes the orbital margin can be intact and the force of injury can be transmitted to the floor and medial walls of the orbit, causing blowout fractures into the adjacent sinuses. Therefore, in the presence of orbital emphysema, a blowout fracture should be suspected.

— *Maxilla:* fractures of midfacial bones. These fractures tend to follow a certain pattern. There are three common patterns, which are named after the person who described them—Le Fort I, II and III fractures.

o Le Fort I is the lowest and almost horizontal fracture through the maxilla, causing separation of the lower part of the maxilla. The fracture line extends from the inferolateral aspect of the nasal aperture horizontally across the lower part of the anterolateral and posterolateral walls of the maxilla. It then passes almost horizontally across the lower part of the medial and lateral pterygoid plates, reaches the medial wall of the maxillary antrum and extends to the inferolateral aspect of the nasal aperture, thus completing a circle.

o Le Fort II fracture separates the midfacial bones from the cranium and the lateral aspect of the face. The medial part of the fracture line is across the nasal bone, nasal septum, frontal process of the maxilla and lacrimal bone, and runs posteriorly along the ethmoidal bone. Laterally the fracture runs obliquely downwards from the inferior orbital margin (near the zygomaticomaxillary suture) along the anterolateral wall of the maxilla and then slightly ascends up the posterolateral wall of the maxilla to the inferior orbital fissure.

o Le Fort III is the highest of the fractures and is bilateral, causing complete separation of the midfacial bone from the base of the skull. The fracture line passes across the nasofrontal region to the ethmoid and runs posteriorly to the inferior orbital fissure. It also involves the pterygoid plates. Laterally the fracture involves the lateral wall of the orbit and the zygomatic arch.

o The Le Fort fractures may occur in combination. The above description is useful for surgical planning.

3 **Lower third.** This includes the mandible. Common sites of fractures are the alveolar process (weakest part), condyles, angle of the mandible, body (usually the fracture is around the canine tooth because of maximum convexity). Bilateral fractures are common. Fractures of the body on one side and the angle on the other side are also common.

CT findings in head injury

If CT is available, it is the quickest way of detecting intracranial trauma. It has been reported that about 10–15% of patients with head injury with no neurological signs were found to have abnormal CT findings. In contrast, about 75% of patients with neurological signs demonstrated abnormal CT findings.

The lesions described in the following sections may be seen in CT.

Haematomas and contusions (acute and delayed)

Haematomas appear as high-density areas (white) on CT without contrast. Haematomas are fairly homogeneous, but contusion shows patchy dense and low-density areas. Low-density areas are due to oedema. Fresh blood appears as dense areas due to haemoglobin. (In anaemic patients it may be isodense with the rest of the brain or even hypodense if the haemoglobin level is low.)

Most haematomas become isodense in 1–3 weeks and in some cases get even smaller and hypodense. The isodense haematomas may be missed unless other signs of mass effect are looked for.

Delayed haematomas may appear from 2–7 days after trauma. Haematomas and associated oedema usually cause space-occupying effects—midline shift, compression on ventricles, cisterns etc.

Subdural haematomas

These usually appear as dense areas and follow the brain surface with a concave inner border and convex outer border. They tend to be diffuse and extend along the subdural space. Thin haematomas (e.g. less than 5 mm) and haematomas near the vertex may be difficult to identify. However, indirect evidence such as midline shift may help. Beware of bilateral subdural haematomas, which may not cause any shift.

- Acute haematomas (occurring 0–1 week after trauma) are usually dense.
- Subacute haematomas (occurring 1–3 weeks after trauma) may be isodense.
- Chronic haematomas (more than 3 weeks after trauma) are usually hypodense.
- Acute-on-chronic haematomas show mixed density.

Epidural haematomas

These are caused by traumatic separation of the dura from the inner table, causing damage to the middle meningeal arterial branches, venous branches or diploic veins. An epidural haematoma is usually seen as a biconvex density under the inner table of the skull. The biconvex appearance is due to firm adhesion of the dura to the inner table. For this reason the epidural haematomas are demarcated by sutures.

Oedema

Oedematous areas appear as low-density areas in the CT. They may be focal, patchy or diffuse. Due to the oedema there may be space-occupying effects, such as compression on the adjacent ventricles and midline shift.

Note: Oedema may have other causes such as infarction. Therefore it should be differentiated. A history of trauma and the site of involvement may be helpful.

Intraventricular and subarachnoid haemorrhage

These may occur with some head injuries and appear as dense areas within the ventricles, basal cistern, sylvian fissures, interhemispheric fissure or cerebral sulci. Resolution of the haemorrhage within the ventricular system and subarachnoid space is fairly quick and may disappear within a week.

Fractures and displaced or depressed bony fragments

These can be seen in CT when viewed with bone windows. The CT is useful to identify soft-tissue contusion and foreign bodies in the scalp or in the intracranial region. It is also useful to identify any traumatic pneumocephalus.

Posttraumatic changes

- Acute or delayed hydrocephalus is caused by blood in the subarachnoid space causing some obstruction to the CSF pathways.
- Ischaemic infarction appears as low-density areas.
- Posttraumatic atrophy is seen in almost one-third of patients with severe head injury. Due to the atrophy there may be

compensatory dilation of the ventricles usually adjacent to the site of atrophy.

• Posttraumatic abscess may be seen in penetrating injury or fracture, or as a complication following surgery. It appears as a low-density area with ring enhancement after contrast injection. This ring enhancement is usually surrounded by a large area of oedema. The lesion will also produce a space-occupying effect.

The use of CT in facial trauma

In some cases plain tomography is performed to demonstrate facial fractures. However, CT of facial bones in coronal, axial and sagittal planes is very useful, not only to demonstrate the fractures but also to show the extent and degree of depression of fragments and associated haematomas, especially in the adjacent sinuses, orbits, etc.

Angiography in cerebral trauma

This has been almost eliminated by CT scanners. However, it is indicated if there is suspicion of vascular damage such as occlusion of an artery or injury to an AV malformation.

MRI in head injury

Even though MRI is superior to CT in detecting small haematomas, especially near the bones, CT is preferable as the initial investigation not only because the examination time is shorter but also because sometimes haematomas that are less than 1–2 days old may not be shown by MRI. CT shows acute haemorrhages well.

Head injury in children—CT appearance

Appearance of haematoma is almost the same as in adults. However, haemorrhagic contusions are less common than in adults due to greater pliability of the skull.

The paediatric brain may demonstrate acute generalised oedema causing narrowing of ventricles and subarachnoid space. Oedema is less marked in adults.

ACUTE SEVERE HEADACHE AND COLLAPSE

Sudden onset of severe headache or sudden collapse may be caused by intracranial haemorrhage.

- The haemorrhage could be from: aneurysm, AV malformation, capillary bleed in hypertension, bleeding disorders or bleeding from a tumour.
- The haemorrhage may be intracerebral, subarachnoid or intraventricular.

In these cases CT is rewarding. Blood appears as dense areas. Valuable clues as to the site of bleeding and the cause may be shown by CT. However, in most cases angiograms (CT or DSA) will be required to show the exact site and cause of bleeding. Multiple vessel studies are necessary as there may be multiple aneurysms. An angiogram will also show the site of the lesion and, in cases of AV malformation, the feeding vessels to the malformation. Angiograms are not necessary in cerebral parenchymal haemorrhage.

In suspected **subarachnoid haemorrhage**, CT scan is performed before lumbar puncture. If haemorrhage is marked, or hydrocephalus or space-occupying effect is detected, lumbar puncture is avoided. However, in cases where no haemorrhage is detected, lumbar puncture could be performed. This is because very small haemorrhages may not be shown by CT. Small amounts of blood are not enough to change the CSF density, or in some (anaemic) patients the haemoglobin content may not be enough to change the CSF density.

SYNCOPE AND SEIZURES

Of the many causes of syncope only a few need radiological assistance for diagnosis or confirmation.

- Syncope caused by reduced cardiac output may need echocardiography, cardiac catheterisation and angiography.
- Syncope is rarely caused by cerebrovascular disease (e.g. transient ischaemic attacks, subclavian steal, vertebrobasilar insufficiency). In these cases Doppler ultrasound or angiography will be useful.
- In cases of seizures, CT of the head may be required to exclude any underlying pathology.

STROKE

Transient ischaemic attacks (TIAs) may represent an early warning sign of impending stroke. Therefore arteriography (DSA) of the neck vessels and cerebral arteries is performed in cases of TIA.

Even though arteriography gives a more definite answer, ultrasound examination of the neck vessels (Duplex and colour Doppler studies) could be performed initially.

In all patients with stroke, CT should be the initial radiological examination. However, if MRI is available, it is preferred to CT as MRI is better at detecting early infarction (within a few hours of vascular occlusion). CT sometimes gives negative results within the first 24–48 hours.

Emergencies in the neck

Major emergencies are trauma, foreign bodies and croup and laryngeal inflammation in children.

TRAUMA

Cervical spine injuries are common and can be life-threatening. They range from nerve root compression and paralysis to death. Therefore, X-ray or CT evaluation of the cervical spine is important in trauma.

Plain X-ray views

1 The first film to obtain is a 'brow up—shoot through' lateral view. (Patient in supine position; movement of neck should be avoided.) Film should be well penetrated. All the cervical vertebrae and possibly the upper thoracic vertebrae should be demonstrated. Demonstration of the lower cervical and upper thoracic spine may be difficult in most patients. Swimmer's lateral projection or a lateral film with shoulder traction could be useful. Sometimes the patient's condition may not permit this. Alternative ways to demonstrate this area are tomography in lateral projection or CT scan if available.

2 If no abnormality is seen in the first film, do an open-mouth AP view of the odontoid process to exclude fracture of odontoid process. In suspicious cases the rest of the views are done only after expert examination of the film: a radiologist should be consulted if available.

3 If no abnormality is seen in the above two views, do the rest of the views (i.e. AP and two obliques). Patients must move the neck themselves.

4 Lastly, if there are no neurological signs, a flexion and extension view (functional view) could be done. Do not force

the neck—the patient must move the neck. In suspicious cases the oblique and functional views should be done under the supervision of the attending doctor.

5 If no abnormality is seen in the above and the symptoms are still suspicious of fracture, tomography of selected areas could be done. If CT is available, it will be useful to show the vertebrae in transverse plane and to detect haematomas. If a helical or multiple-slice scanner is available, high-resolution images could be obtained in the sagittal and coronal planes as well as 3D images.

Clues for interpretation of X-rays

1 For proper interpretation one should be familiar with the normal appearance of the vertebrae, facetal joints, disc spaces and the soft tissues around the spine.

2 Lateral and odontoid process views should be inspected first.

3 Look for fracture lines or deformities in each vertebral body, neural arch and the facets. Look for dislocation or subluxation of facetal joints and any malalignment of vertebrae.

4 Loss of lordosis and scoliosis may indicate bony injury or soft-tissue injury.

5 If the disc is damaged the space may be narrow.

6 Soft tissues anterior to the spine (prevertebral soft tissue) should be inspected for swelling (haematomas). Normal AP distance of the prevertebral soft tissue in the retropharyngeal region (at the anteroinferior angle of C2) is about 6–7 mm in adults and children. Retrotracheal soft tissue at the level of the anteroinferior angle of C6 is about 14–15 mm in children and about 15–20 mm in adults (these measurements are upper limit of normal). Haematoma may be due to fracture or rupture of the anterior spinal ligament.

7 To identify upper cervical subluxation in the lateral view, draw a line along the anterior cortical margin of the spinous processes from C1–C3 (posterior cervical line). If there is more than 2 mm displacement, it is diagnostic. This is usually seen in odontoid fracture or hangman's fracture.

Note: In children slight anterior subluxation of the body of C2 on C3, especially in the flexion view, is normal. In these cases note the posterior cervical line, which will be normal.

8 Look for common fractures. Fractures are common at the C1–C2 articulation, odontoid process and from C5–C7.

9 *Pitfalls:* In the AP view of the odontoid process, watch for superimposed shadow of an incisor tooth which will look like a fracture. Also look for a separate ossification centre of the odontoid process. (In some cases tomography of the odontoid process may be needed to identify the fracture.)

10 CT can be performed to determine the state of soft-tissue structures around the spine.

11 CT is also useful in cases of suspected instability at the fracture and also to identify suspected bony fragments within the vertebral canal.

12 CT (in bone windows) will demonstrate the neural arches and facetal joints. This will be useful to identify fractures or dislocation at the joints. Modern CT scanners can image the spine in various anatomical planes.

13 MRI is more sensitive than CT in demonstrating the spinal cord.

Classification of cervical spine injury

Cervical spine injuries can be classified according to the type of injury—flexion injury or extension injury. However, in many instances the patient is unconscious or cannot describe the injury. As far as treatment is concerned, it is important to decide whether the fracture is stable or unstable. The X-ray findings are useful in making this decision.

Flexion injury

The various kinds of flexion injury are described below in order of severity.

• **Hyperflexion sprain.** Partial damage to posterior ligaments including interspinous ligaments. Flexion lateral view may demonstrate widening or fanning of the space between adjacent spinous processes.

• **Unilateral or bilateral facetal dislocation.**
   — In lateral view, look for anterior displacement of one vertebral body on the other by less than 50%.
   — In AP view look for malalignment of spinous processes (especially in unilateral dislocation). Facets may be

locked (i.e. inferior articular facet of the vertebra above is locked in front of the superior facet of the vertebra below).

- **Anterior wedging of vertebral bodies or compression fractures.** If the neural arches are not fractured this may be a stable fracture.
- **Comminuted fracture of vertebral body ('teardrop' fractures).** In these fractures look for any fragments in the vertebral canal. These fragments could cause damage to the spinal cord. CT scan would be useful in these cases to identify any fragments in the canal.

Extension injury

The various kinds of extension injury are described below in order of severity.

- **Hyperextension sprain.** This causes damage to the anterior longitudinal ligament. Due to hyperextension there may be protrusion or bulging of the disc posteriorly. There may also be some haematoma and swelling from the ligamentum flavum. The disc bulging and the swelling from the ligamentum flavum can cause compression on the spinal cord. In these cases the X-ray may be normal. CT scan or MRI would be useful in these patients.
  — Sometimes lateral plain X-ray may show soft-tissue swelling (haematoma) within prevertebral tissue.
  — Extension injuries may be associated with fractures of the anterior angles of the vertebral bodies.
  — Extension injuries may not be stable in extended positions of the neck but are stable in flexion.
- **Hangman's fracture.** Fracture of both pedicles of axis with displacement of the body of C2 anteriorly and posterior displacement of neural arch of C2. This is well seen in the lateral view.
- **Jefferson bursting fracture.** This fracture is unusual and is caused mainly by vertical compression injury causing bilateral fractures of anterior and posterior arches of C1. In the open-mouth AP view there will be lateral displacement—both lateral masses of C1.

- **Fracture of odontoid process.** Look for fracture line (not to be confused with superimposed shadows and separate ossification centres). Also look for alignment in lateral view—posterior cervical line.

Stable fractures
- Unilateral fracture of lamina pedicle or lateral mass
- Unilateral facetal fracture or dislocation
- Wedge fracture
- Burst fracture—disc forced into fractured end plates of body
- Fracture of spinous process

Unstable fractures
- Bilateral fracture of lamina
- Bilateral dislocation of facets
- Comminuted fracture body (any fracture dislocation)
- Hangman's fracture
- Fracture of odontoid process

FOREIGN BODY IN NECK—PHARYNX AND UPPER OESOPHAGUS

Most swallowed foreign bodies lodge at the level of cricopharyngeal muscle or in the upper oesophagus. Commonest foreign bodies are fish bone, meat or chicken bone, large pieces of meat and coins.

Lateral film of the neck is the most useful view. Film of soft-tissue exposure may be necessary to identify faintly calcified bones. Radio-opaque materials are fairly easy to detect. Superimposition of calcified hyoid, thyroid, cricoid and laryngeal cartilages will be a problem. However, an understanding of their normal expected anatomical position will help to distinguish a foreign body. Pattern of calcification of cartilages (irregular) will also help. Swallowed bone may have a linear cortex. In difficult cases a barium swallow may help to identify the foreign body. Swallowing cottonwool soaked in barium (usually under fluoroscopic control) will occasionally help. This may get caught on the foreign body (FB).

CT is also useful to locate smaller FBs not shown by X-ray.

EPIGLOTTITIS AND CROUP

Young children may develop severe acute inflammation of the epiglottis and larynx. In most cases where the condition is severe, radiological examination is postponed until the patient's condition is stable.

A lateral view of the neck (soft-tissue exposure) is the best view. Rarely, a single midline tomogram in lateral projection may be necessary.

- A swollen epiglottis will look like a thumb—the swollen aryepiglottic fold may also be seen.
- In croup usually the subglottic region from the vocal cord to the level of the inferior border of the thyroid cartilage shows mucosal swelling which causes narrowing of the airway. Vocal cords will also be affected. The need for radiology is debatable. However, if the patient's condition permits, it will be useful to perform an AP and lateral view of the neck. Swollen vocal cords, obliteration of laryngeal ventricles and narrowing of the subglottic airway by swelling can be easily seen.

Helical CT scan of larynx and trachea with sagittal and coronal-reconstruction would be useful if clinically reasonable.

Emergencies in thoracic and lumbar spine
INJURY AND ACUTE DISC PROLAPSE OR RUPTURE
Views

- If the patient is immobilised, a 'shoot through' lateral view is initially performed.
- Lateral film of the thoracic spine is obtained while the patient is breathing. This is to 'blur' the superimposed ribs.
- Swimmer's lateral or lateral tomography may be required for demonstration of upper 3/4 thoracic vertebrae.
- AP view is fairly easy to obtain.
- In cases of suspected ligamentous rupture, flexion and extension views in lateral projection are obtained.
- In lumbar spine, if the condition of the patient permits, oblique views are also performed. These demonstrate the laminae and facetal joints well.

- CT scan is useful to demonstrate the integrity of disc and bony elements. They are also useful to detect facetal dislocation, subluxation and any posterior dislodgment of bony fragments into the vertebral canal. It is also useful to demonstrate the soft tissues around the spine.

Interpretation of X-rays

1 Look for:
   - reduction in the height of vertebral body and disc spaces (compression or wedge fractures)
   - fracture lines or displaced fragments in the vertebrae, including transverse process and spinous process (also look for posterior rib fracture in thoracic region)
   - paravertebral haematoma (loss of psoas shadow in lumbar region, displacement of pleural lining in thoracic region, etc.)
   - subluxation, kyphosis, gibbus and scoliosis.
2 Look for any underlying causes of fracture such as secondary deposits, Paget's disease, osteoporosis, etc.
3 Beware of limbus vertebra non-united secondary ossification centres, butterfly vertebra and narrowing of vertebral bodies caused by long-standing scoliosis and kyphosis.

Unstable injury

- Transverse fractures through vertebral bodies and neural arches
- Fracture dislocation
- Rupture of ligaments (in the lateral view, the interspinous distance is wide, especially in flexion view)

Disc prolapse

- Plain X-ray may show disc narrowing—this is not always seen. Therefore, if symptoms persist, CT scan of the disc would be useful to show disc prolapse.
- High-resolution scanners can differentiate disc material, nerve roots, etc.
- MRI scan is superior in demonstrating spinal cord, nerve roots, discs, ligaments and bone oedema from trauma.

Chest emergencies
ROUTINE VIEWS

- PA and lateral—obtained in erect position, both in full inspiration
- If patient cannot stand, erect PA or AP and lateral in sitting position (in full inspiration) are obtained.
- If patient cannot sit or stand, supine AP is obtained. This is unsatisfactory because the patient may not be able to take a full inspiration and the diaphragm appears elevated. It also causes magnification, especially of the mediastinum. Mobile views are AP.

ADDITIONAL VIEWS

- Oblique views for ribs.
- Apical lordotic view to demonstrate lung apices (to get the superimposed clavicle out of the way).
- Inspiration and expiration films to demonstrate pneumothorax.
- Penetrated film to see mediastinum or lung bases.
- Lateral decubitus (patient lying down on one side—right or left—and film obtained with horizontal beam). This demonstrates mobility of pleural fluid on the dependent side.

INTERPRETATION

There are two ways to interpret.

1. An experienced person will use a problem-oriented approach, depending on the clinical information.
2. An inexperienced person should look at a chest film in a routine, systematic manner.
   a. Start looking at the mediastinal shadows. Cast your eyes along the:
      - anterior mediastinal structures—thymus (enlargement in infants; tumour in adults), thyroid (retrosternal), lymph nodes (if enlarged)
      - middle mediastinum—heart, aortic arch and branches, pulmonary artery, superior and inferior venae cavae
      - posterior mediastinal structures—trachea, bronchi, oesophagus, descending thoracic aorta, lymph nodes, (abnormal) neural tissues, look for hiatus hernia, spine.
   b. Look at the hilar shadows.

c Look at the lung parenchyma and other lung markings (pulmonary vasculature and bronchi).
d Look at the pleura.
e Look at the chest wall (including ribs).
f Cast your eyes along the periphery of the film (e.g. the shoulder, under the diaphragm).

TRAUMA
Rib fractures
First, second and third rib fractures are seen only in severe trauma. Commonest are from 4th to 9th ribs. Flail chest is seen when three or more ribs are fractured at two points. These are usually seen from the 4th to 8th ribs. A common site of fracture is usually the lateral angle. Because of this, oblique views are essential. Rib fractures can cause pneumothorax and haemothorax. Fracture of 10th, 11th and 12th ribs can cause damage to the liver, spleen and kidneys.

Lung contusion
Appears as an area of consolidation. It is not always associated with rib fracture. It may not appear immediately (sometimes a day later) and begins to resolve 2–3 days after injury. It usually resolves completely in about 10–15 days.

Rupture of thoracic aorta
Seen in motor vehicle crashes—usually seen near the ligamentum arteriosum. In this region the aorta is relatively fixed. Sudden deceleration and compression injury causes laceration at this relatively fixed portion of the aorta.

In chest X-rays there will be evidence of superior mediastinal widening, shift of the trachea to the right with obscuring of the aortic arch, and there may be haemothorax on the left. CT scan and aortography are the other radiological investigations in these patients.

Rupture of trachea or bronchus
Common findings in chest X-rays are pneumomediastinum, pneumothorax and surgical emphysema. Occlusion of fractured bronchus can cause collapse of the corresponding lung, lobe or segment.

Rupture of diaphragm

Seen in direct blunt trauma and penetrating injury. Sometimes not diagnosed immediately. In an X-ray the outline of the dome may not be normal. It may be elevated; there may be haemothorax or segmental lung collapse. On the left side, the bowel may herniate into the thorax; and on the right side, the liver may herniate. Rupture in blunt trauma is common on the left side.

CT in chest trauma

If a helical or multislice scanner is available, it will be useful for better demonstration of chest in sagittal and coronal planes as well as in 3D format. CT angiography could be performed to demonstrate aorta and great vessels.

BREATHLESSNESS

Asthma and acute-on-chronic airflow limitation (CAL)

- In CAL, chest X-ray shows overinflated lung, flattened domes of diaphragm, widened retrosternal space, hyper-radiolucency, a barrel-shaped chest, a relatively small and elongated heart shadow, prominent main pulmonary arteries and pruning of peripheral pulmonary arteries (associated pulmonary artery hypertension), and thickened bronchial walls (end-on ring shadows and tramline shadows).
- In asthma, overinflation of lungs and bronchial wall thickenings may be seen. Other findings may include atelectasis caused by mucous plugging or consolidation.

  High-resolution CT of 1 mm thickness is useful for investigation of CAL, especially to identify bronchiectasis, emphysematous bullae and interstitial fibrosis.

Radiological appearance in acute heart failure

Heart failure may be divided into left and right heart failure.

X-ray findings in left heart failure

- Distension of upper lobe veins (normally the upper lobe veins are smaller in calibre than the lower lobe veins).
- Interstitial pulmonary oedema. In the early stages the oedema forms around the hilar region, causing blurring of the hilar markings. Septal lines are due to accumulation of fluid along the lymphatics: 'A' lines are long and radiate from

the hilar region to the periphery; 'B' lines are short and are seen in the region of the costophrenic angles.

• Alveolar pulmonary oedema. This is due to filling of the alveolar spaces with exudates. It is seen as haziness radiating from the hilar region and produces a butterfly-wing appearance. In the severe form, the alveolar oedema produces a patchy or cottonwool appearance.

X-ray appearances in right ventricular failure

• Prominence of superior vena cava (SVC) and azygous vein.
• Pleural effusion. In heart failure often more fluid is seen on the right side. In the early stages, pleural effusions are seen in the costophrenic angles as a homogeneous density demonstrating a 'meniscus sign'. The meniscus sign is seen in the erect position. The fluid in the base changes to a haziness in the supine films. This indicates mobility of the fluid. Small fluid collections are first detected in the lateral view—in the posterior costophrenic angles. In the average chest, the posterior costophrenic angle can accumulate about 150–200 mL of fluid without being seen in the PA view. In the early stages fluid can also accumulate in the fissures between the lobes. This appears as thick oblique fissures.

Pleural effusion

Pleural effusion may have various other causes (e.g. tumour). Large pleural effusions can obscure the underlying cause. If the fluid is mobile, a lateral decubitus view would be useful to demonstrate the lung bases. (Alternatively, CT scan could be performed to identify any mass in the lung base.)

Lung collapse

There are two major radiological signs.

1 Density: collapsed portion of the lung appears dense.
2 Signs of loss of volume:
   — shift of fissures—fissures are shifted towards the opacity
   — diaphragmatic elevation
   — mediastinal shift towards the side of collapse
   — splaying out of lung markings on the side of collapse due to compensatory overexpansion of the remaining lung.

CHEST PAIN
Only the causes where radiology plays a part are included in this section.

Myocardial infarction
Chest X-rays are performed to look at the heart size and shape, and also to look for evidence of heart failure. Upper limit of normal cardiothoracic ratio (CTR) is 50% (CTR = transverse diameter of the heart divided by transverse diameter of the chest).

Pericardial effusion
Chest X-ray is also useful to identify pericardial effusion. In the supine position the heart appears globular in shape, and in the erect position it produces a 'tent shape'. The angle between the right atrium and the right diaphragm is lost. On fluoroscopic examination poor pulsation may be demonstrated in cases of pericardial effusion. (For proper demonstration of pericardial effusion, echocardiography or CT scan is more useful.)

Pulmonary embolism
- Within 24–48 hours there may not be any radiological change. However, if large pulmonary arterial branches are blocked, there may be a cut-off sign (i.e. abrupt ending of an arterial branch).
- Raised hemidiaphragm—on the side of infarction.
- After about 24–48 hours an almost triangular density with its base towards the periphery of the chest may appear.
- There may be a small associated pleural effusion.
- Sometimes the main pulmonary artery on the affected side may enlarge.
- Later in the process, in the area of infarction there may be atelectasis or scar formation.
- Nuclear-isotope ventilation–perfusion scans are performed for diagnosis, but sometimes this is not confirmatory. However, a normal chest X-ray and abnormal isotope scan could be indicative of pulmonary embolism.
- Pulmonary arteriography is the best means of establishing or excluding pulmonary embolism. This is rarely performed because of adverse reactions and the cost. However, recently,

with the introduction of multislice scanners, CT pulmonary angiograms are performed. This would be sensitive to detect emboli in pulmonary arteries up to about the 4th or 5th level of branching.

- Doppler study or venogram of the lower limb veins may show the origin of the clot.

Dissecting aneurysm

- In the PA view there may be widening of the superior mediastinum with the ascending aorta bulging to the right.
- The lateral view may show bulging of the ascending aorta anteriorly. A long-standing aneurysm of the ascending aorta can cause erosion of the posterior aspect of the sternum.
- Leakage from the aneurysm into the pericardium causes a large globular heart.
- When the dissection extends into the arch and descending thoracic aorta, the diameter widens towards the left. Sometimes a double aortic knuckle shadow can be seen. Some aneurysms leak into the pleural cavity and appear as a pleural effusion. In some patients uniform haziness can be seen in the left lung, due to blood spread along the bronchi and pulmonary arterial planes.
- CT scan can demonstrate a dissecting aneurysm and its extent.
- In order to demonstrate the exact site of rupture, some surgeons prefer an aortogram.

Pneumothorax

- Usually PA films in expiratory and inspiratory phases are obtained in the erect position.
- A large pneumothorax is well seen in a normal PA film. A small pneumothorax is usually demonstrated in the expiratory film.
- In order to identify the pneumothorax, follow the lung markings towards the periphery. The markings stop well short of the chest wall. A white visceral pleural line can be seen at this level.
- Do not confuse the accompanying shadow caused by intercostal muscles along the ribs for visceral pleura.

- Look for an associated pneumomediastinum (air can leak from bronchi in asthmatics) and subcutaneous emphysema along the chest wall and neck.

FEVER, COUGH AND PAIN
Pleurisy
- Early stages: no radiological findings.
- Later stages: small amounts of pleural fluid may be seen; there may be associated lung consolidation.

Pneumonia
- Bronchopneumonia: patchy shadows.
- Lobar or segmental pneumonia:
  — homogeneous localised shadows
  — air bronchogram may be seen
  — usually no loss of volume of lungs (this helps to differentiate from lung collapse).

HAEMOPTYSIS
Pulmonary infarction
See the section on Pulmonary Embolism earlier this chapter.

Tumour
A mass, either solitary or multiple, can be seen in the hilar region or elsewhere in the lung. If there is any doubt about the diagnosis, CT would be useful. CT may also demonstrate any enlarged lymph nodes.

OTHER ACCIDENTS
Drowning
Pulmonary oedema is seen in cases of near-drowning in both fresh and sea water. Pulmonary oedema may not develop for up to 2 days. Therefore, negative findings in immediate chest X-rays do not exclude later development of oedema.

Inhalation of toxic gases/smoke
- In toxic gas inhalation, pulmonary oedema develops quickly— in about 4–24 hours.

- In smoke inhalation, the oedema may not develop for up to 2–4 days.
- In chest X-rays oedema appears as patchy infiltrates. There may be segmental atelectasis. These changes usually resolve faster.

Ingestion of hydrocarbons (e.g. petroleum)

May develop patchy pneumonic consolidation in lung bases, usually within 1–2 hours. Severity depends on the amount ingested. Takes up to 2 weeks to resolve.

Foreign body

- Radio-opaque foreign bodies in bronchi are easily seen in chest X-rays. Foreign bodies like nuts, seeds and plastics may be difficult to see.
- Radiological signs are usually indirect (i.e. signs of obstruction).
- In children obstruction is usually ball–valve type, causing air trapping.
- PA films are obtained in inspiration and expiration. The inspiratory film may be normal, but in the expiratory film there will be hyperradiolucency and signs of increased volume on the affected side (flat diaphragm and shift of mediastinum to the opposite side).
- Chest screening is very useful to detect air trapping. Normal lungs show normal density and change of volume during breathing in comparison with the affected lung, which shows fixed volume and density.
- In adults, obstruction usually causes collapse of the lung or lobes.

Radiology in abdominal emergencies

Almost all modalities of imaging (plain X-ray, contrast study, CT and ultrasound) are used in abdominal emergencies.

VIEWS

- Routine views: AP in supine and erect position.
- Additional views: lateral decubitus in patients who cannot stand up, to look for fluid levels or free peritoneal gas.

- In some cases an erect chest X-ray is also performed to look for gas under the diaphragm or any pleural fluid in the lung bases.

INTERPRETATION

An inexperienced person finds it difficult to interpret an abdominal X-ray due to superimposition of various organs. This difficulty can be greatly reduced if the film is looked at in a routine manner; for example, as follows.

1 Look at the bowel shadows: these are easily identifiable because of gas and faeces. Stomach, small and large bowel can be differentiated by their anatomical site and their pattern of mucosal folds and wall—valvulae conniventes in jejunal loops and haustral pattern in large bowel. Note any fluid levels and bowel dilation.
2 Look at the four major organs: liver, spleen, kidneys and bladder, for their size, position, outline and density.
3 Look at the psoas shadows and fat planes in the flank and along the pelvic walls.
4 Look for radio-opaque stones (gall and renal) and abnormal calcification (pancreatic, hepatic and abdominal aortic).
5 Look above and below the diaphragm for abnormal gas, fluid or air collections.
6 Look for any abnormal mass causing displacement of adjacent structures.
7 Look at the bony elements (lower ribs, lumbar spine and pelvis).

ACUTE ABDOMEN

In the plain X-ray of the abdomen the main aim is to identify obstruction, perforation or ileus in the bowel shadows. CT is usually the investigation of choice.

Radiological signs of bowel obstruction

- There may be gaseous distension of the bowel up to the site of obstruction. In complete or almost complete obstruction, very little gas is seen in the bowel distal to the obstruction.
- Multiple fluid levels are seen in erect films.
- A step-ladder pattern of air–fluid levels is seen in small-bowel obstruction. In large-bowel obstruction fluid levels are seen around the periphery. In complete obstruction of the large bowel there may be fluid levels in the small bowel as well.

- In gastric outlet or duodenal obstruction, a distended stomach with a large air–fluid level is seen.
- Volvulus. In sigmoid volvulus look for a dilated loop of bowel in the form of an inverted U in the left hypochondrium. In caecal volvulus the base of the dilated caecum usually points to the right iliac fossa. The volvulus can be confirmed by performing a limited dilute barium or diatrizoate (Gastrografin) enema.
- Intussusception. A sharp cut-off of bowel gas pattern is seen. Common intussusception is at the ileocaecal junction. There may be dilated small bowel with multiple fluid levels. Limited barium enema examination may show a coil-spring appearance. In children the barium enema can be therapeutic and in most cases will be able to reduce the intussusception.

Radiological signs of ileus

- **Generalised.** Slight to moderate gaseous distension of small and large bowel with multiple small fluid levels can be seen. Generalised ileus is usually seen in postoperative patients, peritonitis and retroperitoneal conditions.
- **Localised.** The bowel loops in close proximity to an inflammatory area may show slight dilation and some fluid levels. One or two loops may be involved. This is called sentinel loop (e.g. jejunal loops) and transverse colon are involved in pancreatitis and acute deep gastric ulcers. Terminal ileum is involved in conditions such as appendicitis. Hepatic flexure and some small bowel in the right hypochondrium may show fluid levels in cholecystitis. In renal colic there may be sentinel loops on the affected side.

Radiological signs in perforation

- Free peritoneal gas is usually seen under the diaphragm in the erect position. In a lateral decubitus film, free gas may be seen along the flank. The free gas is sometimes seen only after 24 hours.
- Loculated peritoneal gas; for example, in perforation of a duodenal ulcer there may be loculated gas along the inferior liver margin. If there is a collection of gas in the lesser sac, in the plain X-ray there may be a double gas shadow projected over the fundus of the stomach.

- Retroperitoneal gas from perforation of the retroperitoneal portion of the large bowel.

In order to identify the site of perforation, diatrizoate (Gastrografin) contrast may be used (extravasated contrast is absorbed by the bloodstream and excreted by the kidney). In cases of suspected upper GI tract perforation the contrast may be given orally. In cases of colonic perforation it may be given rectally. Not all perforations can be demonstrated by this technique.

GI TRACT BLEEDING AND ISCHAEMIA

1 It is difficult to demonstrate bleeding points by barium study. However, this examination may be useful in demonstrating the presence of oesophageal varices, peptic ulcers, diverticula or tumours. Barium is less used now; endoscopy is preferred.
2 Highly selective coeliac, superior or inferior mesenteric arteriograms may demonstrate bleeding points. Angiography is also useful to demonstrate occluded arteries causing mesenteric ischaemia. A bleeding rate of 1 mL/min is usually required.

PANCREATITIS

1 Plain X-rays may show only indirect evidence such as sentinel loops or calcification in the region of the pancreas.
2 Barium meal may show a widened loop of duodenum due to enlargement of the pancreas.
3 Ultrasound is able to demonstrate the size and texture of the pancreas. It may also demonstrate oedematous change or any pseudocyst formation. However, sometimes it is difficult to demonstrate the pancreas by ultrasound due to obesity of the patient and presence of excessive gas.
4 A CT scan is the ideal examination to demonstrate the pancreas, especially in the obese patient. The sensitivity is such that it can demonstrate inflammatory changes, a small amount of calcification, a mass, a pseudocyst and also the state of surrounding tissues. It is also useful for follow-up study.
5 Skinny needle biopsy under CT or ultrasound control has greatly improved diagnostic ability.
6 Endoscopic retrograde cholangiopancreatography (ERCP) demonstrates the state of the pancreatic ducts.

CHOLECYSTITIS

1 Plain X-ray may demonstrate radio-opaque gallstones and sometimes demonstrates sentinel loops (localised ileus).

2 Ultrasound is the diagnostic tool of choice. It can demonstrate stones, thickness of the wall of the gall bladder and any oedematous change. It can also demonstrate the size of the bile ducts or any stones in the duct. However, demonstration of the lower common bile duct may be difficult.

3 In a post-cholecystectomy patient with symptoms of biliary colic, CT cholangiography could be useful to exclude any retained stones in the bile duct, strictures, etc.

AORTIC ANEURYSM

The majority of aneurysms are asymptomatic. However, these patients usually present to EDs when there is a rupture or leak. Severe rupture is fatal. If a slow leak is suspected, radiological investigation is carried out.

1 Plain X-rays (AP and lateral) show a soft-tissue mass, especially in the posterior abdominal wall. This is usually on the left side of the lumbar spine and is better seen in the lateral view. 50% of aortic aneurysms may have some calcification in the wall of the artery, which is very useful for identification of an aneurysm.

2 Ultrasound or CT scans are non-invasive, easier and quicker methods of diagnosing aneurysms. A CT scan is superior to ultrasound. It can demonstrate the site and length of the aneurysm. It can also demonstrate the diameter of the aneurysm and the presence of clot. CT is the study of choice in many patients, especially in obese patients. With the modern scanners CT aortography gives excellent results which also show the relationship of renal arteries to the neck of the aneurysm. This is useful for surgical planning.

3 Digital angiography is still used by surgeons to demonstrate the aneurysm and the branches of the abdominal aorta. However, this would show only the lumen and not the actual diameter of the aneurysm or the intraluminal clot.

RENAL COLIC

1 Plain X-rays may show radio-opaque calculi and may demonstrate localised ileus. CT is commonly used.
2 An IVP may demonstrate: obstruction (partial or complete), radiolucent stones, state of kidneys and collecting system.
3 If there is a non-functioning kidney and there are no radio-opaque stones, retrograde pyelography would be warranted.
4 Ultrasound may not detect all the stones in the kidney. It would demonstrate hydronephrosis in the case of ureteric obstruction.

HAEMATURIA

Severe cases of haematuria may present to the ED.

1 An IVP may reveal tumour in the kidneys, ureters or bladder.
2 CT is used to demonstrate renal and bladder tumours as well as any extension of the tumour.
3 Ultrasound can be used if CT scan is not available or if the patient is allergic to the contrast medium.

ABDOMINAL TRAUMA

Blunt trauma is more common. Radiological investigations depend on the patient's condition. The investigations include plain abdominal X-ray, IVP, arteriograms, ultrasound and CT.

Renal contusion and laceration

1 Plain X-ray may show: loss of renal outline, loss of psoas shadow, scoliosis with concavity towards the side of injury, localised ileus on the side of injury, fracture of lower ribs, vertebrae (including transverse processes) and pelvic bones.
2 IVP may show: non-functioning kidney or delayed nephrogram; extravasation of contrast from ruptured kidney, ureter or bladder; clots, seen as filling defects within the pelvicalyceal system, ureter or bladder.
3 Arteriogram. If an IVP shows non-function and renal laceration is suspected, an emergency renal arteriogram is performed to assess the state of the renal arteries. (Renal vessel repair should be performed within a few hours.)

4 Ultrasound and CT, if available, are useful. They can demonstrate rupture, contusion and haematoma. CT is superior to ultrasound.

Renal vein thrombosis

1 An IVP shows an enlarged kidney, prolonged nephrographic phase and reduced excretion.
2 Ultrasound with Doppler may assist but helical CT in rapid sequential imaging after contrast injection has about 90% success in detecting renal vein thrombosis. Other findings include prolonged parenchymal enhancement and delayed excretion.
3 MRI is also an excellent method of demonstrating renal vein thrombosis.

Bladder trauma

• May be contusion or rupture (either intraperitoneal or extraperitoneal).
• In these cases a cystogram will be useful to demonstrate the site of the rupture.

Urethral rupture

• Usually seen in males.
• Site of rupture can be demonstrated by a retrograde urethrogram.

Spleen and liver injury

Splenic injury is more common than liver. Sometimes the plain X-ray signs may be non-specific. If there are some signs, further investigations may be necessary to confirm the diagnosis. Radiological signs depend on whether there is capsular damage or not.

Plain X-ray of abdomen and chest

• Elevation of left diaphragm in splenic injury and right in liver injury.
• Left or right effusion in spleen or liver injury, respectively.
• There may be atelectasis at the left or right base.

- There may be fracture of the lower ribs.
- Blurred liver or splenic outline.
- In splenic haematoma, the stomach may be displaced medially and the splenic flexure of colon downwards. In liver injury, the hepatic flexure may be displaced.
- In cases of rupture there may be loss of flank stripes, separation of walls of bowel loops by peritoneal fluid, obliteration of splenic or hepatic outline and general haziness of abdomen.

Ultrasound
- May show fluid (haemoperitoneum). Blood (fluid) is seen in the lateral gutters and pelvic recesses.
- May show contused areas of the organ.

CT
This is the best examination. If CT is not available, ultrasound is performed. CT can demonstrate intracapsular haematomas, laceration and haemoperitoneum.

Angiogram
Selective arteriograms would be useful to study the state of the arteries and also to demonstrate rupture.

Hollow viscus
- Rupture or perforation rarely occurs with blunt trauma, but may be seen in penetrating injury. When it occurs, there may be gas collections in the peritoneal cavity. Sometimes retroperitoneal and mediastinal gas can be seen. This can be detected in plain abdominal and chest X-rays.
- Diatrizoate (Gastrografin) study may be useful to demonstrate the site of perforation but this is not usually required.
- CT is useful to identify free peritoneal air and also any other injury to the adjacent organs.

Some obstetric emergencies
BLEEDING IN PREGNANCY
This can be due to abortion—threatened, incomplete, complete or missed; ectopic pregnancy; placenta praevia; hydatidiform mole; placental separation (abruptio placentae).

All the above causes can be assessed by ultrasound (using transabdominal and transvaginal probes), which is the examination of choice. The fetal viability can also be assessed.

INTRAUTERINE FETAL DEATH
This can be confirmed by ultrasound.

Intrauterine trauma
Ultrasound is also used to assess the fetus after abdominal trauma.

Fractures of pelvis and limbs
Most fractures are easy to recognise on X-rays. However, some are difficult (e.g. hairline undisplaced fractures). In suspicious cases repeat examination by CT in 10–14 days could be performed (e.g. scaphoid fracture). In about 10–14 days some bone absorption occurs adjacent to the fracture line, which makes the fracture visible. In addition, periosteal reaction (callus) may begin to form.

Undisplaced fractures through the epiphyseal plates are also difficult to recognise. These fractures will also demonstrate bone resorption and callus in about 2 weeks' time.

1 In minor fractures, look at the cortical bone for any discontinuity or dents. Also look for any irregularity in the trabecular pattern.
2 In some areas (e.g. femoral neck and scaphoid), tomogram, CT or nuclear scan may be required to demonstrate an undisplaced crack fracture.
3 If suspicious areas are encountered, oblique views should be done (thin fracture lines are visible only when the X-rays pass perpendicular to the fracture line).
4 In oblique fractures of the metaphysis, always look at the depth of the epiphyseal plates, as the fracture might extend along the plate causing widening of the growth plate.
5 In the forearm and leg, if one of the bones is shortened or dislocated, usually the other bone will have a fracture or dislocation. Therefore, in the distal limbs have a good look at the entire length of the bones, especially the proximal and distal ends and the adjacent joints.
6 In young patients look at the location of ossification centres around the joints to identify any dislocation of the epiphysis

(e.g. elbow). If in doubt consult a radiologist or do a comparative view of the opposite joint.

7 In the wrist, do not miss dislocation of carpal bones (e.g. lunate). Try to identify the position of carpal bones in the lateral view.

8 In the joints, look for indirect signs of haemarthrosis (i.e. displacement of adjacent fat pad). If there is haemarthrosis, always look hard to identify any hairline fracture or epiphyseal displacement. If in doubt, X-ray again in 10–14 days.

9 Look for soft-tissue swelling in the X-ray (sometimes the X-ray has to be viewed under bright light). If found, concentrate on this area to identify any fracture.

10 The pelvis is like a ring—in compression injuries it might break in two or more places. Fracture of pelvic bones may be associated with dislocation or subluxation at the sacroiliac joints or pubic symphysis.

Radiation issues

Ionising radiation can be from natural or artificial sources.

• **Natural radiation.** Heat and light are types of radiation that we can feel or see, but there are other kinds of radiation that human senses cannot detect. We constantly receive invisible radiation from the sky (cosmic radiation), earth's crust, air and even food and drinks.

• **Artificial radiation.** From X-rays, nuclear industries and weapons. Unlike natural radiation, these are fully controllable.

• **Measuring radiation.** The radiation dose received by people (whole body) is measured in greys (Gy). The adverse effective dose (absorbed dose that may cause biological effects or cancer) is measured in sieverts (Sv).

RADIATION EXPOSURE AND LIMITS

• Exposure from natural radiation is about 1.5 mSv per year.

• The International Commission on Radiological Protection (ICRP) has set the following limits.

   a For radiation workers, 20 mSv per year.

   b For the general public, 1 mSv per year (over and above the natural radiation).

   c For patients, considering diagnostic benefits over radiation risk, a definite limit for dose from radiological procedures has not been set. However, scientists have calculated the possible radiation dose associated with some radiological investigations, as indicated in Table 48.1. (These figures are a guide only and may vary from patient to patient, as they are highly dependent on the size of the patient and the exposure

Table 48.1 Possible effective doses of radiation associated with some radiological investigations

Examination	Possible effective dose (mSv)
Dental OPG	0.01
Foot/hand (1 film)	0.02
Skull (2 films)	0.04
Chest (2 films)	0.06–0.1
Mammogram (4 films)	0.13
Cervical spine (6 films)	0.3
Abdomen/pelvis (1 film)	0.7
Thoracic spine (2 films)	1.4
Lumbar spine (5 films)	1.8
IVP (6 films)	2.5
Barium meal (11 films fluoro)	2.5–3.8
Barium enema (10 films)	6–7
Coronary angiogram	1.6–5
CT of head	2.5
CT of chest	5–8
CT of lumbar region	5
CT of abdomen	7–10
CT of coronary-angio region (64-slice)	5–10
CT of whole body	15
Lung scan (nuclear)	2–3
Bone scan	3–5
Sestamibi scan	13
Radiotherapy (6 weeks)	2000
Air travel (crew)	3.8/year
Air travel (passengers)	0.05/7 h
Computer/television use	0.01/year

CT, computed tomography; IVP, intravenous pyelogram; OPG, orthopantomogram.

factors used. In CT, the dose also depends on the number of slices as well as the number of examinations [e.g. pre- and post-contrast studies]. Thin slices produce a higher radiation dose due to more overlap between the slices.)

RADIATION RISKS

The following are suggestions and predictions only.

+ Relative risk of radiation:
  — CT of abdomen (10 mSv).
+ Equivalent risks:
  — smoking 140 cigarettes
  — driving 6000 km in a car
  — flying 40 000 km in a jet
  — canoeing for 5 hours.

Risk of cancer per 10 mSv is 0.04% (1 in 2500 CTs of the abdomen). Some others predict that 1 in 100 patients exposed to 100 mSv (10 CTs of the abdomen) may develop cancer or leukaemia and 42 of the same 100 may eventually develop cancer from other causes.

SUMMARY

There has been considerable technical advances in radiological equipment including CT, mainly aimed at reducing the radiation dosage and to improve resolution of images. Some of the radiation dose for CT given in Table 48.1 are lower for the low-dose scanners.

However, it is now known that in diagnostic radiology, CT is a major contributor of radiation.

+ Referring doctors, radiologists and radiographers should be aware that CT is a high-dose procedure. At the same time, doctors and patients must be assured that CT is a highly beneficial X-ray and should not be feared when the benefit of the examination clearly outweighs the risk.
+ Doctors should order CT examination with caution, especially when ordering multiple examinations, CT with and without contrast and CT of the whole body.
+ Imaging professionals should make every effort to reduce radiation as low as reasonably achievable, while obtaining adequate diagnostic information in the image.

Editorial Comment

Technology is galloping. For example, CT coronary angiograms (320-slice), paediatric CT (256-slice)—no need for sedation as so quick—as well as the use of combinations of different modalities (e.g. PET [positron emission tomography]) with CT for tumours, etc. It is hard to keep abreast, but also it means we now see lesions that we are not sure are pathological or need further tests or treatment. Ask, talk to the experts.

Chapter 49
Ultrasound in emergency medicine

Julie Leung

Acknowledgment

The authors wish to acknowledge the content used from the previous edition of *Emergency Medicine* which was provided by Andrew Finckh.

Point-of-care ultrasound (PoCUS) is a core skill in the practice of emergency medicine. It has been shown to enhance the clinician's ability to assess and manage patients with a range of acute illnesses and injuries and improve patient outcomes. The scope of practice continues to expand as emergency physicians identify clinical problems where PoCUS can aid in patient evaluation and guide invasive procedures.

The Australasian College for Emergency Medicine (ACEM) advocates that ultrasound examination, interpretation and clinical correlation should be available in a timely manner 24 hours a day for ED patients. ACEM specifically supports the use of ultrasound imaging by emergency physicians for at least the following indications: traumatic haemoperitoneum, haemothorax, pneumothorax; abdominal aortic aneurysm; pericardial fluid; intra-uterine pregnancy identification; vascular access and other procedures; basic echocardiography in life support; hydronephrosis; biliary tract disease; soft tissue studies and deep vein thrombosis.

This chapter focuses on: the basic physical principles of ultrasound; ultrasound equipment; common applications of PoCUS in the ED; training, credentialling and quality review.

Editorial Comment

Ultrasound in the acute care of patients is increasingly becoming the standard (e.g. IV lines).
Also selected indications, evidence based (e.g. chest-lung, cardiac) as timely diagnostic aids are increasing. All EDs must have a portable ultrasound machine and training. Technology advances will improve the portability and use of ultrasound at the bedside 24 hours a day, 7 days a week.

Basic physical principles

'Ultrasound' is sound whose frequency is above the range of human hearing. The audible human range is 20–20 000 hertz (Hz), while diagnostic ultrasound employs frequencies of 1–20 megahertz (MHz), with the most common range being 3–12 MHz.

Propagation of sound is the transfer of energy, not matter, from one place to another within a medium.

FREQUENCY AND WAVELENGTH

Frequency and wavelength are inversely related: the higher the frequency, the shorter the wavelength. The shorter the wavelength is, the less the tissue penetration but the greater the resolution and, therefore, the clearer the image.

PIEZOELECTRIC EFFECT

Artificially grown crystals are commonly used for modern transducers. These are treated with high temperatures and strong electric fields to produce the piezoelectric properties necessary to generate sound waves.

These properties mean that when a crystal in the ultrasound transducer has a voltage applied to it, the crystal is deformed and produces a pressure (i.e. the transducer sends an ultrasound). Conversely, an applied pressure received by the transducer deforms the crystal to produce a voltage. This voltage is then analysed by the system. In essence, the piezoelectric crystal acts as both speaker and microphone.

IMAGE RESOLUTION

Resolution is the ability to distinguish between echoes. There are three kinds of image resolution.

1 **Contrast resolution** is the ability of an ultrasound system to differentiate between tissues with varying characteristics (e.g. between liver and spleen).

2 **Temporal resolution** is the ability of an ultrasound system to show changes in the underlying anatomy over time. This is particularly important in echocardiography.

3 **Spatial resolution** is the ability of an ultrasound system to detect and display structures that are close together.

INTERACTION OF SOUND WITH TISSUE

Attenuation is the term used to describe the factors affecting the echoes returning to the transducer.

The four main processes in attenuation are as follows.

1 **Reflection.** This occurs at interfaces between soft tissues of differing acoustic impedance. Impedance is the resistance to propagation of sound. The percentage of the sound reflected is dependent on the magnitude of the impedance mismatch and the angle of approach to the interface, for example:

Soft tissue/air interface   99% reflected
Soft tissue/bone interface   40% reflected
Liver/kidney interface   2% reflected

2 **Refraction.** This is the deviation in the path of the beam that occurs when the beam passes through interfaces between tissues of differing speeds of sound when the angle of incidence is not 90°.

3 **Absorption.** This is the transfer of some of the energy of the beam to the material through which sound is travelling. It explains why high-frequency transducers cannot be used for examining deep structures within the body.

4 **Scattering.** This is the reflection of sound off objects that are irregular or smaller than the ultrasound beam. It occurs at interfaces within the sound beam path. The scatter pattern relies on the size of the interface relative to the wavelength of the sound.

ARTEFACTS

Ultrasound systems operate on the basis of certain assumptions relating to the interaction of the sound beam with soft-tissue interfaces. Some artefacts help ultrasound diagnosis. The common types of artefacts include:

* **Acoustic shadowing.** Occurs when beam energy attenuation at a given interface is high, such as when an object of high density blocks signal transmission.
* **Acoustic enhancement.** Occurs when there is an area of increased brightness relative to echoes from adjacent tissues.
* **Edge shadowing.** Results from a combination of reflection and refraction occurring at the edge of rounded structures. It can be falsely interpreted as acoustic shadowing.
* **Reverberation artefact.** Results from repeated reflections of sound between two interfaces. It is usually generated by high-level mismatch interfaces when the echo amplitude is very high.
* **Beam width effect.** Occurs because the ultrasound beam is not a single line, although the system assumes that it is.
* **Velocity artefact.** Occurs because various tissues have velocities that are different from the constant velocity assumed by the system. This results in incorrect placement of an object.
* **Mirror image.** Where a single image is displayed twice due to reflection off an interface.

Ultrasound equipment
TYPES OF TRANSDUCERS (PROBES)

Common transducers include the linear array, curved array and phased array transducers.

* **Linear array transducer** is constructed with multiple small crystal elements arranged in a straight line across the face of the probe. The beam generated by this transducer travels at 90° to the transducer face. This makes the probe ideal for vascular imaging and central line placement.
* **Curved array transducer** is also constructed with multiple small crystal elements, except that the face of the transducer is convex. This results in a wider field of view at the bottom of the image and a narrower image in the near field of view. This is ideal for viewing intra-abdominal structures.

- **Phased (sector) array transducer** gives a large depth of field with a small footprint allowing the ultrasound to view deep structures through a small acoustic window.

CHOICE OF EQUIPMENT

The ultrasound requirements of individual EDs vary, depending on how the device will be used (Table 49.1). For example, the ED that intends to limit studies to FAST and abdominal aorta scans will have different requirements from the one that wishes to perform ultrasounds to assess a first trimester pregnancy, locate a foreign body, assess testicular blood flow or obtain central venous access. Both present and future needs of the ED need to be determined. Staff who become competent in the basic applications of ultrasound may wish to extend their skills with time.

Table 49.1 Choice of equipment

Type	Essential	Optional	Specialised
Ultrasound system	Variable send-and-receive focusing Support for flat linear and curved linear transducers Measurement calipers Internal memory	Small-footprint intercostal probe Data disc Cineloop facility	Colour/amplitude mapping M-mode obstetric biometry software package Sector size control Pulsed Doppler control Continuous-wave Doppler control Transoesophageal echo facility
Transducers	Multifrequency (2.5–5.0 MHz) curved array Multifrequency (7–10 MHz) linear array (for foreign body and central line access)		Transvaginal probe Cardiac probe Transoesophageal probe
Peripherals	Video recorder hard copy device		

Once the ultrasound needs and budgetary limitations of the ED have been determined, the following features of the ultrasound equipment should be considered:

- machine portability and stability
- machine size—a larger machine may offer more features but be impractical in a resuscitation situation and difficult to store when not in use
- ability to upgrade machine without replacing expensive items
- servicing of machine, including transducers and peripherals.

There are many manufacturers providing machines suitable for PoCUS. Trial of these machines prior to purchase is an effective way of determining suitability in individual EDs.

Common applications in the ED
FOCUSED ASSESSMENT FOR SONOGRAPHY IN TRAUMA (FAST/EFAST)

The FAST/eFAST scan is a useful diagnostic test in the evaluation of the patient with blunt abdominal trauma (see Figure 49.1). FAST/eFAST can determine the presence of free intraperitoneal fluid, pericardial fluid, pleural fluid and pneumothorax. It is up to 90% sensitive and 99% specific for traumatic haemoperitoneum and 92–98% sensitive and > 99% specific for pneumothorax. Ideally the FAST/eFAST examination is performed in 5 minutes or less. The curvilinear low-frequency probe should be used and will suffice for all windows.

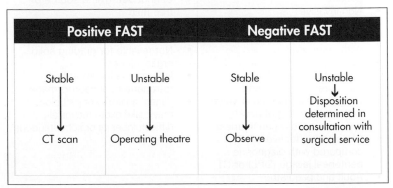

Figure 49.1 Blunt trauma algorithm

The advantages and disadvantages of FAST/eFAST are shown in Box 49.1.

FAST/eFAST involves the following minimum views.

1 The hepatorenal interface (Morison's pouch) and the right diaphragm. The transducer is placed at the right midaxillary line between the 11th and 12th ribs. The liver, kidney and diaphragm are viewed. The tip of the liver is often the first place for free blood to collect in the supine patient.

2 The splenorenal interface and left diaphragm. The transducer is placed at the left posterior axillary line between the 9th and 10th ribs. The spleen, kidney and diaphragm are viewed.

3 The pouch of Douglas (retrovesical or retrouterine). Ideally the bladder is full. The transducer is placed approximately 1 cm superior to the pubic symphysis. The examination is performed in both transverse and longitudinal planes.

4 Subxiphoid or intercostal views of the pericardium. With a subxiphoid view, the transducer is advanced to the xiphoid

---

Box 49.1 Advantages and disadvantages or limitations of FAST/eFAST

Advantages	Disadvantages
• Safe to operator and patient	• Positive examination requires presence of free intraperitoneal fluid (minimum of 600 mL)
• Rapid	
• Acceptable in the pregnant patient	• Cannot determine source of free fluid
• Non-invasive	• Not reliable for excluding hollow visceral injury
• Easily performed/easily learned	
• Can be performed concurrently with resuscitation	• Not reliable for grading solid organ injuries
• Can be performed in a resuscitation area (i.e. monitored environment)	• Not reliable for excluding retroperitoneal haemorrhage
• Repeatable (of particular value in the monitoring of non-operative solid organ injuries)	• Patient anatomy or pathology may make exam technically difficult (obesity or subcutaneous emphysema)
• More cost-effective when compared with diagnostic peritoneal lavage (DPL) or CT	
• Adult and paediatric applications	

process and the beam is directed at the left shoulder. The transducer is variously tilted, swept and rotated to obtain a four-chamber view and view the pericardial space. An effusion can be suspected when an anechoic area is seen between the liver edge and the right atrium or ventricle. A collapsed right ventricle offers evidence of pericardial tamponade. Clotting blood can be difficult to distinguish from anterior pericardial fat.

5 Lung ultrasound. Ultrasound has been shown to be more sensitive than chest X-ray in the diagnosis of pneumothorax in trauma patients. Ideally the linear array probe (5–10 MHz) is used. For assessment of pneumothorax the probe is placed over the anterior thorax in a sagittal orientation in the midclavicular line. Ultrasound can only detect a pneumothorax which is directly under the probe, so several sites on the anterior chest should be examined. Absence of lung sliding, the presence of the 'stratosphere' sign instead of the normal 'seashore' sign on M-mode image and the presence of a lung point (transition point of pneumothorax) should make one suspicious of a pneumothorax.

Other views include the bilateral paracolic gutters.

FAST/eFAST is also useful in penetrating thoracoabdominal trauma to detect pericardial effusion/cardiac tamponade, pneumothorax/haemothorax and haemoperitoneum. However, there are limitations such as detection of bowel injuries.

ABDOMINAL AORTIC SCAN

The ability to detect abdominal aortic aneurysm (AAA) can improve patient outcomes, as mortality has been shown to decrease if the diagnosis is made prior to or shortly after rupture. Ultrasound is an excellent tool for detecting the presence of AAA but can be limited in terms of the ability to assess for rupture.

This study involves scanning the aorta in both transverse and longitudinal planes continuously from the diaphragm to the aortic bifurcation. It includes measurement of the maximum aortic diameter in both planes.

A segment of the abdominal aorta > 3 cm is considered an aneurysm, or if the dilated segment is 1.5 times greater in diameter than the adjacent normal segment.

If an aneurysm is present several additional items need to be assessed, including:

- proximal edge, especially relationship of aneurysm to origin of renal arteries
- distal extent, especially relationship to origin of common iliac arteries
- presence of thrombus
- presence of dissection
- true aneurysmal diameter (outside to outside edge)
- residual lumen diameter
- presence of haematoma surrounding aorta in rupture
- presence of free intraperitoneal fluid.

Indications for ultrasound to detect AAA include presence of syncope, shock, hypotension, abdominal pain, abdominal mass and flank pain or back pain, especially in the older patient.

The presence of an AAA on ultrasound in the unstable patient confirms the need for a laparotomy for presumed rupture.

BASIC ECHOCARDIOGRAPHY IN LIFE SUPPORT (BELS)

BELS is a brief, time-limited examination in the shocked or arrested patient. It is used to: assess for pericardial effusion and tamponade; detect the presence of cardiac activity; allow a global assessment of contractility; provide an estimate of left ventricular (LV) and right ventricular (RV) size; and assess central volume status.

This study images the heart with four views. Ideally the patient should be positioned on the left side with the left arm above the head. This may not be possible during resuscitation. The sector array probe on a cardiac preset should be used.

1 Parasternal long axis view: the probe is placed to the left of the sternum with the probe marker pointing towards the patient's right shoulder, and then moved from the 2nd to 5th intercostal space to search for the best acoustic window. It provides an excellent view of the left atrium, left ventricle and aortic outflow tract and allows assessment of LV systolic function, presence of a pericardial effusion, RV and LV dilation and wall thickness.

2 Parasternal short axis view: the probe is rotated clockwise 90° from the parasternal long axis position. The probe marker should point towards the patient's left shoulder. It provides

an ideal view for assessing global LV function and the relative shapes and sizes of the two ventricles.

3 Apical four-chamber view: the probe is placed in the region of the apex beat with the probe marker at 3 o'clock and the face of the transducer is angled up towards the base of the heart. The apex of the heart should be centred in the screen with the intraventricular septum perpendicular and the lateral wall visible. It offers information about all four chambers and their relative sizes.

4 Subcostal/subxiphoid view: the probe is placed below and slightly to the right of the xiphisternum with the marker in the 3 o'clock position and tilted anteriorly. All four chambers should be visible.

In addition the IVC is imaged in longitudinal and transverse planes and IVC collapsibility can be assessed.

BELS is unable to rule out more subtle pathology such as valve disease or segmental wall motion abnormalities.

Other applications

+ **Pregnancy.**
  — First-trimester pelvic ultrasound to establish the location of the pregnancy and fetal heart rate in the symptomatic pregnant patient or the asymptomatic patient with risk factors for ectopic pregnancy. A ruptured ectopic pregnancy should be the main consideration in the pregnant patient with an empty uterus and fluid in the pouch of Douglas or free intraperitoneal fluid on ultrasound.
  — Second- and third-trimester pelvic ultrasound for detection of fetal cardiac movement, location of placenta and the evaluation of the pregnant trauma patient.
+ **Assessment of above-calf DVT.**
+ **Lung ultrasound:** can be used in the diagnosis of pleural fluid, pneumothorax, pulmonary oedema, pneumonia, abscess and pulmonary contusion. It also aids in procedural guidance for thoracocentesis and intercostal catheter placement. In the critically unwell patient it is useful in the assessment of cardiac arrest, respiratory distress and shock and fluid status.

- **Shock.**
  - A structured ultrasound protocol evaluating the heart, IVC, abdomen, aorta and lungs can provide valuable information which can guide the clinician during the initial evaluation and stabilisation of undifferentiated shock. This provides the opportunity for improved clinical treatments and patient outcomes.
  - There are various protocols such as the RUSH and FALLS protocols. The RUSH (Rapid Ultrasound in SHock) protocol evaluates the pump (heart: pericardial effusion, tamponade, LV contractility, RV strain), tank (lungs: pleural/peritoneal fluid, pulmonary oedema, tension pneumothorax; IVC) and pipes (vessels: AAA, aortic dissection, DVT) in sequential order.
- **Biliary ultrasound:** cholecystitis and cholelithiasis are best imaged with ultrasound.
- **Renal ultrasound:** ultrasound images the kidneys well and can be a sensitive bedside test for hydronephrosis.
- **Procedural uses** (see Table 49.2): this includes use for vascular access, insertion of nerve blocks and drainage of ascites or pleural fluid. Ultrasound may localise the percutaneous insertion/incision site before the procedure (static guidance) or may provide real-time guidance of the procedure with needle, catheter or other device (dynamic guidance).
- **Localisation of foreign bodies.**

Table 49.2 Procedural applications for ED ultrasound

Application	Strengths and uses	Limitations
Central and peripheral venous access	Body habitus Anticoagulation Lack of anatomical or palpable landmarks	Vessels may be difficult to visualise without Doppler technology
Bladder size and aspiration	Avoids dry taps Avoids urethral catheterisation	
Abscess location and aspiration	Soft-tissue infection without clear fluctuance	Other sonolucent structures
Thoracocentesis and paracentesis	Localisation of fluid and avoidance of viscera	

Table 49.2   Procedural applications for ED ultrasound (cont.)

Application	Strengths and uses	Limitations
Pericardiocentesis	Ultrasound-guided pericardiocentesis offers a safer therapeutic alternative in the presence of pericardial tamponade than traditional 'blind' methods	
Foreign-body localisation	Excellent visualisation in fluid and uniform surrounding tissue	
Nerve blocks	More effective than blind techniques with decreased complications and lower amounts of anaesthetic required to achieve an effective block	
Lumbar puncture (LP)	Reduces number of failures of LP in difficult patients	
Arthrocentesis	Useful especially in aspirating deeper and more difficult joints such as the hip and ankle	

Training, credentialling and quality review
INITIAL TRAINING
Accurate training and experience are vital to accurate ultrasound examination. The format of courses instructing individuals in ED ultrasound depends on the number of primary applications being taught.

CREDENTIALLING PROCESS AND MAINTENANCE OF STANDARDS
The ACEM has determined the credentialling process that outlines the minimum standards deemed sufficient to maintain a level of competency in ED PoCUS. This includes the satisfactory completion of an introductory course and the performance and recording of a requisite number of accurate proctored ultrasound examinations.

For example, the FAST/eFAST module involves the performance of at least 25 accurate trauma examinations, with 50% of them clinically indicated and at least five positive for intraperitoneal, pleural or pericardial fluid. A bedside practical exit exam is then required.

Once a level of proficiency is attained in each module, ongoing maintenance of credentials is essential. This includes ongoing annual ultrasound training and the performance of a specific number of ultrasound examinations for each module.

Individual institutions can adopt or adapt these standards as determined by local needs.

DOCUMENTATION

The results of ED ultrasound examinations that are used to facilitate patient care decisions should be documented in the patient's clinical record.

The following are basic items that should be documented:

- type of examination (e.g. FAST/eFAST)
- reason for examination (e.g. blunt abdominal injury)
- views obtained
- adequacy of views obtained—if inadequate, state reasons
- findings and interpretation—normal, abnormal or indeterminate.

Findings incidental to the examination should also be documented and the patient informed of them.

A patient undergoing an ED ultrasound should be informed that the exam is a focused one directed at determining the presence of specific pathologies or to answer a specific clinical question. Radiologists still provide expertise in comprehensive examinations.

QUALITY REVIEW AND QUALITY IMPROVEMENT

A process of measuring and documenting performance, accuracy and image quality is essential as part of a continuous quality improvement process. Periodic review of images with radiology staff will allow the identification of errors in clinical interpretation or failure to obtain appropriate images. Tracking clinical outcomes of patients by obtaining reports of follow-up imaging procedures or surgical findings can also be used to monitor the clinical interpretation of ultrasound studies.

Online resources

Australian College for Emergency Medicine (ACEM). ACEM Policy on the use of focused ultrasound in emergency medicine.
www.acem.org.au

Australian College of Emergency Physicians (ACEP). ACEP Policy Statement. Ultrasound guidelines: emergency, point of care, and clinical ultrasound guidelines in medicine. (June 2016)
www.acep.org

International Federation for Emergency Medicine. Point of care ultrasound curriculum guidelines. (May 2014)
www.ifem.cc

Emergency Care Institute NSW. UTEC Point of Care Ultrasound Training.
www.aci.health.nsw.gov.au/networks/eci/clinical/clinical-resources/clinical-tools/ultrasound-in-the-ed

Intensive Care Network. Focused cardiac ultrasound course.
www.intensivecarenetwork.com/courses/fcus/

Ultrasound Podcast.com
www.ultrasoundpodcast.com

Ultrasound Village
www.ultrasoundvillage.com

Chapter 50
X-ray and CT common misses

John Raftos

X-ray
GAMEKEEPER'S/SKIER'S THUMB (AVULSION OF THE ULNAR COLLATERAL LIGAMENT)

Caused by forced radial deviation of the thumb. Avulsion of the ulnar collateral ligament requires open reduction and internal fixation to prevent joint instability. Look for an avulsed fragment from the ulnar corner of the base of the proximal phalanx of the thumb. Always test patients with thumb injuries for integrity of the ulnar collateral ligament. (See Figure 50.1.)

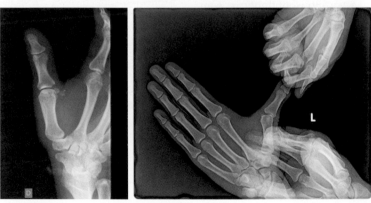

Figure 50.1 Gamekeeper's thumb

POSTERIOR GLENOHUMERAL DISLOCATION

In posterior shoulder dislocation, the humeral head may appear in anatomical position in anteriposterior (AP) plain radiographs. Clinically the patient will have difficulty moving the shoulder joint. Look for the 'light bulb' sign seen here. CT scan whenever there is a doubt about the integrity of the joint. (See Figure 50.2.)

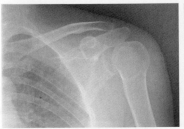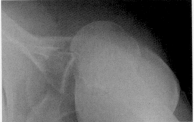

Figure 50.2 Posterior glenohumeral dislocation

FEMORAL NECK FRACTURE

Fractures of the femoral neck may not be evident on plain radiographs. Any patient with hip pain and difficulty mobilising but apparently normal radiographs of the femoral neck should have CT or MRI imaging to exclude occult fracture. (See Figure 50.3.)

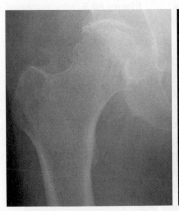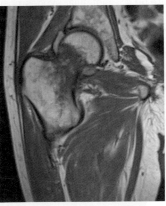

Figure 50.3 Femoral neck fracture

TIBIO FIBULAR SYNDESMOSIS INJURY AND MAISONNEUVE FRACTURE

Always inspect the AP radiographs of patients with ankle injuries for widening of the tibiofibular syndesmosis. Always palpate the proximal fibula in patients with ankle injuries for a possible Maisonneuve fracture. If you find a fracture of the upper fibula, always image the ankle for possible fracture or tibiofibular diastasis. (See Figures 50.4 and 50.5.)

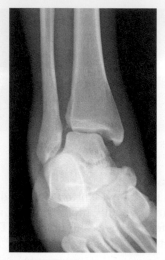

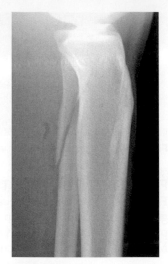

Figure 50.4 Tibiofibular syndesmosis injury

Figure 50.5 Maisonneuve fracture

LATERAL TIBIAL PLATEAU FRACTURE

Lateral tibial plateau fractures are caused by valgus injuries of the knee, most commonly with significant force as in pedestrian bumper bar injuries but also in simple falls from standing. The plain images may show no apparent fracture but will usually show a lipohaemarthrosis. If a patient with a knee injury has a significant lipohaemarthrosis and is unable to bear weight, then CT is indicated and will reveal the lateral tibial plateau injury. (See Figure 50.6.)

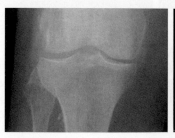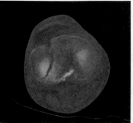

Figure 50.6 Lateral tibial plateau fracture

RETRO-ORBITAL HAEMATOMA

This relatively common complication of blunt head/facial/orbital trauma often does not cause obvious proptosis and the pain and visual loss it causes may be masked in intoxicated or unconscious patients. All patients with periorbital haematoma should therefore have a CT scan including the orbits which should be inspected for evidence of retro-orbital haematoma and proptosis. Urgent lateral canthotomy is indicated for raised intraocular pressure. (See Figure 50.7.)

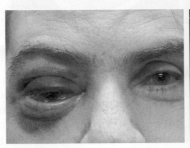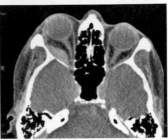

Figure 50.7 Retro-orbital haematoma

CT
ISODENSE SUBDURAL HAEMATOMA

Isodense subdural haematomas are usually detected because of asymmetry but not all isodense subdurals are asymmetrical. (See Figure 50.8.)

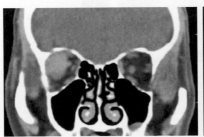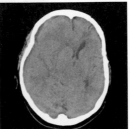

Figure 50.8 Isodense subdural haematoma

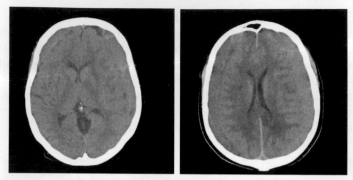

Figure 50.8—cont'd

SMEAR SUBDURAL HAEMATOMA

A small subdural haematoma soon after a head injury has the potential to rapidly increase in size and to become life-threatening in an anticoagulated patient. Great care is needed to detect the smallest amount of subdural blood in this patient group and to promptly reverse anticoagulation. (See Figure 50.9.)

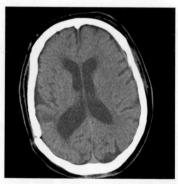

Figure 50.9 Smear subdural haematoma

Chapter 51

Test ordering: blood results, CSF analysis, pleural fluid analysis, ascitic fluid analysis and joint fluid analysis, choosing wisely

Farzad Jazayeri

Diagnosis has been described in many different ways: like solving a puzzle, a mystery or putting a name to a complaint. Diagnosis is the process of trying to understand the nature of a patient's problems to clarify their prognosis and treatment options. It is mostly challenging due to patient's variability, physician variability and system complexity.

We start our trip from complaint to diagnosis through the process of history, physical examination, hypothesis and synthesis diagnostic tests, and then likely diagnosis.

Usually the differential diagnosis list is made based on history, and physical examination and the investigations are done to:
* risk-stratify the patients
* confirm the diagnosis
* rule out the life threats
* narrow the differential diagnosis.

So it is very important to do the test in the context of potential diagnosis.

Blood results

The most common blood tests are haematology, biochemistry, serology, blood culture and clinical pharmacology.

Interpretation of blood results should always be in clinical context of the patient; for example, completely normal WBC count and inflammatory markers will not rule out appendicitis as the cause of pain in a patient with right iliac fossa pain.

HAEMATOLOGY
FBC
Definitions

Haemoglobin—oxygen-carrying molecule in whole.

Haematocrit—packed cell volume, expressed as a percentage.

RBC count—the number of RBCs in a microlitre volume.

MCV—mean corpuscular volume is the average volume of the patient's RBCs; normal RBC has a volume of 80 to 96 femtolitres.

MCH—mean corpuscular haemoglobin is the average haemoglobin content in a RBC. Low values are seen in iron deficiency and thalassaemia, while increased values occur in macrocytosis of any cause like B_{12} deficiency.

MCHC—mean corpuscular haemoglobin concentration is the average haemoglobin concentration per RBC.

RDW—red cell distribution width is a measure of the variation in RBC size on the peripheral blood smear, normally 11.5–14.5%. A high RDW implies a large variation in RBC sizes, and a low RDW implies a more homogeneous population of RBCs. An increased RDW indicates the presence of cells of widely differing sizes, but it is not diagnostic of any particular disorder.

Reticulocyte count—the reticulocyte count usually is a percentage of all RBCs, 0.5–2.5%, and it helps to distinguish among the different types of anaemia:

High reticulocyte count reflects an increased erythropoietic response to continued haemolysis or blood loss.

A stable anaemia with a low reticulocyte count is strong evidence for deficient production of RBCs (i.e. a reduced bone marrow erythropoietic response to the anaemia).

Haemoglobin
Polycythaemia: high levels of Hb and divides into two groups.

Relative: caused by reduce plasma volume; for example, dehydration.

Absolute: due to increased red blood cells, divided into primary caused by abnormal RBC progenitors, polycythaemia vera and secondary caused by circulating factor causing blood cell production, usually due to hypoxia or erythropoietin producing tumour.

Anaemia

The WHO definition of anaemia is a haemoglobin (Hb) concentration < 120 g/L in females and < 130 g/L in males.

Acute

>   Most common cause is due to haemorrhage, external or internal.
>
>   Patients usually are symptomatic.

Chronic

>   Mostly gradual onset and usually patients remain asymptomatic and can tolerate lower levels of Hb.

Approach to anaemia can be morphological or kinetic.

>   The kinetic approach has three independent mechanisms.
>>   Decreased RBC production.
>>>   Lack of nutrients, bone marrow disease, bone marrow suppression or low levels of trophic hormones.
>>   Ineffective production.
>>>   Thalassaemia, myelodysplastic syndrome.
>>   Increased RBC destruction.
>>>   Haemolytic anaemia, microangiopathic haemolytic anaemia (MAHA), or hypersplenism and blood loss.

Morphological approach.

>   The causes of anaemia can also be classified according to measurement of RBC size.
>>   **Macrocytic anaemia:** MCV exceeds 100 fL; for example: liver disease, alcoholism, reticulocytosis, hypothyroidism.
>>   **Microcytic anaemia:** MCV is less than 80 fL.
>>   The three most common causes of microcytosis in clinical practice are iron deficiency, alpha or beta thalassaemia minor and less often anaemia of chronic disease.
>>   **Normocytic anaemia:** MCV is normal.
>>   For example, anaemia of chronic disease, haemolysis and blood loss.

White cell count

Normal 4–11 × 10⁹/L

Five types: neutrophils, eosinophils, basophils, monocytes and lymphocytes

Leucocytosis

Elevation of white cell count which could be caused by rise of any of the subgroup of leucocytes.

Can be caused by a broad range of aetiologies from infection to strenuous physical activity, so lacks sensitivity.

Neutrophils:

Infection (usually bacterial), inflammation, trauma, severe pain, vomiting or in general acute stress response of any type.

Lymphocytosis:

Infection, usually viral such as EBV and other viral infections, post-splenectomy, stress, seizure and leukaemia (usually WBC > 30 000 with presence of blasts)

Eosinophilia:

Allergic reaction, drug reaction and asthma

Leucopenia

WBC < 4000

Infection, bacterial (brucellosis, TB), viral (HIV, measles), chemotherapy and alcohol use

Neutropenia

Neutrophil count = WBC (cells/microL) × (per cent [polymorph neutrophil {PMNs} + bands]/100)

Generally, count < 1.5×10^9 considered neutropenic

Important due to increased risk of life-threatening infection with reduction in neutrophil count

Causes: severe infection, chemotherapy, bone marrow suppression due to infiltration or malignancy

Platelets

Normal 150–350 × 10^9

High

Reactive: trauma, infection, surgery, post-splenectomy in the absence of myeloproliferative or myelodysplastic disease and will return to normal

Essentially caused by myeloproliferative neoplasm

Low

Bone marrow disorders: drug-induced, nutritional deficiency

Malignancy, radiation, infection and sepsis

Increased platelet destruction: ITP

Increased platelet consumption: thrombotic thrombocytopenic purpura (TTP), DIC, haemolytic uraemic syndrome (HUS) (these patients more at risk of thrombosis than bleeding)

Dilutional: fluid resuscitation

Redistribution/splenomegaly, portal hypertension and congestion of spleen

Functionally abnormal

Renal failure

Liver failure

Myeloproliferative disorders

Paraproteinaemia, multiple myeloma

Medication, aspirin, Plavix

Biochemistry

Renal function

Abnormal high creatinine or eGFR usually classified to renal, pre-renal or post renal.

A simplified guide to the aetiology of renal failure is BUN/ Cr ratio—pay attention to unit of measurement (common mistake):

Urea(BUN): Cr ratio in SI units of mmol/L: micromol/L (providing urea is >10 mmol/L)

Pre-renal > 100:1

Normal or post renal 40–100:1

Renal < 40:1

Liver function test:

Aminotransferase

ALT

More specific to liver

AST

Presence in liver and bone

Gamma-glutamyl transferase (GGT)

Liver and biliary epithelial cells

Alkaline phosphatase (ALP)

Presence in bone and liver; hepatic cause of elevation is usually associated with elevation of other liver enzymes, specifically GGT, and it is suggestive of intrahepatic or extrahepatic biliary obstruction

Assessment of the function of the liver
Albumin
Bilirubin
PT and INR
AST/ALT ratio
Most liver injuries cause higher elevation of ALT compared to AST; if this ratio is > 2:1 it is suggestive of alcoholic liver disease, especially with the presence of elevated GGT

Patterns of liver test abnormalities

Hepatocellular pattern
Disproportionate elevation in the serum aminotransferases compared with the alkaline phosphatase
Serum bilirubin may be elevated
Cholestatic pattern
Disproportionate elevation in the alkaline phosphatase compared with the serum aminotransferases
Serum bilirubin may be elevated
Mixed pattern

COAGULATION

Indications

Severe haemorrhage and
Screening for DIC, ITP, TTP
Sepsis
Anticoagulation therapy
Presence of thrombosis
Assessment of the function of the liver
History of bleeding and easy bruising
Family history of abnormal bleeding
Snake envenomation

Prothrombin time (PT)

- Measures the effectiveness of the extrinsic clotting pathway
- Particularly sensitive to low levels of fibrinogen as it measures time of clotting from exposure of fibrinogen to tissue factor

International normalised ratio (INR)
- Also measures extrinsic clotting pathway

Activated partial thromboplastin time (APTT)
- Measures the effectiveness of the intrinsic pathway (XII, XI, IX and VIII)
- Primary role is in the assessment of unfractionated heparin therapy and haemophilia A and B

Thrombin time (TT)
- Primary use is to determine the presence of an anti-coagulant effect of dabigatran
- Sensitive to hyperfibrinogenaemia
- Unaffected by warfarin therapy or Factor Xa inhibitors
- Normal range 13–16 seconds

D-dimer

Is a fibrin degradation product. It is used as part of Wells scoring risk assessment for DVT and recently for YEARs scoring system. The other areas that it has been used are aortic dissection, snake bite and DIC screening.

Lipase

Increases in many conditions but the common use of lipase is for diagnosis of pancreatitis in conjugation with history and imaging studies. The specificity increases but sensitivity decreases with increase in the level of lipase for diagnosis of pancreatitis. The mostly accepted level for diagnosis of pancreatitis is 3–4 times rise above upper limit of normal.

The level of rise of lipase dose not correlate with the severity of pancreatitis. It is not included in any severity scoring systems.

Troponin

Rise or fall of troponin is one of the criteria in universal definition of myocardial infarction.

Troponin can rise in patients with either pulmonary embolism or stroke. In both scenarios the prognosis of the patient with increased troponin appears to be worse.

UEC
Sodium
> Mainly extracellular ion
>
> Normal sodium level 135–145 me/L
>
> High or low levels of sodium mostly cause neurological symptoms

Hyponatraemia:
> \> 125 mmol/L asymptomatic
>
> 115–125 mmol/L lethargy, confusion, anorexia, nausea and vomiting
>
> < 115 mmol/L muscle cramps and weakness, convulsions and coma

Hypernatraemia
> 146–149 mmol/L mild
>
> 150–169 mmol/L moderate
>
> \> 169 mmol/L severe
>
> Level above 160 has high mortality

Potassium
> Normal range 3.5–5.0 mmol/L.
>
> Mainly intracellular ion.
>
> Levels will change due to blood acidity. Patients usually asymptomatic at the levels between 3.0 and 6.0 mmol/L but with worsening levels symptoms such as weakness, constipation, fatigue, feeling of heart racing and in extreme cases it can cause cardiac arrhythmias and cardiac arrest.

CRP
> Acute phase reactant, sensitive for inflammation but not specific. It starts to rise 2 hours post inflammatory process and peaks at 48 hours. Very high levels, usually above 100, may be indicative of bacterial infection.
>
> It can be used as an index for progress and response to treatment.

CSF analysis
CEREBROSPINAL FLUID
Produced by choroid plexus, 400–600 mL per 24 hours

Normal volume in adult 125–150 mL

NORMAL CONTENT

Pressure in adult lying lateral decubitus is 60–200 mm of
water

Colourless

Acellular; however, up to 5 WBCs but less than 3
polymorphonuclear leucocytes/microL and 5 RBCs are
considered normal in adults

Protein < 38 mg/dL

Glucose 60–80% of same time blood sugar

TEST TO ORDER

Microscopy, culture, CSF and blood, and sensitivity

Cell count

Should be done very quickly after the LP as delay will reduce
the count. Traumatic LP will affect the cell count number.
Recent study on paediatric population has suggested the
correction factor of 877:1 (877 RBC for 1 WBC).

Antibiotic treatment prior to LP is likely to affect Gram culture
but will not change the biochemistry of the CSF.

CSF glucose

CSF to blood glucose ratio.

Low glucose levels are suggestive of bacterial meningitis
especially if < 1.0 mmol/L. Viral meningitis usually has
normal glucose, but low glucose has been reported with
mumps, HSV, HZV and enterovirus meningitis

Protein

High levels indicate infection, SAH or traumatic LP. In viral
meningitis it is typically high but < 150 mg/dL and if
levels > 220 mg/dL it is more likely to be a bacterial
infection (likelihood of viral infection < 1%)

PCR

HSV, Enterococcus, N. meningitis, S. pneumonia and
H. influenzae type b.

This can be useful when the patient was given antibiotics
prior to CSF collection.

CSF culture

Reported sensitivity 50–80% (depends on the number of viable
bacteria in the sample) and specificity of 97%.

Blood culture

Approximately 60–80% of patients with bacterial meningitis have positive blood culture.

Xanthochromia.

Indicated if LP is performed for suspected SAH. It starts to appear 2–4 hours after entrance of blood into CSF but to increase the sensitivity 12 hours of gap between the onset of headache and LP is recommended.

Pleural fluid analysis
PLEURAL FLUID
Pleural fluid is formed at a rate of approximately 100 mL/day

NORMAL CONTENT
Clear, ultrafiltrate of plasma
Protein < 2%
WCC < 1000 mm^3
Glucose level similar to plasma
pH 7.60 due to bicarbonate gradient
Tests to order

Protein

LDH

Glucose

pH

Microscopy

Culture

Divided into two groups

1 **Transudates**: protein < 30 g/L. Result from imbalances in hydrostatic and oncotic pressures in the chest, as occur with congestive heart failure (CHF).

2 **Exudates**: protein > 30 g/L. Result from infection, malignancy, immunological responses, lymphatic abnormalities and non-infectious inflammation.

Diagnostic criteria: the Light's Criteria Rule is a traditional method of differentiating transudates and exudates that measures serum and pleural fluid protein and LDH

Light's Criteria Rule: if any one of the following three criteria present the pleural fluid is exudate

Pleural fluid protein/serum protein ratio greater than 0.5, or
Pleural fluid LDH/serum LDH ratio greater than 0.6, or
Pleural fluid LDH greater than two-thirds the upper limits of
the laboratory's normal serum LDH.

Glucose: a low pleural fluid glucose concentration (< 3.33 mmol/L),
or a pleural fluid/serum glucose ratio less than 0.5, narrows
the differential diagnosis of the exudate to the following
possibilities
Rheumatoid pleurisy
Complicated parapneumonic effusion or empyema
Malignant effusion
Tuberculous pleurisy
Lupus pleuritis
Oesophageal rupture

pH: pleural fluid pH should always be measured. Differential
diagnosis for pleural fluid with pH < 7.30, with normal blood
pH, is the same as pleural fluid with low glucose level as
mentioned above.

The mechanisms responsible for pleural fluid acidosis
(pH < 7.30) include:
increased acid production by pleural fluid cells and bacteria
(empyema)
decreased hydrogen ion efflux from the pleural space.

Ascitic fluid analysis

Presence of fluid within the peritoneal cavity is ascites, most
commonly due to portal hypertension secondary to liver
cirrhosis. Other causes include malignancy, heart failure and
constrictive pericarditis.

Abdominal paracentesis is central to determining the cause of
ascites and in ruling out or confirming spontaneous bacterial
peritonitis (SBP). In patients with SBP, mortality increases by
3.3%/h of delay in performing a paracentesis.

Initial tests that should be performed on the ascitic fluid include
the following.
Appearance assessment.
Clear: uncomplicated ascites.

Bloody: malignancy, traumatic tap and cirrhosis.

Cloudy: infection.

Serum-to-ascites albumin gradient determination (SAAG).

Cell count and differential: most important test and should be performed on every sample. Antibiotic treatment should be considered in any patient with a neutrophil count $\geq 250/mm^3$.

Total protein concentration has been mainly replaced by SAAG calculation but the total protein concentration may also help differentiate uncomplicated ascites from cirrhosis or from cardiac ascites, both of which have a SAAG ≥ 11 g/L. But in cirrhosis, the total protein is < 25 g/L, whereas in cardiac ascites it is ≥ 25 g/L.

Measurement of total protein, glucose and lactate dehydrogenase (LDH) in ascites may also be of value in distinguishing SBP from bowel perforation into ascites. If neutrophil count ≥ 250 cells/mm^3 and patient has two out of the three criteria patient should be assessed for perforation and peritonitis.

Total protein > 11 g/L.

Glucose < 2.8 mmol/L.

LDH greater than the upper limit of normal for serum.

Additional tests that may be performed to aid in confirming a particular diagnosis include the following.

Gram stain.

Positive in suspected bowel perforation but has low sensitivity and specificity.

The Gram stain is most helpful in ruling in free perforation of the bowel into ascites.

Culture, aerobic and anaerobic blood culture bottles.

Positive in infection, bowel perforation.

Glucose.

Concentration of glucose normally equal to the blood unless it has been consumed by bacteria or WBC (malignancy, infection, bowel perforation).

Lactate dehydrogenase concentration.

Increase in malignancy, infection, bowel perforation.

LDH ascitic fluid/serum (AF/S) ratio.

Is approximately 0.4 in uncomplicated ascites due to cirrhosis. In SBP, the ascitic fluid LDH level rises and the ratio approaches 1.0. If the LDH ratio is more than 1.0, extra LDH is present in the peritoneal cavity, usually because of infection, bowel perforation or tumour.

Amylase concentration.

Increase in pancreatic ascites or bowel perforation.

AF/S ratio of amylase is approximately 0.4(6). The ascitic fluid amylase concentration rises above this level in the setting of pancreatitis or bowel perforation into ascites. In pancreatic ascites, the ascitic fluid amylase concentration is approximately 2000 IU/L and the AF/S ratio is approximately 6.0.

Cytology and possibly carcinoembryonic antigen level.

In suspected malignancy.

Bilirubin concentration.

If ascetic fluid is brown or in suspected bowel or biliary perforation.

CLASSIFICATION OF ASCITES BY THE SERUM-TO-ASCITES ALBUMIN GRADIENT

High albumin gradient (SAAG ≥11 g/L)

Cirrhosis

Alcoholic hepatitis

Heart failure

Massive hepatic metastases

Heart failure/constrictive pericarditis

Budd-Chiari syndrome

Portal vein thrombosis

Idiopathic portal fibrosis

Low albumin gradient (SAAG < 11 g/L)

Peritoneal carcinomatosis

Peritoneal tuberculosis

Pancreatitis serositis

Nephrotic syndrome

Joint fluid analysis

Synovial fluid analysis is helpful for determining the underlying cause of arthritis, particularly for septic or crystal-induced arthritis.

The white cell count, differential count, cultures, Gram stain and crystal search using polarised light microscopy are the most useful studies.

ROUTINE COMPONENTS OF SYNOVIAL FLUID ANALYSIS

Colour

Colourless, clear fluid is normal, while increasing amounts of plasma and nucleated cells contribute to the yellow or yellow-green appearance of inflammatory or septic fluids. Bright red, rusty or chocolate-brown fluids are indicative of fresh or old blood.

Viscosity

As joint fluid is expelled from the syringe and allowed to drop into a suitable receptacle, normal fluid will produce a long string-like extension as it falls. Release of proteolytic enzymes into inflamed synovial fluid typically causes a decrease in viscosity. However, frankly purulent (septic) effusions may also be viscous.

Gram stain

Fast and easily done, provide information regarding the potential cause and may identify the cause that normally won't grow in a routine culture media.

Cell count

Normally acellular. Inflammation and infection cause an increased number of leucocytes. Bacterial infection usually causes purulent fluid with WBC count of > 50 000 cells/mm^3 with usually more than 75% PMNs.

Crystal analysis

Monosodium urate crystals (MSU)

MSU crystals are brightly birefringent and are needle-shaped suggestive of gout.

Calcium pyrophosphate dihydrate crystals (CPPD)

CPPD crystals have a rhomboidal or rectangular shape and positive birefringence. However, compared with MSU crystals, the birefringence is weaker, and some CPPD crystals may not appear birefringent and their presence is suggestive of pseudogout.

CATEGORIES OF JOINT EFFUSIONS
Noninflammatory: WBC approximately < 2000 cells/mm^3; for
example, osteoarthritis, avascular necrosis or a meniscal tear.
Inflammatory: $2000 < \text{WBC} < 50\,000$ cells/mm^3; for
example, septic arthritis, crystal-induced arthritis (e.g. gout,
pseudogout) or spondylarthritis.
Septic: WBC $> 50\,000$ cells/mm^3; for example, septic arthritis
due to bacteria, mycobacteria or fungus.
Haemorrhagic: large numbers of red blood cells; for example,
haemophilia, anticoagulation, trauma or tumour.

Choosing tests wisely
There are many tests ordered by medical practitioners that are
deemed unnecessary. Some experts estimated the cost of unnecessary tests to be about $200 million a year.

There are many causes of ordering unnecessary tests, but one
of the most important causes is uncertainty about the diagnosis.
Uncertainty is common in medicine; often we are not sure what
test to order or we are not sure what is the potential cause for patient symptoms, so to feel safe, we resolve this by ordering more
unnecessary tests.

Some causes of overuse might include the following.
1 Indication creep
    A test is developed for a certain purpose but gradually its
    indication extends to unnecessary conditions. For example,
    CRP is an inflammatory marker useful mainly in progress and
    response to treatment but at times is ordered for almost any
    febrile illness. Blood culture is useful to identify the specific
    cause for sepsis in very sick patients but it is often ordered for
    well but febrile or even non-febrile patients.
2 Fear of litigation and missing the diagnosis
    The concern of missing a diagnosis, potential legal con-
    sequences and not providing the necessary treatment for the
    patients is another cause for overuse of tests in the emer-
    gency department. This is also known as 'defensive medicine'.
    For example, ordering a brain CT scan in a patient with no
    indication, just based on fear of missing an unlikely intrac-
    ranial bleed.

3 Patient demand and patient satisfaction

Some doctors believe that by ordering more tests they may appear more caring and increase the patient satisfaction. For instance, a patient with simple symptoms and signs of upper respiratory infection does not need any tests but at times full blood count and a chest X-ray is done to increase patient satisfaction.

There has been a greater emphasis on the appropriateness of laboratory testing since the initiation of Choosing Wisely. Choosing Wisely was launched in 2012 by the American Board of Internal Medicine Foundation with a goal of avoiding wasteful or unnecessary medical tests, treatments and procedures.

Following that, Choosing Wisely Australia was launched in 2015. It is an initiative that brings the community together to improve the quality of healthcare through considering tests, treatments and procedures where evidence shows they provide no benefit or, in some cases, lead to harm.

Led by Australia's colleges, societies and associations and facilitated by NPS MedicineWise, Choosing Wisely Australia challenges the way we think about healthcare, questioning the notion 'more is always better'.

Chapter 52
Nursing and allied health advanced practice and adjunct roles

Wayne Varndell and Julie Gawthorne

Acknowledgement

The authors wish to acknowledge the content used from the previous edition of *Emergency Medicine* which was provided by Barbara Daly, Sarah Hoy, Kirsty McLeod and Gordian Fulde.

Advanced practice in Australia has developed significantly over the past few decades with many roles now highly specialised and requiring post-graduate qualifications. Emergency nursing and other allied health professionals such as physiotherapists are no exception with the scope, skill and knowledge extending to meet the needs of patients and the healthcare system. The introduction of ED key performance indicators including waiting times, length of stay, transfer of care and patient satisfactions have all been influential in advancing nursing and allied health practice. To meet these indicators EDs have developed new models of care, and advanced nursing and allied health roles have become an integral part of these new models.

This chapter will discuss the various advanced nursing roles in EDs including triage, nursing and allied health advanced practice and clinical roles. Due to the diversity of Australian EDs, the specific function of these roles will differ depending on the location and size of the ED.

The triage nurse

The term 'triage' is derived from the French word 'trier' meaning to sort or pick out. In the ED the patient's journey begins at triage. Many patients present simultaneously and the role of triage is to obtain a brief clinical assessment that determines clinical urgency and the time and sequence in which patients receive emergency care.

The triage assessment is a systematic, focused assessment that should take no longer than five minutes. The assessment should include the patient's presenting complaint, associated clinical signs and symptoms, general appearance, physiological observations and relevant medical history. Depending on the patient's chief complaint the triage assessment may include vital signs, the Glasgow Coma Scale (GCS) and a pain score. Patient age, mechanism of injury and comorbidities will also form part of the triage assessment and influence decision-making.

Following an assessment, the triage nurse will allocate a triage category. In Australasian EDs a standardised triage system called the Australasian Triage Scale (ATS) is used. The ATS was developed to assess urgency, prioritise care, achieve greater consistency within practice and create equity in funding models.

The ATS has five categories with category one being the most urgent to category five being the least urgent. The ATS applies to both adult and paediatric presentations. The triage category is at the discretion of the triage nurse; however, a number of EDs have specific mandatory triage categories for certain presentations. All triage categories have maximum waiting times and key performance indicators (Table 52.1).

Triage is a dynamic and ongoing process in which patients are continually reassessed. If a patient's condition changes while they are waiting for treatment or if additional relevant information becomes available that impacts on the patient's urgency, the patient should be re-triaged. For example, if a patient's level of pain increases compared with initial triage assessment, or they become tachycardic or hypotensive, the patient will be re-triaged to a higher category.

The triage nurse is a qualified experienced registered nurse who demonstrates and maintains clinical expertise in emergency nursing. To work at triage, nurses are required to have completed local triage training programs. Most training programs incorporate the Emergency Triage Education Kit (ETEK) as well as a supervised practical component. The level of training and experience will differ depending on the location and size of the hospital. For example,

Table 52.1 ATS categories, descriptions, waiting times and performance thresholds

Triage category	Maximum waiting time	Description of category	Performance indicator (%)	Example
1	Immediately	Immediately life threatening	100	• Cardiac arrest • Major trauma • Severe respiratory distress • Severe haemodynamic compromise. BP < 80 mmHg • Decreased LOC (GCS < 9)
2	10 minutes	Imminently life threatening OR Time critical treatment OR Very severe pain	100	• Acute stroke • Cardiac chest pain • Suspected sepsis • Decreased LOC GCS (9–12) • Severe localised trauma – major fracture, amputation • Severe pain requiring analgesia • Acute behavioural disturbance—violent, aggressive, severe agitation
3	30 minutes	Potentially life threatening OR Situational urgency OR Humane practice	80	• Abdominal pain • Moderate respiratory distress • Moderate limb injury—deformity, pain, altered neurovascular status • Head injury with LOC • Moderately severe pain • Risk self-harm, situational crisis, thought disordered, potentially aggressive

Continued

Table 52.1 ATS categories, descriptions, waiting times and performance thresholds (cont)

Triage category	Maximum waiting time	Description of category	Performance indicator (%)	Example
4	1 hour	Potentially serious OR Situational urgency	70	• Abdominal pain—no risk factors • Musculoskeletal injury • Laceration requiring suturing • Minor head injury—no LOC • Minor limb trauma
5	2 hours	Less urgent	70	• Minimal pain • Minor wound/injuries • Scheduled visit—wound review, medication, result review • Social issues—accommodation, money

Australian College of Emergency Medicine, Australian Triage Scale. Retrieved from: www.acem.org.au

there are often 3–4 triage nurses per shift in busy metropolitan hospitals as opposed to 2 nurses on shift for a whole hospital in rural or remote areas.

Following the patient assessment, the triage nurse is responsible for allocating patients to the most appropriate assessment and treatment area in the ED, such as to the fast track treatment area or waiting room. The patient may also follow a variety of treatment paths and interact with any of the following ED staff and teams:

- emergency nurse practitioner
- advanced practice nurse
- emergency physiotherapy practitioner
- aged service emergency team
- clinical nurse consultant
- clinical nurse specialist
- nurse educator
- clinical nurse educator
- emergency department navigator.

EMERGENCY NURSE PRACTITIONER (ENP)

An emergency nurse practitioner is an advanced practice registered nurse who has undertaken further higher degree study (e.g. Master of Nurse Practitioner degree) and is endorsed and authorised by the Nursing and Midwifery Board of Australia to complete independent, autonomous assessment, diagnosis and management of patients, including prescribing of medications and referral within their speciality area. The introduction of the emergency nurse practitioner role to the ED has had a positive impact on the quality of care, patient satisfaction, waiting times, leadership and reducing hospital readmissions.

ADVANCED PRACTICE NURSE (APN)

Advanced practice nurse is a term used to define a level of nursing practice that uses comprehensive skills, experience and knowledge in nursing care. In the ED setting this may include ordering and interpretation of investigations, diagnosis, procedures, prescribing and discharging patients.

APN roles can have different tittles in different EDs and may include the clinical initiatives nurse (CIN), advanced practice nurse (APN) and advanced clinical nurse (ACN). For the purpose of this chapter the term APN will be used to describe all extended practice nursing roles except the nurse practitioner.

APNs work within a defined scope of practice that includes specific protocols and standing orders protocols under the supervision of an ED consultant or registrar. The APN's primary focus is patients waiting to be seen, particularly those in the waiting room. APNs are responsible for initiating treatment and diagnostics, escalating care when required and expediting flow through the ED. See the examples in Boxes 52.1 and 52.2.

Examples of APN practice include:

+ administration of analgesia, including opioids
+ administration of medication (e.g. antiemetics, bronchodilators, antihistamines)
+ ordering radiology
+ ordering pathology
+ wound management including suturing
+ fracture management including plastering
+ ultrasound-guided vascular access
+ insertion of fascia iliaca blocks.

Box 52.1   Example 1: Patient presenting with an ankle fracture

- A 25-year-old male presents to ED with a painful left ankle following inversion injury playing basketball.
- Triage assessment indicates pain and tenderness at the posterior edge of the lateral malleolus and base of the fifth metatarsal. The ankle is swollen and deformed and the patient is unable to bear weight. The left ankle is neurovascularly intact, and the patient describes pain severity as 7/10. Triage category 3 is allocated by the triage nurse.
- The patient is referred to the APN who performs a set of vital signs that are within normal limits, applies rest/ice and elevation, inserts an IV and administers 2.5 mg morphine for pain and an antiemetic for nausea as per nurse-initiated protocols. A left ankle and foot X-ray are ordered according to Ottawa ankle rules.
- The patient's ankle X-ray is attended.
- The APN views the X-ray with the ED registrar and ED physiotherapist. The X-ray shows a fracture to the left lateral malleolus.
- The APN applies back slab plaster as per standing order.
- After orthopaedic review, the patient is discharged home for follow-up in the fracture clinic with a patient information handout on ankle fracture management, plaster cast care and pain management.

> **Box 52.2   Example 2: Accute care of an 80-year-old female presenting with recurrent falls**
>
> • An 80-year-old female presents via ambulance to the ED with recurrent falls. The patient's neighbour found her on the floor with a painful right hip, unable to bear weight.
> • Triage assessment indicates a painful right hip, shortening and external rotation of the right leg. The patient's GCS is 14; she is confused regarding day/date/time. Vital signs are within normal limits. The right leg is neurovascularly intact. The patient is unable to recall her medical history. Triage category 3 is allocated and a referral made to the APN.
> • The APN starts the patient on a fractured neck of femur (NOF) pathway and orders right hip and pelvis and chest X-ray. An IV cannula is inserted and bloods taken for pathology (FBC, UECs, LFTs, group-and-hold). Analgesia is given as per nurse-initiated pain protocol. An ECG and pressure risk assessment are performed and the patient remains nil by mouth.
> • The patient's pain has not improved and the APN inserts a fascia iliaca block as per protocol for pain ongoing pain management. An IDC is inserted.
> • The medical officer decides there is a need for further investigations in ED (e.g. if head injury is present or if the patient is on warfarin, need to consider CT of brain).

APNs are experienced registered nurses who are required to complete a local education package that includes theoretical and practical components and competency-based assessment.

EMERGENCY PHYSIOTHERAPY PRACTITIONER

An emergency physiotherapy practitioner is a physiotherapist who has undertaken further post-graduate study to assess and manage acute musculoskeletal injuries using a range of diagnostic investigations such as X-ray and ultrasound, movement and manual therapy to diagnose and manage acute injuries and injury prevention and rehabilitation education. Emergency physiotherapy practitioner roles have been identified as an effective strategy to improve access, follow-up and quality of service for patients presenting to EDs with musculoskeletal conditions; adding to the emergency department team through their specialist expertise and skills. Emergency physiotherapy practitioners work autonomously as a primary contact clinician within an endorsed scope of practice, or collaboratively as part of the emergency care team in more complex musculoskeletal injuries to enhance patient outcomes.

AGED SERVICE EMERGENCY TEAM (ASET)

The aged service emergency team is led by a clinical nurse consultant specialising in aged care. ASET is a multidisciplinary team including a nurse, a physiotherapist, a social worker and, in some areas, an occupational therapist.

The specific objectives of this team include:

- undertaking a comprehensive assessment of elderly patients over 70 years of age presenting to the ED
- aiming to prevent avoidable admissions by setting up services or accessing respite care
- identifying potential admission for patients who are considered at risk
- commencing treatment for patients being admitted by providing physiotherapy and social work input while in the ED
- encouraging health promotion by providing information on social and educational activities available for older people in the community
- improving communication between hospital and community workers, and hospital and residential care staff, regarding patients presenting to the ED.

An example of how the ASET functions is described in Box 52.3.

CLINICAL NURSE CONSULTANT (CNC)

The clinical nurse consultant is an experienced registered nurse with at least five years' experience in emergency nursing and postgraduate qualifications. CNCs provide expert clinical advice to patients, carers and other healthcare professionals within a defined specialty. The domains of the ED CNC include clinical leadership, research, education and service planning. The CNC provides expert, highly complex clinical care, and is responsible for delivering, driving evidence-based practice in the ED and identifying, implementing and evaluating clinical practice changes and research activities. CNCs provide clinical leadership, and are involved in policy and practice development at local, state and

---

Box 52.3 Example 3: Further care of an 80-year-old female with a fractured hip

Patient presents via ambulance to the ED with recurrent falls. Patient found on the floor by neighbour with painful right hip, unable to weight bear.

Triage assessment indicates painful right hip, shortening and external rotation of right leg. Patient is confused regarding day/date/time. Unable to confirm past medical history. Vital signs within normal limits. Triage category 3 is allocated. Referral made to APN and ASET nurse.

APN orders right hip X-ray, chest X-ray, IV cannula is inserted, bloods taken for pathology (FBC, renal profile, group-and-hold), analgesia given as per nurse-initiated narcotic protocol, ECG, intravenous fluids, pressure risk assessment, patient remains nil by mouth.

ASET nurse undertakes comprehensive assessment including:

— Pre-morbid mobility assessment to identify level of independence. This also includes history of falls and potential causes. This may lead to a referral to other specialty teams, e.g. dizziness may require investigation by neurology team.

— Ability to perform activities of daily living (ADLs).

— Community services usage and frequency of services.

— Current home support, e.g. family, contact numbers, need for respite care.

— Mental status is assessed via Abbreviated Mental Test Score (AMTS) and Confusion Assessment Method (CAM) diagnostic algorithm. Both these tests are performed with involvement of the patient's family.

Early linkage to community care packages is made to ensure safe and timely discharge of the patient back to the community after acute admission. Early involvement of the GP is an important aspect of the discharge planning process.

Medical staff continue treatment and management of the patient in conjunction with ED nurses and the ASET.

Once clinical work-up is complete, referral to orthogeriatric team for admission for fractured right pubic ramus.

Medical officer decides the need for further investigations in ED—e.g. if head injury present or if the patient is on warfarin, need to consider CT of brain.

---

national levels. CNCs are representative on peak professional organisations including editorial boards and emergency associations.

CLINICAL NURSE SPECIALIST (CNS)

The clinical nurse specialist is a registered nurse with 2–4 years' post-registration experience and who is a senior member of the emergency nursing team that has undertaken postgraduate study and supervised practice. In addition, the clinical nurse specialist provides advanced and complex patient care and assists in managing and leading the ED. There are two classifications of CNS. Grade 1 holds relevant post-graduate qualifications, supporting and contributing to quality improvement, mentoring of staff in relation to expert practice, and actively contributing to emergency nursing practice. In addition to grade 1 criteria, CNS grade 2 has extended autonomy in relation to decision-making and operates within a designated scope of practice to provide primary case management of a complete episode of care.

NURSE EDUCATOR

A nurse educator is a registered nurse who has completed further clinical education or postgraduate qualifications relevant to the clinical area, who assesses, plans, implements and evaluates nursing education, both post-registration speciality courses and tertiary-level programs. The nurse educator also provides clinical supervision and preceptorship, and supports the development and growth of nurses including clinical supervision and, more broadly, the emergency care team. In addition to the responsibilities of theoretical and clinical teaching, the nurse educator contributes to the leadership and research activity and translation of best clinical practice. Globally, there is an urgent requirement for more agile and skilled nurses; the nurse educator is critical to maintaining and advancing nursing practice standards, optimising patient outcomes and the recruitment and retention of nursing staff.

CLINICAL NURSE EDUCATOR

A clinical nurse educator is a registered nurse who has undertaken further vocational study in teaching and assessment in the workplace and (ideally) holds postgraduate qualifications relevant to the clinical area. The clinical nurse educator is integral to the success of the nursing team, and includes a variety of critical responsibilities, including orientation of new staff, providing training and continuing education, assessing staff competency in local work practices, updating policies and procedures and clinical supervision. The principal difference between a nurse educator and clinical nurse educator is the designing of education and postregistration courses to meet professional, service and organisational needs.

EMERGENCY DEPARTMENT NAVIGATOR

The emergency department navigator is a senior registered nurse with significant experience in emergency department operations. Traditionally, patient flow in the emergency department has been led by the nurse in charge and senior medical officer. Increasing demand for emergency care, overcrowding and prolonged length of stay imperil patient and staff safety and reduce delivery of timely quality care. This has led to the development of the navigation role. The core purpose of the emergency department navigator is to enhance the patient's journey through the department in a timely and safe manner, by using departmental resources optimally, improving team collaboration and communication, and problem-solving. The initial examination of the role has demonstrated positive impact on patient and staff safety, throughput and department efficiency, communication and cost saving.

Editorial Comment

Future professional and career roles for nurses must continue to progress due to the enormous healthcare needs of the community. We are in a time of re-engineering the patient journey (e.g. the 4-hour rule) linked to funding and key performance indicators (KPIs). This affects EDs, all hospital clinical services, ambulance services and community GPs and health workers. Thus, the imperative to more efficiently but also safely process the patient must be met by many changes. Core (apart from inpatient bed availability) to all of this is front-loading—senior doctors and nurses starting decisions and diagnosis soon after triage. Also, reorganising the ED into teams and areas (fast-track, etc.) relies heavily on nurses having advanced skills, training and supervision. With these measures, it is even more vital that the nursing, medical and administrative ED staff meet weekly to solve and improve issues to ensure that staff actually lead the changes and process.

Resources

Australasian College of Emergency Medicine. Guidelines on the implementation of the Australasian Triage scale in emergency Departments. 2016.

Nursing and Midwifery Board of Australia. Advanced nursing practice and speciality areas within nursing. Fact Sheet. 2016.

Agency for Clinical Innovation. Impact of Physiotherapy Care in the Emergency Department. ACI; 2014 (cited December 2017); Available from: https://www.aci.health.nsw.gov.au/ie/projects/physiotherapy-in-ed

Thompson J, Yoward S, Dawson P. The Role of Physiotherapy Extended Scope Practitioners in Musculoskeletal care with Focus on Decision Making and Clinical Outcomes: A Systematic Review of Quantitative and Qualitative Research. Musculoskeletal Care 2017;15(2):91–103.

Hodge A, Varndell W. Professional Transitions in Nursing: A Guide to Practice in the Australian Healthcare System. Sydney, Australia: Allen & Unwin; 2018.

Fulbrook P, Jessup M, Kinnear F. Implementation and evaluation of a 'Navigator' role to improve emergency department throughput. Australasian Emergency Nursing Journal: 2017; 20(3):114–121.

Chapter 53
Emergency medicine in a rural setting

Alan Tankel

Definitions

There are a number of different definitions of what constitutes a rural emergency department in Australia. For example, Gosford, Wollongong and Geelong are regarded as rural/regional centres by the Australasian College for Emergency Medicine (ACEM) but as major cities by the Australian Statistical Geography Standard (ASGS) while Darwin, Townsville and Hobart are regarded as major cities by ACEM but as rural/regional centres by ASGS.

Using the ACEM definition, 31% of the population lives in rural/regional Australia while 37% of Australia's ED presentations in 2014/15 were outside of metropolitan areas. Whichever definition we use, this represents a significant proportion of the population who are entitled to the same access to healthcare as every other person in Australia and New Zealand.

Challenges

There are many challenges when practising emergency medicine in rural settings. These include the relative isolation and lack of access to specialist advice and care. However, with the increasing use of technology, the capacity to get a specialist opinion via telehealth or other online technology is improving all the time.

Many of Australia and New Zealand's rural and regional centres are also responsible for more remote facilities that have variable access to medical and, more remotely, nursing cover throughout any particular day.

In many rural settings, you may be the first provider of healthcare to a severely injured multi-trauma patient or a potentially critically ill septic patient. This can be very challenging but, at the same time, very rewarding.

Clinicians who choose to work in these communities must have the knowledge and skill set to perform a relevant history and examination and to be able to organise appropriate investigations which may include point-of-care testing (POCT) and transporting other investigations for analysis elsewhere, when elsewhere may be several hours away depending on the level of remoteness.

POCT is becoming increasingly more available, helping reduce the number of patients who are transferred unnecessarily to larger centres for basic investigations or treatment. However, there is a limited range of investigations that are available for POCT and there will be a range of important investigations that will still need to be sent to larger centres, with potentially significant delays in accessing the results of these investigations. POCT will help ensure that patients who require care at a higher level than can be delivered locally are transferred for the necessary care if that is indicated and that is their desire.

The lack of access to imaging modalities such as ultrasound, CT, MRI and, in more remote environments, simple X-rays means that clinicians working in those areas must have the ability to decide which patients require transfer for those investigations and which patients are safe to be managed locally based on their clinical assessment. Point-of-care ultrasound (PoCUS) is becoming increasingly more available and may be used effectively to influence these decisions.

Transferring certain patients, particularly elderly and very young patients, to larger centres can have a significant impact on the family unit as carers may have significant work or financial commitments such as being the manager of the only grocery store in town or the local pharmacy or post office. Separating elderly patients from their routine environment can be particularly distressing and disorientating for them and not necessarily in their best interest.

Many rural and remote ED depend on short-term or fly in/fly out (FIFO) medical staffing. This has a potentially negative impact on continuity and standardisation of healthcare in those areas. It takes time for FIFO staff to get to know their local environment and to understand what is available and, more importantly, what is not available locally.

Practising emergency medicine in a relatively resource-poor environment requires individuals who have a willingness and an ability to practise without the infrastructure in terms of specialty and subspecialty support that may be available in a tertiary or major metropolitan facility.

Education

ACEM has developed the Emergency Medicine Certificate (EMC) and Emergency Medicine Diploma (EMD) which are both designed to develop the skills of those who will work in any part of rural, regional or remote Australia and New Zealand.

There are also many short courses available aimed at increasing procedural and ultrasound skills as well as critical care and trauma skills.

A knowledge of envenomation (snakes, spiders, marine) is essential and will be expected in many of the more remote parts of Australia as well as in our regional centres. See Chapter 44 Envenomation.

Stabilisation for retrieval

(See Chapter 8 Patient transport, retrieval and pre-hospital care.)

There will always be patients who require transfer for care that cannot be delivered locally. This may be in relatively stable patients who are being transferred for straightforward investigations or treatment and do not require retrieval or even transport by ambulance. However, there will always be a group of patients that do require retrieval who are critically ill or who are potentially critically ill.

Clinicians need to know how to prepare patients optimally for transfer and ensure that their patient is receiving the best possible care given the resources that are available.

The patient may need to be intubated to optimally manage a severe head injury. There is clear evidence that the duration of hypoxia and hypotension in head-injured patients significantly influences long-term outcomes. Early intubation allows the patient to be appropriately sedated and ventilated which may help reduce intracranial pressure and support safe management of the patient while awaiting retrieval.

The patient may require insertion of a chest drain, an indwelling urethral catheter (IDC), a nasogastric tube, central and arterial lines or an intraosseous needle. As the senior or only clinician available, you may need to be able to safely administer a variety of relatively unfamiliar medications albeit with advice from your local retrieval service (e.g. sedation, inotropes).

A basic understanding of splinting of fractures is essential to reduce pain and to reduce bleeding, particularly in long-bone fractures. These are relatively simple techniques to learn and there are proprietary brands on the market that can be used.

It is arguably even more important to know when not to perform a particular procedure. Examples in trauma include knowing when not to insert a nasogastric tube (e.g. if there is any blood or CSF coming from the ears, nose or mouth which may represent a base of skull fracture) or when not to insert an indwelling urethral catheter (e.g. if there is blood at the meatus, blood in the scrotum or a high-riding or impalpable prostate). In those cases, insertion of an orogastric tube or a suprapubic catheter may be required.

Managing expectations

For those who wish to spend any part of their working lives in rural, regional and remote Australia or New Zealand, there will be an expectation that you are able to function effectively in that environment and have a skill set that may not be required in a tertiary or major metropolitan setting.

Clinicians may be expected to have the ability to provide procedural sedation safely for the management of a variety of conditions (e.g. lacerations, fractures, burns). Experience and familiarity with regional nerve blocks (e.g. Bier's, wrist, fascia iliaca, femoral, foot) would clearly be advantageous. The ability to perform these procedures safely and appropriately reduces the need to transfer patients unnecessarily, improves patient (and family/carer) satisfaction as well as providing personal satisfaction and maintaining your own skill set.

It is important, wherever you are, to always advocate for your patients but you may also need to advocate for your colleagues in terms of maintaining and improving clinical and educational resources.

Teamwork is essential in all clinical environments but particularly in smaller communities where each individual member of staff, both clinical and non-clinical, are dependent on each other. It is important to understand your own personal limitations as well as the limitations of the environment you are working within.

Rewards

With optimal care, you may be able to ensure your head-injured patient is able to live independently and return to work as opposed to requiring lifelong care in an institution with no prospect of ever being a functioning member of society again. At the other end of the scale, you may be able to offer optimal care for a child with burns from a spilled boiling kettle or for a simple fracture from a fall.

Rural emergency medicine provides the opportunity to practise high-quality emergency medicine at a time when there is rapidly advancing technology. Learning to be self-sufficient, understanding your limitations and the limitations of your workplace may be more challenging, but it is also infinitely more rewarding.

Online resource

Australasian College for Emergency Medicine
   https://acem.org.au/

Chapter 54
Caring for Indigenous patients
Pauline Deweerd, Mark Byrne and Bonita Byrne

Providing practical health services to Aboriginal people
Pauline Deweerd

Central to providing care to Aboriginal and Torres Strait Islander patients is an awareness of the implications of: the cultural identity; the powerful role of traditional beliefs about sickness and death; the role of the family, community and traditional healers; and the impact of experiences with western civilisation that spans generations.

Aboriginal and Torres Strait Islander people have poorer access to medical care, domiciliary nursing care, palliative care, allied healthcare, bereavement and home care support in comparison with the non-Indigenous counterparts. This is likely to be due to the result of a range of factors including a lack of culturally respectful care shown by healthcare services, geographic isolation, difficulty in accessing services or lack of understanding of the roles that services can play, as well as mistrust of government agencies due to past experiences of injustice.

The key step to providing culturally safe care and competent care is an acknowledgment that difference between cultures exists; these require respect and that our usual ways of relating to people can cause them to feel uncertain, unsafe or offended.

At every visit to the ED, all patients should be asked if they are Aboriginal and/or Torres Strait Islander. This will enable medical staff to assist in informing referral processes to culturally related and specific services. This also relates to services available within the hospital such as Aboriginal health workers/liaison officers or social workers.

Being aware of a patient's cultural background is also beneficial if there are language barriers, including support for patients if they don't understand medical jargon. It is also important in keeping large extended family at ease through regular communication.

Relationship with family and community

Family and community are highly valued—family may be extended and involve complex relationships of obligation, support and avoidance. It can become too much or too hard, particularly where there are factions or family breakdowns.

Elders in the community are the respected holders of knowledge.

Relationship with the home

'Country', or traditional homelands, is central for many Indigenous people. Patients will often use the regional terms to describe themselves. For example, Koori (New South Wales [NSW]), Goori (Victoria and some parts of NSW), Murri (Queensland and some parts of NSW), Nungar (South Australia), Yolngu (Northern Territory [NT]) and Noongar (Western Australia [WA]).

The wish of many Aboriginal people is to go home to their country—especially at end of life.

Communication styles

- Be direct, maintain eye contact and explain what you are doing throughout the whole treatment.
- Establish early with the patient who is the right person to assist in decision-making. Consenting may take longer than usual consenting procedures.
- Arrange family meetings, especially for those family members who have travelled in from distances (rural, remote and regional areas).
- Identify who is the next of kin.
- Involve your Aboriginal health workers or social workers in family meetings.
- Build the relationship and get the trust of the patient, families and carers.
- Ask the patient what would they liked to be called—Elders can be called Uncle or Aunty with permission (respect).
- Use interpreters if you need (especially those with limited education).
- Offer to involve the family in providing the direct care.

- Consider larger rooms if a large number of the patient's family and community are present.
- Provide open spaces (where available).
- Don't judge Aboriginal patients who are involved in substance abuse—guide and offer assistance. Medical teams do not know the background of the patients and what has caused them to take these substances.
- Listen to the needs of the patients.
- All medical staff need to undertake cultural awareness training.
- Attend regular in-services delivered by Aboriginal staff/people to get a greater understanding of Aboriginal culture.
- Build on your understanding of the culturally appropriate services available to assist patients.
- Not all Aboriginal people smoke, drink or are involved in substance abuse.
- If staff in an ED need any assistance to support their Aboriginal patients, they need to contact their Aboriginal health/liaison workers.

Indigenous patients
Mark Byrne and Bonita Byrne

EPIDEMIOLOGY
Indigenous Australians are the most disadvantaged across all socioeconomic denominators. These disadvantages stem from colonisation and land dispossession.

Aboriginal health not only includes physical health but also encompasses social, emotional and cultural wellbeing.

Aboriginal and Torres Strait Islanders comprise 2.4% of the total Australian population. Most (69%) live outside the major urban centres, with 1 in 4 Indigenous Australians living in remote areas compared with only 1 in 50 non-Indigenous Australians.

Over 50% of Indigenous Australians live in NSW (29%) and Queensland (27%). Although only 12% of all Indigenous Australians live in the Northern Territory (NT), they represent 29% of the total population of the NT.

HEALTH STATUS
Aboriginal history has continued implications for healthcare, and the health status of Indigenous Australians is worse than that of other

Australians. Life expectancy is worse than in many underdeveloped nations: 53% of men and 41% of women die before the age of 50.

Aboriginal patients may have chronic conditions at a younger age and, therefore, age-based risk stratification is often not applicable among Indigenous Australians.

Cardiovascular disease is the leading cause of death for Indigenous Australians, with respiratory, endocrine and external causes the other major causes.

Indigenous Australians also have higher rates of mortality from all major causes of death. Mortality rates for Indigenous males and females for endocrine, nutritional and metabolic diseases are around 7-fold and 11-fold higher than those for non-Indigenous males and females.

CULTURAL ISSUES

Providing affordable, culturally appropriate facilities and transport will improve access and attendance.

Mandatory training should be available so that all health staff can be educated in Aboriginal culture, with emphasis on the local community.

Treating Indigenous patients as individuals and avoiding cultural stereotyping is essential.

Cultural and communication barriers can affect the patient–doctor interaction. Finding a balance between medical priorities and social needs is essential.

Aboriginal health workers

An Aboriginal health worker or Aboriginal liaison officer is an invaluable resource and should be consulted when appropriate.

There are over 130 Aboriginal community-controlled health services and Aboriginal medical services throughout Australia that are also excellent local resources.

Communication

Many Indigenous Australians have difficulty in understanding and/or being understood by a health provider. Therefore, culturally appropriate communication is essential for effective patient management.

For example, in the Northern Territory, 70% of the Aboriginal population speaks a language other than English at home. This has implications in relation to providing information on appropriate care, obtaining informed consent, explaining diagnosis and treatment and reinforcing compliance.

Eye contact is often avoided and should be understood within its cultural context.

Aboriginal people have strong family ties and kinships, and the inclusion of the extended family in decisions is appropriate.

Many Aboriginal people have a fear of hospitals, which they may associate with death. Be patient, and make allowances if compliance is to be achieved. Further, consider alternatives to admission such as daily reviews and ambulatory IV antibiotics.

Where possible, a doctor of the same gender should see an Indigenous patient, as there is men's business and women's business. This includes not placing men and women in the same room.

Provide written information and instructions each and every time, prior to discharging. Use everyday language, without jargon, and take the time to make sure the patient understands the information. Arrange prompt follow-up and provide written information to the referral service.

Allow time and space for the extended family during grieving and when a death has occurred.

Alcohol and substance abuse

Indigenous Australians are less likely to drink alcohol than other Australian people. However, there is a higher prevalence of dangerous drinking levels among Aboriginal people.

Alcohol and substance abuse is a major contributing factor to the poor health and wellbeing status of many Aboriginal people. It has a causal and a non-causal relationship with domestic violence, mental health, suicide, road deaths, imprisonment, sexually transmitted infections and sexual abuse.

Alcohol abuse has a major impact on Indigenous communities. The immediate management of alcohol-related ED presentations is no different than in the wider community.

Illicit drug use, including marijuana, amphetamines, heroin and inhalants such as glues, aerosols and petrol, is also a major problem in many communities.

Proactive and opportunistic provision of culturally appropriate intervention is the role of all primary-care medical staff, as even small reductions in alcohol consumption have benefits for both the individual and the wider community.

Despite widespread alcohol and substance abuse, a non-judgmental, non-stereotypical attitude is essential. Individual assessment is paramount, and making assumptions based on Aboriginality is inappropriate.

Editorial Comment

Especially for those emergency doctors working in the many city or rural hospitals that see and treat these groups, it is important and rewarding to actively become familiar with and good at caring for these patients (e.g. by doing courses, rural rotations, locum work); there are simple but important differences of engagement and communication that are not intuitive and are important to be aware of. We all know that there are health challenges to improve many aspects of Indigenous health, thus leading to decreased morbidity and mortality. There should be access for the health professional to involve liaison workers who can support, work and follow-up with family, elders and other agencies. Care must not end with only an ED visit.

Online resources

Australian Indigenous HealthInfoNet
www.healthinfonet.ecu.edu.au

Chapter 55
Students' guide to the emergency department

Sascha Fulde and Tiffany Fulde

The emergency department (ED) can be the highlight of a student's day or the place where you feel most out of place, or both at the same time. Hopefully, this chapter will outline some practical tips for getting the most out of this wonderful resource.

Advantages of the ED

As the place where almost all patients enter the hospital, the ED is a short-case heaven. In addition, you can see patients before they've been overrun by a thousand other students and doctors. Just think: by the time a patient gets up to a ward, they've most likely had the same questions asked and been poked in the sore spot by the ED intern, ED registrar, the intern on the admitting team and then the registrar, plus at least one nurse. They've had a stressful time, feel unwell and, ultimately, probably just want to be left alone; whereas in the ED they haven't been examined that many times. They're prepared to be undressed, poked and prodded because they recognise that that is what happens when they come to an emergency department. A student can often be useful: either confirming examination findings, sometimes finding something someone missed, either on history or examination; or just alleviating some of the patient's worry by spending some time with them while they're waiting for the results of investigations. Even if you're only doing an examination, it makes the patient feel that something is happening and that they're being taken care of. The patient is also in the mind-set where they really want to talk about their story and those niggly details of symptoms as it's pretty much all they can think about. Thus the ED is a fantastic resource for a medical student.

When patients present to the ED, they're much more likely to present in a way that is useful to a student. First, as no one knows what is wrong with them, you actually get a chance to test your clinical and diagnostic skills. Second, they present in the same way that short and long cases are often presented in exams. The complaints are also often at a level which you will be expected to know. For example, you are much more likely to see a patient with chest pain than one with a phaeochromocytoma.

LEARN TO HANDLE EMERGENCIES

As a student my biggest fear was that I would actually kill some-one! My second biggest fear was failing exams. And the third was, how do I actually save someone's life? I'm not just talking about the big trauma cases, but also the smaller practical proce-dures. This is one of the greatest things the ED can teach you. By spending time there and talking to the doctors, you learn how to actually prioritise management and the basic couple of things that you need to do right now before you stop and work out the clinical management guidelines. You can also learn how to actu-ally do them.

FIND PATIENTS FOR TUTORIALS, CASE HISTORIES AND PRESENTATIONS

Although the hospital is full of patients, it can often be hard to find patients that fit the requirements of the task you're trying to do—for instance, finding an interesting surgical case to present in a surgical tutorial or even for a bedside tutorial. As staff in the ED have seen all the patients that have entered the hospital, they are wonderful at knowing what patients are around and worth chasing up.

FITS WELL WITH PROBLEM-BASED LEARNING (PBL) COURSES

At the beginning of a PBL course it can often be difficult to ap-proach medicine on the wards, as you have only learnt informa-tion on certain specific disorders or systems. This can make it overwhelming to approach a general medical or surgical term. However, in the ED the patients present in the same way as a case in a scenario, and this allows you to approach things you haven't seen before.

One of the strengths of PBL, which is that you focus on individual areas, can sometimes be slightly frustrating. By only focusing on one clinical vignette, you can sometimes feel like you don't know much about broader medicine. By hanging around the ED for even only a short period of time, you can very quickly start to counteract that and learn a lot across a broad range of areas.

PROVIDES A PLACE TO INTEGRATE A LOT OF KNOWLEDGE

Whatever level you're at in your training, the ED provides a great place to pull both your clinical skills and your esoteric knowledge together and practise what you've been learning. It's always easier to remember something when you've seen a patient with it and seen how they were managed.

GET A WIDE RANGE OF CLINICAL MATERIAL

With increasing specialisation of medicine and increasing numbers of students, often you only get to experience a limited number of different departments. For instance, you may never have had the opportunity to do a cardiology term. The ED is the place where you can compensate for this deficit. All the acute cardiology patients will come through the ED, so you can see how they are managed.

SEE MILD PATIENTS THAT GET DISCHARGED

The ED also has a range of severity of patients, so you get to see the simple sprains, cuts and bruises before they are discharged.

SEE GREAT SIGNS BEFORE THEY ARE TREATED

Often you trail around the hospital trying to find a patient to practise your examination signs on, only to find that while many people are unwell, they've already been treated (e.g. 'Mrs X had shifting dullness but we tapped it last night').

In the ED you can see these signs often when they are at their peak before the arrhythmia is treated or the blood pressure lowered.

AVOIDING BEING BARRED

As a student, you're always going to be refused by some patients. Even though you know it's not personal, this is often demoralising. In contrast, it's always exciting to go and visit a patient you saw when they first presented in the ED and have them recognise you and happily let you repeat your examination to see their improvement.

The ED also provides an excellent opportunity to learn about the unspoken professional etiquette between different doctors. At some stage all doctors, whether interns or the most senior consultants, come to and interact in the ED. This allows you to learn a lot about the finer negotiations; for instance, of getting staff up late at night.

Use it as a light at the end of the tunnel

Little encounters that you can have in the ED allow you to pretend to be a real doctor, even if only for a few seconds—not just a nurse or a cannulating technician doing a cannula or a blood pressure, but a real doctor. This not only reminds you what you're working for, but why you're working so hard. It really allows you to put all the hard decisions you're making into perspective. It can be even more important to remind yourself that there is a light at the end of the tunnel. This can be really motivating, either because being a doctor is exciting or because it makes you realise you're not quite knowledgeable enough yet.

How do you get the most out of it?
SO HOW DO YOU ACCESS THIS GEM?

First you must get access either by your swipe card or the keypad access code. This is crucial. Emergency department staff are usually very happy to have you there, but it's much easier if you just appear at the doctor's desk. If you have to constantly ask to come and go, you're probably much less likely to be there regularly.

Go to the ED regularly. If you become a familiar face to staff, they very quickly go out of their way to help you meet your learning goals or just to be friendly. A good tip is to leave the hospital via the ED. This forces you to see whether there are any interesting patients when you know you've got nowhere better to be. Even if you only see one patient a day, you'll start to become part of the hospital team.

The ED can get very busy. When this happens, people often get stressed. If you are around, do not automatically skulk back to the student room or ask if you can intubate the patient! Ideally, find a way to be involved while getting in as few people's way as possible. This can involve standing at the outer edge as resuscitation is going on, or going and seeing one of the low-triage-category patients by yourself to start with.

ATTACH YOURSELF TO A REGISTRAR

As the ED is usually very busy, you can also get a lot out of it by attaching yourself to a consultant or registrar and becoming their assistant. By doing the little tasks like chasing results, you can really help them out. This often engenders a lot of goodwill, which means that you get good teaching along the way and opportunities to do practical procedures if you're interested.

FOLLOW YOUR PATIENTS UP

When you have seen a patient in the ED, make sure you take the opportunity to follow them to the next step in their treatment. For instance, watch their surgery or check on them in the medical ward in a few days' time. Most teams are more than happy for you to be included in care when you explain that you saw the patient in the ED. Thus, you get to see many aspects of medicine and surgery.

DON'T COME IN HORDES

Although it's often less confronting to come in a group or with a partner, it'll be easier to get accepted by staff and patients if you come by yourself. It's also better to come alone, as this is how you're ultimately going to be in exams and it really allows you to realise your strengths and weaknesses and work on them.

ASK THE NURSES *FIRST*

Before doing anything, first ask a nurse. This is very important. Even if you have a doctor's permission and the nurse is busy, wait until they are finished and then ask their permission. Nurses often end up coordinating care, so they know whether they've had time to give the pain relief that the doctor has prescribed so that the patient can handle talking to you.

FIND THE THINGS THAT ARE USEFUL TO YOU AS A STUDENT BUT THAT NO ONE ELSE CARES ABOUT

There are many things happening in a hospital that are commonplace, barely thought-about activities but that can be really useful to a student. For instance, most people who come into the ED get an ECG and some blood tests. If you regularly look up the results and try to interpret them, whether you know the patient's history or not, you can become very good at interpreting results. This is easy to do and doesn't need any doctor's or nurse's help—you simply look them up and then check how the doctor interpreted them.

Another useful skill you can learn is to practise writing up notes. After seeing a patient, if you practise putting the salient points down on paper you can then compare your notes with the registrar's and see how good you were at getting all the points and putting them down in a clear format.

ASK ABOUT TEACHING

Most EDs have compulsory teaching sessions for interns, RMOs (residents) and registrars. They are often more than happy for a few students to attend. These sessions are usually filled with teaching on diseases that are of interest to you and will often make it into exams. So just ask some of the registrars and interns who organise the tutorials, if and when they're on and whether you can attend.

PRACTISE PROCEDURES—ALWAYS TAKE A BLUEY

The ED is a really good place in which to practise the basic procedures that you're expected to be able to do as an intern. There is always someone who needs bloods taken or a cannula or catheter, and people are usually happy to oversee you doing one. One important thing is to always check that you have all the equipment you need before you start a procedure. When you're doing anything you're a bit unfamiliar with, always take a bluey (a plastic protective sheet) so you don't make a mess of the sheets—this alienates the patient and makes the nurses cross. Also, always take a set of cotton balls and tape just in case something goes wrong— you can patch almost anything up.

If you have the chance, practise procedures on models. Many EDs have simulation centres or plastic models to practise procedures on. These can be fantastic for your first couple of times or if it's been a while since you've done one.

HAVE A SLIGHTLY THICK SKIN

Unfortunately, at some point as a student you're likely to get in trouble for something. While it's important to be considerate and do your best to avoid it, at some point you will get on someone's bad side. When this happens, just apologise and try to make it right. Then don't let it get to you. It happens to everyone.

FIND A FRIENDLY FACE AND TAKE ADVANTAGE OF THEM!

In every department there are a few really incredibly nice people. When you find them, make friends and then ask them about all those niggly things you need help with. They understand how hard it can be to be a student and they're more than happy to help, but you need to ask them. The worst they can say is 'no'.

TAKE MORE RESPONSIBILITY

When you're in more senior years, take more responsibility. You can use time in the ED as a pre-intern term. Go in at nights and help out. You can see some of the most interesting, diverse patients after dark. Plus, people appreciate your dedication and usually try to help you get the most out of it. You can even clerk patients from beginning to investigations and then take the write-up, just needing a signature, to your supervising doctor. This will help you, and hopefully save them a little time even if they then go back and check it.

Summary

Ultimately, make sure you enjoy both being a medical student and your life outside of medicine. Don't let the stress of medicine or all the advice above distract you from enjoying your time as a student. We hope that you learn a lot from this book and that this chapter has helped to inspire you to head into the ED.

Editorial Comment

It is our responsibility, privilege and delight to help and supervise our future colleagues, especially senior students who quickly and enthusiastically take up a workload. A very good system is to 'buddy' them with a doctor—even nights and weekend shifts; they love it. Also remember that you will be asked questions and that demonstration and teaching really improves and keeps your practice up-to-date.

The ED is often the most desired term, as students sense the joy and terror of being the first to deal with unknown, unexpected and potentially very ill patients—all this among a great gang of healthcare professionals.

It is usually final-year students that are attached to the ED. They are going to be interns in months—maybe at your hospital! So, even more so, time spent teaching them intern skills is very worthwhile.

Chapter 56
A guide for interns, residents, medical officers working in emergency medicine

Tiffany Fulde and Richard Sullivan

Introduction

As for many interns about to start work in emergency medicine, this may seem like the most daunting term in your year as an intern, but don't be alarmed—for most junior doctors it is one of the most rewarding periods, and the term where an intern feels most useful as a doctor. You will learn a lot during this term through the variety of people and presentations you see, and you will gain confidence in initiating management and recognising sick patients. You will improve your procedural skills and your communication with colleagues and patients, and you will work closely with a large team of health professionals. By the end of the term, ward and after-hours work will seem more manageable, and the term can be a big turning point for your year.

Emergency medicine does have a more rapid turnover than other parts of the hospital, and a greater focus on service provision, but with a good approach you should be able to balance this with your educational needs and enjoy your term.

Day 1—getting started

On your first day, make sure you take a moment to familiarise yourself with your surroundings. Introduce yourself to the team, including the registrars and consultants, other junior doctors, nurses, ward clerks, physiotherapists, social worker, pharmacists and anyone else who is part of your emergency department (ED) team. The more familiar you are with the team and the more familiar they are with you, the easier the transition to a new term will be.

Orientation to the ED is very important. Most hospitals arrange a formal session of orientation to the department, including its layout, preferred documentation, use of IT for orders and results, electronic medical records (EMRs) and triage, and any relevant policies and clinical protocols/pathways. If you haven't had any orientation, ask the most senior staff in the department how the department works—especially the layout, where to pick up patients and where to take them to be seen, how to click patients off on the computer or list, and with whom you should discuss patient care. Each ED is set up differently—some are divided into acute and subacute, or fast-track, areas; others have mental health or paediatric areas. It is important to familiarise yourself with the way your ED works each time you start a new rotation. This will make your job a lot easier.

Always remember that everyone knows how daunting it can be for a new intern in the ED. You should never be afraid to ask questions—the more questions you ask, the more you will learn and the better you will be at your job. So ask questions of everyone around you—there is no such thing as a stupid question.

Working up a patient

Once you have familiarised yourself with the department and who you will be working with, it will be time for you to dive in and start seeing a patient. If you are unsure, you can ask the registrar who they would like you to see first; otherwise, take the next patient on the list.

Generally, interns are expected to see the lower triage categories (categories 3–5). If you would like to see a higher-priority patient, tell the registrar or consultant before seeing the patient. You should try to see more-complex and higher-category patients as you progress through the term.

You should do the initial work-up and then report back to your registrar or consultant, and discuss further management. Prior to this discussion, try to formulate differential diagnoses and a potential management plan; this will be the best way to learn and gain confidence to work more independently. As you progress through the term, you may be able to initiate more investigations and management independently, but you should always discuss your patients with someone more senior. The timing of this discussion depends on how sick the patient is, and on your experience—the earlier the better if the patient is deteriorating, or if you are unsure. Some special cases will always require early involvement of senior doctors, for example paediatric presentations.

ASSESSING THE PATIENT

Once you have 'clicked off' your patient, take a look at the history on the triage sheet, and start thinking of likely differentials and what further information you will need from your history, examination and investigations. Make sure you have an appropriate environment in which to assess the patient.

- Do they need monitoring?
- Are they likely to be violent or abscond?
- How mobile are they?
- Will they need a bed?
- Will you need to perform any invasive investigations/ examinations (e.g. internal or rectal examinations will need a private area)?
- Do you need any special equipment (e.g. slit lamp)?

You can discuss these with the triage nurse and the nurse in charge to ascertain where you should see the patient. If you have to wait for an ideal environment, see if there is anything you can start doing in the meantime (e.g. initial history, bloods, X-rays or ECG).

In the ED, assessment and management of patients often occur simultaneously, and initial management may precede a full history. Some management and investigations may have been started at triage, for example analgesia and antiemetics or X-rays in suspected fractures. You should develop a systematic approach to identify the main complaint and start treatment as appropriate (e.g. bronchodilators in an asthma attack) before returning to take a full history and ensuring nothing gets missed. You will become more skilled at performing a multitude of tasks simultaneously during your ED term, but keep it simple at the start. Remember your training; and if you are stuck, go through the process of ABCDE and go back to the first principles of history, examination and investigations.

Also, think about possible sources for more information: old notes, notes from other hospitals, referral letters and family members and friends may all be useful sources. It may take you a while to get all this information, so the sooner you request it, the better.

It is very important that if you are ever worried about a patient at any stage during your work-up, do not hesitate to go immediately to a registrar or consultant and request help—they expect it, and welcome early recognition of a deteriorating patient. A key skill for junior doctors is to recognise your own limitations, and seniors will respect you for this. Ensuring your own safety and patient safety is particularly important as an ED doctor.

2 INVESTIGATIONS

- Most patients in the ED will require bloods, and many ED doctors and nurses will advise you to place a cannula while you are taking bloods—that way you have access if you need it, and you will save the patient having an extra needle later on. As a general rule, a 20-gauge cannula should suffice. This is a great way to practise your cannulation skills.
- In most cases, if you are taking bloods you should take at least one purple tube, one lime or gold, and one blue. You may not need to order tests for all of these tubes, but this will enable you to add on most common tests if you need them and avoid the need for further venepuncture as you work through your likely differentials. Consider whether blood cultures may be necessary.
- Similarly, if the patient requires radiology, try to order all tests at the same time (e.g. chest X-ray and foot X-ray) to avoid multiple trips to radiology and unnecessary delay.
- As a general rule for a junior, you should talk to a senior doctor before arranging more-extensive investigations (i.e. other than bloods, X-rays, ECG, spirometry). Various departments will have different policies regarding the ordering of CT scans and this should be discussed with someone more senior. If a test is urgent, make sure you communicate this clearly, usually both on the order form and via phone.
- Make sure you chase results for each test you have ordered (or hand-over that they need to be chased) and discuss these results with a senior doctor.

3 DISCUSSION

Once you have taken your history and done your examination (+/− bloods and basic radiology), it is probably time to run over the case with a registrar or consultant (*remember to speak to someone earlier if you are worried about a patient, even if the history and examination is not complete*). The purpose of this conversation is to come to an agreed working diagnosis or problem list, and an agreed management plan.

Communication with the registrar and the consultant is a useful skill to develop and will help you when making referrals over the phone to other teams (which most doctors find more difficult than face-to-face).

- Practice being succinct, and present only the findings which are relevant to the diagnosis and management of your patient.
- It is very useful to start the conversation with an overarching statement which summarises the case and your thoughts on disposition and management, as this helps frame the conversation for the listener (e.g. 'I have just seen a 49-year-old man with intermediate-risk chest pain who I think requires admission for stress testing and monitoring'. Then go into further detail of the history).
- It is important that you know the patient's vitals before you begin the conversation, and make sure you include what has already been done for the patient.
- You might try to finish your presentation with how you would like to manage the situation and ask if anything else needs to be done or if you have left anything important out.
- If you are really concerned, do not hesitate to ask for a senior review.

At all times, remember that *patient safety comes first*. If the senior doctor asks you something you do not know or forgot to ask, never pretend that you know the answer or make up information—the senior can usually tell, but more importantly this may give a false impression of how your patient is and what should be done. As an intern you are still learning, and it is okay not to know all the answers.

4 FURTHER REFERRAL

Following the discussion with your senior, you should have a clear plan for the patient, whether it is further assessment, investigations or examination, or management. Make sure you continue to monitor your patient, and chase any outstanding investigations.

- If you think the patient is likely to be discharged, you might start your discharge planning, including letter, scripts and follow-up appointments or referrals to extra services. Liaise with social work and physiotherapy if necessary, and consider how the patient is going to get home: will they need transport or a family member to collect them, are they safe to go by themselves or will they need extra help? Try to arrange these things early so that there is no delay when the patient is ready for discharge. There is often an aged-care service in the emergency team which can assist with this process, so liaise closely with them. Some hospitals offer a 'hospital in the home' program; if so, consider whether the patient is suitable for this. If given the option of home- or hospital-based treatment, most patients would choose home.

- If you think the patient is likely to require admission, you might start to organise your referral to the appropriate team's registrar. It is a good idea to be prepared with the patient's notes and investigation results easily accessible. Consider which team you are referring to, and why: What is the problem you think they should manage? Is the patient known to a particular doctor or team? Do you have all the relevant information? You may not need to wait for every investigation result before calling the registrar, unless it is integral to the diagnosis. For example, if the patient has appendicitis clinically, you don't necessarily need to wait for the WCC—but you would probably wait for a beta-hCG in a female patient.

As with your earlier discussion with your senior ED doctor, try to synthesise your **referral information** and keep your findings relevant to the problem and team you are speaking to. Think about what information that team cares about—it might be slightly different to what the ED thinks is the most important information. A concise opening sentence about the presentation, followed by an explanation of the diagnosis including relevant history, examination and investigations and the patient's current situation, is usually all that is required. Try using the principles of ISBAR to aid your communication (see Box 56.1).

Box 56.1   ISBAR model for clinical hand-over

I   Introduction
  - *Identify yourself, your role and your location.*
  - *Identify the patient.*

S   Situation
  State the patient's diagnosis/reason for admission and current problem.

B   Background
  What is the patient's history?

A   Assessment
  What are the most recent observations? What is your assessment?

R   Recommendation
  What do you want the person taking over care of the patient to do? When should this occur?

Don't be rattled if you are asked questions or met with scepticism, as this can be quite common with ED referrals. Make sure you communicate clearly and calmly; if you run into serious obstruction, notify your senior who will advise you what to do.

Sometimes it may be appropriate to refer to a team for further assessment or management before the principal diagnosis has been decided. Do not be afraid to be upfront about this during your referral, but explain why you think the patient should be seen at this stage. For example, 'This 30-year-old man has presented with lower left quadrant abdominal pain. I am not entirely sure of the cause, but the patient has required ongoing morphine and I am concerned about [*insert diagnosis*] and would like a medical/surgical opinion regarding admission and further investigation'. While such referrals may be met with resistance, medicine often requires doctors to be prepared to deal with uncertainty, and not all patients will fit a clear diagnosis. This is particularly true in the ED. Patients may often require admission to further investigate and observe the development of symptomatology.

Once you have made your referral, make sure you **document** any recommendations by the team, and arrange any investigations or management they have requested. It is also important to follow-up on the patient to ensure their condition has not changed, that they have been seen by the registrar and to ensure that a plan is being implemented.

- If the patient is to be admitted, make sure they are ready for the ward, including charting all medications.
  — Some medications given in the ED are not able to be given on the ward (e.g. IV morphine), so make sure there are appropriate alternatives available.
  — Think about when the patient is likely to be reviewed next, and make sure they have everything they need arranged until then (e.g. IV fluids, cannula).
  — Order any necessary tests and make sure that anything that is time-critical is clearly handed over to the ward resident (e.g. serial troponins).
  — If the registrar has not already done so, notify the nurse in charge that the patient requires a bed.
- If the patient is to be discharged, ensure you have a clear plan for necessary follow-up from the registrar.
  — For all patients who are to be discharged, make sure you have cleared them with a senior doctor before discharge.
  — All patients will need a discharge letter, including a clear outline of any outstanding investigations you would like their GP to follow-up, and any further follow-up arrangements.
  — If the patient requires medications on discharge, you should ensure that they have a prescription (script) and will be able to fill this within an appropriate time (e.g. if discharging after-hours, are there any pharmacies open or do you need to provide a take-home pack? Can the script wait until morning?). You should also have a care for whether patients are unable to fill their prescription (e.g. due to financial burden). Clarify your approach in these situations with someone senior.
  — Make sure you advise the patient of any special instructions on discharge, including warning signs for re-presentation, medication and timing of follow-up. If something is particularly important to follow-up, do not hesitate to call the GP as well as providing a letter.

5 PATIENTS AND PATIENCE

One of the most important parts of your job is to communicate to the patient and inform them about the hospital process. Try to keep the patient updated as regularly as possible on their progress. Often patients do not know how the hospital works, or do not understand the need to refer to an inpatient team and for another doctor to see them before a decision on admission is made. It is also useful to advise patients on expected delays before certain test results may be available. All these discussions go a long way in assisting the patient to have a better experience in the department.

Also remember that patients and their families are often in a stressful and unfamiliar environment. Try to be patient with demanding patients—they may not understand the multiple demands on your time or that they are a lower priority than patients who are more unwell. Try to explain and reassure and be empathetic to their concerns. If you do, these interactions can be the most rewarding part of your job.

Further into the term/learning opportunities
RESUSCITATION/TRAUMA

Early in the term, the resuscitation bay may seem an intimidating place. Throughout your term, try to get involved as much as you can when patients are brought through for resuscitation or trauma calls. Begin by observing the process and the teamwork; then, when you feel comfortable, ask the team leader if you can be involved. A good place to start is as the procedures team-member: your job will be to place a large cannula, usually 18-gauge is sufficient, and take blood, including for blood gases. Often an extra set of hands—for log-rolls or cardiac compressions—is really useful as well. It is a very different experience to be involved in managing a high-acuity situation, and a great learning opportunity. Get involved however you can.

As you progress through your term, you should also be proactive in seeing the higher-triage-category patients that come into these areas. When you first pick up the high-acuity patients in the resuscitation bay you may feel anxious about being alone with a very sick patient, but you will be surprised how many consultants and registrars are looking over your shoulder and are ready to support you. Don't be afraid to call out for extra help if you need it.

These experiences are invaluable, and will give you confidence in handling a patient that is deteriorating, which will help you significantly in the future when you are the first to see a deteriorating patient on the wards. Touch base with a senior sooner than with lower-category patients, and remember 'ABCs' if stuck.

2 FORMAL TEACHING AND EDUCATIONAL OPPORTUNITIES

It is greatly recommended that you attend any educational opportunities available. Most EDs provide a formal teaching program for junior medical officers. You should be supported to attend these by other staff, and you should make an effort to attend as many of them as possible. Discuss with seniors if there are any topics in particular you would like more exposure to. These sessions will help to ensure that you are familiar with the main ED presentations and skills, as you are unlikely to see the full variety in one term, and will make your work easier when managing these presentations for the first time.

A lot of teaching in the ED occurs 'on the job'. This can provide a lot of learning and experience in a variety of areas, including clinical assessment, investigation interpretation and management options. Take every opportunity to further your procedural and clinical skills under supervision, then with increasing independence as appropriate. Wound closure and suturing, plastering and fracture management and use of special equipment such as slit lamps are common ED skills that you should become proficient in. If you have the opportunity, try to gain exposure and experience in more-complex procedures, such as lumbar punctures or chest drain insertion.

Always work within your experience level, and if you are unsure ask someone more senior to supervise you.

3 FOLLOW-UP

A great opportunity to consolidate your learning is by following up on the patients you have seen in the ED who get admitted. If you have time before or after your shift, check what happened to your patients after admission, what the ultimate diagnosis was, what further investigations were useful and what management was implemented. This will give you a longitudinal view of patient care and a broader context for patient care in the ED. It will also help you to reflect on and evaluate your assessment and management in the ED. This can improve your diagnostic skills, build your confidence by seeing the things you did effectively and improve your management of future presentations.

Miscellaneous
CHERRY-PICKING

Patients on the ED waiting list are ordered according to the priority in which they need to be seen. If you do not follow this order and choose instead to see only the patients who are interesting or easy for you, also known as 'cherry-picking', you are performing a very great disservice—not just to the patient, but to the other doctors on your team and, importantly, to yourself. It is really important for your learning that you take all opportunities for exposure to a wide range of presentations and management. The ED is a unique environment in which to see a variety of undifferentiated and multisystem presentations. Challenge yourself: this is the time in your career where you are most supported and supervised—it is the best time to learn. Also, look after your colleagues—*you* wouldn't appreciate being left to see all the complicated or less-desirable presentations!

HAND-OVER BETWEEN SHIFTS

Hand-over is essential for the continuity of patient care and for patient safety, and also has implications for your own welfare. Internship can be a very stressful period and it is important that you try to leave on time and have a life outside of the workplace. As you approach the end of your shift, you should start preparing to hand over the care of your patients. If you can do this well, it will help your patients, your colleagues and yourself.

There are multiple ways to perform clinical hand-over, and each department will differ in its procedures. In some departments patients may be reassigned by a senior doctor or during a ward round, but often you will have to seek someone out on the later shift to take your patients.

Ideally you would facilitate the other doctor's taking over care as much as possible by preparing as much as you can of the plan. For example, if the patient is likely to be discharged but needs to wait for a test result, try to write the discharge letter before you hand over so that the other doctor need only add the result; or, if the patient is likely to be admitted, chart the medications.

If possible, it is usually preferable for the person who has assessed the patient to make the referral to the registrar, as they know the patient best. If the work-up is incomplete, you may need to clarify that you are handing over to a certain ED doctor and agree with the registrar that the ED doctor will call again with further information once available.

It is important to communicate to the person taking over care what has been done and what they need to do for the patient. Try to make hand-over brief, clear and simple. Emphasise what you would like the person to do. For example, 'This is a 65-year-old man who had a simple mechanical fall with nil evident injuries. He is on warfarin for AF, and has an INR in therapeutic range. Could you please chase the CT head and if normal can you please discharge this patient—the summary is already written but just needs updating with the CT result'. Take care not to hand over irrelevant details, as the plan may get lost in the intricacies of the story (which you have already gone over with the senior), and usually all the information the listener needs or wants is what they have to do. That message will be diluted if you delve too deeply into the story, so leave that to your discussion with the senior when you are working out a plan.

Sometimes it is not possible to have your patients 'parcelled up' neatly before your shift ends—the department could be very busy, or there might be too much uncertainty regarding the patient's diagnosis and plan. Try to help your colleague as much as possible, but it is important to recognise your own limits. Just do the best you can. With this in mind, try to be understanding when someone else hands you over a patient who is incompletely worked up. Also, if you see someone from the earlier shift struggling to get out or over their time, offer them a hand. This will come back to you next time you're trying to end your shift.

If there is reluctance to take over patients who are incompletely worked up, the flow-on effect is that ED doctors are often reluctant to pick up new patients in the last hour of their shift, especially patients who are more complex or who may have delays with investigation, keeping them at work after their shift has ended. If you find yourself in this situation, there is still a lot you can do to help the department and your colleagues. You can try to see a patient who you think will be quick, and likely to go home; or ask if anyone needs a hand, and help start the work-up for patients who are waiting—put in cannulas and take bloods, order X-rays or chart medications. You can apply this at any stage: if your patient-load prevents you picking up a new patient but you have time while you wait for results, see if there is any way to help out.

Remember that you are part of a team—try to support each other, and if you are consistently finding it difficult to leave close to time or having problems with patient hand-over, ask a senior for advice and support.

BREAKS AND DEBRIEFING

As your day in the ED will usually be less structured than during other terms, it is often difficult to schedule regular breaks. Periods when the department is busy with many patients waiting, and when you have many patients or patients who are unwell and slightly unstable, are particularly difficult times and ED interns often feel compelled to skip their breaks. You may actually reach the end of your shift and realise that you forgot to eat lunch or dinner if you have been particularly busy.

Make sure you take the time to eat, have a drink and sit down. You will actually perform better after your break, which can make you more efficient and effective and ultimately save you time—and, importantly, it will help prevent you burning out and getting tired later in the term.

If you are finding it hard to have a meal, some of the best times to take a break are around the time the new staff arrive for their shift, and also when you are waiting for pathology or radiology results. When you go for a break, let someone on your shift know, and give a quick update to the nurses looking after the same patient about the progress. If you are worried about a patient, consider where you take your break. Can you stay in a more accessible area?

During your ED term you will inevitably experience situations that will be challenging, emotional and possibly even confronting. If you feel you need to take some time out, do not hesitate to go to the coffee room and have a 10-minute break to have a tea or coffee. Let someone know before you go; you will find that most people in the department will understand.

If you do encounter such situations, it is important that you debrief with someone afterwards—even days later, if you need time to digest things. Talk to someone you feel comfortable with—either at work or outside—about any events that you found difficult; it will help you cope and learn. Listening to others talk about their experiences can also be very positive. Sharing your experiences through the term with other interns and residents can be particularly helpful in understanding common challenges and realising that others may be having a very similar experience to your own.

You may also like to discuss things with someone more senior in the department; gaining feedback on how you are going, and how you might approach things differently, can be very productive and a central component to your development.

PERSONAL SAFETY AND PERSONAL PROTECTIVE EQUIPMENT (PPE)

Your workplace should be a safe environment. Unfortunately, the ED—more than most parts of the hospital—is a place where you encounter more-frequent risks, and you will need to be alert to potential dangers and be proactive in taking precautions to minimise these.

Due to the nature of presentations in the ED, including wounds, patients who present with vomiting, bleeding and so on, as well as the nature of management which includes a greater number of procedures, you will be at an increased risk of exposure to body fluids.

- Familiarise yourself with the PPE available, where to find it and local PPE protocols, and adopt universal precautions. For example, during procedures, treat every patient as though they had a known blood-borne pathogen (even if they appear low-risk).
- If you are exposed, notify a senior immediately. Your ED will have a protocol for management of post-exposure prophylaxis. Always err on the side of caution: even if you feel it was low-risk, make sure you discuss this with a senior colleague.
- As always, hand hygiene is important and should be performed with all patients. It is often forgotten, however, that multi-resistant organisms can be present in the ED and you should continue to use additional precautions (e.g. gown and gloves) if seeing a patient with previous infection

or colonisation, to minimise risk of cross-infection to other patients. Remember to ask about recent travel.

In the ED you will also see aggressive patients, patients under the influence of alcohol or other substances, and mental health patients. You will need to adjust your approach to these patients according to the risk they present.

- Many EDs keep a record of patients who have previously been aggressive, via an alert on the triage system or EMR. Ask someone how to access this, and before you go to assess the patient, check if they have any alerts registered. This can be a useful indicator of their behaviour.

- Assess every patient for risk, including changeability. Ask the triage staff how the patient behaved at assessment and in the waiting room. Be careful where you see these patients, and if you are uncomfortable ask a colleague to accompany you. You may need to consider calling security to search the patient for weapons before you assess them. The ED nursing staff are particularly valuable in advising you of patient risk. The nurses may well have already treated the patient and be familiar with their pattern of behaviour.

- Take whatever precautions are appropriate for the environment (some hospitals may offer personalised duress alarms, for example), and make sure you familiarise yourself with the hospital protocol for aggressive or violent patients, including physical and chemical sedation.

- Again, you should always err on the side of caution. If you are concerned, ask for advice and seek help early.

ONLINE RESOURCES AND EMRS

- **Electronic and online resources** are incredibly useful tools, and will hopefully be readily available in your ED. Familiarise yourself with what's available and how to access these.
  - These references are very handy while you are seeing patients, to refresh your knowledge of detailed management, such as medication regimens, and to provide advice and direction in cases you have not seen previously. This is particularly helpful in the ED due to the wide variety of presentations you will see—you will inevitably see things you are unfamiliar with or have forgotten. E-resources are

also useful to reinforce your learning after you have seen a patient.

— Some useful resources include the online Therapeutic Guidelines, Australian Medicines Handbook, MIMS, UpToDate and BMJ Best Practice (see 'Online resources'; many hospitals have subscriptions where necessary). There are also videos of procedures you can access from various websites to consolidate your learning.

• **Electronic medical records (EMRs)** can give you access to previous discharge summaries, medications and pathology, which can provide helpful information against which to compare a patient's current condition and establish a baseline. If you have access to these capabilities, try to take advantage of their use and also keep them as up-to-date and accurate as possible for future reference.

These tools will help you to maximise your own learning and efficiency and improve patient outcomes.

DOCUMENTATION

In a rushed environment, writing good notes might seem a lower priority than starting management and chasing investigations. It is actually equally—if not more—important to document what you have done and who you have discussed your patients with. If you are busy, it is easy to forget or confuse details, and documentation should be part of a consistent, systematic approach. Some find it useful to jot down some rough notes while taking the patient history, then write more-detailed notes away from the patient. This may be especially useful if your ED uses EMRs and the patient is not yet logged on to the system. Find a system that works for you.

Accurate and detailed notes are particularly important in the ED. You may be asked to complete legal documentation months after you have seen a patient if their injuries are part of a court case (e.g. if you have seen an assault victim). As the treating doctor, it is your notes and your opinion that will be used. Months later you will not remember each patient, so make sure that you document relevant details (e.g. size and depth of wounds—consider drawing the location). Ask for guidance on how to complete any requests for medicolegal documentation from senior doctors, medical records and your medical indemnity association as you see fit.

NIGHTS/AFTER-HOURS

Night shifts can be tiring, but also a lot of fun, allowing you to bond with the rest of the ED team. In some hospitals, interns do not do night shifts in the ED.

The main difference on a night shift, and some after-hours shifts, is that certain services may not be available. It is usually difficult to get some tests done after-hours, for example CT and ultrasound. Discuss with the senior whether these tests are urgent, and whether someone should be called in. If it can wait until morning, make sure you order the test and get everything ready (e.g. if the patient needs a cannula) so that the test can be performed as early as possible in the morning. Similarly, you may change your approach to referring patients to other teams at unsociable hours—can the phone call wait until early morning, or is it urgent?

During nights and after-hours there are often fewer people around in the ED. While this can make the ED feel calmer, you should be aware of increased risk to your safety in isolated areas. Do not take patients into areas where they may be unsupervised (e.g. subacute areas, unless there are appropriate staff around). It could endanger you, and your patient could deteriorate unnoticed.

WORK–LIFE BALANCE

Your ED term may be the first time you've done shift work. Shift work can be tiring and the odd hours can be antisocial and even isolating, so it's important to take care of yourself. On the plus side you may well find you have more time away from work. In many hospitals, ED shifts are 10 hours long, meaning 4 shifts a week. You also won't be doing the ward overtime shifts, which will give you more free time.

Make the most of these opportunities—whether it's for study or extra courses, time away or catching up on things you've been putting off; enjoy the increased flexibility. If you are looking to go away, you might even be able to swap shifts with someone in order to have up to 5 days off in a row without taking any extra leave; look into this early.

Intern year is a great time to enjoy yourself, and to learn, without the pressures of medical school exams or assessments. Although there may be many challenges in your ED term, there will be many rewards and opportunities both within and outside the hospital.

All the best!

Quick/general tips

- If in doubt, ask someone.
- Try to order all the tests you may need at the start (e.g. take one of each tube you may need for bloods).
- Carry some extra gauze and some tape.
- Always discuss your patient with a registrar or consultant. If you are worried, make sure you speak to someone more senior sooner.
- Every female is assumed pregnant until a beta-hCG has proven otherwise. Order a beta-hCG.
- Use the resources available—Therapeutic Guidelines, MIMS, Australian Medicines Handbook and clinical protocols.
- Make the most of the nursing and allied health staff. Keep them informed and involved in the patient's plan and progress.
- Look after your own safety.
- Never discharge someone without clearing the patient with a registrar or consultant.
- Adopt universal precautions, and if in doubt err on the side of caution.
- Always follow-up any investigation you have ordered, including ECGs.
- Triage is a guide—if you are concerned about a patient deteriorating, you may need to see them sooner.
- Don't be ashamed if you do not know something: be honest, and you will learn for next time.
- Try not to be disheartened if you meet any obstruction or criticism. Try to learn from the experience, and understand the multiple factors at play in the situation. Remember you are part of a team, and ask for help if needed.
- If you're stuck remember your ABCs, and go back to the basics of history and examination.
- Look after each other. You are part of a team: ask for help when you need it, and offer help to others when you can.
- Have fun!

Online resources

Australian Medicines Handbook
  https://shop.amh.net.au
BMJ Best Practice
  http://bestpractice.bmj.com/best-practice/welcome.html
MIMS
  www.mims.com.au
Therapeutic Guidelines
  www.tg.org.au
UpToDate
  www.uptodate.com

Chapter 57
So it's your first night shift 'in charge'—how to manage the department

Sascha Fulde

Most registrars find the transition from working supervised to being 'in charge' to be a very stressful time in their career. It is usually the first time when a junior doctor is truly on their own, and the fact that this usually happens overnight gives an added level of complexity. Over the years, I've adopted strategies from many wonderful doctors and developed several strategies of my own to help you survive your first 'in charge' shift.

Reprioritise your responsibilities

Most people recognise that when you're the doctor 'in charge' your responsibilities increase. This often feels like the most overwhelming factor. The key here is to recognise that you can't do everything and that you need to have a clear idea of what order you need to do tasks in. So you need to prioritise your responsibilities. This may seem obvious, but this prioritisation will enable you to rank what you need to do when you inevitably become time pressured during your shift.

Key responsibilities are as follows.
- Deal with the emergencies, emergently.
- Make sure no-one dies (who shouldn't).
- Manage the department.
- Oversee junior staff.

DEAL WITH THE EMERGENCIES, EMERGENTLY

As the most senior clinician on the floor, you will need to keep an eye on the very sick. This means you should 'eyeball' every very sick person that comes in. This does *not* mean that you should personally manage all seriously ill patients. You will often find that your junior staff can take histories, chart medications and make referrals on complex patients, particularly if you are there to ensure the resuscitation occurs swiftly and effectively. If you have a junior doctor present with you at the bedside, for the first 5–10 minutes of a critically ill patient's care, you can often rapidly diagnose and commence resuscitation. This makes good use of your added experience, when dealing with very sick patients, while not tying you up for too long. You will also often be able to request consultations from on-site registrars where necessary (e.g. surgical, obstetric and intensive care registrars) or call in necessary teams (e.g. retrieval teams) or specialist proceduralists (e.g. ENT). This means that other senior staff will be on hand early on in the patient's care and can take responsibility for the patient's care, freeing you up to move on to your next task. That said, you will often need to double back in 15–20 minutes and check that the patient is being cared for appropriately. It's also helpful to ask the nurse to come and alert you if there are any problems.

MAKE SURE NO-ONE DIES

It sometimes seems like a 'sick' patient appears out of nowhere from your 'blind spot'. Anyone who has been in this situation will share that feeling of your stomach sinking as a colleague says, 'I think [patient X] is unstable'. One way to approach the ED is to look for potentially sick patients among the patients in the department and waiting room. Some ways to do this are as follows.

- Every time you log in to the computer system, scan the list for patients with abnormal vital signs. If you find someone with abnormalities you can't explain, prioritise that patient (allocate a medical officer to see or ask a senior nurse to check on them).
- Look through the list every 1–2 hours and identify high-risk presenting problems, especially problems that could be mimics (e.g. renal colic and AAA).
- Make sure you prioritise paediatric patients as children often present as stable until they acutely decompensate and become very unwell.
- Don't forget the patients in the waiting room or your short stay unit. These patients end up being largely your responsibility

and are often undifferentiated. Try and take a good handover of admitted patients, particularly what is outstanding and make a time in your shift to step into the unit and check no-one has deteriorated.

MANAGE THE DEPARTMENT

Doctors often worry about their level of knowledge or procedural skills before being 'in charge' but one of the most important skills is being able to take a step back and look globally at the department to see what resources you can use and are being used currently. The first step is making sure you don't become too involved in seeing *all* the patients yourself. Your time is limited and going to be pulled in many different directions. After that, it is a balancing act. You need to balance seeing new high-acuity patients, reviewing other doctors' patients, and rapid assessments of patients waiting, including commencing investigations and management. This is a skill that you would get better at managing over time.

OVERSEE JUNIOR STAFF

This is a role you will be familiar with; however, it will be a larger portion of your responsibility as you are now ultimately responsible for all patients that present on your shift. However, you are not expected to suddenly 'know all the answers'. Remember if you are unsure for any reason, keep the patient in the department, short stay unit or waiting room as appropriate.

Keys to success

As is always the case in the ED, remember that you're not alone— you are part of a team. While you're now the most senior player, you have a lot of support that you can call on. The first key is to understand the team you have. When I start a night shift, I like to consider who I have as part of my emergency team. This means who are my senior nurses who can help offload and guide me, and who are my junior doctors. It's really important to find out what experience they have and then consider how best to use those skills. If you have a very junior intern it may be helpful to get them to accompany you and take the bloods and document while you take the history, perform the examination and manage the patient. The next step is to remember who you have as help within the hospital. Don't forget you may have other registrars in the hospital (e.g. intensive care unit / high-dependency unit, anaesthetics, paediatrics, medical or surgical registrars). Depending on your relationship with staff in the hospital it may be helpful to call them at the beginning of a shift and explain that you're doing your first set of nights 'alone' and would they mind if you called them for informal advice if you are worried or stuck. It can also be helpful to alert them that if you call for help—you're actually going to need them to come quickly (it's an actual call for help). Lastly, don't forget your support out of hospital—mainly your Fellow Australian College of Emergency Medicine (FACEM) on call and also any specialist teams you have available to you. No one has ever got into trouble for asking for too much help and your FACEM will want to know if you are worried about a patient or concerned about how the department is functioning. If in doubt, call—we are there to support you.

Other tips and tricks

- Handover is crucial. Pay attention and ask questions—what's the plan, what's outstanding/do you need me to do, if this happens what would you like me to do.
- Look at the patient list and anticipate needs—balance timing and resources.
  — Prioritise those that are unsorted.
  — Prioritise those that are likely to be able to go home if seen now—but not if they are seen at day or evening off when resting.
- Have good resources: hard copy, your own notes or online.
- Do a round at 5 am.
- Check in with the nurse unit manager (NUM). They are in charge as well and often are aware of other issues that you need to know about. I will check in regularly and also do a round with the NUM at 5 am.
- Remember that this is one of those major life stresses. Everyone finds it hard. This means it is extra important to look after yourself. Eat well and sleep well. Try and prioritise being prepared for the extra responsibility at work, and try and avoid major changes in the rest of your life—this is not the month to move to a new house etc.
  Good luck on your first set of nights—you've got this!!

Chapter 58
So you had a bad shift . . .

Sascha Fulde

It happens to us all. By the time you leave the department you're already several hours late, you haven't eaten, drunk or sat down for 12 hours, your brain is numb from all the decisions you've made and you still have that churning feeling in your gut that things didn't go right or there's too much left undone . . .

Based on many years of experience, there are several things we recommend you do.

- Go home—emergency medicine is a team sport and you have done your relay in the race. You now need to rest and recuperate so you are back to peak for your next shift.
- Prevent as much as possible—plan to protect yourself. Try and structure your life so you can arrive at work on time, rested, fed and watered. We all have days where your garage door breaks and you're locked in the garage, only to get out and discover a flat tyre. However, planning to arrive at work stressed and overwhelmed is adding an unnecessary level of difficulty that (as per Murphy's Law) will definitely mean you have a very difficult shift. This means if at all possible on the days you're working, ensure that you don't also plan to arrive from a 24-hour flight from overseas, stay up all night with friends or 'Marie Kondo'-style sorting your cupboards etc.
- Develop a plan before you need it. Have a plan of what you're going to do to look after yourself before you need it. This can be for the hours after your shift to several days post, but think what works for you. Are you someone who likes to talk it through and who is your person to talk to? Are you someone who needs to be distracted? Does exercise provide the mental breath of fresh air that you need? Think of what it is before you feel like this and have a 'bad shift plan' that you put in place.

- On your next day off or evening off when resting—try and reflect on what went wrong. If it was in relation to a patient, reflect on what went well and what didn't and why. Then think about what you would do differently next time. If the whole shift was a mess of impending disaster, reflect on what strategies you tried, what worked and what didn't and how you would like to work next time. If it's all a blur or you can't work out what you could do differently—ask someone. Ask to speak to the FACEM who was on, your mentor or someone you trust and ask what they would have done. This is often really useful to reassure that you tried everything you could and that it is just how things go.
- Try and balance your life. When work is hard make sure that your days off are refreshing. Give some thought to whether that takes the form of going on adventures, long walks with your dog or spending time with friends and family or by yourself. Try and remind yourself that there is a whole other world out there, and in addition to being an incredible emergency doctor, you are an amazing, interesting person.
- Remember that even the best doctor in the world has made and continues to make mistakes. In my experience, the true legends know this and continually endeavour to do better and be better. You can only do this by being **kind** to yourself and continuing to practise and learn.

Chapter 59
Useful resources: FOAM resources, podcasts and online emergency medicine material

Sascha Fulde

FOAM Podcasts

Free Open Access Medical (FOAM) Education is an incredible resource. One of the most inspiring elements of emergency medicine is the vibrant community of doctors devoted to excellent patient care and education. Below is a short list of some of our personal favourite resources. This is far from an exhaustive list, but are some of our favourites.

PODCASTS
Topic review

- Emergency Medicine Cases (https://emergencymedicinecases.com/podcasts/main-episodes/)
  — A podcast in multiple formats: long format (over 1 hour), Quick Hits (approximately 30 minutes; brief coverage of many topics), Journal Jam and Best Case Ever (10 minutes; discussion of a guest's best case).
  — A key feature of this podcast is the ability to sign up for 'just the nuggets', a series of six follow-up emails that reinforce key messages by using spaced repetition.
- Core EM (https://coreem.net)
  — Short (approximately 10 minutes) episodes covering key topics.
- FOAMcast (http://foamcast.org)
  — Thirty minute discussion of Emergency Medicine Core Content based on the textbooks *Rosen's Emergency Medicine* and *Tintinalli's Emergency Medicine*.

- Pediatric Emergency Playbook (http://pemplaybook.org)
  — A practical discussion of management of paediatric emergency topics, both common and rare (approximately 30 minutes).
- ERCAST (https://www.hippoed.com/em/ercast/)
  — American podcast focusing on common topics (30 minutes)
- Resuscitation Conference Podcast (https://www.resus2019.com/updates)
  — Recorded lectures from an annual conference focusing on topical resuscitation topics (30 minutes).
- SMACC (https://www.smacc.net.au/past-talks/the-talks-smaccdub/)
  — Recorded lectures from SMACC conference.
  — Large portfolio of short-form talks (20 minutes) that cover many emergency topics.
- CRACKCast (https://canadiem.org/crackcast/)
  — Each episode covers one chapter from *Rosen's Emergency Medicine*.
  — A good revision source for exams (30 minutes).
- Simulcast (http://simulationpodcast.com)
  — Australian podcast discussing all things simulation education (30 minutes).

Journal discussion

- The Resus Room (https://theresusroom.co.uk/march-2019/)
  — Discussion of recent interesting papers from the United Kingdom (approximately 30 minutes).
- The Skeptics' Guide to Emergency Medicine (http://thesgem.com)
  — Interview with an expert about a paper using a structured approach (30 minutes).
- The St Emlyn's virtual hospital (https://www.stemlynsblog.org/podcasts/)
  — Covers a variety of topics including clinical practice, current evidence and philosophical topics (20 minutes).

- The Medical Journal of Australia (https://www.mja.com.au/podcasts)
  — Interviews an author of an interesting article from the MJA this month.
  — Not always emergency focused, but current and Australian.
- Feminem (https://feminem.org/podcast/)
  — Short episodes (less than 30 minutes) that aim to inspire women and men, interviewing interesting practitioners with a focus on gender equality in emergency medicine.
- Annals of Emergency Medicine (https://www.annemergmed.com/content/podcast-archive)
  — Monthly summary of important articles in the Annals of Emergency Medicine journal (40 minutes).

Other
Paid
- ECG weekly (https://ecgweekly.com)
  — Weekly 15 minute video by Dr Amal Mattu.
  — Excellent discussion of ECGs.
- Em:Rap (https://www.emrap.org)
  — Operating for 18 years, one of the original producers of emergency medicine education in an audio format.
- EMA (https://www.emrap.org/ema?episode-guide-publish-date=%5B567954000000%2C1552610400000%5D)
  — Monthly episode showing review and summary of current literature pertaining to emergency medicine content.

We hope you enjoy these recommendations and find them as useful as we do. If you have any extra recommendations please feel free to let us know.

Chapter 60
Career, lifestyle and success

Gordian Fulde and Sascha Fulde

Career

What do you want to be?

A question disliked the more you grow up!

Once you have graduated in medicine, it is normal to not really know where you want to go next.

SOME HINTS

The most important is **_HAVE NO REGRETS_**—that is, if after a good term or an interest is kindled, go for it! It doesn't matter if the exams are hard or if lots of others have the same interest and so on.

- If you try and it does not work out, you will not be bitter; but if you don't try, later it can lead to massive regrets.
- It is okay to change choices, especially when a new, good opportunity presents itself.

HOW TO GET YOUR NOSE IN FRONT

- Talk to people—bosses, registrars who are in that field—to ask their advice and show you are interested. When possible, attend unit education and other meetings, offer to help with audits and so on.
- Get the information and start plans regarding college requirements and exams (you want these for any career interview).
- Choose and ask one or two people to be your mentor/role model. Keep in contact!

PUBLISH OR PERISH

Yes, publishing is valuable. Some hospitals and colleges will not give you a job if you do not have publications.

- Try to choose a project you find interesting.

- Try to choose co-investigators who have a track record of success.
- Try to be the first or second author.
- Check it is doable (around your time/commitments) and can be written up in a reasonable timeframe (i.e. has a good hypothesis).
- Do not get disheartened if it gets rejected or needs rewrites.
- Try to make sure it is a reputable peer-reviewed journal.
- Consider specialist journals.
- It allows you to discuss in detail your research, a common interview question.

EXAMS: HOW TO PASS—FIRST TIME

- Allow 12 months of serious study.
- Data—old papers, trial exams—is a must.
- Talk to and get notes/tutorials from recent successful candidates.
- If possible, talk to examiners.
- You **MUST** form study groups and have at least one study buddy that you meet regularly (if you study alone, you will do poorly).
- Go to as many courses and tutorials as you can.
- Practise—practise each part of multiple-choice questions (MCQs), Vivas, essays, objective structured clinical examination (OSCE) and so on (e.g. each shift get quizzed by each registrar, consultant).
- Bug them—you only really learn and retain by practising, especially things you do not think you know well.

JOBS

Do your homework. Find out, ask about a possible role, possible new hospital/department. It is essential for the questions: What do you do? Why this job? Make an appointment to visit the department; it is a really smart thing to do for both you and them.

INTERVIEWS

Again, do your homework, practise interview questions and be prepared for the 'left-field questions' which are now common in all industries (e.g. Who is your favourite action hero and why?)

Try to relax, smile and be yourself. Try to think that if you were the interviewer, what would you be looking for?

Daily stuff to stay out of hassles and do well!

* Mistakes—we all make them.
  — University, job orientation and common sense have taught you the fundamentals, but even a good doctor makes mistakes and has a bad day!
  — Manage it how you would advise a friend to sort it. Get advice. But always be honest, do not be afraid to apologise and have open disclosure (with admin, medical defence advice when necessary). Never try to cover up—in general life the cover-up gets people in more trouble than the original event.
* Getting consults and arranging tests.
  — Yes, it is mostly online now but we mainly are still dealing with humans. So take every opportunity to talk on the phone, go around to X-ray and explain what you think the patient needs. Even better, ask their advice regarding tests, apologise for hassling/urgency, tell them why and so on.
  — It works, and say thank you especially to this invisible army of nurses, radiographers, clerical support, allied health, secretaries and so many more who make it all happen.

TRIBALISM AND TEAMS

* Humans tend to group and not be nice to other groups (e.g. professionals, sport clubs, nations).
* So they have to keep neutral. Remember the old saying, if you cannot say anything nice, do not say anything at all—it works.
* As part of a team, you are there to work well, learn and gain experience. Even if that term is not exciting/sexy, it probably has a lot to offer and probably represents a big slice of overall general patient care—get the most out of it.
* Also be aware that high-profile, very clever specialities can breed arrogance. Again, learn and ask questions.
* Sometimes in a term the workload and hours become excessive (e.g. other staff on leave, no relief person for their exams, sick leave).
* Once again, use a structural approach.

- Keep a record of the workload and overtime. Is there a simple solution? First, talk to your senior. If you are worried it may cast a shadow on your term assessment, it can be difficult. However, if there is a group of you (especially if there are straightforward solutions such as a better roster) maybe go to administration as a group.
- As an admin tip, it is often cheaper to employ another staff member than to pay lots of overtime.

BULLYING, HARASSMENT AND DISCRIMINATION

Bullying is repeated, unreasonable behaviour directed towards someone that creates a risk to their health and safety. It also impairs their ability to do their job.

If bullying occurs document:

- repetitive verbal abuse, threats or yelling
- unjustified criticism
- physical or mental intimidation
- behaviour such as excluding, ignoring, isolating or belittling
- giving people impossible tasks or timeframes
- deliberately withholding information that is vital for effective work performance
- spreading false rumours or lies or backstabbing.

See www.fwc.gov.au/documents/documents/factsheets/guide_antibullying.pdf

Sadly bullying, harassment, discrimination as well as the bad effects on any individual are quite prevalent and often complex.

Very early

- Talk to someone!
- Seek help and advice!
- You are not alone!
- It is not acceptable!
  Help is available at:
- Doctor's Health Advisory Service (http://dhas.org.au):
- NSW and ACT–02 9437 6552
- NT and SA–08 8366 0250
- Queensland–07 3833 4352
- Tasmania and Victoria–03 9280 8712 http://www.vdhp.org.au
- WA–08 9321 3098

- New Zealand–0800 471 2654
- Medical Benevolent Society (http://www.mbansw.org.au/)
- AMA lists of GPs willing to see junior doctors (http://www.doctorportal.com.au/doctorshealth/)
- Lifeline on 13 11 14
- beyondblue on 1300 224 636
- beyondblue Doctors' health website: https://www.beyondblue.org.au/about-us/our-work-in-improving-workplace-mental-health/health-services-program

Lifestyle

It is very important. Medicine and hospital life can break you. It is essential to pick up warning signs early. For example:

- always exhausted
- no time for friends
- no time to do fun things
- saying no to many things you used to do
- grumpy, cynical
- depressed
- sleep disturbances
- dangerous 'escapes' such as alcohol and drugs (these do not fix anything but just make it a lot worse)
- your pot plants all die
- patients, consults, tasks become irritations/problems
- becoming unpleasant to others (e.g. nurses, allied health)
- grizzling all the time.

PREVENTION AND REMEDIES

Have and keep a good routine (the hospital will always be there).

- Exercise (e.g. walking, short morning exercise routines).
- Healthy diet (avoid overeating, unhealthy food—too easy if time poor or tired for night shifts).
- Sleep—enough is a MUST! Nights, late and early shifts. Your mind and body need any deficit paid back! Batteries all need recharging.
- Fun—make the effort, set a day, a time, it is a priority to know what you like. Do not let ages go by, procrastinating this includes hobbies, interests (e.g. a dog), time with a friend.

- Friendships and family are vital, essential. Yes, they take time and can be inconvenient but without talking to and spending time with them, you will struggle more with your work and be at risk of mental or physical health issues. These are the ones who you can turn to and will support you.
- If you are in trouble, talk to your mentor or GP, or seek professional help (you are not alone or the only one).
- All hospitals have access to free confidential counselling.
- In the end it is about healthy, rational self-esteem, not feeling worthless.
- You are a doctor! Really cool!
- Wow, how lucky are you to be able to help people, be listened to, be trusted and even respected. Whose shoes would you really rather be in? People want your advice.
- Your patients are worse off than you.
- What you do really matters, even the annoying little tasks like chasing results, somebody else's discharge summary, dealing with so many people—some will be annoying so recognise this quickly and always be professional—it is a passing parade.
- Healthcare/medicine is one of the industries that is not threatened by robots and artificial intelligence—it is a future growth area for employment.

SUCCESS

The key to success!

- Appreciate how fortunate you are.
- Be positive.
- Be nice to those around you (e.g. smile, say g'day, learn their names, definitely say thank you, praise, say well done, if someone swaps a bad shift for you—coffee or chocolates are in order not just be prepared to pay back).
- Treat other people as loved ones.
- Mind games—yes, quiet ones are the best.
- Shit happens!
- Think it, do NOT say it!
- Do not whinge all the time—it is too easy to do this.

- Have some mantras in your head so you do not feel guilty to say no (e.g. 'a lack of planning on your behalf does not constitute an emergency on mine').
- If you come to me with a problem and have not thought of possible solutions, you really have a problem.
- Corollary—you yourself are in a good position to offer solutions. When dealing with administrative duties and so on, discuss them—it really works.
- In clinical situations (I call it the social work approach—it is excellent), ask the patient (or others) their thoughts on issues . . . and listen!
- Always be honest (e.g. explain to patients you do not know—medicine is full of uncertainty—but discuss strategy; choices—make sure they ask questions; shared decision-making).
- It is okay to 'bail' and walk away (politely) if not comfortable, and get assistance, advice (e.g. aggressive patients, feeling harassed [including sexual], bullied or just beyond your capabilities to easily cope with). Remember the action of holding your hand up with your palm facing away—'Stop'. It works, so use it! Do not stay and fight, always keep notes and always go and talk to someone even outside of the workplace. All hospitals have access for free confidential counselling.
- Develop areas of special interests, get involved, study, keep updated, take opportunities to give a tutorial and talk to others (medical, nurse, students etc.).
- If you can, advocate it (e.g. basic life support, become an instructor and teach it to community groups or how to use an AED).

Chapter 61
Career in emergency medicine: workplace-based assessment

Sascha Fulde and Marian Lee

Choosing emergency medicine
Sascha Fulde

So you are considering a career in emergency medicine? Good!

Please also read Chapter 60 Career, Lifestyle and Success.

Often there are many possibilities and you are trying to navigate which one. That is normal, and often fate (e.g. job opportunities, training location) leads to confounding factors.

One useful technique to assess each option is to get a page for each and draw a line down the middle, making one side for positives, the other for negatives. It really helps clear the issues and you may even be able to rank them.

Talk to people, such as directors of emergency medicine training (each hospital has one) and bosses you get on with (especially if to use as a reference) if still choosing (also at interviews). Phrase it 'seriously considering' and have reasons why.

Most importantly, as soon as emergency medicine becomes an interest, look at the Australian College for Emergency Medicine (ACEM) website and even ring them. Do not wait until applying for hospital/training jobs as there are conditions that need to be met even in PGY2 (postgraduate year 2). There are prerequisites that need to be known and discussed before interviews in PGY1. All colleges keep changing their regulations so ask, look up, talk to them... early.

Finally, and probably most importantly, if you are interested find out and give it a go. If it does not end up being the one, you will not have any lifelong regrets.

The different facets of workplace based assessment

Marion Lee

Workplace based assessment (WBA) has been used in facilitating training in many workplaces, and recently it has been introduced, implemented and embedded in the ACEM training program at the specialist (FACEM) and the non-specialist (Certificate and Diploma) levels. What are the rationales for its use? Who stands to benefit from it? Is it worth the effort and time?

WBA IS A LEARNING TOOL

WBA is a term that embraces a number of tools specific to the learner's workplace. It recognises that learning takes place by doing the work required. In emergency medicine, the WBA tools selected are those that are able to assess the performance of the work required of a trainee in the emergency department. These tools enable assessments to occur with minimal to no alteration to the day-to-day work. Implicit is the authenticity of the assessments to the work required. There is no deconstruction of the work in order for it to be assessed. It is an assessment of the integrated performance of the trainee—the observable end result of the multiple layers of learning needed to deliver the work required of an emergency medicine trainee. Hence, WBA is context specific and done in real-time with minimal to no alteration or manipulation of the environment in which work is normally done.

From the assessor's perspective, what you see is what you assess. It is the outcome of training, visible as the quality of patient care delivered. This is the most significant criterion capturing the interest of the stakeholders: the workplace (hospital), ACEM and the public. Assessments in the workplace aim to assess what is important—work performance. However, this is only part of the story of WBAs.

As tools, WBAs have two utilities. It is evident that it is an assessment of learning. It tells the assessor what the trainee has learned—the visible integration of the multiple layers of learning (described variously by Miller's pyramid of learning and Bloom's taxonomy of learning). A point of emphasis is that WBA is not able to assess the layers of learning. It doesn't give the full story of what determines the observed behaviours. However, the observed performance informs the feedback that occurs after the assessment. This is how WBA is useful for learning and it needs to be recognised as a learning tool.

How best to utilise WBA for learning? This requires both parties to be engaged with the WBA as a means of providing relevant feedback. The data resulting from the WBA provide a platform for useful feedback for the trainee. The value of the data lies in its specificity to the context, because the observed behaviour originates from a situation that the trainee and assessor have just experienced. Hence, it provides a shared experience for exploring the thinking behind the behaviour/action. The assessor may enquire about the rationale behind the observations. The trainee gets to explain the actions. Essentially, the assessor provides an evaluation—feedback, followed by the process of feed-forward. The latter is where the assessor promotes learning by referring the trainee to calibration points and discusses strategies with the trainee as to how to get there. The interactions after an assessment is the most valuable part of the WBA process. Recognising this aspect of WBA is paramount to understanding and utilising WBA as a means for learning.

If one accepts that WBA is a means for learning, then the question is how good is it for learning. The feedback and feed-forward process are dependent on the efforts of both the trainee and the assessor. The latter needs to be informed in regards to the standard that the trainee needs to achieve. The trainee needs to be able to see and understand the calibration points or milestones. The expected learning outcomes or standards of practice are derived from the body that both parties belong to—ACEM. The ACEM Curriculum Framework is the document that embodies the standards required at each level of training.

The Curriculum Framework is an extensive document that outlines progressive milestones in the training towards the FACEM. WBA is mapped onto the progressive training milestone outlined in this document. It enables trainees to be self-directed in their training. For assessors, it is a reference for gauging expectations and a transparent measure of performance. In essence, the Curriculum Framework ensures both parties are pursuing the same ultimate outcomes.

WBA AS AN ASSESSMENT TOOL

One really cannot get away from the fact that an assessment is an assessment. WBA, as depicted above, is a tool for learning because the feedback is formative. However, WBA has a dual role in the ACEM training program as it is also a summative feedback tool as it is used as an assessment tool to determine progression through the training program. How does this duality work?

Implementing a WBA program requires certain logistics to be incorporated. This is to ensure WBA causes minimal interruption to the workplace. Multiple WBA tools and more than one assessor are essential to achieving the main outcome, which is to provide multiple opportunities to obtain a summary of the quality of the trainee's work. A trainee would have a collection of WBAs composed of various WBA tools. A different assessor evaluates the trainee at multiple points in their training period. This collection, at a pre-determined time, is reviewed as a whole. This evaluation is done remotely in time and place, by a group of assessors who can see and track the trainee's performance in the various assessment criteria over the course of training. That is, the progression in performance. The key point is the demonstration of progression towards the pre-determined milestones. The conclusive evaluation/summative feedback is based on whether the training outcomes have been met. Hence, any single WBA is not going to define a trainee's performance but the overall picture provided by the set of WBAs over a defined period of time would be used to arrive at the conclusion.

If no single WBA is going to define a trainee's performance at work, then it means that a single WBA cannot fail a trainee. Each WBA is a learning tool due to the benefits of feedback and feedforward. The performance over time, shown in the set of WBA, assessed by various Emergency Consultants would be like pixels in the screenshot that is viewed by a separate group of assessors tasked with the role of providing a summative evaluation. This analogy to a pixelated picture illustrates the concept that a more accurate picture is gained by more pixels or a larger set of WBAs. What is mandated in the ACEM training program is the minimal number per set of WBA at different stages in the training program. It is an arbitrary value based on multiple factors. The number is grounded in what is achievable at the workplace and the estimated minimum amount of data required to inform a progression decision. A strategic approach by trainees would be to disregard the number required and concentrate on the number necessary to portray an authentic picture of their clinical performance. If this is understood then it follows that the number required is arbitrary and doing as many as is necessary during a training period would be in their favour. Hence, by owning the WBA as a tool for learning, trainees can ensure they submit a picture that truly reflects their progression in training.

THE RATIONALE BEHIND THE WBA MENU

Another aspect of WBA to reveal is the rationale for the various WBA tools. As mentioned previously, WBA is based on observed behaviours. The latter are visible outcomes of the integration of multiple layers of learning. Specifically, the behaviours are observed actions and communication—what is done, how it is done, what is said and how it is said and to whom. Hence the assessments are not based on inferences; meaning that what is not seen or heard cannot be assessed. It makes sense that multiple types of WBAs are required to capture the complex behaviours that make up clinical practice. The tools selected by ACEM are those that, as a set, enable an evaluation of the domains of practice defined by ACEM. The collection of WBA tools embraces all the domains of practice whereas each individual tool does not.

Also on the menu of WBAs are the assessors. The program encourages the partnering of the trainee with multiple emergency physicians as assessors. This provides the trainee with opportunities to be exposed to the diversity of perspectives within the uniformity that exists within the FACEM.

WBAS PROVIDE A STRUCTURE FOR LEARNING HOW TO ASSESS

A lot has been revealed about WBA. From a long-term perspective, WBA provides the structure for one to learn to assess objectively, feedback specifically and feed-forward effectively. This is true for trainees and assessors. In fact, there is a natural evolution for trainees to become WBA assessors in time and take their turn in facilitating the learning of future emergency medicine trainees

CONCLUSION

The multiple facets of WBA have been presented to capture the curiosity of the reader and (hopefully) transform it into an enduring interest. The most important point is to recognise WBA as a tool for learning as well as a method to assess what has been learned. As it is conducted in the place where work is done, it is in a prime position to demonstrate actions/behaviours that are the integrated outcomes of learning. It is also a way of assessing what really matters. As to its more intimidating aspect of being an assessment of what is learned, one must remember that for the ACEM training program, the individual assessments are data points to populate the final picture of clinical performance on which the summative decision is based. The more assessment points available, the more evidence based the decision. Hence WBA enables the trainee to be self-directed in learning and by owning it, determines the outcome of the final assessment.

Chapter 62
Administration and governance in the ED

John Vinen

Overview

Successful management of the ED requires an effective leadership and management team to coordinate the multiple processes involved in all aspects of clinical care and the administrative processes required to support the clinical care. These skills are necessary for the clinical leads, clinicians and all the members of the ED team to attain and to have the training, resources, facilities, attributes and sense of mission that are required for safe, efficient and effective clinical care.

Managing the emergency department

The ED is a busy, complex and dynamic environment with physical, temporal and economic restraints requiring an efficient, effective and responsive administrative structure that has clearly defined professional and administrative roles and responsibilities and a defined continuous management process based on the ED's business plan.

There are four domains to support safe and quality care: 1. consumer participation; 2. clinical effectiveness; 3. effective workforce; and 4. risk management. All domains need to be incorporated into every aspect of ED management.

The need for effective and responsive ED management will continue to increase due to increasing workload, the need to improve patient safety, the requirement to maximise efficient patient flow, increasing complexity of medical care, increasing costs, technological advances, networked services, the need to move to evidence-based care, the legal environment and public expectations.

In order to manage all of the requirements, EDs require an effective responsive administrative structure, governance processes, teamwork, leadership processes and committed staff.

Business plan

The ED business plan is an essential multipurpose plan developed and reviewed annually by the ED administrative group to inform ED staff and hospital management about the agreed financial and performance plan for the forthcoming financial year.

The business plan is monitored monthly and if desired outcomes are not achieved, remedial action needs to be taken.

Administration

The administrative structure needs to be based on administrative, professional, training and operational requirements with common objectives which need to include:

- high-quality patient care focus
- patient safety
- staffing recruitment, credentialling, orientation and retention
- training/supervisory requirements
- teamwork/training
- workload
- process of patient care
- models of care
- staff allocation to clinical teams/areas/functions
- patient flow
- clinical risk management (CRM), quality assurance (QA) and audit
- results review
- rosters and shift management
- liaison (internal and external).

Administrative structure

The ED administrative structure needs to reflect the size and complexity of the individual ED with basic structural requirements included in all ED's management structure:

- administrative group (overall management)
- administrative support

- clinical leadership group (clinical leadership and teaching/training skills)
- clinical support (including team leaders/shift managers [nursing and medical])
- clinical teams
- director of emergency medicine training (DEMT)
- term supervisors.

Governance

Clinical governance is defined by the Australian Council on Healthcare Standards as: 'the system by which the governing body, managers, clinicians and staff share responsibility and accountability for the quality of care, continuously improving, minimising risks and fostering an environment of excellence in care for consumers.'

EDs require clinical and administrative leadership for effective governance, an effective process of patient care in order to ensure timely, efficient and safe delivery of care for patients. The ED medical and nursing managers are responsible for the effective communication and coordination of care across the ED aimed at the ability to produce effective change where change is required. For clinical governance to be successful there must be a willingness from all staff to make it work.

An ED clinical governance team needs to be established and meet regularly, led by a senior clinician with multidisciplinary membership. Minutes and action points and outcomes need to be kept. With careful leadership the clinical governance team can be a major team-building process within the department and an opportunity to improve the quality of patient care.

Failure to learn from an error in the care of patients represents a failure of clinical governance by not ensuring:

- there is adequate staff in terms of numbers, training and seniority 24 hours a day, 7 days a week, every day of the year
- staff have the required training, skills and supervision
- the environment meets the clinical requirements
- an effective audit/QA/CRM process
- changes are made (including to guidelines) following review of an incident/adverse event.

Clinical risk management (CRM)

CRM involves:

- administrative structure
- policies and procedures
- staffing, recruitment, credentialling, orientation, education and training, continuing professional development
- audit, incident monitoring, review and introduction of corrective strategies.

CRM is achieved by:

- effective leadership and joint responsibility
- a committed representative ED management team
- shared vision and values
- a systematic approach to establishing, maintaining and improving the quality of patient care within a clinical care setting
- establishing and fostering an open, fair and equal culture
- recruitment
- comprehensive orientation of all new staff
- credentialling
- training
- ensuring that risk management systems and processes are incorporated into everyday practice, learn from mistakes, share knowledge, implement solutions and monitor success
- a robust quality assurance (QA) and incident audit and review process
- implementing methods of assessing clinical effectiveness and quality of service delivery
- learning from others, looking for innovative and effective ways of delivering better quality care
- being aware of local and national governance agenda.

Clinical governance requires the application of a framework made up of components which together ensure clinical services are safe. These include:

- the ED's organisational and clinical structure
- policies and processes
- the way the quality and performance of the service are measured and managed
- how to analyse data and to whom data is reported

- how to continually improve care while at the same time continuing to provide ED services.
  Guiding quality assurance, the framework specifically:
- focuses on best practice and evidence-based clinical guidelines
- establishes principles that outline accountabilities
- assists ED staff to review and continually improve services
- defines the infrastructure and staffing required for effective service delivery while at the same time coordinating, monitoring, evaluating and reporting service quality
- building capacity within the system to identify and respond to risks and opportunities.

Emergency department models of care (applicable to EDs that are level 3 and above)

The varying urgency, clinical (and other) requirements means that numbers in each subset of patients' multiple models of care are required in the ED. They are:

- Resuscitation (triage category 1 and some patients from the other triage categories including those whose condition deteriorates)
- Acute care (triage category 2 and some patients from the other triage categories including those whose condition indicates the need to be in an acute care area and those who require close observation)
- subacute care
- fast track
- short stay area/clinical decision unit
- mental health unit
- waiting room.
  Clinical team-based models:
- trauma team
- paediatric resuscitation team
- sexual assault team (can involve staff from outside the ED)
- hospital medical emergency team
- external medical team.

EDs caring for adults and children also require a paediatric model of care (MOC)

To effectively operate multiple MOCs, the staffing levels and skill mix requirements need to be determined based on analysis of activity data and the volume of patients who will be treated in each MOC.

The skill mix and expertise of staff need to match the requirements of each model to deliver care—providing the right skills in the right place to make the right decisions.

The introduction of multiple MOCs will only be possible in EDs busy enough to effectively utilise multiple MOCs. Smaller EDs may only be able to implement one or possibly two MOCs.

The number, skill mix, qualifications and expertise of staff needs to meet the requirements of each model in order to deliver timely, efficient and safe care on a 24-hour, 7-day-a-week basis.

Smaller EDs will only be able to establish a small number of team-based MOCs with emphasis on clinical team MOCs.

Teams and teamwork

Emergency medicine is a team-based speciality where teamwork is essential for the delivery of safe, efficient and effective care.

Working in well-formed functional teams has many advantages in the delivery of emergency care including clear understanding of individual roles and responsibilities, training under supervision, effective leadership, skill mix, complementary skills, common purpose, common goals, shared commitment and support. Leadership and team training is essential.

The rostering process, leave requirements and regular medical term changeover mean that team membership needs to be dynamic, with frequent changes in team membership. This will need to be carefully managed if the teams are to remain effective, with a team meeting at the beginning of each shift so that each team member knows who the team leader is, who the other team members are and their roles.

Patient care process (PCP)

An essential component of all MOCs is an efficient, effective and safe process of care.

The requirements of the PCP (Figure 62.1) are:
- patient reception/triage (ambulatory and ambulance arrivals)
- allocation to the appropriate clinical area
- rapid initial assessment/commencement of treatment

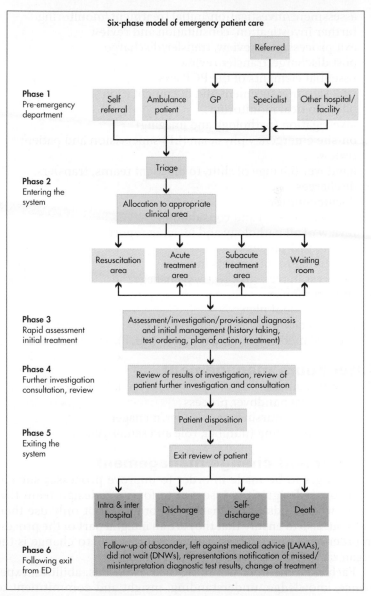

Figure 62.1 Six-phase model of emergency patient care

- assessment/investigation/initial treatment/monitoring
- further investigation, consultation and review
- exit process. exit review, transfer/discharge
- post discharge/transfer review.
  Essential elements of the PCP are:
- vital sign measurement and documentation
- physiological monitoring
- investigation (pathology and imaging)
- on-site emergency physician (EP) supervision and patient review
- handover (change of shift, to inpatient teams, transfers, discharges)
- documentation
- specialty referral and consultation
- review of all pathology and imaging reports
- audit/CRM process.
  Additional requirements include:
- a process in place to effectively manage the after-hours periods
- surge response
- major incident plan
- overcapacity plan
- external medical emergency team (MET).

After-hours management

Each shift requires:
- an effective handover process
- medical and nursing team leader/manager
- adequate staffing (number, role and seniority).

Project and change management

For changes to be made in order to improve processes such as workflow redesign, it is essential to form a redesign team that 'owns' what needs to be changed in order to not only use their skills but also to ensure that they are an integral part of the process in order to ensure success. The biggest obstacle to change is the organisation's culture and individual attitudes.

Each team member will bring their own skills, abilities, experience, knowledge, understanding, insight and commitment to support the common goal.

The redesign team will need to know what and why change is required, what the outcome needs to be and how to get there (a 'vision statement').

For change to be successful it is essential to have effective leadership, staff involvement, realistic expectations, adequate resourcing and time to achieve what needs to be achieved.

Teaching, training and skills acquisition

One of the major responsibilities of ED management is to maximise staff opportunities to learn and develop clinical and administrative skills for both training and accreditation purposes.

Staff working in the ED are required to have administrative and management responsibilities in order for the ED to function. Without these skills the ED patient safety will be put at risk and the ED will be inefficient, with increased waiting times and poor patient flow.

The best way to learn administrative and management skills is by experience-based mentoring by experienced ED managers.

The ED is an ideal learning environment due to the number, variable presentation and range of medical conditions (many of which present with undifferentiated symptoms and signs) and the ready availability of experienced professionals from whom to learn.

Learning and acquiring skills can be challenging owing to the workload, shift work, limited time available, frequent interruptions and the need for repetitive teaching in order to ensure that all staff receive the required training.

Acquisition of administrative skills includes:

♦ time management
♦ communication skills
♦ building internal and external relationships.

The ED does not operate in isolation, with an essential requirement that input and output are managed effectively with good working relationships with all involved.

INTERNAL RELATIONSHIPS

These relationships include support services such as imaging, pathology, medical records and inpatient.

An effective working relationship with inpatient medical teams needs to be developed and maintained in order to ensure timely patient consultation and seamless transfer of care to inpatient teams and joint management of patients where required.

EXTERNAL RELATIONSHIPS

Strong and effective working external relationships are essential to manage inputs into the ED by referring doctors (general practitioners, specialists, other hospitals/medical services) and police and ambulance services.

ORGANISATIONAL SUPPORT

Organisational support (administrative and financial) is essential for the ED to deliver timely, effective high-quality patient care. Effective patient flow is a hospital-wide responsibility requiring continuous organisational management.

Administrative pearls
- Patient safety depends on a well-functioning ED.
- Effective governance is the key to success.
- Good time management protects both you and the patient.
- Using evidence-based guidelines will improve outcomes.

The future

EDs and hospitals need to rapidly move to the '24-hour hospital' concept where ED resources, support services and inpatient services are available 24 hours a day rather that largely in business hours as is currently the case.

EDs are leading the way with 16-hour 7-days-a-week emergency physician rostering while the rest of the hospital largely operates on traditional on-call rosters with EDs commonly required to 'baby sit' patients in the ED because they are 'too sick' to go to a ward bed after-hours.

How to write a Clinical Practice Guideline

Clinical Practice Guidelines are designed to guide clinical decision-making to minimise variation and ensure correct decisions are made resulting in safe and appropriate care.

Clinical Practice Guidelines must be evidence-based and where there is no evidence consensus-based from a recognised creditable source with references.

Clinical Practice Guidelines 'time out' and must be kept up to date with at a minimum an annual review.

Guidelines also need to take into account that many medical conditions including life-threatening conditions commonly present as an 'undifferentiated' illness and that many medical conditions present in an 'atypical' way, with confounding factors and the presence of comorbid and more than one medical illness present.

Where up-to-date jurisdictional, specialty, professional college hospital and recognised organisations' guidelines are available, they should be used rather than developing 'local' Clinical Practice Guidelines.

Clinical Practice Guidelines need to be readily available, easily findable and readily accessible (including during periods of IT system downtime).

They need to be practical and usable (refer to the National Blood Authority's massive blood transfusion [MTP] template at https://www.blood.gov.au/system/files/documents/pbm-mtp-template_0.ppt).

All staff need to be made aware of what Clinical Practice Guidelines are available at orientation.

Where a Clinical Practice Guideline needs to be developed, the following principles need to be followed:

- Define what the guideline is for.
- Define who the intended users are.
- Decide on the format (free text, pathway, algorithm, flow chart, protocols, etc.)
- Structure: the title should define the clinical topic and intended users, followed by the author(s), their qualifications and roles with institutional affiliations listed. The date of publication and revision should be specified. The process on which the guideline was based needs to be documented (simplification of a published evidence-based guideline, group consensus after literature review, individual recommendation based on clinical experience, or some other technique).

- Follow the process outlined in the following.
  — Graham R, Mancher M, Wolman DM. Clinical Practice
    Guidelines We Can Trust. The National Academies
    Press. 2011. https://www.nap.edu/read/13058/chapter/1.
    Accessed 24 January 2018
  — Counselman FL, Babu K, Edens MA et al. The 2016
    Model of the Clinical Practice of Emergency Medicine.
    JEM 2017;52:846–9. http://www.jem-journal.com/
    article/S0736-4679(17)30108-7/fulltext. Accessed 24
    January 2018

Online resources

Australian Commission on Safety and Quality in Health Care. Safety
    and Quality Improvement Guide Standard 1: Governance for
    Safety and Quality in Health Service Organisations (October 2012).
    https://www.safetyandquality.gov.au/publications-and-resources/
    resource-library/nsqhs-standards-safety-and-quality-improvement-
    guide-governance-safety-and-quality-health-service-organisations

Emergency Department Models of Care July 2012. http://www.health.
    nsw.gov.au/Performance/Publications/ed-model-of-care-2012.pdf

Agency for Clinical Innovation. https://www.aci.health.nsw.gov.au/.

ACEM Statement on Hospital Emergency Department Services for
    Children. https://acem.org.au/getattachment/7827788e-b979-
    42ae-8dd7-c394a3526280/Statement-on-Hospital-Emergency-
    Department-Service.aspx. Accessed 24 January 2018

RACP Standards for the Care of Children and Adolescents in Health
    Services. 2008. https://www.racp.edu.au/docs/default-source/
    advocacy-library/standards-for-the-care-of-children-and-
    adolescents-in-health-service.pdf. Accessed 24 January 2018

Graham R, Mancher M, Wolman DM. Clinical Practice Guidelines We
    Can Trust. The National Academies Press. 2011. https://www.nap.
    edu/read/13058/chapter/1. Accessed 24 January 2018

Scott IA, Chew DP, Branagan M. Editorial. Raising the bar on guideline
    utility and trustworthiness. IMJ 2017;47:613–16. http://onlinelibrary.
    wiley.com/doi/10.1111/imj.13444/full. Accessed 24 January 2018

Campbell SG, Sinclair DE. Strategies for managing a busy emergency
    department. CJEM 2004;6:271–6. https://www.cambridge.org/

core/services/aop-cambridge-core/content/view/
S1481803500009258. Accessed 7 February 2018

Kayden S, Anderson PD, Freitas R et al. (Editors) Emergency
Department Leadership and Management. Cambridge University
Press; 2014.

Rice MM. Emergency department administration and management.
Emerg Med Clinics N Am 2004;22:XV–XVII. http://www.emed.
theclinics.com/article/S0733-8627(03)00116-0/pdf. Accessed
8 February 2018

Croskerry P, Cosby KS (Editors) Patient Safety in Emergency Medicine.
Lippincott Williams & Wilkins; 2009.

NSW Health. Emergency Department Workforce Analysis Tool.
2nd Edition. http://www.health.nsw.gov.au/workforce/Publications/
edwat-ed2.pdf. Accessed 8 February 2018

Craig S, Dowling J. 'Registrar in charge shifts': Learning how to run a busy
emergency department. EMA 2013; DOI: 10.1111/1742-6723.12042.
http://onlinelibrary.wiley.com/doi/10.1111/1742-6723.12042/full.
Accessed 8 February 2018

Chapter 63
Rules, confidentiality, legal matters

John Raftos, Lesley Forster and Gordian Fulde

General principles

All of our interactions with patients and with our hospitals are governed in some way by laws, rules and regulations.

Editorial Comment
Although these topics are not foremost in the hearts of health carers, they are ignored at your peril as they are essential parts of what we do. The quality and length of time with the patient has been proven to be the main factor contributing to dissatisfaction (complaints, lawsuits). EDs are undergoing re-engineering of patient flow—the '4-hour rule'. There will be definite improvements for patients but also definite negative aspects, especially during any change. As with any clinical system issue, identify it and use your governance system (e.g. clinical review issue reporting) to document it; this allows actions, improvements and responsibility to be logged.

Codes

Know them! Especially red, blue and black (Figure 63.1).

Confidentiality

With photos, clinical material, emails and phone, the patient's confidentiality is paramount. As a guide, no photos, no X-rays, ECG or material pertaining to any patient can be taken, used or transmitted without appropriate comment or permission.

Yes, it is happening all the time between doctors and the hospital for the sole purpose of patient care. Even beware presenting

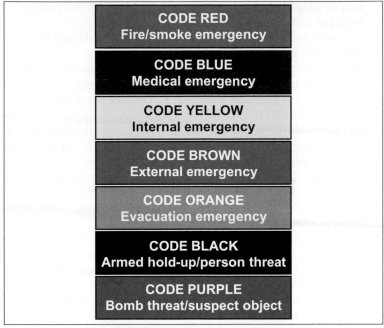

Figure 63.1 Emergency codes

such material at clinical meetings, when publishing, in trial exam questions—even if deidentified. Ideally, it should all be encrypted. Know the current law and regulations—ask your administration, preferably get a written reply.

Never, never send any material to anybody who is not entitled to it especially on social media or to friends. Standard policy can be found at https://ama.com.au/sites/default/files/documents/ FINAL_AMA_Clinical_Images_Guide.pdf

Doctors are bound by confidentiality in patient care. A doctor must never give out any information about any patient to any other person, including the patient's family and friends, without the patient's consent. In New South Wales, the only exceptions to this rule are the:

- *Traffic Act 1909*, under which the doctor is obliged to take a blood sample for alcohol testing following traffic accidents and to supply the patient's name and address to the police with the sample

- *Coroners Act 2009*, under which the doctor is obliged to report any unexplained death to the coroner
- *Public Health Act 2010* (Infectious Diseases), under which the doctor is obliged to report the presence of certain infectious diseases and the patient's contact details to the Ministry of Health.

Occasionally the public interest may override a doctor's duty of confidentiality. If, say, a patient confides to a doctor an intention to commit a serious criminal offence such as homicide or sexual assault, then it would be appropriate for the doctor to provide a relevant third party, usually the police, with that information. Faced with such a situation, you should consult the ED consultant or medical administrator on duty for advice.

There are other circumstances where the situation is not quite so clear and judgment must be made as to what constitutes a serious criminal offence. It is probably accepted, for example, that a doctor does not need to notify police of a patient's involvement in minor criminal activities, such as personal use of illicit drugs, especially when there is no risk of harm to others.

Some occasions arise where there is no clear answer; for example, if a patient who is known to be involved in drug trafficking presents to the ED. In such a case you should discuss with the ED consultant on duty, medical administration and even with your medical indemnity organisation whether to make the very serious decision to override the duty of confidentiality.

For guidance, the St Vincent's Hospital policy regarding internally concealed drugs is shown in Box 63.1.

Requests for information

Telephone requests for information about a patient are governed by the rules of confidentiality. As a general principle, no information should be given to any person without the patient's consent.

If a friend or relative telephones and asks for information about a patient, the patient's consent should be obtained before any information is given. If the patient is responsive/competent, then the patient can speak directly to the relative or friend. If the patient is not responsive/competent or not in a position to speak

---

Box 63.1   St Vincent's Hospital policy and procedure for management of patients with internally concealed drugs

These patients may present of their own accord or may be brought in by the police.

Some drugs (e.g. heroin and cocaine) may cause death if leakage occurs. This is much less likely with hashish. Mechanical problems such as obstruction may occur with any ingested packets.

Medical management should proceed as appropriate. Drug screens and other investigations are performed if medically indicated. Abdominal and chest X-rays, CT may be required. Close observation and supportive therapy are indicated. Specific antidotes such as naloxone may be required. Decontamination may be needed if packet rupture and toxicity have occurred (toxicity may occur by diffusion without packet rupture). GlycoPrep (or similar) may be used to hasten transit. Laparotomy may be indicated to relieve mechanical obstruction or to urgently remove leaking packets which cannot be otherwise retrieved.

If, in the judgment of the treating doctor, the amount of substance is small (i.e. unlikely to be intended for large-scale trafficking but rather intended for individual use) and the patient was not brought in by the police, then it is not mandatory that the police be contacted. Where large quantities are involved, the following steps should be taken:

+ Contact the emergency department director.
+ Contact medical administration.
+ A decision will then be taken regarding the need to contact police. The police will be contacted where the patient has obviously been involved in drug trafficking.
+ Medical management should never be impeded and remains first priority.
+ Patients should not be forcibly restrained.
+ Consent issues for medical procedures and treatment apply in the same way as with all patients.
+ The safety of Hospital staff should not be compromised.
+ Packets recovered are the responsibility of the police, if they are present. If the police are not present, recovered packets should be placed in a signed sealed bag, labelled and locked in the S.8 cupboard (checked in by two registered nurses). A check should be made between shifts to ensure that the seals remain unbroken. This must be documented in the S.8 book and in the patient's medical record. The packets should then be passed on to the police when they arrive.
+ Ensure that the documentation in the medical record is comprehensive and precise, as the history may be called in evidence.

Reproduced with permission.

on the telephone, then no information should be given over the telephone and the caller should be advised to come to the hospital to see the patient for more information.

Social workers and emergency services personnel will often find a critically ill patient's contact information in their belongings or telephone. In this circumstance it is reasonable to telephone the apparent next of kin to advise them that their relative is at the hospital.

Distressing information should not, generally, be given over the telephone. Relatives of very ill patients should be asked where possible to come to the hospital, where any information can be given thoughtfully and sympathetically.

As a general rule, the results of tests (e.g. pregnancy, HIV, sexually transmitted infections) which have been performed in the department should not be released over the telephone. The patient should return to the ED or receive the results from the local doctor. In this way, mistakes and even medicolegal complications can be avoided.

Medical certificates

These are legal documents.
- Stick to facts you can defend.
- Keep it brief; medical certificates go to the employer.

Police statements

Many of our patients have been involved in accidents, assaults or other incidents that may require police involvement.

If police are present in the ED and ask about a patient's condition or injuries, then you can use a broad descriptive term, such as 'stable', but you should not give a description of injuries or comment on prognosis without the patient's consent. If police telephone the ED asking for information about a patient, you should not give any information in the first instance. If the situation is covered by the Traffic Act or the Coroner's Act, you can at times ring the police station or refer all other enquiries to medical administration.

Police may require a formal statement from you, to be used in court, about a patient you have treated. The correct procedure for this is that the police should make a formal request to medical administration who will then ask you to complete a standard police statement form. You should refer to your contemporaneous notes and only write down objective facts and never opinions. You should ask a consultant to review your statement before you submit it. Remember that an appropriately worded statement will save you from spending a day at court.

Editorial Comment
It is helpful to have your own copy of your notes and statements.

Patient care incidents

No matter how wise and diligent we are in our work, we are all involved in incidents in which an apparent error has occurred or a patient has had an unexpected outcome. The appropriate professional response to such incidents is to critically analyse, learn and change practice. If you are involved in an incident that you think has adversely affected patient care, you should immediately discuss it with the consultant on duty, write a detailed personal note about the incident as soon as possible after it has occurred, take a personal copy of the records and, if necessary, contact your medical indemnity organisation for advice. You should keep notes that you have written about an incident confidential and in a safe place and reveal them only to your medical indemnity organisation. You should not formally respond to any request for information without discussion with a consultant and/or your medical indemnity organisation.

Root cause analysis

If the hospital perceives that an apparent patient care incident has caused a real or potential adverse outcome, then it will conduct an investigation into the incident in the form of a root cause analysis (RCA). The aim of an RCA is not to blame or punish but to discover institutional causes for the incident and to institute change to prevent recurrence. If you are involved in the care of a patient that is subject to an RCA, then one of the investigators may contact you and ask for details of patient care. You may already have perceived that there has been a problem, contacted your medical indemnity organisation and made a personal note of events. Depending on advice from your medical indemnity organisation, you should then discuss the matter with the RCA investigator. As is the case with any investigation, you should provide only the facts as you remember them or as they are recorded in the notes. You should not express opinions or comment on the actions or any other person.

Physical examination / intimate examination

Most physical examination involves touching patients in a way that would not occur in a normal social context. On that basis, you should always describe to a patient what you are going to do and ask for their consent to do it, using expressions such as:

'I'd like to examine your abdomen for tenderness, if that's okay with you.'

More intimate examinations, such as those of the perineum, genitalia, rectum and female breast, have the potential for misinterpretation. Consequently, you should always have a chaperone, usually a nurse, present when these examinations are performed and you should record in the notes that the patient consented to the examination and the name of the chaperone.

Personal appearance, behaviour and deportment

Doctors are in a privileged position and interact with patients who are often physically and emotionally distressed. The doctor–patient relationship allows patients to reveal information and to undergo painful and distressing procedures that are not a part of the normal social relationship. A part of that relationship is the professional appearance and behaviour of the doctor. We should dress and behave as the patient would expect a doctor to do. It should go without saying that we should always be neatly and professionally dressed. Our hair, hands and nails should be clean and neat. We should treat the patient with dignity, respect and empathy.

Medicine is a compassionate profession. We deal with patients from all strata of society and from many different backgrounds. We should treat our patients as we would expect ourselves and our family to be treated; that is, with care and compassion and never with blame, criticism or disrespect.

The following are hints for a happy and successful life in the ED.

+ Talk to all the staff—try to know their first names.
+ Be friendly, listen and be quick to praise or say thank you.
+ Be prepared to apologise—none of us is perfect.
+ Don't complain. You are privileged to be able to work as a doctor. Be happy and show your colleagues that you are.
+ Do not fight (even if it is a just cause) with the rest of the hospital, ambulance crew, GPs, etc.
+ Look at it from their point of view!
+ Avoid conflict.

Results of investigations

Important diagnoses can be delayed or missed with potentially serious consequences for the patient. Delay in management of a lung mass reported incidentally on a chest X-ray may be the difference between life and death.

If, as a doctor, you order an investigation, then you have an obligation to review the results of that investigation, even if the result is not available for some time after your shift ends. Failure to review an investigation result is a breach of the duty of care that you owe to the patient.

EDs all have failsafe mechanisms for ensuring that abnormal investigation results are reviewed. These include the medical imaging registrar or consultant ringing the ED consultant on duty for significantly abnormal images and the ED consultant checking hard copy of all imaging results. None of these mechanisms is foolproof, however, and the patient's interest is always best served by the doctor who ordered the investigation reviewing its result.

Notifiable diseases

Notification by medical practitioners of certain diseases is mandatory. In practice, notification is usually made by the pathology laboratory on a positive test result.

Public Health Act 2010 notifiable diseases
URGENT: BY PHONE AS SOON AS POSSIBLE

+ Avian influenza
+ Botulism

- Cholera
- Variant Creutzfeldt-Jakob disease (vCJD)
- Diphtheria
- Foodborne illness ($\geq$ 2 linked cases)
- Gastroenteritis (in an institution)
- Haemolytic uraemic syndrome
- Haemophilus influenzae type b
- Legionnaires' disease
- Lyssavirus
- Measles
- Meningococcal disease
- Middle East respiratory syndrome coronavirus (MERS-CoV)
- Paratyphoid
- Plague
- Poliomyelitis
- Rabies
- Severe Acute Respiratory Syndrome (SARS)
- Smallpox
- Typhoid
- Typhus (epidemic)
- Viral haemorrhagic fevers
- Yellow fever

ROUTINE: BY PHONE OR MAIL

- AIDS
- Acute rheumatic fever
- Acute viral hepatitis
- Adverse event following immunisation
- Creutzfeldt-Jakob disease (CJD)
- Leprosy
- Pertussis
- Rheumatic heart disease (< 35 years of age)
- Syphilis
- Tetanus
- Tuberculosis

Mandatory blood alcohol and drug testing

In Australia, as in many countries, the treating doctor/nurse in an ED must perform a venepuncture and obtain a blood alcohol sample, if (refer to your own state legislation) the patient presents within 12 hours of an accident, and as a result of the accident, and the accident was on a public road, and the patient could have directly contributed to that accident (i.e. pedestrian, driver, motorcycle rider, horse rider, bicycle rider, scooter rider, skateboarder). If a patient refuses blood sampling for the Traffic Act, the police must be notified. Blood samples for the Traffic Act must be taken with supplied police kits. There are also kits for public transport accident victims (e.g. a passenger in a bus who fell) and for boat drivers who are also subject to mandatory testing.

DRUG TESTING

At times the police will bring someone to the ED for alcohol and drug testing when it is suspected that they have been intoxicated in control of a vehicle. Each state has its guidelines and conditions, along with kits and instructions for supervision of the passing of urine for testing. Legislation compels the ED to take samples for police alcohol and drug testing in these circumstances. Other testing (e.g. DNA sampling) should be undertaken by police doctors and not the ED.

Sexual assault forensic testing

(See Chapter 35 Sexual Assault and Domestic Violence.)

Sexual assault forensic tests should only be performed at designated sexual assault crisis units with trained staff and protocols. The patient must be stable and all serious conditions should have been diagnosed and adequately treated before they can be safely directed to a sexual assault crisis unit.

Coroner's investigations
THE DECEASED PATIENT

- Is it a coroner's case? (See Box 63.2.)
- Looking after a grieving family appropriately is a top priority—it is hard, it hurts; but it is vital.

The coroner has a specialist police unit that will investigate potentially suspicious deaths. Investigations are usually precipitated by a complaint, usually by family, to the coroner about a patient's treatment in hospital before their death. The coroner will then ask the Coronial Investigation Unit to take on the case. Police

---

Box 63.2 The circumstances which necessitate that a death be notified to the coroner*

A 'coroner's case' is clearly defined as follows.
1. Sudden death of unknown cause (i.e. unable to write death certificate).
2. Death from a violent or unnatural cause or in suspicious or unusual circumstances.
3. Death within 1 year and 1 day of an accident to which the death is or may be attributable.

Note: If the patient is 65 years or more and the accident was attributable to their age, contributed substantially to their death, was in no way suspicious or unusual and was not caused by an act or omission of another person, a death certificate may be written. If, however, the accident occurred in a hospital or nursing home, the death is always a coroner's case, regardless of a patient's age.

4. Death of a patient within 24 hours of an anaesthetic, general *or* local, administered in the course of a medical, surgical or dental operation or procedure, other than a local anaesthetic administered solely for the purpose of facilitating a procedure of resuscitation from apparent or impending death.
5. Death of a patient who has not been attended by a medical practitioner within the period of 3 months immediately prior to the death.
6. Death in an admission centre, mental hospital, residential centre for handicapped persons or similar facility or while in the custody of a police officer or in other lawful custody.

*If there is any doubt whether or not a death is a coroner's case, medical administration should be contacted.

---

investigators will attend the hospital and take statements from all staff involved in the patient's care. If you are asked to make such a statement, you should ask an ED consultant and your medical defence organisation for advice. Your statement should contain only facts that you clearly remember and/or are recorded in the notes. You should not expand on the facts or offer opinions. Your statement should be reviewed by your consultant and medical defence organisation before it is submitted. Any personal notes that you may have made about the case should remain confidential in a safe place. If you are asked to appear at the Coroner's Court, you should ensure that you have legal representation provided by your medical defence organisation.

How to avoid a lawsuit

The assumption that good doctors are not sued is, sadly, not true.

Good doctors are sued even when they do everything right and, in reality, even good doctors have bad days.

A successful civil action against a doctor must involve both negligence and injury. Negligence is usually defined as a departure from what would be widely accepted by peer professional opinion in Australia to be competent professional practice or a departure from an acceptable standard of care. Negligence itself is not compensable unless there is objective injury directly caused by the negligence (there are no punitive damages in Australia). It is the financial hardship caused by the injury that the civil legal system compensates. So, if an intravenous drug user presents with back pain and the doctor fails to consider the possibility of a spinal infection, and the patient becomes paraplegic, the court will compensate the patient for lifetime loss of income, pain, and so on. Civil actions are not punitive; that is, their intention is not to punish the doctor but to compensate the patient. If you become involved in a civil action, as most of us will, do take the opportunity to reflect on your practice, but do not feel that you are a bad doctor. Most doctors involved in civil actions are good doctors who have been involved in a particularly difficult case or who have had a bad day.

To minimise the risk of a complaint or a civil action, treat your patients and their relatives the way you would want to be treated in the same circumstances. Be open and friendly, concerned and, above all, talk to them and tell them what is happening. Explain delays in advance and apologise if the system is not working well. The attitude of your other staff (nurses, clerks) is equally important—if the department is rude and uncommunicative, there will be complaints and civil actions.

Make your patients and their relatives feel that you value them as people and that you will spend the time and thought needed to make them well. Patients do not expect to be cured, but they do expect that everyone will treat them courteously and compassionately.

Personal care

Involvement in patient complaints and lawsuits is personally challenging and can lead the doctor involved to question their ability.

Anxiety, sleeplessness, depression and substance abuse are all potential sequelae of the stress involved in such situations. All doctors should have a general practitioner. If you find yourself distressed by a complaint or lawsuit, then you should see your GP for help. You should discuss your feelings with family, friends and/or a senior colleague. Your medical indemnity organisation should have the facilities to provide counselling if needed. You should be mindful of the risks of alcohol and drug use when you are emotionally vulnerable—they do not solve any problems, they just make them worse.

Consent

There has been a change in the legal definition of informed consent following the *Rogers v Whitaker* decision. Courts now believe that, in giving informed consent, a patient must be informed of all material risks. A risk becomes 'material' if the judge believes that a reasonable person in the patient's position would be likely to attach significant importance to it in deciding whether or not to have treatment. In this context, emergency doctors should not obtain a patient's consent for procedures that they will not personally perform. If a specialist team plans to perform a procedure on a patient, then it is their responsibility to obtain consent for that procedure. It is neither safe nor reasonable to obtain consent for a procedure with which you are not intimately familiar.

ED doctors must obtain informed consent and documentation for any invasive procedure that they will perform personally (e.g. lumbar puncture, central line insertion, chest tube insertion). Written consent should be obtained and signed by the patient and a witness.

Procedural mistakes

As we often hand over patients, take care to avoid doing the wrong test or the wrong procedure on the patient we do not know (e.g. 'The patient in bed 5 needs a CT or an LP'). We should, as is now routine in operating theatres, use the 'Time out' routine (see Box 63.3).

Reports and records

Comprehensive records, written when you saw the patient, are the keystone of safe practice. The better the records, the better your

---

Box 63.3   Emergency department pre-procedure 'time out'

Immediately prior to the commencement of the procedure, the
procedure team MUST STOP all activity and verbally confirm the:
- presence of the correct patient and consent
- correct site has been marked (if applicable)
- correct procedure to be undertaken is documented
- availability of any special equipment.

---

chance of a successful defence in the case of a potential criminal
or civil action.

It does not matter what you did—if you did not write it down,
you did not do it! Conversely, if you did write it down, you did do it!

Going to court

The important rules in court appearances are to:
- talk to a senior colleague before you go
- have legal representation provided by your medical defence
  organisation if necessary
- stay calm
- pause to gather your thoughts before you answer
- keep it simple.

The best answers are 'yes' or 'no'. Do not attempt to expand
answers or to explain. Do not 'second-guess' where the questioner
is heading.

If you do not understand a question, ask for an explanation.

Do not try to beat the barristers at their own game—you cannot, any more than they can intubate someone.

Do not get angry—if you do, you will look bad and the lawyer
will have won.

Tell the truth, but say no more than you have to.

Doctors out-of-hours or away from their workplace

Recent regulatory decisions have changed our potential obliga-
tions away from our usual place of medical practice.
- If a doctor in hospital is about to leave at the end of a shift,
  the doctor has a common law duty to attend to an emergency.
- If a doctor is at a theatre, sports event or similar, not as a
  doctor, and a call is made 'Is there a doctor here?', the doctor

may or may not have a duty of care towards the patient (we are not discussing moral duty here, just legal duty).

- If a doctor is not working, but is somewhere that he/she is known to be a doctor (such as a favourite restaurant or an aeroplane seat) or can be identified as a doctor (e.g. by a sticker on the doctor's car), then the doctor probably has a legal duty of care.
- If a doctor drives past the scene of an accident, are they obliged to stop and render assistance? Recent cases suggest that a doctor may be open to regulatory action if it is identified that they failed to render assistance.

We should probably always accept our moral duty to provide care.

Standards of behaviour out-of-hours/ mandatory reporting

Remember that, under current legislation, doctors have a duty to report apparently impaired colleagues to Australian Health Practitioner Regulation Agency (AHPRA), the medical regulatory authority. With this in mind, doctors should be careful to ensure that they are not in a position of presenting to an ED as a result of alcohol or drug use or for any other reason that may bring their ability to practise safely into question.

Duty of care: patients who refuse treatment

The practice of emergency medicine has always been, and still is, based on the principle that it is always desirable to preserve life, and that all individuals want their lives to be preserved.

This tenet is now being challenged by euthanasia laws in several Australian states and by the increasing use of Advanced Care Directives and Not for Resuscitation / Limitation of Care Orders. This raises questions for ED doctors who must balance their own obligation to treat to maintain life with the patient's 'right' to decline.

If a patient presents critically ill with a potentially life-threatening condition but verbally indicates that they do not want to be treated, then the doctor is obliged to test the patient's competence to make that decision. The doctor must assure themself that the patient is competent to make that decision and that their judgment is not clouded by illness, drug use or mental illness. In this situation, active treatment should continue while the ED doctor consults with their consultant, mental health services and the medical administrator on call to determine the patient's competence.

Written Advanced Care Directives and Not for Resuscitation / Limitation of Care Orders are increasingly common and are always open to interpretation because their wording cannot cover every clinical situation. If a patient presents with a potentially life-threatening illness and has an existing Advanced Care Directive or Not for Resuscitation / Limitation of Care Order, then they should initially be treated actively. The doctor should then have an objective discussion with the patient and/or their next of kin/guardian before a decision not to provide medical care is made. If a Not for Resuscitation / Limitation of Care Order exists and the patient and/or next of kin/guardian agree that resuscitation is not wanted because of terminal illness or poor quality of life, then it would usually be seen to be reasonable to withhold resuscitation.

Insurance

As an employee of the hospital, technically you are covered by the hospital's insurer but you are not covered for:

- professional matters
- alleged misconduct
- informal consultations or opinions (e.g. given to your neighbours)
- cross-suits initiated by the hospital against you as an individual
- emergencies that may arise outside the hospital.

Therefore, it is advisable to have personal medical indemnity cover.

Media

You are not permitted to talk to the media or represent the hospital unless given permission by hospital administration.

Complaints

Complaints are a part of life in every business and should always be seen as a way to improve service. The ED should investigate every complaint objectively and change practice if there is evidence of an institutional problem. We should respond to each complaint promptly and be ready to apologise when appropriate. An early telephone call to the complainant will show our concern and will often resolve the matter without the need for further action.

If it appears that a complaint is substantiated and may involve significant injury, then the staff involved should be notified along with the hospital's internal complaint investigation service and the hospital's insurer.

Index

Index

Index

advanced practice nurse (APN), 1043–1045
  practices, 1044, 1044b, 1045b
  roles of, 1043–1044
AEDs *see* automatic external defibrillators
AF *see* atrial fibrillation
after-hours shifts, 1086
age, burns, 135
aged care assessment team (ACAT), 398
aged service emergency team (ASET), 1046, 1047b
AGEP *see* acute generalised exanthematous pustulosis
agitation, poisoning and overdose, 289
AIDS dementia, 446–447
aircraft, retrieval, 140
air embolism, 475
airway, 16
  adjuncts, 20–22
  assessment, 17–31
  management, 20–22
  manoeuvres, 20
airway adjuncts
  face masks, 21–22, 22f
  nasopharyngeal airway (NPA), 21
  oropharyngeal airway, 20–21
  self-inflating bag, 22, 23f
  suction, 21
airway, breathing and circulation (ABCs), 507
airway emergencies, paediatric patients, 648–649
  croup, 982
airway management, 16
  advanced life support, 8
  airway adjuncts, 20–22
  airway manoeuvres, 20, 20f
  assessment, 17–31
    difficult bag-mask ventilation, 17–18
    difficult intubation, 18

difficult surgical airway, 18–20
basic life support, 1
drugs in, 28, 29t
endotracheal, 88–90, QR68
intubation
  difficult, 18
  endotracheal, 16, 23–27
  hypothermia, 903, 908
  preparation for, 27–31
shock, 108
trauma primary survey, 71–72
ventilators, 31–36
see also ventilation
airway obstruction
  foreign body, 14, 15f, 793–794
  diagnostic imaging, 981
AKI *see* acute kidney injury (AKI)
alanine aminotransferase (ALT) test, 302
alcohol
  acute intoxication, 323–324
    complications of, 322
    treatment of, 324
  chronic alcohol abuse, complications of, 322–323
  clinical effects of, 323, 323t
  epidemiology, 321
  hazardous use, assessment and management of, 328–329
  impact on emergency department, 321–322
  related seizures, 327
  safe drinking levels, 322
  standard drinks, 322
  Wernicke's encephalopathy, 327–328
  withdrawal
    management of, 326–327
    predictors of, 326b
    scale, 325, 325–326t
    syndrome, 324–325

alcohol withdrawal, 394
  management of, 326–327
  predictors of, 326b
alcohol withdrawal scale (AWS), 325, 325–326t
alcohol withdrawal syndrome, 324–325
alert response phase, 934–935
alkalinisation, urinary, 409, 439
alkalosis
  metabolic, 355–357t
    acetazolamide for, 380
    correction factors for, 358t
    NAGMA, 379–380
    urinary Cl and, 380b
  respiratory, 355–357t, 381–382
    causes, 381
    clinical effects, 382
    management, 382
alpha$_1$-blockers, for renal/ureteric calculus, 596
ALS *see* advanced life support
alteplase, for stroke, 268
altered consciousness
  circulatory status and, 74
  electrocardiogram (ECG), 196–209, 197f, 198t, 199f, 201f, 203f, 204b, 204t, 205f, 207f, 208f
altered mental status
  neurological emergencies examination, 262–264
  history, 262
  investigations, 264
  management, 264–265
alveolar gas equation, QR26
alveolar osteitis, 803–804
amaurosis fugax, 768
ambulances, retrieval, 139–140
amethocaine (tetracaine), ophthalmic, 760, 773
AMI *see* acute myocardial infarction

Index

Index

Index

Index

Index

Index

Index

Index

Index

Index

Index

Index

Index

Index

Index

Index

Index

Index

Index

necrosis, 423
  acute tubular, 384
Necrotic arachnidism, 879
necrotising fasciitis, 423
  clinical features, 423, 854
  diagnosis, 854
  differential diagnosis, 854
  management, 424, 854
needle aspiration
  for peritonsillar abscess,
    790, 790b
  for priapism, 592
needle-stick injuries,
    415–417
  community, 417
needle thoracostomy, 51–53
negligence, 1135
Neisseria meningitidis, 420
neonatal jaundice, 679
neonatal rash, 677
neonates
  assessment of, 728, 729t
  see also Newborns and
    infants
neoplasia, 800
neoplastic diseases,
    haemoptysis with, 240
neostigmine, for myasthenia
    gravis, 284
nephrostomy
  with ESWL, 583
  for renal/ureteric calculus,
    597
nerve agents, 942
nerve injuries
  hand
    carpal tunnel syndrome,
      756
    digital nerves, 558–559,
      748
    function–screening
      tests, 744
    upper limb palsies, QR60
neurogenic pulmonary
    oedema, 244
neurogenic shock, 117
  management, 117
neuroleptic malignant
    syndrome (NMS), 829–
    831t, 909

neurological deficit,
    paediatric, 650
neurological emergencies
  altered mental status,
    262–264
  history, 262
  investigations, 264
  management, 264–265
  Bell's palsy, 282–283
  Guillain-Barré syndrome,
    283
  headache, 274–275
    acute narrow-angle
      glaucoma, 275
    encephalitis, 278–279
    giant cell arteritis
      (temporal arteritis),
      281
    lumbar puncture (LP), 277
    meningitis, 275–277,
      276t
    migraine, 279–281
    other causes, 282–283
    subarachnoid
      haemorrhage
      (SAH), 272–274
  ischaemic stroke, 267–270
    CT, 268
    investigations, 268
    management checklist,
      269–270
    mechanical clot
      retrieval, 269
    neurological impairment
      patterns, 267
    spontaneous
      intracerebral
      haemorrhage, 270–
      272
    thrombolysis, 268
    transient ischaemic
      attack (TIA), 270
  lumbar puncture (LP) in,
    277–278
    additional
      considerations, 278
    complications, 277
    indications, 277
    interpretation, 277–278
    preparation, 277

myasthenia gravis, 283–
    284
  periodic paralysis, 284
  seizures
    history, 265
    investigations, 266
  status epilepticus, 266–
    267
  stroke
    CT, 976–977
    TIAs, 976
  trigeminal neuralgia,
    281–282
neuropathic pain, 628
neuropathy, peripheral, 454
neurosurgical emergencies
  blunt cerebrovascular
    injury, 513
  headache in, 503–504
  herniation syndromes,
    506
  management
    airway, breathing and
      circulation, 507
    analgesia, 512
    measures to reduce ICP,
      512
    surgical intervention,
      512
  non-traumatic
    complications of
      ventricular
      drainage devices,
      526–527
    epidural abscess,
      527–528
    space-occupying lesions,
      525–526
    spontaneous
      intracerebral
      haemorrhage, 525
    subarachnoid
      haemorrhage, 522–
      525
    primary *versus* secondary
      brain injury, 503–504
  traumatic
    cervical spine and spinal
      cord injuries,
      515–521

Index

non-steroidal anti-inflammatory drugs (NSAIDs)
after ESWL, 583
for dry socket, 804
for migraine, 280
ophthalmic, 773
pain management with, 632, 632t
for rib fracture, 98
for TMJ dysfunction, 809
non-variceal bleeding, 488
noradrenaline
for acute pulmonary oedema (APO), 249
for Fournier's gangrene, 588
for septic shock, 114
norfloxacin
prolonged QT interval and torsades de pointes caused by, 198t
for pyelonephritis, 605
for traveller's diarrhoea, 426
normal anion gap metabolic acidosis (NAGMA)
evaluation, 379, 380
management, 379, 380
metabolic alkalosis, 379–380
renal causes of, 379b
urine osmolal gap, 379
normal values, QR87
normochloraemic, 377
normocytic anaemia, 467, 1025
norovirus, 426
nose emergencies
acute sinusitis, 783–784
epistaxis, 784–785, 785b, 786b, 786f, 787f
equipment, 774b
foreign bodies, 786–788
fractured nasal bones, 788
Not for Resuscitation (NFR), geriatric patients, 389
Not for Resuscitation/Limitation of Care Orders, 1138, 1139

notifiable diseases, 1131
routine, 1132
urgent, 1131–1132
NSAIDs *see* non-steroidal anti-inflammatory drugs
NSTEACS *see* non-ST-elevation acute coronary syndrome
NSW immunisation schedule, 688f
NSW Rape Crisis hotline, 706
nuclear hazards, 941
see also Chemical, biological and radiological hazards
nuclear magnetic resonance (NMR), 959–964
nucleic acid testing (NAT), for CMV, 458
nucleoside reversion transcriptase inhibitors (NRTIs), 452, 453, 455
nucleotide reverse transcriptase inhibitors, 453
Numeric Rating Scale (NRS), 628
nurse educator, 1048
vs. clinical nurse educator, 1048–1049
nurse unit manager (NUM), 1092
nursing and allied health roles, 1039
advanced practice nurse, 1043–1045
ASET, 1046, 1047b
clinical nurse consultant, 1046–1047
clinical nurse educator, 1048–1049
clinical nurse specialist, 1047–1048
emergency department navigator, 1049
emergency nurse practitioner, 1043
emergency physiotherapy practitioner, 1045–1046
nurse educator, 1048
triage nurse, 1039–1049, 1041–1042t

nystatin
for candidiasis, 447–448

O

obstetric emergencies, diagnostic imaging of
bleeding in pregnancy, 998–999
intrauterine fetal death, 999
intrauterine trauma, 999
obstructive shock, 106, 107t
management, 117–118
pericardial tamponade causing, 118
pulmonary embolism causing, 119
tension pneumothorax causing, 118–119
OCP *see* oral contraceptive pill
octopus envenomation, 881
odontoid process fracture, cervical spine, 981
oedema
CT, 974
see also Acute pulmonary oedema
oesophageal candidiasis, 447
oesophageal disruption, trauma management, 98
oesophagitis, 491–493
oesophagus
foreign body in, 792–793
diagnostic imaging of, 981
rupture as chest pain cause, 161
OIs *see* opportunistic infections
olanzapine, 827
dosage and administration route, QR8
poisoning and overdosage, QR65
prolonged QT interval and torsades de pointes caused by, 198t
olecranon fractures, 549
oliguria, 439

Index

Index

Index

Index

Index

Index

Index

Index

Index

Foreign Body Airway Obstruction (Choking)

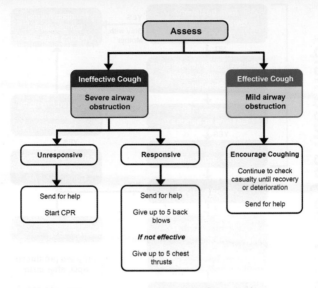

Assess

Ineffective Cough

Severe airway obstruction

Effective Cough

Mild airway obstruction

Unresponsive

Responsive

Encourage Coughing

Continue to check casualty until recovery or deterioration

Send for help

Send for help

Start CPR

Send for help

Give up to 5 back blows

If not effective

Give up to 5 chest thrusts

January 2016

AUSTRALIAN RESUSCITATION COUNCIL

NEW ZEALAND Resuscitation Council WHAKAHAUORA AOTEAROA

Newborn Life Support

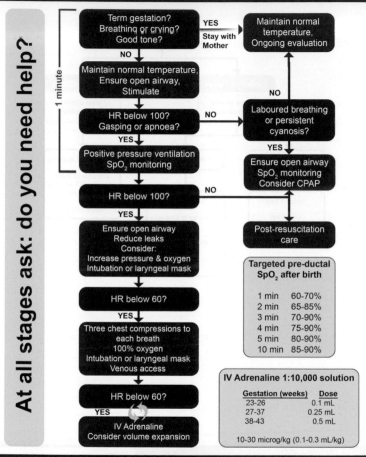

At all stages ask: do you need help?

Term gestation?
Breathing or crying?
Good tone?

YES — Stay with Mother → Maintain normal temperature, Ongoing evaluation

NO

Maintain normal temperature,
Ensure open airway,
Stimulate

HR below 100?
Gasping or apnoea? — **NO** → Laboured breathing or persistent cyanosis?

YES

Positive pressure ventilation
SpO₂ monitoring

Laboured breathing or persistent cyanosis? — **NO** ↑

YES

Ensure open airway
SpO₂ monitoring
Consider CPAP

HR below 100? — **NO** →

YES

Ensure open airway
Reduce leaks
Consider:
Increase pressure & oxygen
Intubation or laryngeal mask

Post-resuscitation care

HR below 60?

YES

Three chest compressions to
each breath
100% oxygen
Intubation or laryngeal mask
Venous access

HR below 60?

YES

IV Adrenaline
Consider volume expansion

1 minute

Targeted pre-ductal SpO₂ after birth

1 min	60-70%
2 min	65-85%
3 min	70-90%
4 min	75-90%
5 min	80-90%
10 min	85-90%

IV Adrenaline 1:10,000 solution

Gestation (weeks)	Dose
23-26	0.1 mL
27-37	0.25 mL
38-43	0.5 mL

10-30 microg/kg (0.1-0.3 mL/kg)

January 2016

AUSTRALIAN RESUSCITATION COUNCIL

NEW ZEALAND Resuscitation Council
WHAKAHAUORA AOTEAROA

Advanced Life Support for Adults

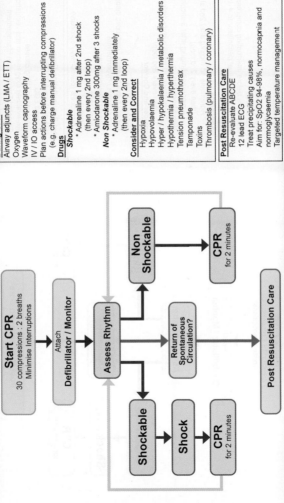

Start CPR
30 compressions : 2 breaths
Minimise interruptions

Attach
Defibrillator / Monitor

Assess Rhythm

Shockable → **Shock** → **CPR** for 2 minutes

Non Shockable → **CPR** for 2 minutes

Return of Spontaneous Circulation?

Post Resuscitation Care

During CPR
Airway adjuncts (LMA / ETT)
Oxygen
Waveform capnography
IV / IO access
Plan actions before interrupting compressions
(e.g. charge manual defibrillator)

Drugs
Shockable
  * Adrenaline 1 mg after 2nd shock
    (then every 2nd loop)
  * Amiodarone 300mg after 3 shocks
Non Shockable
  * Adrenaline 1 mg immediately
    (then every 2nd loop)

Consider and Correct
Hypoxia
Hypovolaemia
Hyper / hypokalaemia / metabolic disorders
Hypothermia / hyperthermia
Tension pneumothorax
Tamponade
Toxins
Thrombosis (pulmonary / coronary)

Post Resuscitation Care
Re-evaluate ABCDE
12 lead ECG
Treat precipitating causes
Aim for: SpO2 94-98%, normocapnia and normoglycaemia
Targeted temperature management

AUSTRALIAN RESUSCITATION COUNCIL

NEW ZEALAND
Resuscitation Council
WHAKAHAUORA AOTEAROA

January 2016

Advanced Life Support for Infants and Children

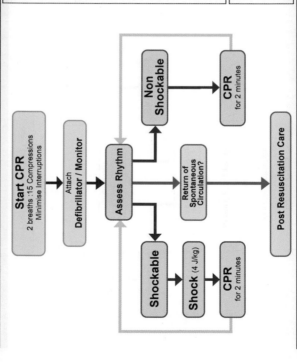

Start CPR
2 breaths :15 Compressions
Minimise Interruptions

Attach
Defibrillator / Monitor

Assess Rhythm

Shockable

Shock (4 J/kg)

CPR
for 2 minutes

Non Shockable

CPR
for 2 minutes

Return of Spontaneous Circulation?

Post Resuscitation Care

During CPR
Airway adjuncts (LMA / ETT)
Oxygen
Waveform capnography
IV / IO access
Plan actions before interrupting compressions
(e.g. charge manual defibrillator to ≤ J/kg)

Drugs
  Shockable
    * Adrenaline 10 mcg/kg after 2nd shock
      (then every 2nd loop)
    * Amiodarone 5mg/kg after 3 shocks
  Non Shockable
    * Adrenaline 10 mcg/kg immediately
      (then every 2nd loop)

Consider and Correct
Hypoxia
Hypovolaemia
Hyper / hypokalaemia / metabolic disorders
Hypothermia / hyperthermia
Tension pneumothorax
Tamponade
Toxins
Thrombosis (pulmonary / coronary)

Post Resuscitation Care
Re-evaluate ABCDE
12 lead ECG
Treat precipitating causes
Re-evaluate oxygenation and ventilation
Targeted Temperature Management

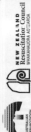

NEW ZEALAND
Resuscitation Council
WHAKAHAUORA AOTEAROA

AUSTRALIAN
RESUSCITATION
COUNCIL